Adjuvant Therapy fc

Cancer Treatment and Research
Steven T. Rosen, MD, *Series Editor*

Leong, S.P.L. (ed.): *Atlas of Selective Sentinel Lymphadenectomy for Melanoma, Breast Cancer and Colon Cancer*. 2002. ISBN 1-4020-7013-6.
Andersson, B., Murray D. (eds.): *Clinically Relevant Resistance in Cancer Chemotherapy*. 2002. ISBN 1-4020-7200-7.
Beam, C. (ed.): *Biostatistical Applications in Cancer Research*. 2002. ISBN 1-4020-7226-0.
Brockstein, B., Masters, G. (eds.): *Head and Neck Cancer*. 2003. ISBN 1-4020-7336-4.
Frank, D.A. (ed.): *Signal Transduction in Cancer*. 2003. ISBN 1-4020-7340-2.
Figlin, R. A. (ed.): *Kidney Cancer*. 2003. ISBN 1-4020-7457-3.
Kirsch, M., Black, P. McL. (eds.): *Angiogenesis in Brain Tumors*. 2003. ISBN 1-4020-7704-1.
Keller, E.T., Chung, L.W.K. (eds.): *The Biology of Skeletal Metastases*. 2004. ISBN 1-4020-7749-1.
Kumar, R. (ed.): *Molecular Targeting and Signal Transduction*. 2004. ISBN 1-4020-7822-6.
Verweij, J., Pinedo, H.M. (eds.): *Targeting Treatment of Soft Tissue Sarcomas*. 2004. ISBN 1-4020-7808-0.
Finn, W.G., Peterson, L.C. (eds.): *Hematopathology in Oncology*. 2004. ISBN 1-4020-7919-2.
Farid, N. (ed.): *Molecular Basis of Thyroid Cancer*. 2004. ISBN 1-4020-8106-5.
Khleif, S. (ed.): *Tumor Immunology and Cancer Vaccines*. 2004. ISBN 1-4020-8119-7.
Balducci, L., Extermann, M. (eds.): *Biological Basis of Geriatric Oncology*. 2004. ISBN
Abrey, L.E., Chamberlain, M.C., Engelhard, H.H. (eds.): *Leptomeningeal Metastases*. 2005. ISBN 0-387-24198-1.
Platanias, L.C. (ed.): *Cytokines and Cancer*. 2005. ISBN 0-387-24360-7.
Leong, S.P.L., Kitagawa, Y., Kitajima, M. (eds.): *Selective Sentinel Lymphadenectomy for Human Solid Cancer*. 2005. ISBN 0-387-23603-1.
Small, W., Jr., Woloschak, G. (eds.): *Radiation Toxicity: A Practical Guide*. 2005. ISBN 1-4020-8053-0.
Haefner, B., Dalgleish, A. (eds.): *The Link Between Inflammation and Cancer*. 2006. ISBN 0-387-26282-2.
Leonard, J.P., Coleman, M. (eds.): *Hodgkin's and Non-Hodgkin's Lymphoma*. 2006. ISBN 0-387-29345.
Leong, S.P.L. (ed.): *Cancer Clinical Trials: Proactive Strategies*. 2006. ISBN 0-387-33224-3.
Meyers, C. (ed.): *Aids-Associated Viral Oncogenesis*. 2007. ISBN 978-0-387-46804-4.
Ceelen, W.P. (ed.): *Peritoneal Carcinomatosis: A Multidisciplinary Approach*. 2007. ISBN 978-0-387-48991-9.
Leong, S.P.L. (ed.): *Cancer Metastasis and the Lymphovascular System: Basis for Rational Therapy*. 2007. ISBN 978-0-387-69218-0.
Raizer, J., Abrey, L.E. (eds.): *Brain Metastases*. 2007. ISBN 978-0-387-69221-0.
Woodruff, T., Snyder, K.A. (eds.): *Oncofertility*. 2007. ISBN 978-0-387-72292-4.
Angelos, P. (ed.): *Ethical Issues in Cancer Patient Care, Second Edition*. 2008. ISBN 978-0-387-73638-9.
Ansell, S. (ed.): *Rare Hematological Malignancies*. 2008. ISBN 978-0-387-73743-0.
Gradishar, W.J., Wood, W.C. (eds.): *Advances in Breast Care Management, Second Edition*. 2008. 978-0-387-73160-5.
Blake, M., Kalra, M. (eds.): *Imaging in Oncology*. 2008. ISBN 978-0-387-75586-1.
Bishop, M.R. (ed.): *Hematopoietic Stem Cell Transplantation*. 2008. ISBN 978-0-387-78579-0.
Stockfleth, E., Ulrich, C. (eds.): *Skin Cancer after Organ Transplantation*. 2008. ISBN 978-0-387-78573-8.
Fuqua, S.A.W. (ed.): *Hormone Receptors in Breast Cancer*. 2008. ISBN: 978-0-387-09462-5.
Green, D., Kwaan, H.C. (eds.): *Coagulation in Cancer*. 2009. ISBN: 978-0-387-79961-2.
Stack, M.S., Fishman, D.A. (eds.): *Ovarian Cancer, Second Edition*. 2009. ISBN: 978-0-387-98093-5.
Goldman, S., Turner, C.D. (eds): *Late Effects of Treatment for Brain Tumors*, 2009. ISBN: 978-0-387-77102-1.
Castiglione, M., Piccart, M. (eds): *Adjuvant Therapy for Breast Cancer*, 2009. ISBN: 978-0-387-75114-6.

Adjuvant Therapy for Breast Cancer

Edited by

Monica Castiglione, M.D., M.H.A
University of Geneva
Geneva, Switzerland

And

Martine J. Piccart, M.D., Ph.D.
Jules Bordet Institute
Brussels, Belgium

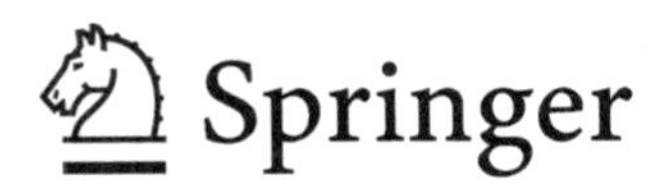

Editors
Monica Castiglione
University of Geneva
ISPM/RGT
Boulevard de la Cluse 55
1205 Geneva
Switzerland
monica.castiglione@bluewin.ch

Martine J. Piccart
Universite Libre Bruxelles
Inst. Jules Bordet
1000 Bruxelles
Belgium
martine.piccart@bordet.be

Series Editor:
Steven T. Rosen, M.D.
Robert H. Lurie Comprehensive Cancer
Center
Northwestern University
Chicago, IL
USA

ISSN 0927-3042
ISBN 978-1-4614-1716-3 e-ISBN 978-0-387-75115-3
DOI 10.1007/978-0-387-75115-3
Springer Dordrecht Heidelberg London New York

Printed on acid-free paper

Springer is part of Springer Science + Business Media (www.springer.com)

Acknowledgments

We would like to thank all contributors for their enthusiasm

We would like to thank Laura Walsh – who always believed in the project – for her patience (a typical feminine characteristic!) and for her continuous support.

We would like to thank the team at Springer for editorial work

Contents

Contributors

Stefan Aebi, MD Breast and Gynecological Cancer Center, Departments of Medical Oncology and Gynecology, University Hospital, Inselspital, Berne, Switzerland, stefan.aebi@insel.ch

Anne-Catherine Andres, PhD Department of Clinical Research, University of Bern, Bern, Switzerland, anne-catherine.andres@dkf.unibe.ch

Laura Biganzoli, MD "Sandro Pitigliani" Medical Oncology Unit, Hospital of Prato-Istituto Toscano Tumori, Prato, Italy, lbiganzoli@usl4.toscana.it

Frances M. Boyle, MBBS, PhD, FRACP Pam McLean Centre, University of Sydney, Sydney, Australia, franb@med.usyd.edu.au

Shelly M. Brock, MSN, ARNP-C Division of Hematology/Oncology and Breast Clinic, Mayo Clinic, Jacksonville, Florida, USA

Monica Castiglione, MD, MHA University of Geneva, ISPM/RGT, Boulevard de la Cluse 55, 1205 Geneva, Switzerland, monica.castiglione@bluewin.ch

Amy Jo Chien, MD University of California San Francisco, Helen Diller Family Comprehensive Cancer Center, San Francisco, California, USA, amyjo.chien@gmail.com

Diana Crivellari, MD Division of Medical Oncology C, Centro di Riferimento Oncologico, Aviano (PN), Italy, dcrivellari@cro.it

Nancy E. Davidson, MD University of Pittsburgh Cancer Institute, University of Pittsburgh School of Medicine, Pittsburgh, Pennsylvania, USA, davidna@jhmi.edu

Silvia Dellapasqua, MD Medical Senology Research Unit, Division of Medical Oncology, European Institute of Oncology, Milan, Italy, silvia.dellapasqua@ieo.it

Leisha A. Emens, MD, PhD Department of Oncology, The Johns Hopkins University, Baltimore, Maryland, USA, emensle@jhmi.edu

Lesley Fallowfield, BSc, D.Phil Brighton and Sussex Medical School, University of Sussex, East Sussex, UK, l.j.fallowfield@sussex.ac.uk

Prudence A. Francis, MB, BS, FRACP Breast Medical Oncology, Peter MacCallum Cancer Center, Melbourne, Australia, prue.francis@petermac.org

Lucia Fratino, MD Onco-Geriatric Program, Oncological Department, Centro di Riferimento Oncologico, National Cancer Institute, Aviano (PN), Italy, lfratino@cro.it

M. Gardner, MD Centre René Huguenin, St Cloud, France

Pia Ursula Huguenin, MD+ Radiation Therapy Department, Kantonsspital Graubünden, Chur, Switzerland

Valerie Jenkins, BSc, D.Phil Brighton and Sussex Medical School, University of Sussex, Brighton, UK, val@sussex.ac.uk

Stella Kyriakydes, BA Psychology, MED Psychology Past President of EUROPA DONNA Cyprus, 28 Prodromou street, Engomi, Nicosia, Cyprus, cysky@cytanet.com.cy

Sibylle Loibl, MD, PhD Ambulantes Krebszentrum Frankfurt, Germany, German Breast Group, Departments of Medicine and Research, Neu-Isenburg, Germany, sibylle.loibl@germanbreastgroup.de

Ulrike Nitz, MD Niderrhein Breast Centre, Mönchengladbach, Germany, ulrike.nitz@wsg-online.com

Nina Oestreicher, PhD, MS Genentech, Inc., South San Francisco, CA; School of Pharmacy, University of California San Francisco, CA, USA, hill.nina@gene.com

Olivia Pagani, MD Institute of Oncology of Southern Switzerland (IOSI), Ticino, Switzerland, olivia.pagani@ibcsg.org

Frances M. Palmieri, RN, MSN, OCN Division of Hematology/Oncology and Breast Clinic, Mayo Clinic, Jacksonville, Florida, USA, palmieri.frances@mayo.edu

Ann H. Partridge, MD, MPH Dana-Farber Cancer Institute, Brigham and Women's Hospital, Harvard Medical School, Boston, MA, USA, ahpartridge@partners.org

Edith A. Perez, MD Division of Hematology/Oncology, Internal Medicine, Mayo Clinic, Jacksonville, Florida, USA, perez.edith@mayo.edu

Louise Picard, PhD Faculté des sciences sociales, École de service social, Pavillon Charles-De-Koninck, Université Laval, Québec (Québec) Canada GIK 7P4, louise.picard@svs.ulaval.ca

Martine Piccart, MD, PhD Jules Bordete Institute, Brussels, Belgium, martine.piccart@bordet.be

Annabel Pollard, MAPS Peter MacCallum Cancer Centre, Clinical Psychology & Psych-Oncology Research Unit, Victoria, Australia, annabel.pollard@petermac.org

Kathy Pritchard, MD, FRCPC Department of Medicine, University of Toronto, Sunnybrook Research Institute, Sunnybrook Odette Cancer Centre, Toronto, Canada, kathy.pritchard@sunnybrook.ca

Meredith M. Regan, ScD IBCSG Statistical Center, Department of Biostatistics and Computational Biology, Dana-Farber Cancer Institute and Harvard Medical School, Boston, MA, USA, meredith_regan@dfci.harvard.edu

Angelika Reiner-Concin, MD Department of Pathology, Danube Hospital, Vienna, Austria, angelika.reiner@wienkav.at

Kathryn J. Ruddy, MD Dana-Farber Cancer Institute, Brigham and Women's Hospital, Harvard Medical School, Boston, MA, USA, kruddy@partners.org

Hope S. Rugo, MD University of California San Francisco, Helen Diller Family Comprehensive Cancer Center, San Francisco, California, USA, jfaison@medicine.ucsf.edu ?

Tiina Saarto, MD Department of Oncology, Helsinki University Central Hospital, Helsinki, Finland, tiina.saarto@hus.fi

Rosalba Torrisi, MD Research Unit of Medical Senology, Department of Medicine, European Institute of Oncology, Milan, Italy, rosalba.torrisi@iso.it

M. Tubiana-Hulin, MD Centre René Huguenin, St Cloud, France, m.tubiana@stcloud-huguenin.org

Pinuccia Valagussa, BS Fondazione Michelangelo, Michelangelo Operations Office, Milan, Italy, pinuccia.valagussa@istitutotumori.mi.it

Janette Vardy, MD, PhD, FRACP Sydney Cancer Centre, Concord Repatriation General Hospital, Department of Medical Oncology, The University of Sydney, Cancer Institute NSW, Concord, Australia, jvardy@med.usyd.edu.au

Introduction

Breast cancer is still the most frequently diagnosed cancer in women. Despite a continuous increase in incidence, mortality has decreased dramatically and great steps have been made in the knowledge of this malignant disease.

Large amounts of literature on the subject are available; just during the last 12 months more than 12,000 new articles have been reported in PubMed and innumerable other publications have appeared in the scientific as well in the lay press.

Why another book? In the arena of immediate information transfer, why should somebody be interested in a new volume?

Because... knowledge on breast cancer is evolving constantly; new laboratory and translational research results are allowing us a better understanding of the disease separating different types of breast cancer. With increasing insight into the disease, increasing focus on molecular, genetic, pathologic, biologic, polymorphisms, genomic, proteomic ... aspects of breast cancer, we run the risk of forgetting the woman behind the disease, the woman facing the disease, the woman living with the disease, the family around the woman.

Because... despite the fact that we are moving toward targeted therapies for the individual patient, the current reality is unfortunately not yet there.

Because... we wanted a book in which the woman with breast cancer is at the center.

Because... we wanted a practical book reporting on the current aspects of the disease, with special emphasis on clinical aspects.

Because... we wanted a book accessible to educated patients looking for information on the disease.

Because... we wanted a book written by women scientists for scientists on this typically feminine disease.

So, some may ask: Is it necessary to have a "feminine" perspective to a particular disease? Obviously not! You do not need to be a man for better care of a prostate cancer patient and you do not need to be a woman for better care of patients with breast cancer. However, men and women still look at things differently. Despite the criticisms of some friends, in our opinion the chapters, besides having an excellent scientific content, also have a special feminine flavor.

We would like to acknowledge one of the contributors, Dr. Pia Huguenin, who prematurely died just after completing her chapter. She was a talented physician, and a sweet, courageous person and we remember her with love.

Bern,
Brussels,
December 2008

Monica Castigllione-Gertsch
Martine Piccart-Gebbhard

Part I
Basics

History of Adjuvant Therapy

Pinuccia Valagussa

Breast cancer is a significant public health problem in virtually all industrialized societies. In many developed countries it is the most common life-threatening malignancy and the second most frequent cause of cancer-related mortality. After peaking in the 1990s, and despite a gradual increase in incidence [1], the overall mortality for breast cancer has been declining in the United States and in some European countries [1, 2].

The fact that so many women with breast cancer are cured, i.e., that their risk of dying from all causes is similar to that of a normal population of the same age, is probably due both to the more frequent detection of smaller cancers with better prognosis as well as to a better understanding of the biology of the disease and to the use of effective adjuvant treatment modalities [2].

For most of recorded history, breast cancer was recognized as almost universally fatal. For this reason, the available treatments – largely surgical, including oophorectomy as well as mainstay local control procedures – were intended to be palliative [3].

A major shift occurred in the late nineteenth century with the popularization of a theory of cancer spread that suggested a curative role for local surgery [4]. According to this hypothesis, first proposed by William Steward Halsted around 1880, breast cancer spread first by direct extension into contiguous tissues and then, by an orderly progression through the lymphatic circulation, to the rest of the body. Were this hypothesis correct, total resection of the primary cancer and the immediate lymphatic drainage could provide a cure if the disease had not yet spread beyond this anatomical location. By the end of the nineteenth century, improvements in surgical technique had made it possible to resect local disease with a wide margin, including axillary lymphadenectomy, in an attempt to catch all cells before they could infiltrate locally or break through the nodal filter. In the 1898, in New Orleans, the American Surgical Association established that this surgical intervention was to be considered the standard of care for breast cancer patients.

P. Valagussa (✉)
Operations Office, Fondazione Michelangelo, Milano,

M. Castiglione, M.J. Piccart (eds.), *Adjuvant Therapy for Breast Cancer*,
Cancer Treatment and Research 151, DOI 10.1007/978-0-387-75115-3_1,

The operation described above, known as Halsted's radical mastectomy [4], was indeed able to decrease both local and distant failure rates compared with historical series. Postoperative irradiation was added years later to improve prognosis further, but even such an extended local regional approach failed to cure a large proportion of breast cancer patients.

During the 1960s, Bernard Fisher, an American surgeon, and his brother Edwin, a pathologist, conducted a series of seminal studies which began to dismantle the concept of anatomical importance in the spread of cancer. Their laboratory experiments revealed for the first time that regional lymph nodes were not an effective barrier to tumor cell dissemination. Evidence indicated that regional nodes were of biological rather than anatomical importance in cancer, and the observed findings led to the conclusion that the lymphatic and blood vascular systems were so interrelated that it was impractical to consider them as independent routes of neoplastic cell dissemination [5]. The laboratory studies provided a matrix upon which an alternative hypothesis, i.e., biological rather than anatomical and mechanistic, could be formulated. Bernard Fisher synthesized that hypothesis in 1968 [6] and selected breast cancer to test in a series of controlled clinical trials conducted by the National Surgical Adjuvant Breast and Bowel Project (NSABP).

The Guiding Principles of Adjuvant Therapy

The experimental foundations of systemic adjuvant therapy were derived to a great extent from studies performed by investigators at the Southern Research Institute [7, 8]. Their observations of the survival of mice with transplantable solid tumors of varying age and size subjected to resection led them to postulate a great variability in metastatic body burden at the time of surgery. Because of this, empirical considerations had to be utilized in the selection of drugs, treatment schedule, and duration of treatment. Surgical cure rates in solid tumors of mice also showed a relationship to the size of the tumor. Of interest was the "break" point in survival curves, after which no further recurrences were noted. These break points appeared at similar times after surgery, although the percentage of survival was different in each case, indicating that the biology of the tumor was similar in the various animals, but the tumor cell burden accounted for the variability experienced. A corollary to this was that definitive conclusions about therapeutic effectiveness must be withheld until this "break" point is reached, since it is the patients with large tumor burdens who are least likely to benefit from adjuvant chemotherapy and who make up the first portion of the survival curves. As for selection of drugs and treatment schedules, they must be effective to achieve a net reduction in cell burden by the next cycle; it is apparent that the optimal treatment intensity must generally be identical to the intensity that yields the optimal results in advanced disease.

Martin et al. [9] demonstrated that both drug combinations and surgery were essential in making an optimal impact on the survival of mice with mammary tumors. However, since the tumor burden is generally lower if therapy is started in adjuvant situations, the duration of treatment needed to assure eradication is likely to be briefer. The emergence of drug resistance is also likely to advance in parallel with the progress of the disease and constitutes a major element in adjuvant therapy failure. As a corollary to these studies, it was assumed that with lower tumor burdens the emergence of primary resistant cells would occur to a lesser degree.

Starting from the mid-1970s, hormones began to receive renewed attention as potential adjuvant treatments [10, 11]. In carcinogen-induced mammary tumors in mice, demonstration that the antiestrogen compound tamoxifen was able both to delay the appearance of tumors and to decrease their overall frequency has been of great interest not only for its relevance in adjuvant treatment of breast cancer but also because of its possible inhibition of carcinogenic influences.

Trials with Endocrine Therapy

Many clinicians have always thought that the complex problem of breast cancer could be interpreted, and therefore managed, through hormonal mechanisms. Adjuvant endocrine therapy dates back to 1889 when Schnizinger suggested that ovariectomy be done before or at the time of mastectomy.

A number of attempts with adjuvant ovarian ablation followed, but failure to implement correct methodology and apparently minimal therapeutic effects led to loss of interest in this modality. Later, between 1948 and 1974, a total of nine randomized trials were activated, consisting of either surgical or radiotherapeutic ablation alone. A detailed overview of the ovarian ablation studies activated before 1990 was published in 1996 by the Early Breast Cancer Trialists' Collaborative Group (EBCTCG) [12]. In women aged under 50 years, ablation of functioning ovaries significantly improved long-term survival, at least in the absence of chemotherapy. In contrast, in women aged 50 or over when randomized, most of whom would have been menopausal, there was only a non-significant improvement. Subgroup analyses on hormonal receptor status were not feasible because this assay was not available in many of these old trials.

The benefits achieved in the premenopausal subset renewed interest in this modality of treatment because of the availability of medical ovarian suppression which became the subject of new trials around the end of the 1990s. All these new trials will be discussed later in this book.

Mainly because of minimal toxicity, the antiestrogen tamoxifen has most often been for many decades the drug of choice in trials of adjuvant endocrine therapy. The first study to randomly test tamoxifen for 2 years vs no further treatment after locoregional therapy was launched by Nolvadex Adjuvant Trial Organization in the early 1970 and was chaired by Michael Baum [13]. Patients were eligible to participate in this study regardless of menopausal, nodal, and receptor status. Subsequently, because preliminary results from clinical trials showed that the treatment benefit was higher with extended duration of tamoxifen, and because the drug has a good safety profile, tamoxifen began to be administered for longer periods, mainly to patients with hormonal receptor positive tumors.

The EBCTCG meta-analysis [14] convincingly showed that tamoxifen administered for 5 years to women with estrogen receptor (ER) positive tumors reduces the risk of recurrence and death, with absolute improvements in 10 year survival of 12.6% for node-positive and 5.3% for node-negative patients. These benefits are independent of patient age, menopausal status, progesterone receptor status, and the use of adjuvant chemotherapy. By contrast, no advantage was demonstrated in women with ER-negative tumors for whom tamoxifen is no longer recommended.

The optimal duration of tamoxifen administration is still undefined, even if it is well known that 5 years of treatment are superior to shorter periods. Prolonging of the duration (10 years or indefinitely) did not provide evidence of clinical benefit in two trials [15, 16]. Currently, two large randomized trials are trying to answer this question of optimal duration. The "Adjuvant Tamoxifen Longer Against Shorter" (ATLAS) study has randomized 15,254 patients with ER-positive or unknown breast cancer between tamoxifen given for 5 years and tamoxifen given for 10 years. Similarly, the "adjuvant Tamoxifen Treatment, offer more?" (aTTOm) study was closed to accrual in 2006. Preliminary results from both trials [17, 18] suggest tamoxifen, when delivered beyond 5 years, continues to decrease breast cancer risk, but endometrial risk was also increased in postmenopausal women. At the time of the present writing, the median observational time of the both studies prevents any firm conclusions on mortality rates.

Tamoxifen is quite well tolerated, and the most common side effects consist of hot flushes and vaginal discharge; however, a two- to threefold higher risk of uterine cancer and thromboembolic events in postmenopausal patients has been reported. However, the benefits obtained with tamoxifen clearly outweigh its side effects [14].

A revolutionary change in the adjuvant treatment of postmenopausal patients with breast cancer has occurred since the publication of the results (reported later in this book) of the first large adjuvant trials that investigated the use of third generation aromatase inhibitors as replacement for or in sequence with tamoxifen. These generations of drugs have been shown undisputedly to improve breast cancer outcome, and several other drugs are being considered.

Trials of Chemoendocrine Therapy

The combination of chemotherapy and endocrine therapy is empirically based on the assumption that each modality exerts its effect on different tumor cells and that the toxicities are different. However, there are theoretical arguments suggesting that the simultaneous administration of these two therapies may not be optimal, because an interaction between the different mechanisms of action may occur, at least with given chemotherapy agents and tamoxifen [19]. On the other hand, tamoxifen demonstrated an additive effect when it was combined with doxorubicin and cyclophosphamide in vitro [20].

The EBCTCG meta-analysis [14] and several adjuvant trials have shown that, in tumors with positive hormone receptors, the combination of chemotherapy and endocrine therapy significantly increases the benefits in terms of disease-free and overall survival achieved with either modality alone.

Trials with Chemotherapy

The first trials of adjuvant chemotherapy in the treatment of breast cancer were launched in the 1950s. They mainly consisted of single agent chemotherapy, in some studies given for a short period of up to 2 months after mastectomy (perioperative chemotherapy). Their results were difficult to interpret because of lack of accurate methodology in some of the studies, which also included only a few dozens of patients [21].

The modern generation of prospective randomized adjuvant treatments began with the studies started in the United States in September 1972 [22] and in Milan in June 1973 [23], respectively. Both studies had similar eligibility criteria for patient selection (tumors with positive axillary nodes) and the experimental arms (single agent phenylalanine mustard or L-PAM in the American study; cyclophosphamide, methotrexate and fluorouracil or CMF in the Italian study) were first tested and found effective in clinically advanced disease.

The preliminary results of the two trials [22, 23] raised unexpected hopes and controversies. A decade of countless debates on the role of adjuvant chemotherapy, made people aware that there was no single or simple solution for a complex biological problem such as breast cancer. Today, more than 30 years after the first publications, we should all recognize that, beside demonstrating that adjuvant chemotherapy can achieve a long-lasting [24] and humanly worthwhile benefit in patients with moderate and high-risk breast cancer, they contributed immensely to a better understanding of a complex discipline involving almost all the techniques and knowledge of biology, epidemiology and therapeutics. Last, but not least, they have also contributed in the crossing of medical compartments and to the adoption of a correct methodology in cancer research.

Following these first two studies, numerous prospective randomized trials were designed over the years to answer specific questions: single agents vs combination chemotherapy; optimal treatment duration; addition of new classes of drugs such as anthracyclines, taxanes and, more recently, targeted monoclonal antibodies; use of sequential drug regimens; use of high-dose and dose-dense regimens. Available results are summarized in the EBCTCG paper published in 2005 [14].

It is beyond the scope of this introductory chapter to list all these studies which will be discussed in the following sections, but a few comments are needed. With the aim of further improving the prognosis of operable breast cancer patients, in the early 1980s many research groups designed and carried out randomized trials including tests on anthracyclines. The international overview [14] confirmed that anthracyclines were able to achieve a modest but humanely worthwhile benefit in decreasing the annual odds of recurrence and death compared with so-called CMF-like regimens. Of note, the many anthracycline-containing regimens used in the studies that were part of the international effort consisted mainly of the substitution of either methotrexate alone or of both methotrexate and fluorouracil with either doxorubicin or epirubicin. The anthracyclines were given at different doses and the regimens were administered at various intervals and for a different number of cycles. Although many individual trials failed to observe a true benefit for the anthracycline regimen, the arithmetic construction on which the meta-analysis is based (i.e., the summing up of many individual trials to increase the statistical power) allowed researchers to assess that there was a reduction in the risk of disease relapse and death of approximately 10%, corresponding to an absolute difference of approximately 3%.

The treatment results observed after sequential doxorubicin and CMF in a poor-risk subset [25] could probably be explained by an increased density of doxorubicin that was delivered within 9 weeks, whereas in the alternating regimen it was spread over 27 weeks. The concept of dose density has been confirmed by the National Cancer Institute's Breast Intergroup INT C9741 trial [26], in which patients who received the dose-dense regimens had a significantly improved early treatment outcome compared with their counterparts.

The role of sequential non-cross-resistant regimens was tested in many other trials. Of note, the joint efficacy analysis of the National Epirubicin Adjuvant Trial and of the Scottish Cancer Trials Breast Group [27] reported a highly significant benefit in favor of the sequential administration of epirubicin for four cycles followed by CMF compared with CMF alone, supporting the hypothesis that single-agent anthracyclines given first, before CMF, can indeed ameliorate treatment outcome. The addition of taxanes after delivery of doxorubicin and cyclophosphamide contributed to improving therapeutic results compared with the non-taxane regimen both in the adjuvant and neo-adjuvant settings.

In summary, the long-term results of available trials indicate that the sequential delivery of two effective non-cross-resistant regimens such as doxorubicin and CMF is a valid, safe, and reproducible treatment approach to attain an improved outcome. Although we await more mature results of the modern adjuvant taxane studies, we can conclude that doxorubicin and/or taxane-containing regimens represent a recommended treatment option for moderate- to high-risk patients with operable breast cancer [28], in whom the significant improvement in the reduction of the odds of recurrence and death is not counterbalanced by an increased risk of life-threatening sequelae.

Concluding Remarks

Approximately 30 years ago, delivering systemic adjuvant therapy to patients who were free of identifiable metastatic disease because some of them might eventually develop distant disease was a revolutionary departure from prior treatment approaches [6]. Long-term experience with conventional adjuvant systemic therapies has demonstrated that this treatment modality, by suppressing micro-metastases regardless of their anatomical location, can effectively decrease the risk of disease relapse and death.

Randomized clinical trials are an important tool by which to set the standard of care for early breast cancer, but the low event rates in a stage of disease that is potentially curable require large sample sizes and long follow-up to demonstrate improvements in patients' outcome. In all clinical trials what is measured is indeed an 'average' effect and the experience gained through the past three decades has led us to a growing recognition that not all breast cancers with seemingly similar clinical and morphological features have the same behavior. Because of this heterogeneity, adjuvant systemic therapy involves the possibility both of over-treating certain patient subsets who have truly localized disease cured by surgery and of an ineffective treatment for other patients' subsets whose cancer is not sensitive to the delivered drug treatments.

As both physicians and investigators, our ultimate goal is to tailor treatment approaches, so that only patients who are at risk of disease relapse will receive adjuvant systemic treatments with drugs that can achieve complete eradication of metastatic cells [28]. Over the past few decades, hundreds of biochemical markers have been tested and individual markers in individual studies raised great promise in their abilities to predict either breast cancer prognosis or treatment responsiveness. Unfortunately, and because of the biases inherent to many of the research designs (e.g., specimen assessment, use of continuous or discrete values, lack of definition of inclusion criteria, adequacy of statistical power, analysis, and data interpretation) the results of many of these studies failed to be reproducible between different research groups and, at times, also within the same research group when the same markers were tested on independent case series or after a prolonged period of observation. So, we continued our clinical studies by using the old standards of tumor stage, grade, and axillary involvement for predicting prognosis and of hormone receptor status and, in the past few years, of HER2 expression for predicting sensitivity to endocrine therapy and trastuzumab treatment, respectively. However, the many studies of single markers published over the past three decades have made amply clear that there is no single marker that provides reliable prognostic information for an individual patient, nor can it predict response or resistance to specific treatments with a high degree of accuracy.

Recently, the development of molecular genetic techniques has allowed the identification and analysis of molecular factors that have an important role in normal cell growth and differentiation. Such factors have also been shown to influence the behavior of tumors with respect to cellular differentiation, growth rate, metastatic pattern, and response to therapy. We now trust that the development of innovative tools, such as micro-array analysis or real time reverse transcription polymerase chain reaction (RT-PCR), can shed some light on the complex interplay of tumor markers, prognosis, and responsiveness. As reported later in this book, the ability to assess multiple markers simultaneously provides an added dimension to our biological understanding of tumor behavior, and profiles based on multiple, independent markers of prognosis or response appear to have higher precision than any single marker.

Intuitively, patients with a good prognostic signature could be spared systemic adjuvant chemotherapy. However, it must be kept in mind that the definition of good prognosis, either through gene expression profiles or more conventional guidelines, does not take into consideration the personal estimates of each individual patient with breast cancer, who may regard her own risk of disease relapse, albeit low, worthy of systemic treatment. In fact, balancing the long-term benefits and risks associated with an adjuvant treatment, it can be concluded that some months of adjuvant chemotherapy and/or some years of tamoxifen produce worthwhile effects for a wide range of women with early breast cancer. Furthermore, recurrent disease usually translates into a fatal outcome and surely impairs the quality of life of the patients. Thus, predictors of good prognosis must have a very low rate of false-negative prediction (i.e., the overwhelming majority of patients with a good prognosis profile should in fact remain relapse-free) in order for the predictor to be clinically useful.

An even more appealing way of using molecular markers is in fact the possibility to select, among effective available drug regimens, the one with the highest probability of cure for the individual patient. The ability to predict who will or will not respond to a given drug or drug regimen has important implications regarding clinical decision-making and treatment recommendations. Although predictive accuracy may not be an all or nothing phenomenon, patients can be spared treatments that are devoid of efficacy, but are associated with toxicity. Furthermore, delivering treatments that are associated with a more pronounced anti-tumor activity against tumors with specific molecular features will lead to improved benefit, making for the patients the real difference between cure and palliation.

All of the observations reported in recent years in the medical literature need to be confirmed in large validation trials, performed with statistical rigor and reported clearly and with unbiased statistics. An important goal for the next generation of genetic profiles will also be to test whether the predictive accuracy is specific to a defined drug therapy or whether it simply predicts response to a variety of regimens with different drug associations. Only if there is a regimen-specific predictive accuracy will we have in our hands a powerful tool to tailor treatment to individual patients.

As investigators, we will continue our studies in future years, raise and test hypotheses, and accept or reject them based on the findings obtained. As physicians, we want to provide our patients with the most effective therapy and minimal toxicity and we want to do so as soon as such therapy becomes available. How can innovative approaches based on very preliminary findings be used for the care of patients with early breast cancer, a disease where long-term follow-up data are required to judge the cost/benefit of the delivered treatments? Overly cautious interpretation of pilot studies could delay implementation of potentially more effective treatments in routine clinical practice. Conversely, overly enthusiastic interpretation of such studies may lead to inappropriate use, causing more harm than good for patients.

The major lesson learned over the past few decades is that good ideas and good hypotheses are insufficient for changing our routine treatment strategy. Selecting optimal treatment from all existing options and alternatives should be based on more than provocative outcome statistics of early data. Evidence in support of new therapies and new technologies must come from well-designed, well-conducted and analyzed clinical trials before such therapies and technologies can be adopted into standard practice. We can be of more help to our patients by fully informing them about ongoing clinical trials and supporting their participation in these studies.

References

1. Jemal A, Siegel R, Ward E. Cancer statistics. *CA Cancer J Clin.* 2006;56:106–30.
2. Peto R, Boreham J, Clarke M, et al. UK and USA breast cancer deaths down 25% in year 2000 at ages 20–69 years. *Lancet.* 2000;355:1822.
3. Kinne D. Primary treatment of breast cancer. In: Harris JR, Helman S, Henderson IC, et al., eds. *Breast Diseases.* Philadelphia, PA, Lippincott; 1991:347–73.
4. Halsted WS. The results of radical operations for the cure of carcinoma of the breast. *Ann Surg.* 1907;46:1–19.
5. Fisher B, Fisher ER. The interrelationship of hematogenous and lymphatic tumor cell dissemination. *Surg Gynecol Obstet.* 1966;122:791–98.
6. Fisher B. The evolution of paradigms for the management of breast cancer: A personal perspective. *Cancer Res.* 1992;52:2371–83.
7. Skipper HE, Schabel FM Jr. Tumor stem cell heterogeneity: Implication with respect to the classification of cancers by chemotherapeutic effect. *Cancer Treat Rep.* 1984;68:43–61.
8. Griswold DP Jr. Body burden of cancer in relationship to therapeutic outcome: Consideration of preclinical evidence. *Cancer Treat Rep.* 1986;70:81–6.
9. Martin DS, Fugman RA, Stolfi RL, Hayworth PE. Solid tumor animal model therapeutically predictive for human breast cancer. *Cancer Chemother Rep.* 1975;5:89–109.
10. Henderson IC. Adjuvant endocrine therapy. In: J Allegra, ed. *Management of Breast Cancer through Endocrine Therapies.* Amsterdam: Excerpta Medica; 1984:38–57.
11. Pritchard KI. Current status of adjuvant endocrine therapy for resectable breast cancer. *Semin Oncol.* 1987;14:23–33.
12. Early Breast Cancer Trialists' Collaborative Group. Ovarian ablation in early breast cancer: Overview of the randomised trials. *Lancet.* 1996;348:1189–96.
13. Nolvadex Adjuvant trial organization. Controlled trial of tamoxifen as single adjuvant agent in management of early breast cancer. Analysis of six years. *Lancet.* 1985;1:836–40.
14. Early Breast Cancer Trialists' Collaborative Group. Effects of chemotherapy and hormonal therapy for early breast cancer on recurrence and 15-year survival: An overview of the randomised trials. *Lancet.* 2005;365:1687–717.

15. Fisher B, Dignam J, Bryant J, et al. Five versus more than five years of tamoxifen for lymph node-negative breast cancer: Updated findings from the National Surgical Adjuvant Breast and Bowel Project B-14 randomized trial. *J Natl Cancer Inst*. 2001;93:456–62.
16. Stewart HJ, Prescott RJ, Forrest AP. Scottish adjuvant tamoxifen trial: A randomized study updated to 15 years. *J Natl Cancer Inst*. 2001:93:456–62.
17. Peto R, Davies C and the ATLAS investigators. ATLAS (Adjuvant Tamoxifen, Longer Against Shorter): International randomized trials of 10 versus 5 years of adjuvant tamoxifen among 11,500 women: Preliminary results. In: Program and Abstracts of the 30th Annual San Antonio Breast Cancer Symposium; San Antonio, Texas (abstract 48).
18. Gray RG, Rea DW, Handley K, et al. aTTom adjuvant Tamoxifen – To offer more?: Randomized trial of 10 versus 5 years of adjuvant tamoxifen among 6,934 women with estrogen receptor-positive (ER+) or ER untested breast cancer – preliminary results. Proc Am Soc Clin Oncol, 26, 2008 (abstract 513).
19. Osborne CK. Effects of estrogen and antiestrogens on cell proliferation. In: Osborne CK, Ed. *Endocrine Treatment in Breast and Prostate Cancer*. Boston, MA: Kluwer; 1988:11–129.
20. Berman E, Adams M, Duigou-Osterndorf R, et al. Effect of tamoxifen on cell lines displaying the multidrug-resistant phenotype. *Blood*. 1991:77:818–25.
21. Bonadonna G, Valagussa P, Veronesi U. Results of ongoing clinical trials with adjuvant chemotherapy in operable breast cancer. In: Heuson JC, Mattheiem WH, Rozencweig M, eds. *Breast Cancer Trends in Research and Treatment*. New York, NY: Raven Press; 1976:239–58.
22. Fisher B, Carbone P, Economou SG, et al. L-Phenylalanine mustard (L-PAM) in the management of primary breast cancer: A report of early findings. *N Engl J Med*. 1975; 292:117–22.
23. Bonadonna G, Brusamolino E, Valagussa P, et al. Combination chemotherapy as an adjuvant treatment in operable breast cancer. *N Engl J Med*. 1976:294:405–10.
24. Bonadonna G, Moliterni A, Zambetti M, et al. 30 years' follow up of randomized studies of adjuvant CMF in operable breast cancer: Cohort study. *BMJ*. 2005;330:217–23.
25. Bonadonna G, Zambetti M, Moliterni A, et al. Clinical relevance of different sequencing of doxorubicin and cyclophosphamide, methotrexate, and fluorouracil in operable breast cancer. *J Clin Oncol*. 2004;22:1614–20.
26. Dang C, Hudis C. Adjuvant taxanes in the treatment of breast cancer: No longer at the tip of the iceberg. *Clin Breast Cancer*. 2006;7:51–8.
27. Poole CJ, Earl HM, Hiller L, et al. Epirubicin and cyclophosphamide, methotrexate, and fluorouracil as adjuvant therapy for early breast cancer. *N Engl J Med*. 2006;355:1851–62.
28. Bonadonna G, Hortobagyi GN, Valagussa P. Individualized therapy of breast cancer: A dream or a reality? In: Bonadonna G, Hortobagyi GN, Valagussa P, eds. *Textbook of Breast Cancer. A Clinical Guide to Therapy*. 3rd ed. London New York: Taylor & Francis; 2006:395–99.

Prognostic and Predictive Factors

Laura Biganzoli

Prognostic factors are key elements for medical oncologists to select, among the group of patients with early breast cancer, those who are candidates for an adjuvant treatment based on their risk of tumor relapse. Predictive factors drive the decision of which type(s) of treatment should be given.

If we perform a literature search on prognostic and predictive factors in breast cancer we immediately realize how redundant is the number of markers that have been/are being evaluated and a dedicated book would be needed to review all of them critically. So, for the purpose of writing this chapter, I have decided to start from markers whose roles have been established to be relevant for patient care by an international panel of breast cancer experts [1].

Prognostic Factors

Three risk categories have been defined for patients with operated breast cancer by the St. Gallen Consensus's Panel. These categories are defined by patient's age, tumor size, axillary nodes status, histologic and/or nuclear grade, HER2/neu status, and presence or absence of peri-tumoral vascular invasion.

Age

Despite controversial data available on the value of age as a prognostic factor, the prognosis of breast cancer in very young women is generally considered to be unfavorable. Park and colleagues retrospectively evaluated the 10-year outcome of 1,098 breast cancer patients divided into 2 age groups (<35, n = 183, and >35 years) [2]. Age was observed to be an independent prognostic factor in

L. Biganzoli (✉)
"Sandro Pitigliani" Medical Oncology Unit, Hospital of Prato,
Tuscany Cancer Institute, Prato, Italy

M. Castiglione, M.J. Piccart (eds.), *Adjuvant Therapy for Breast Cancer*,
Cancer Treatment and Research 151, DOI 10.1007/978-0-387-75115-3_2,

the multivariate analysis with women aged 35 years or younger presenting a shorter loco-regional recurrence-free distant relapse, and overall survival. When the data was matched for stage and lymph node status, patients ≤ 35 years continued to show a poorer 10-year distant relapse free survival. Similar results were produced by Aebi and colleagues who evaluated the outcome of adjuvant therapy in a population of young (<35 years) premenopausal patients treated in four randomized trials [3]. Ten-year disease free survival and overall survival were worse in younger than in older (≥ 35 years) patients. Of interest, younger patients with estrogen receptor (ER) positive tumors had a poorer disease free survival than patients with ER negative tumors. In contrast, among older patients the DFS was similar irrespective of ER status. These data have been recently confirmed. Saghir et al. showed that young age had a negative impact on the survival of patients with positive axillary lymph nodes and positive hormonal receptors [4]. According to Colleoni and colleagues, compared with less young, very young patients with endocrine responsive and node-negative breast cancer have a worse prognosis [5].

Tumor Size

Tumor size is one of the most important independent prognostic factors for overall and recurrence free survival in breast cancer. Mirza and colleagues reviewed the literature looking for the role of prognostic factors in patients with node negative tumors entered in studies with sample size >200 patients and a follow-up in excess of 5 years [6]. In multivariate analysis, tumor size was an independent prognostic parameter for overall survival, being the second strongest factor after axillary lymph node status. A positive correlation has been found in several studies between tumor size and the frequency of axillary nodes involvement [7]. According to the St. Gallen experts, tumors larger than 2 cm indicated intermediate- or high-risk allocation, even in the absence of other adverse prognostic features [1]. The risk allocation of tumors below 1 cm in size and negative nodes remained controversial.

Axillary Nodes

Nodal status is the most powerful independent prognostic factor in breast cancer. There is evidence that overall survival decreases as the number of positive nodes increases [8, 9]. According to the St. Gallen experts, involvement of four or more nodes in the axilla by itself indicated high-risk, but patients with one to three nodes involved required HER2/neu overexpression or amplification to be included in the high-risk group, with other patients with one to three nodes included in the intermediate-risk category [1]. Although nodal micrometastases were prognostically relevant in several studies [10, 11], the panel considered that neither they nor isolated tumor cells in lymph nodes should influence risk allocation.

Tumor Grade

The histological grade of breast carcinomas has long provided clinically important prognostic information. Elston and colleagues showed that patients with grade 1 tumors have a significantly better survival than those with grade 2 and 3 tumors [12]. Gene expression grade index appeared to reclassify patients with histologic grade 2 tumors into two groups with high vs low risks of recurrence [13]. Debate exists about the real role of grade 2 in defining patients' prognosis, i.e., intermediate risk.

HER2/neu Status

Several studies, mainly retrospective, have evaluated the prognostic role of HER2 overexpression or gene amplification in early breast cancer [14]. Of the 81 studies considering 27,161 patients reviewed by Ross et al., 73 (90%) of the studies and 25,166 (92%) of the cases found that either HER-2/*neu* gene amplification or HER-2 protein overexpression predicted breast cancer outcome on either univariate or multivariate analysis. In 52 (71%) of the 73 studies that featured multivariate analyses of outcome data, the adverse prognostic significance of the HER-2 gene, message, or protein overexpression was independent of all other prognostic variables. Thirteen (16%) of the studies reported prognostic significance on univariate analysis only (in eight studies, multivariate analysis was not performed). Only 8 (10%) of the studies encompassing 1,995 (8%) of the patients, showed no correlation between HER-2/*neu* status and outcome. According to the St. Gallen panellists, HER2 status should be regarded as useful for patient care, with overexpression indicating a worse prognosis [1].

Peritumoral Vascular Invasion

The prognostic significance of involvement of lymphatic or microvascular spaces in the primary tumor has been variably described [15–18]. There are data coming from retrospective studies indicating this to be an independent prognostic factor in both node-positive and node-negative patients [19, 20]. The St. Gallen panelists agreed that the presence of peritumoral vascular invasion defined intermediate risk for patients with node-negative disease but its value for patients with positive axillary lymph nodes was considered uncertain [1].

Others

Among the many putative prognostic factors, the detection of bone marrow metastasis, the expression of UPA/PAI-1 by the primary cancer, and the recognition of simultaneous multiple gene expression patterns, or "signature" appear to be particularly promising.

The presence of tumor cells in the bone marrow of primary breast cancer patients at surgery has been shown to be an independent prognostic indicator of relapse [21]. This prognostic factor was not considered adequate by the St. Gallen panelists because of the absence of a standardized examination for detecting these cells.

UPA/PAI-1 over-expression, as determined by a highly validated and accurate ELISA in relatively large cancer sections, appears to be strongly prognostic. As shown by Harbeck et al., high levels indicates dire prognosis [22]. In contrast, patients with low UPA/PAI-1 and ER showed a particularly good prognosis [23].

Data in breast cancer have demonstrated the ability of microarray-based expression profiling to predict disease-free survival and overall survival from profiles in breast cancer surgical specimens [24–29]. Different microarray platforms have been used. Recently Hu and colleagues utilized a microarray data set combining method to create a large validation test set of over 300 tumors, and used it to validate a newly derived gene list for breast cancer prognostication and prediction [30]. When the new intrinsic gene set was used to cluster hierarchically this combined test set, tumors were grouped into LumA, LumB, Basal-like, HER2+/ER−, and Normal Breast-like tumor subtypes demonstrated by Perou et al. in previous datasets. These subtypes were associated with significant differences in relapse-free and overall survival. Multivariate Cox analysis of the combined test set showed that the intrinsic subtype classifications added significant prognostic information that was independent of standard clinical predictors. From the combined test set, the authors developed an objective and unchanging classifier based upon five intrinsic subtype mean expression profiles (i.e., centroids), which is designed for single sample predictions (SSP). The SSP approach was applied to two additional independent data sets and consistently predicted survival in both systemically treated and untreated patient groups. According to the authors this study validates the "breast tumor intrinsic" subtype classification as an objective means of tumor classification that should be translated into a clinical assay for further retrospective and prospective validation.

Predictive Factors

In the following paragraphs, an overview of the different predictive markers already tested or under evaluation in patients with early breast cancer, for both hormonal therapy and chemotherapy, will be presented. For each marker, the level of evidence reached so far will be stated. Table 1 reports the type and grading of evidence for recommendations.

Table 1 Type and grading of evidence for recommendations

Level	Type of evidence
I	Evidence obtained from meta-analysis of multiple well-designed controlled studies; randomized trials with low false-positive and low false-negative errors (high power)
II	Evidence obtained from at least one well-designed experimental study; randomized trials with high false-positive and/or negative errors (low power)
III	Evidence obtained from well-designed quasi-experimental studies; such as nonrandomized controlled single-group pre-post, cohort, time, or matched case-control series
IV	Evidence from well-designed non-experimental studies, such as comparative and correlation descriptive and case studies
V	Evidence from case reports and clinical examples
Category	**Grade of evidence**
A	There is evidence of type I or consistent findings from multiple studies of types II, III, or IV
B	There is evidence of types II, III, or IV and findings are generally consistent
C	There is evidence of types II, III, or IV, but findings are inconsistent
D	There is little or no systemic evidence
NG	Grade not given

Predictive Markers for Adjuvant Hormonal Therapy

The last overview performed by the EBCTCG (R. Peto, 2006, unpublished) provides data regarding the predictive power of ER when the efficacy of adjuvant tamoxifen given for approximately 5 years is evaluated. From these data it may be concluded that the activity of tamoxifen is strictly dependent on the ER status, and that there is a correlation between the level of ER positivity and the efficacy of tamoxifen. To date, ER is the only firmly established factor known to predict the efficacy of adjuvant hormonotherapy with level I/category A evidence. Nevertheless, about one-third of ER and/or PgR-positive tumors do not respond to endocrine therapy, clearly indicating the need for additional predictive markers.

With the exception of ER and PgR, the proto-oncogene HER-2 and its encoded protein have been the most extensively evaluated markers. Preclinical data suggest that HER-2 overexpression may be associated with decreased efficacy of tamoxifen, and even with a potential detrimental effect [31]. Several clinical studies, both in the metastatic and the adjuvant settings, have addressed this issue and provided contradictory results (Table 2) [32–37]. De Placido et al. [33] published the results of a retrospective study in which the activity of adjuvant tamoxifen was correlated with the expression of HER-2. They concluded that tumors overexpressing the HER-2 protein, measured by IHC, are less responsive to tamoxifen. Updates of the Swedish Breast Cancer Group study [34] and a study from a Spanish group [35] have been published, supporting the association between HER-2 overexpression and resistance to tamoxifen.

Table 2 HER-2/neu and adjuvant

Group (reference)	Study arms	No. of patients (in clinical trial)	Percentage with HER-2 Measured (%)	Methods of HER-2 evaluation	Results
GUN (De Placido) [33]	TAM No TAM	433	57	IHC	HER-2 is a strong predictor of adjuvant TAM failure, independently of ER
Swedish group (Stal) [34]	TAM 2 years TAM 5 years	871	66	DNA amplification assay (slot blot) flow cytometry	HER-2 overexpression decreases the benefit of prolonged adjuvant TAM treatment
Spanish group (Climent) [35]	Radical mastectomy Breast-conserving surgery (TAM assignment not rando)	283	88	IHC	Patients treated with adjuvant TAM had significantly longer DFS and OS when HER-2 was negative
CALGB 8541 (Berry) [36]	CAF 600/60/ 600 mg/m^2 CAF 400/40/ 400 mg/m^2 CAF 300/30/ 300 mg/m^2 (TAM assignment not rando)	999	65	IHC, FISH, differential PCR	In ER + /node-positive patients, the efficacy of adjuvant TAM does not depend on HER-2 status
Danish group (Knoop) [37]	TAM No TAM	1716	88	IHC	The study does not support the hypothesis that HER-2 status could predict benefit from adjuvant TAM, in ER + early stage BC

Rando, Randomized; GUN, Gruppo Universitario Napoletano; CALGB, Cancer and Leukemia Group B; IHC, immunohistochemistry; FISH, fluorescence in situ hybirdization; PCR, polymerase chain reaction; ER, estrogen receptor; CAF, cyclophosphamide + doxorubicin + 5-fluorouracil; OS, overall survival; BC, breast cancer

From Di Leo A, Cardoso F, Durbecq V, Giuliani R, Mano M, Atalay G, Larsimont D, Sotiriou C, Biganzoli L, Piccart MJ. Predictive molecular markers in the adjuvant therapy of breast cancer: state of the art in the year 2002. *Int J Clin Oncol*. 2002;245–53. Table 4. With kind permission of Springer Science and Business Media

On the other hand, the Cancer and Leukemia Group B (CALGB) and the Danish Breast Cancer Cooperative Group reported two trials in which no such association was found [36, 37].

Several facts could account for these conflicting results: (1) all the studies are retrospective; (2) the actual number of HER-2-positive patients who received adjuvant tamoxifen is low in all the studies; and (3) there is lack of standardization of methods for assessing HER-2 overexpression across different laboratories. More recently, early results from the TransATAC study suggest that in the adjuvant setting HER-2 and hormone-receptor positive breast cancer tends to be less sensitive to tamoxifen and aromatase inhibitors than HER-2 negative and hormone-receptor positive disease. The magnitude of anastrozole superiority over tamoxifen seems to be independent of the primary tumor HER-2 status [38]. This recent finding contrasts the main conclusions from two previously reported neoadjuvant studies, suggesting an increased superiority of aromatase inhibitors over tamoxifen in the presence of HER-2 and hormone-receptor positive disease [39, 40]. Of note, the two neoadjuvant studies correlated HER-2 status with objective response rates to neoadjuvant hormonotherapy [39, 40], while in the TransATAC study, disease-free survival was the main clinical outcome correlated with the primary tumor HER-2 status [38]. This difference between TransATAC and the two neoadjuvant studies might explain the apparent discordance.

The level of evidence regarding HER-2 as a predictive marker for adjuvant tamoxifen is, therefore, level II, category B.

Overexpression of the anti-apoptotic molecule bcl-2 is usually associated with high ER concentration and, contrary to expectation, has been associated with a higher likelihood of response to tamoxifen. In a total of 205 tumor samples from ER-positive metastatic breast cancer patients, high bcl-2 expression correlated with a better clinical response to tamoxifen (62% vs 49%; $p = 0.07$) and longer survival [41]. In the adjuvant setting, in 81 patients treated with tamoxifen, a significantly better relapse-free survival was found among those with bcl-2-positive tumors than in those with bcl-2-negative disease ($p = 0.02$) [42]. In another retrospective study, the interaction between bcl-2 and response to tamoxifen was evaluated in 289 patients with ER- and/or PgR-positive early breast cancer. This is the only study in which a "control" group of patients who did not receive treatment with tamoxifen exists, although the assignment to each group was not randomized. Despite the relatively small number of patients in each subgroup, there was a trend towards a greater benefit of tamoxifen in ER+/bcl-2-positive patients, as opposed to ER+/bcl-2-negative patients [43].

The potential predictive role of other markers, such as the β isotype of ER, *p-53* mutations, the proliferation marker Ki67, and intra-tumoral aromatase activity (for aromatase inhibitors) is still under evaluation.

The National Surgical Adjuvant Breast and Bowel Project (NSABP) group has recently reported the results of a retrospective study evaluating the prognostic value of a recurrence score for hormone-receptor positive early breast cancer patients treated with tamoxifen in the adjuvant setting [44] . The level of expression of 16 cancer related genes was measured by reverse-transcriptase-polymerase-chain-reaction (RT-PCR) in 668 archival samples from patients treated with adjuvant tamoxifen 20 mg daily for 5 years in the context of the NSABP B-14 trial. A prospectively defined algorithm led to the calculation of a recurrence score and allowed for the segregation of the study population into three distinct cohorts with different clinical outcomes. The Kaplan-Meier estimates of the rates of distant recurrence at 10 years in the low-risk, intermediate-risk, and high-risk groups were 6.8%, 14.3%, and 30.5%, respectively [44]. In a multivariate Cox model, the recurrence score provided significant predictive power that was independent of age and tumor size. In addition, the recurrence score was also predictive of overall survival. Of note, the 16 genes allowing for the determination of the recurrence score are involved in proliferation, invasion, HER-2, or hormone-receptor pathways [44].

The same group has recently reported the results of a second retrospective study in which node-negative ER positive patients were treated with either adjuvant tamoxifen or same treatment combined with a CMF-like adjuvant chemotherapy. The results of this study show that the benefit deriving from chemotherapy seems to be confined to the group of patients with a high recurrence score [45]. An adjuvant therapy clinical trial is ongoing in the U.S. to test the predictive value of the 16-gene signature in a prospective setting.

Predictive Markers for Adjuvant Chemotherapy

HER-2 as a Predictive Marker

The 2006 EBCTCG overview has confirmed the superiority of an anthracycline-based regimen over CMF in the adjuvant treatment of early breast cancer patients. The benefit is, however, modest and is associated with a definite increase in toxicity. This is the typical clinical situation in which the use of a predictive marker might help in selecting those patients for whom the benefits of the more aggressive treatment might be substantial and justify the increased toxicity.

HER-2 has been investigated in this setting, Data suggesting that HER-2-positive tumors might be resistant to adjuvant treatment with CMF (with or without prednisone) comes from three retrospective studies (Table 3) [46–48]. In two of these trials, when patients were divided into two subgroups according to the expression of HER-2, as measured by IHC in primary tumor samples, it was observed that adjuvant CMF (plus prednisone) was more effective than no adjuvant treatment only in the subset of HER-2-negative patients [46, 47]. In the third trial, all patients benefited from adjuvant CMF, but the magnitude of the benefit was superior in HER-2-negative patients [48]. However, in a study reported by the Milan group, HER-2 failed to show any predictive activity in a population of node-positive breast cancer patients randomly allocated to

Table 3 HER- and adjuvant CMF/CMF-like chemotherapy

Group (reference)	Study arms	No. of patients (in clinical trial)	Percentage with HER-2 Measured (%)	Methods of HER-2 evaluation	Results
Intergroup Group 0011 (Allred) [46]	Observation CMFP	677	100	IHC	After CMFP, only HER-2 negative patients had longer DFS and OS, showing clear benfit from CT; no benefit in HER-2 positive patients
IBCSG trial V–Ludwig (Gusterson) [47]	N–: PeCT vs. Not N+: CMFP vs. Not	2504	60	IHC	Tumors that overexpress HER-2 overexpression decreases are less responsive to CMF-containing adjuvant CT
ICRF study (Miles) [48]	Follow-up CMF	391	70	IHC	All patients benefited from CMF, but benefit was greater in HER-2-negative (median Os, 7.3 [follow-up group] vs 12.7 years [CMF group]) than in HER-2-positive (median OS, 4.4 [follow-up group] vs 6.1 years [CMF group] patients
Milan trial (Menard) [49]	Follow-up CMF	386	87	IHC	Clinical benefit of CMF in patients with HER-2-positive, as well as in those with HER-2-negative tumors

PeCT, Perioperative cyclophosphamide + methotrexate + 5-fluorouracil (CMF); CMFP, postoperative CMF + prednisone; IBCSG, International Breast Cancer Study Group; ICRF, Imperial Cancer Research Fund; CT, chemotherapy

From Di Leo A, Cardoso F, Durbecq V, Giuliani R, Mano M, Atalay G, Larsimont D, Sotiriou C, Biganzoli L, Piccart MJ. Predictive molecular markers in the adjuvant therapy of breast cancer: state of the art in the year 2002. *Int J Clin Oncol.* 2002;245–53. Table 5. With kind permission of Springer Science and Business Media receive CMF or no treatment [49]. Albeit based on a limited number of patients, this study is in contradiction with the previous ones. Therefore, regarding the predictive value of HER-2 for CMF-like chemotherapy regimens, the evidence is level II, category C.

Three retrospective studies performed by the National Surgical Adjuvant Breast and Bowel Project (NSABP), the Belgian Adjuvant Study Group, and the Milan group [50–52], evaluated the predictive value of HER-2 in a population of node-positive breast cancer patients, randomly assigned to receive CMF or anthracycline-based chemotherapy. These reports suggest reduced CMF efficacy in patients overexpressing the HER-2 oncoprotein, and all three studies agree in defining the HER-2-positive subgroup as the most sensitive to anthracycline-based adjuvant chemotherapy. Two other retrospective studies [53, 54] generated similar results regarding HER-2 overexpression and responsiveness to anthracyclines. Additionally, an Intergroup Study, presented at the 1998 ASCO meeting, showed that, in tumors overexpressing HER-2, chemo-endocrine therapy with cyclophosphamide, doxorubicin, 5-fluorouracil (CAF), plus tamoxifen seemed to yield better results than tamoxifen alone [55].

More recently, the Canadian group (NCI-C) has reported the results of a retrospective study exploring the predictive value of HER-2 gene amplification in a population of node-positive pre-menopausal patients treated in the context of the MA-5 phase III trial with either CMF or CEF [56]. This study suggests that the superiority of CEF over CMF is seen only in the population of HER-2 positive patients [56]. Conversely, the Danish group (DBCG) has not found a similar interaction between HER-2 and anthracyclines in their study comparing CMF and CEF in the adjuvant treatment of breast cancer patients [57]. Taken together, these studies provide level II, category C evidence concerning clinical practice recommendations.

Topoisomerase II Alpha (Topo IIα)

The topo IIα gene is located next to the HER-2 gene on chromosome 17q12-q21, and its amplification may lead to overexpression of the topo IIα protein. Because this enzyme is inhibited by anthracyclines and is the main target of these drugs, its overexpression may render the cells more sensitive to topo IIα inhibitors [58, 59]. Studies have shown that topo IIα amplification only occurs with concurrent HER-2 amplification, and it is possible that the predictive value of HER-2 regarding anthracycline-based chemotherapy is explained by the concomitant amplification of the *topo IIα gene* [58, 60–62]. Preclinical data also indicate that intra-tumoral topo IIα levels may explain some forms of resistance to anthracyclines observed in in vitro systems [63].

Table 4 shows the results of those studies that have explored the predictive value of topoisomerase IIα gene aberrations in a population of early breast cancer patients treated in the context of phase III trials with an anthracycline or non-anthracycline-based adjuvant chemotherapy [57, 64–66]. Based on the results of these retrospective studies, we have to conclude that the level of evidence for topo IIα gene amplification is II category B.

Table 4 Phase III trials in which topo II gene has been tested as a predictive marker

Study (year)	Design	No. topo II Evaluable pts.	HER-2 Status	% topo II Gene amplification	% topo II Gene deletion	Results
Di Leo et al. [64] (2002)	→ CMF → HEC → EC	61	+	38	13	HEC + EC > CMF if topo II amplified HEC + EC = CMF if topo II non-amplified
Knoop et al. [37] (2005)	→ CMF → FEC	773	+/–	12	11	FEC > CMF if topo II amplified or deleted FEC = CMF if topo II normal
O'Malley et al. [65] (2006)	→ CMF → FEC	443	+/–	11	6	FEC > CMF if topo II amplified or deleted FEC = CMF if topo II normal
Slamon et al. [66] (2006)	→ AC → DT → DPT → AC → D	2990	+	35	5	AC → DT = DPT = AC → D if topo II amplified AC → DT = DPT > AC → D if topo II non-amplified

CMF = cyclophophamide-methotrexate-fluorouracil; HEC = standard doses epirubicin-cyclophosphamide; EC = moderate doses epirubicin-cyclophosphamide; AC → DT = doxorubicin-cyclophosphamide → docetaxel-trastuzumab; DPT = docetaxel-carboplatin-trastuzumab; AC → D = doxorubicin-cyclophophamide → docetaxel; FEC = fluorouracil-epirubicin-cyclophophamide

Factors preventing the use of topo IIα gene amplification as a marker predicting the activity of anthracyclines in the adjuvant setting are: (1) the fact that also topo IIα gene deletion seems to predict response to anthracyclines and this is hard to explain biologically [57, 65]; (2) the lack of correlation between gene status and topo IIα protein levels evaluated by IHC [67–69]; (3) the lack of reproducibility studies showing an acceptable level of inter-laboratory agreement when topo IIα gene status is evaluated on the same samples in different laboratories.

Markers Predicting the Activity of Taxane-Based Regimens

Taxanes have been evaluated in the adjuvant setting only recently. Therefore, most of the available results regarding possible predictive factors were obtained in the context of metastatic or neoadjuvant breast cancer studies. Three randomized studies have suggested that tumors overexpressing HER-2 might be more sensitive to a taxane-based than to anthracycline-based regimens (Table 5) [70–72]. Based on these results, the level of evidence is II category B. More clinical evidence is needed to implement the results of these retrospective studies into clinical practice.

In a clinical study of neoadjuvant chemotherapy, *p-53* mutated tumors showed a high response rate when treated with taxanes, but a low response rate when treated with anthracyclines [73]. This and other in vitro and in vivo

Table 5 HER-2/neu and taxanes

Group	Design	Setting	No. pts.	HER-2 technique	Results
TAX 303[70]	→ A → TxT	Advanced	176	IHC/FISH	HER-2+ TxT > A HER-2– TxT = A
UCLA[71]	→ EC → ET	Advanced	297	FISH	HER-2+ ET > EC HER-2– ET = EC
CALGB[72]	→ AC → AC→T	Early	1,500	IHC/FISH	HER-2 + AC → T > AC HER-2- AC → T = AC

EC = Epirubicin-Cyclophosphamide; ET = Epirubicin-Paclitaxel; A = Doxorubicin; TxT = Docetaxel;
AC = Doxorubicin-Cyclophophamide; T = Paclitaxel; FISH = fluorescence in-situ hybridization;
IHC = immunohistochemistry

studies have raised the hypothesis that *p-53-m*utated tumors might be less sensitive to anthracyclines, while retaining sensitivity to taxanes [74]. To test this hypothesis, a large multicenter international prospective trial has been opened under the auspices of B.I.G. (Breast International Group) and coordinated by the EORTC.

The most attractive markers as far as taxane treatment is concerned are probably the microtubule-associated parameters (MTAP). These are a specific target for taxanes because these drugs interact with microtubules. Preclinical data suggest that mammary and pancreatic tumors with exquisite responsiveness to docetaxel in in vitro models have the highest expression of the *Tau* gene (MTAP-2 family) and of the α-tubulin protein [75]. Assessment of MTAP-2 expression by IHC in paraffin-embedded samples is feasible, making possible retrospective studies correlating MTAP-2 levels and docetaxel activity in both the metastatic and adjuvant settings.

The M.D. Anderson group has evaluated the predictive value of TAU protein in the context of a neoadjuvant phase II trial in which breast cancer patients were treated with a paclitaxel-based chemotherapy. The results of this retrospective study seem to suggest that TAU protein down-regulation is associated with a 44% pathologic complete response (pCR) rate, while in the TAU overexpression group pCR rate is 17% [76]. The same group has produced similar results in a pre-clinical study where TAU gene has been down-regulated and this has produced increased sensitivity of breast cancer cells to paclitaxel but not to epirubicin [76].

Of note, proteins associated with the mitotic spindle regulation have been suggested as markers predicting sensitivity or resistance to taxanes also in two different phase II neoadjuvant studies in which response to single-agent docetaxel or to paclitaxel-based sequential chemotherapy has been correlated with gene expression profiles evaluated by gene microarray technology on pre-treatment primary tumor samples [77, 78].

Although data exist on p-53 gene mutation or MTAP expression and resistance to taxanes, current levels of evidence do not recommend the use of these tools in clinical practice (level II C for p-53, level III B for MTAP).

Markers Predicting the Activity of Anti-HER-2 Therapies

The identification of patient candidates for anti-HER-2 therapies either in the early or in the metastatic setting is by far the most relevant information provided by HER-2 testing of breast cancer samples. Large phase III trials have unequivocally proved the efficacy of anti-HER-2 agents such as trastuzumab and lapatinib in patients carrying HER-2 positive tumors [79–84].

The identification of molecular markers complementing HER-2 scores with the aim to define better the profile of anti-HER-2 compound sensitive tumors is certainly a relevant research area. Different events seem to play a role in the onset of clinical resistance to anti-HER-2 compounds. Among these, activation of the insulin-like growth factor 1 (IGF-1) pathway, PTEN deficiency, PI3K gene mutations, compensatory signalling from other HER family members, and polymorphism of the FC receptor, have been suggested as potential markers of resistance [85]. Ongoing clinical studies will likely clarify the role of these markers in predicting the likelihood of response of HER-2 positive tumors to anti-HER-2 therapies.

Conclusions

Hormone receptor expression for adjuvant hormonotherapy and HER-2 over-expression for anti-HER-2 compounds are the only predictive markers for which level I category A evidence justifies use in routine clinical practice.

The significant translational research efforts carried out in the past decade in this field have led to the generation of some fascinating hypotheses. New techniques now exist to test a number of these hypotheses. In particular, the use of cDNA micro-arrays will permit a better biological characterization of breast cancer, and perhaps even a new classification of the disease, based on distinct molecular profiles, which may be of prognostic and/or predictive value. It is now time to test these hypotheses in a new generation of prospective predictive marker studies, some of which are already ongoing, and the results of which are eagerly awaited. Their outcome may radically change the therapeutic approach to early breast cancer in the future.

References

1. Goldhirsch A, Glick JH, Gelber RD, et al. Meeting highlights: International expert consensus on the primary therapy of early breast cancer 2005. *Ann Oncol.* 2005;16:1569–83.
2. Park WB, Kim SI, Kim EK, et al. Impact of patient age on the outcome of primary breast carcinoma. *J Surg Oncol.* 2002;80:12–8, 2002.
3. Aebi S, Gelber S, Castiglione-Gertsch M, et al. Is chemotherapy alone adequate for young women with oestrogen-receptor-positive breast cancer? *Lancet.* 2000;355:1869–74.
4. El Saghir NS, Seoud M, Khalil MK, et al. Effects of young age at presentation on survival in breast cancer. *BMC Cancer.* 2006;6:194 [Epub ahead of print]
5. Colleoni M, Rotmensz N, Peruzzotti G, et al. Role of endocrine responsiveness and adjuvant therapy in very young women (below 35 years) with operable breast cancer and node negative disease. *Ann Oncol.* 2006;17:1497–503.
6. Mirza AN, Mirza NQ, Vlastos G, Singletary SE. Prognostic factors in node-negative breast cancer: A review of studies with sample size more than 200 and follow-up more than 5 years. *Ann Surg.* 2002;235:10–26.
7. Shetty MR, Reiman HM Jr. Tumor size and axillary metastasis: A correlative occurrence in 1244 cases of breast cancer between 1980 and 1995. Eur J Surg Oncol. 1997;23:139–41.
8. Carter CL, Allen C, Henson DE. Relation of tumor size, lymph node status, and survival in 24,740 breast cancer cases. *Cancer.* 1989;63:181–87.
9. Fisher ER, Costantino J, Fisher B, Redmond C. Pathologic findings from the National Surgical Adjuvant Breast Project (Protocol 4). Discriminants for 15-year survival. National Surgical Adjuvant Breast and Bowel Project Investigators. *Cancer.* 1993;71(6):2141–50.
10. Cserni G, Gregori D, Merletti F, et al. Meta-analysis of non-sentinel node metastases associated with micrometastatic sentil nodes in breast cancer. *Br J Surg.* 2004;91:1245–52.
11. Colleoni M, Rotmensz N, Perruzzotti G, et al. Size of breast cancer metastases in axillary lymph nodes: Clinical relevance of minimal lymph node involvement. *J Clin Oncol.* 2005;23:1379–89.

12. Elston CW, Ellis IO. Pathological prognostic factors in breast cancer. I. The value of histological grade in breast cancer: Experience from a large study with long-term follow-up. *Histopathology*. 1991;19:1403–10.
13. Sotiriou C, Wirapati P, Loi S, et al. Gene expression profiling in breast cancer: Understanding the molecular basis of histologic grade to improve prognosis. *Natl Cancer Inst*. 2006;98:262–72.
14. Ross JS, Fletcher JA, Linette GP, et al. The Her-2/neu gene and protein in breast cancer 2003: Biomarker and target of therapy. *Oncologist*. 2003;8:307–25, 2003
15. Pinder SE, Ellis IO, Galea M, et al. Pathological prognostic factors in breast cancer. III. Vascular invasion: Relationship with recurrence and survival in a large study with long-term follow-up. *Histopathology*. 1994;24:41–7.
16. Kato T, Kameoka S, Kimura T, et al. The combination of angiogenesis and blood vessel invasion as a prognostic indicator in primary breast cancer. *Br J Cancer*. 2003;88:1900–8.
17. Hasebe T, Sasaki S, Imoto S, et al. Histological characteristics of tumor in vessels and lymph nodes are significant predictors of progression of invasive ductal carcinoma of the breast: A prospective study. *Hum Pathol*. 2004;35:298–308.
18. Schoppmann SF, Bayer G, Aumayr K, et al. Prognostic value of lymphangiogenesis and lymphvascular invasion in invasive breast cancer. *Ann Surg*. 2004;240:306–12.
19. Davis BW, Gelber RD, Goldhirisch A, et al. Prognostic significance of peritumoral vessel invasion in clinical trials for adjuvant therapy for breast cancer. *J Clin Oncol*. 1999;17:1474.
20. de Mascarel I, Bonichon F, Durand M, et al. Obvious peritumoral emboli: An elusive prognostic factor reappraised. *Eur J Cancer*. 1998;34:58–65.
21. Slade MJ, Coombes RC. The clinical significance of disseminated tumor cells in breast cancer. *Nat Clin Pract Oncol*. 2007;4:30–41.
22. Harbeck N, Kates RE, Schmitt M, et al. Urokinase-type plasminogen activator and ist inhibitor type 1 predict disease outcome and therapy response in primary breast cancer. *Clin Breast Cancer*. 2004;5:348–52.
23. Harbeck N. Pooled analysis validates predictive impact uPA and PAI-1 for response to adjuvant chemotherapy in breast cancer. *Breast*. 2005;14(l):S27.
24. Sorlie T, Perou CM, Tibshirani R, Aas T, Geisler S, Johnsen H, et al. Gene expression patterns of breast carcinomas distinguish tumor subclasses with clinical implications. *Proc Natl Acad Sci U S A*. 2001;98(19):10869–74.
25. Sorlie T, Tibshirani R, Parker J, Hastie T, Marron JS, Nobel A, et al. Repeated observation of breast tumor subtypes in independent gene expression data sets. *Proc Natl Acad Sci U S A*. 2003;100(14):8418–23.
26. van 't Veer LJ, Dai H, van de Vijver MJ, He YD, Hart AA, Mao M, et al. Gene expression profiling predicts clinical outcome of breast cancer. *Nature*. 2002;415(6871):530–6.
27. van de Vijver MJ, He YD, van't Veer LJ, Dai H, Hart AA, Voskuil DW, et al. A gene-expression signature as a predictor of survival in breast cancer. *N Engl J Med*. 2002;347(25):1999–2009.
28. Huang E, Cheng SH, Dressman H, Pittman J, Tsou MH, Horng CF, et al. Gene expression predictors of breast cancer outcomes. *Lancet*. 2003;361(9369):1590–6.
29. Sotiriou C, Neo SY, McShane LM, Korn EL, Long PM, Jazaeri A, et al. Breast cancer classification and prognosis based on gene expression profiles from a population-based study. *Proc Natl Acad Sci U S A*. 2003;100(18):10393–8.
30. Hu Z, Fan C, Oh DS, et al. The molecular portraits of breast tumors are conserved across microarray platforms. *BMC Genomics*. 2006;7:96.
31. Osborne CK, Bardou V, Hopp TA, et al. Role of the estrogen receptor coactivator AIB1 (SRC-3) and HER-2/neu in tamoxifen resistance in breast cancer. *J Natl Cancer Inst*. 2003;95:353–61.
32. Carlomagno C, Perrone F, Gallo C, et al. c-erb B2 overexpression decreases the benefit of adjuvant tamoxifen in early-stage breast cancer without axillary lymph node metastases. *J Clin Oncol*. 1996;14:2702–8.

33. De Placido S, De Laurentiis M, Carlomagno C, et al. Twenty-year results of the Naples GUN randomized trial: predictive factors of adjuvant tamoxifen efficacy in early breast cancer. *Clin Cancer Res.* 2003;9:1039–46.
34. Stal O, Borg A, Ferno M, et al. ErbB2 status and the benefit from 2 or 5 years of adjuvant tamoxifen in postmenopausal early stage breast cancer. *Ann Oncol.* 2000;11:1545–50.
35. Climent MA, Seguì MA, Peirò G, et al. Prognostic value of HER-2/neu and p-53 expression in node-positive breast cancer. HER-2/neu effect on adjuvant tamoxifen treatment. *The Breast.* 2001;10:67–77.
36. Berry DA, Muss HB, Thor AD, et al. HER-2/neu and p-53 expression versus tamoxifen resistance in estrogen receptor positive, node-positive breast cancer. *J Clin Oncol.* 2000;18:3471–9.
37. Knoop AS, Bentzen SM, Nielsen MM, et al. Value of epidermal growth factor receptor, HER-2, p-53, and steroid receptors in predicting the efficacy of tamoxifen in high-risk postmenopausal breast cancer patients. *J Clin Oncol.* 2001;19:3376–84.
38. Dowsett M, Allred DC, on behalf of the TransATAC investigators. Relationship between quantitative ER and PgR expression and HER2 status with recurrence in the ATAC trial. *Breast Cancer Res Treat.* 2006;100:S21(Abstract 48).
39. Ellis MJ, Coop A, Singh B, et al. Letrozole is more effective neoadjuvant endocrine therapy than tamoxifen for ErbB-1- and/or ErbB-2-positive, estrogen receptor-positive primary breast cancer: Evidence from a phase III randomized trial. *J Clin Oncol.* 2001;19:3808–16.
40. Smith IE, Dowsett M, Ebbs SR, et al. Neoadjuvant treatment of postmenopausal breast cancer with anastrozole, tamoxifen, or both in combination: The immediate preoperative anastrozole, tamoxifen, or combined with tamoxifen (IMPACT) multicenter double-blind randomized trial. *J Clin Oncol.* 2005;23:5108–16.
41. Elledge RM, Green S, Howes L, et al. bcl-2, p-53, and response to tamoxifen in estrogen receptor-positive metastatic breast cancer: A southwest oncology group study. *J Clin Oncol.* 1997;15:1916–22.
42. Gasparini G, Barbareschi M, Doglioni C, et al. Expression of bcl-2 protein predicts efficacy of adjuvant treatments in operable node-positive breast cancer. *Clin Cancer Res.* 1995;1:189–98.
43. Cardoso F, Paesmans M, Larsimont D, et al. Potential predictive value of Bcl-2 for response to tamoxifen in the adjuvant setting of node-positive breast cancer. *Clin Breast Cancer.* 2004;5:364–9.
44. Paik S, Shak S, Tang G, et al. A multigene assay to predict recurrence of tamoxifen-treated, node-negative breast cancer. *N Engl J Med.* 2004;351:2817–26.
45. Paik S, Tang G, Shak S, et al. Gene expression and benefit of chemotherapy in women with node-negative, estrogen receptor-positive breast cancer. *J Clin Oncol.* 2006;24:3726–34.
46. Allred DC, Clarck GM, Tandon AK, et al. HER-2/neu node-negative breast cancer: Prognostic significance of overexpression influenced by the presence of in-situ carcinoma. *J Clin Oncol.* 1992;10:599–605.
47. Gusterson BA, Gelber RD, Goldhirsch A, et al. Prognostic importance of c-erbB2 expression in breast cancer. *J Clin Oncol.* 1992;10:1049–56.
48. Miles DW, Harris WH, Gillett CE, et al. Effect of c-erbB2 and estrogen receptor status on survival of women with primary breast cancer treated with adjuvant cyclophosphamide/methotrexate/fluorouracil. *Int J Cancer.* 1999;84:354–9.
49. Menard S, Valagussa P, Pilotti S, et al. Response to cyclophosphamide, methotrexate, and fluorouracil in lymph node positive breast cancer according to H ER2 overexpression and other tumor biological variables. *J Clin Oncol.* 2001;19:329–35.
50. Paik S, Bryant J, Tan-Chiu E, et al. HER2 and choice of adjuvant chemotherapy for invasive breast cancer: National Surgical Adjuvant Breast and Bowel Project Protocol B-15. *J Natl Cancer Inst.* 2000;92:1991–8.

51. Di Leo A, Larsimont D, Gancberg D, et al. HER-2 and topoisomerase as predictive markers in a population of node positive breast cancer patients randomly treated with adjuvant CMF or epirubicin plus cyclophosphamide. *Ann Oncol.* 2001;12:1081–9.
52. Moliterni A, Ménard S, Valagussa P, et al. Her2 overexpression and doxorubicin in the adjuvant chemotherapy of resectable breast cancer. *Proc Am Soc Clin Oncol.* 2001;20:23a(Abstract 89).
53. Paik S, Bryant J, Park C, et al. erb B2 and response to doxorubicin in patients with axillary lymph node-positive, hormone receptor-negative breast cancer. *J Nat Cancer Inst.* 1998;90:1361–70.
54. Thor AD, Berry DA, Budman DR, et al. erb-B2, p-53, and efficacy of adjuvant therapy in lymph node-positive breast cancer. *J Nat Cancer Inst.* 1998;90:1346–60.
55. Elledge RM, Green S, Ciocca D, et al. HER-2 expression and response to tamoxifen in estrogen receptor-positive breast cancer: A southwest oncology group study. *Clin Cancer Res.* 1998;4:7–12.
56. Pritchard KI, Shepherd LE, O'Malley FP, et al. HER2 and responsiveness of breast cancer to adjuvant chemotherapy. *N Engl J Med.* 2006;354:2103–11.
57. Knoop AS, Knudsen H, Balslev E, et al. Retrospective analysis of topoisomerase IIa amplifications and deletions as predictive markers in primary breast cancer patients randomly assigned to cyclophosphamide, methotrexate, and fluorouracil or cyclophosphamide, epirubicin, and fluorouracil: Danish Breast Cancer Cooperative Group. *J Clin Oncol.* 2005;23:7483–90.
58. Jarvinen TAH, Tanner M, Rantanen V, et al. Amplification and deletion of topoisomerase IIa associate with ErbB-2 amplification and affect sensitivity to topoisomerase II inhibitor doxorubicin in breast cancer. *Am J Pathol.* 2000;156:839–47.
59. Smith K, Houlbrook 5, Greenall M, et al. Topoisomerase IIa co-amplification with erbB2 in human primary breast cancer and breast cancer cell lines: Relationship to m-AMSA and mitoxantrone sensitivity. *Oncogene.* 1993;8:933–8.
60. Jarvinen TAH, Kononen J, Pelto-Huikko M, et al. Expression of topoisomerase IIa is associated with rapid cell proliferation, aneuploidy, and c-erb B2 overexpression in breast cancer. *Am J Pathol.* 1996;148:2073–82.
61. Jarvinen TAH, Tanner M, Barlund M, et al. Characterization of topoisomerase IIa gene amplification and deletion in breast cancer. *Genes Chromosomes Cancer.* 1999;26:142–50.
62. Isola JJ, Tanner M, Holli K, et al. Amplification of topoisomerase IIα is a strong predictor of response to epirubicin based chemotherapy in HER-2/neu positive breast cancer. *Breast Cancer Res Treat.* 2000;64:31.
63. Nitiss JL, Beck WT. Anti-topoisomerase drug action and resistance. *Eur J Cancer.* 1996;32A:958–66.
64. Di Leo A, Gancberg D, Larsimont D, et al. HER-2 amplification and topoisomerase II alpha gene aberrations as predictive markers in node-positive breast cancer patients randomly treated either with an anthracycline-based therapy or with cyclophosphamide, methotrexate, and 5-fluorouracil. *Clin Cancer Res.* 2002;8:1107–16.
65. O'Malley FP, Chia S, Tu D, et al. Prognostic and predictive value of topoisomerase II alpha in randomized trial comparing CMF to CEF in premenopausal women with node positive breast cancer (NCIC CTG MA.5). *Proc Am Soc Clin Oncol.* 2006;24:11s (Abstract 533).
66. Slamon D, Eiermann W, Robert N, et al. BCIRG 006: 2nd interim analysis phase III randomized trial comparing doxorubicin and cyclophosphamide followed by docetaxel with doxorubicin and cyclophosphamide followed by docetaxel and trastuzumab with docetaxel, carboplatin and trastuzumab in HER2 neu positive early breast cancer patients. *Breast Cancer Res Treat.* 100, 2006, late-breaking abstract 52.
67. Durbecq V, Desmed C, Paesmans M, et al. Correlation between topoisomerase-IIalpha gene amplification and protein expression in HER-2 amplified breast cancer. *Int J Oncol.* 2004;25:1473–9.

68. Mueller RE, Parkes RK, Andrulis I, et al. Amplification of the TOP2A gene does not predict high levels of topoisomerase II alpha protein in human breast tumor samples. *Genes Chromosomes Cancer*. 2004;39:288–97.
69. Callagy G, Pharoah P, Chin SF, et al. Identification and validation of prognostic markers in breast cancer with the complementary use of array-CGH and tissue microarrays. *J Pathol*. 2005;205:388–96.
70. Di Leo A, Chan S, Paesmans M, et al. HER-2/neu as a predictive marker in a population of advanced breast cancer patients randomly treated either with single-agent doxorubicin or single-agent docetaxel. *Breast Cancer Res Treat*. 2004,86:197–206.
71. Konecny GE, Thomssen C, Luck HJ, et al. Her-2/neu gene amplification and response to paclitaxel in patients with metastatic breast cancer. *J Natl Cancer Inst*. 2004;96:1141–51.
72. Hayes DF, Thor A, Dressler L, et al. HER2 predicts benefit from adjuvant paclitaxel after AC in node-positive breast cancer: CALGB 9344. *Proc Am Soc Clin Oncol*. 2006;24:5s (Abstract 510).
73. Kandioler-Eckersberger D, Ludwig C, Rudas M, et al. TP-53 mutation and p-53 over-expression for prediction of response to neoadjuvant treatment in breast cancer patients. *Clin Cancer Res*. 2000;6:50–6.
74. Di Leo A, Tanner M, Desmedt C, et al. p-53 gene mutations as a predictive marker in a population of advanced breast cancer patients randomly treated with doxorubicin or docetaxel in the context of a phase III clinical trial. *Ann Oncol*. 2007;Mar 17 [ahead of print].
75. Veitia R, Bissery MC, Martinez C, et al. Tau expression in model adenocarcinomas correlates with docetaxel sensitivity in tumor-bearing mice. *Br J Cancer*. 1998;78:871–7.
76. Rouzier R, Rajan R, Wagner P, et al. Microtubule-associated protein tau: A marker of paclitaxel sensitivity in breast cancer. *Proc Natl Acad Sci U S A*. 2005;102:8315–20.
77. Chang JC, Wooten EC, Tsimelzon A, et al. Gene expression profiling for the prediction of therapeutic response to docetaxel in patients with breast cancer. *Lancet*. 2003;362:362–9
78. Hess KR, Anderson K, Symmans WF, et al. Pharmacogenomic predictor of sensitivity to preoperative chemotherapy with paclitaxel and fluorouracil, doxorubicin, and cyclophosphamide in breast cancer. *J Clin Oncol*. 2006;24:4236–44.
79. Slamon DJ, Leyland-Jones B, Shak S, et al. Use of chemotherapy plus a monoclonal antibody against HER2 for metastatic breast cancer that overexpresses HER2. *N Engl J Med*. 2001;344:783–92.
80. Piccart-Gebhart MJ, Procter M, Leyland-Jones B, et al. Trastuzumab after adjuvant chemotherapy in HER2-positive breast cancer. *N Engl J Med*. 2005;353:1659–72.
81. Romond EH, Perez EA, Bryant J, et al. Trastuzumab plus adjuvant chemotherapy for operable HER2-positive breast cancer. *N Engl J Med*. 2005;353:1673–84.
82. Joensuu H, Kellokumpu-Lehtinen PL, Bono P, et al. Adjuvant docetaxel or vinorelbine with or without trastuzumab for breast cancer. *N Engl J Med*. 2006;354:809–20.
83. Slamon D, Eiermann W, Robert N, et al. Phase III randomized trial comparing doxorubicin and cyclophosphamide followed by docetaxel with doxorubicin and cyclophosphamide followed by docetaxel and trastuzumab with docetaxel, carboplatin and trastuzumab in HER2 positive early breast cancer patients: BCIRG 006 study. *Breast Cancer Res Treat*. 2005;94:S5 (Abstract 1).
84. Geyer CE, Forster J, Lindquist D, et al. Lapatinib plus capecitabine for HER2-positive advanced breast cancer. *N Engl J Med*. 2006;355:2733–43.
85. Nahta R, Esteva FJ. HER2 therapy: Molecular mechanisms of trastuzumab resistance. *Breast Cancer Res*. 2006;8:215.

New Perspectives for Therapy Choice

Anne-Catherine Andres

Introduction

Carcinogenesis is a multi-step process involving the successive accumulation of genetic mutations which provoke the initiation of uncontrolled growth, allow the cell to progress and lose differentiation capacity and eventually lead to transformation into the invasive, metastatic phenotype. Mutations can either lead to the inactivation of genes involved in growth suppression (tumor suppressor genes) or to the activation of growth promoting genes (oncogenes). Some mutations frequently affect the same gene in different individuals, such as the inactivation of BRCA-1 and -2 in heritable breast cancer [1] or the activation of c-ErbB2 in about 30% of spontaneous breast cancer [2]. Additional mutations, however, are not predictable and can occur in a broad variety of genes. The only prerequisite is that they complement each other and in their concerted action enable carcinogenic growth. The fact that multiple combinations can lead to the development of cancer implies that each tumor possesses individual growth characteristics and, thus, women with similar breast cancer types may respond differently to the various standard treatment protocols. In general, the treatment benefits cannot be reliably predicted for an individual patient and over-treatment with unnecessary side effects or under-treatment with fatal consequences for survival are presently unavoidable. Thus, a major effort has been initiated to achieve individual profiling of cancerous lesions facilitating the choice of the most effective treatment protocol and aiming at the elaboration of new "tailor-made" treatment strategies. In this chapter I will summarize different molecular approaches for tumor fingerprinting and discuss their benefits, pitfalls, and prospects for diagnosis, prognosis, and treatment.

A.-C. Andres (✉)
Department of Clinical Research, University of Bern, Tiefenaustrasse 120, CH-3004 Bern, Switzerland
e-mail: anne-catherine.andres@dkf.unibe.ch

M. Castiglione, M.J. Piccart (eds.), *Adjuvant Therapy for Breast Cancer*, Cancer Treatment and Research 151, DOI 10.1007/978-0-387-75115-3_3,

"Omics" in Cancer Diagnosis and Prognosis

Gene Expression Profiling: Genomics and Transcriptomics

Micro-array based technologies allow screening for the expression of many thousands of individual genes in a given tissue sample. RNA is isolated from the tissue of interest and in the presence of labelled nucleotides reversed transcribed into cDNA. This cDNA (referred to as target) can subsequently be hybridized to chips containing immobilized gene-specific oligonucleotide probes (20–80 nucleotides) (conventionally termed reporter platform) (Fig. 1). Since the human genome sequencing project suggests that the total number of human genes is approximately 25,000 [3], it is possible to analyze simultaneously the expression of all known human genes in one experiment. Usually reporter platforms contain only a selection of genes either customized to address specific questions or are commercially available with random selections or with pathway related subgroups of genes. These analyses allow the detection of the transcribed (switched on) genes in a given sample, not only qualitatively but also quantitatively. This diagnostic approach is referred to as transcriptomics.

In breast cancer, transcriptomics has allowed the identification of the expression profile (signature) of luminal and basal-like breast tumor subtypes and has revealed that c-erbB2 positive tumors represent an intrinsic subtype of breast cancer [4–6]. Moreover, an expression profile has been proposed which predicts clinical outcome, metastasis formation and survival in node-negative patients [7–9]. Classical grading of breast cancer allows the distinction between low and high risk groups with the corresponding treatment consequences. However,

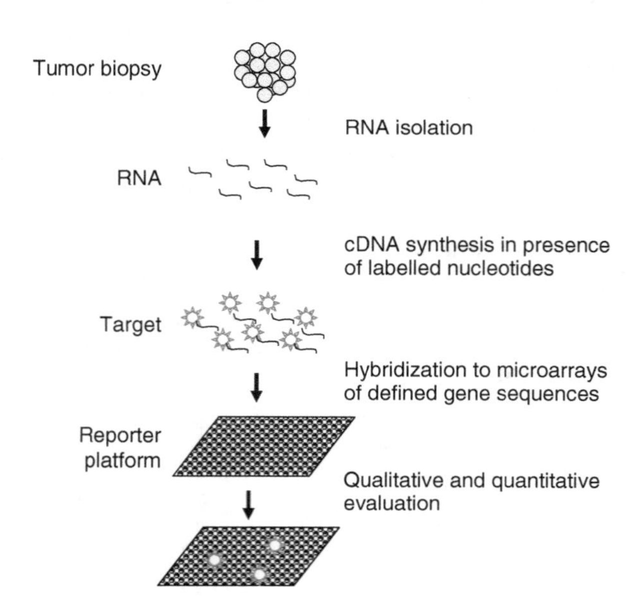

Fig. 1 Schematic representation of the gene expression profiling technique

micro-array technology offers the possibility to characterize also the intermediate groups. An effort in this direction has recently been undertaken for grade 2 breast cancers and has enabled the distinction of two groups, one resembling grade 1 expression profiles and the second corresponding to grade 3 breast cancer [10]. If validated, such refined sub-classifications may allow the avoidance of under- or over-treatment for these intermediate groups of breast cancers.

Transcriptomics has also recently been used to predict response to chemotherapeutic or hormonal treatment. Gene expression profiling of pre-treatment breast tumor biopsies has allowed the characterization of the constellation of gene expression identifying responders to docetaxel, doxorubicine/cyclophosphamide and tamoxifen treatment [11–13]. These promising studies raise the hope that predictive gene expression profiles could indeed be defined for any given adjuvant therapy.

Gene expression profiling has also been applied to characterize tumors from patients carrying a germ-line mutation in the BRCA-1 or BRCA-2 gene. These analyses revealed that BRCA-1 tumors are mainly of the basal subtype whereas BRCA-2 tumors mainly belong to the luminal category [4]. This finding suggests that the genetic background of an individual may influence tumorigenesis and outcome. Transcriptomic analysis has been applied to experimental mouse mammary tumors in different inbred mouse strains exhibiting different rates of metastasis formation and has revealed strain-specific tumor expression profile signatures [14]. These findings demonstrate that indeed the genetic background may predispose an individual to the development of breast cancer and its progression. The assessment of germ line DNA polymorphisms predicting metastasis risk would offer technical advantages over expression profiling on the tumor itself. Genomic DNA preparation entails fewer pitfalls than RNA extraction and the analyses can be made from small biopsies of any tissue of the patient at any time before or during treatment. In humans, however, the genes and polymorphisms associated with increased risk of carcinogenesis and predisposition to metastasis remain in large to be identified [15].

Protein Profiling: Proteomics

Genomics and transcriptomics provide information on mutations in the genetic information (DNA) and on the constellation of genes which are activated and transcribed into RNA. DNA and RNA, however, are only carriers of information which has to be translated into proteins in order to become functional. The total protein content of a cell (the proteome) is a highly versatile and dynamic population and its complexity cannot entirely be predicted from transcriptomics. A variety of control mechanisms and modifications occur post-transcriptionally and post-translationally such as alternative RNA splicing, RNA silencing, RNA and protein stability, co- and post-translational protein modifications which make the qualitative and quantitative prediction of protein constellation (= function) difficult. Proteomics aims at identifying the proteins expressed in a given cell or tissue, cataloguing them and in the best case assigning them to cellular functions.

Three conceptually distinct technologies are mainly used to analyse the constellation of proteins in biological materials: Forward phase arrays (FPA), tissue lysate arrays (TLA) and matrix-assisted or surface-enhanced laser desorption and ionization with time of flight spectrometry (MALDI-TOF, SELDI-TOF).

FPA (Fig. 2a) employs capture proteins which are covalently bound to nitrocellulose filters. These capture proteins are usually a mixture of antibodies directed against a selection of proteins. Protein extracts are prepared from the tissue of interest and incubated with these nitrocellulose filters. If present in the lysate, proteins will bind specifically to the immobilized antibody capture proteins. Binding can be visualized either by directly labelling the protein extracts or by a second reaction with a specific labelled antibody. This method allows the analysis of one tissue sample for a variety of different proteins [16]. In oncological applications, the antibody capture proteins are selected to represent defined proteins involved in signalling pathways controlling cell survival, apoptosis or angiogenesis [17].

In the TLA methodology (Fig. 2b), entire protein extracts of tissue samples are immobilized on nitrocellulose filters and subsequently incubated with a defined, labelled reporter protein. As in FPAs, these reporter proteins are usually antibodies raised against signalling pathway components. The TLA approach enables the immobilization of many protein extracts and thus a variety of different patient samples can be simultaneously analysed for the presence of a given protein. Since the protein arrays have a shelf life of up to 2 years, extracts of the same patient at different stages of diagnosis and treatment can be investigated [18].

The above-mentioned screening methods are so called "low-throughput" in the sense that they allow the search for only a limited number of known, selected proteins, a limitation of the methods. In contrast, MALDI- and SELDI-TOF assays can be used for "high throughput" screening of complex protein mixtures also including unknown proteins (Fig. 2c). Proteins extracted from a tissue of interest are separated by two-dimensional gel electrophoresis according to their charge and size. Selected spots are isolated, proteolytically digested and captured to an energy absorbing matrix (MALDI) or a selective surface (SELDI). Subsequently the bound proteins are ionized by laser energy and fly from the matrix through a vacuum tube onto a detector plate. The time of flight is dependent on the mass and charge of the particle (m/z ratio) which is recorded at the detector plate. Complex bioinformatics and extensive databases allow then the identification of the protein fragments based on these values [19, 20].

To date proteomic approaches are mainly limited to research purposes and are not yet suitable for clinical diagnostics. However, strenuous efforts are currently under way in many laboratories to translate the benefits of these techniques to clinical applications and first trials can be expected soon. For

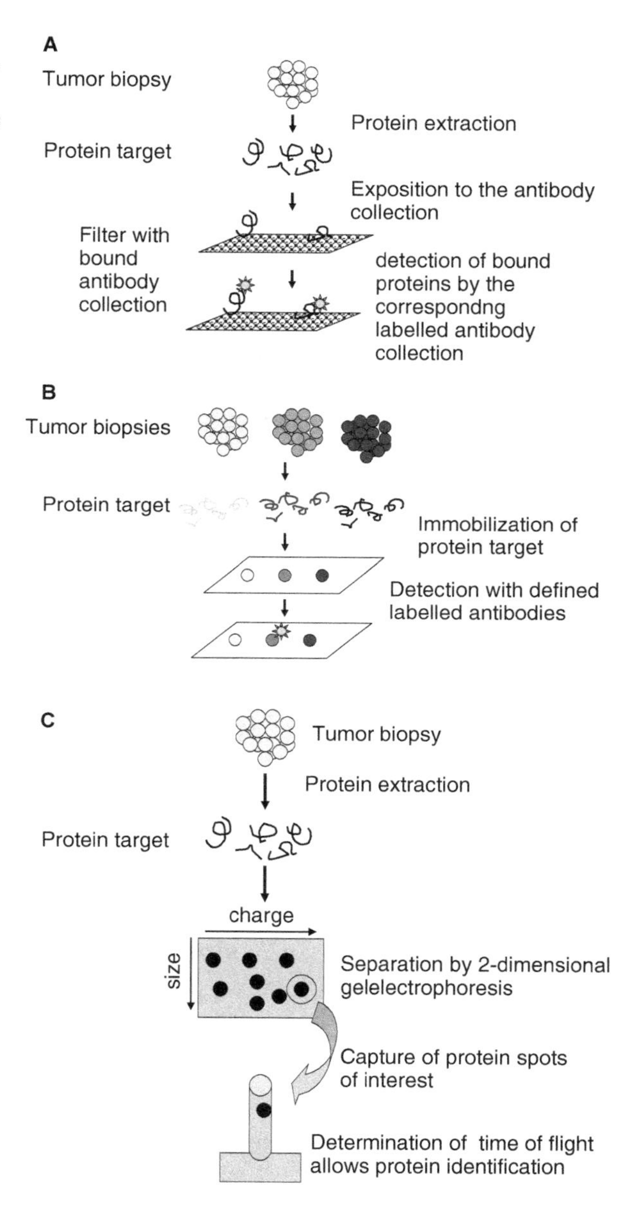

Fig. 2 Schematic representation of proteomic approaches. **a** Forward phase arrays. **b** Tissue lysate arrays. **c** Protein profiling based on the MALDI-TOF or SELDI-TOF technology

breast cancer, the SELDI-TOF technology has been applied to analyse human blood serum. Li et al. have identified three proteins discriminating between stage 0–1 cancer patients and unaffected controls [21]. Moreover, HSP27, 14-3-3 sigma and the mammaglobin/liophilinB complex were identified as breast cancer biomarkers in blood serum [22, 23]. These studies, however, included relatively small patient numbers and need to be confirmed in additional studies.

Profiling of Metabolic Endproducts: Metabolomics

Classically, the functioning of a cell has been considered as a unidirectional process in which the genetic information is processed via RNA to proteins which then lead to changes in the cellular phenotype. It is now acknowledged that cellular processes are much more complex and are networked by complex feed-back loops, often driven by enzymatic end-products, the metabolites. Metabolomics aims at the quantitative assessment of all metabolites present in a given tissue at a given physiological or developmental stage (the metabolome). Metabonomics is similar, however, is restricted to the comparative analysis of pathological conditions. Analysis of the metabolome has several advantages over transcriptomics or proteomics: Firstly, moderate changes in enzyme levels have little influence on metabolite fluxes; however, they have significant effect on the accumulation of metabolic end-products. Secondly, since the metabolites are the most downstream evidences of gene expression, their accumulation effectively amplifies the often modest changes in gene expression and thereby offer increased sensitivity. Thirdly, metabolic pathways are not only regulated by gene expression but also by post-translational regulation often initiated by the metabolic end-product itself [24].

Currently, the most widely used strategies comprise (1) metabolite target analysis which restricts itself to the analysis to metabolites of a particular enzyme system suspected to be affected by a particular biological change, (2) metabolite profiling which is confined to metabolites associated with specific cellular pathways targeted by pharmacological interventions, and (3) true metabolomics or metabonomics which involves qualitative and quantitative profiling of all metabolites in a tissue. Methodologically, the procedures for all three strategies are similar: Tissues of interest are immediately snap-frozen in liquid nitrogen (to arrest all enzymatic activity), extracted by heat-assisted acid, alkaline or ethanol treatment and resolved by high resolution separation techniques such as gas or liquid chromatography mass spectroscopy or nuclear magnetic resonance. As for proteomics and transcriptomics, interpretation of the data requires bioinformatics and data-bases which are still under development [24].

Matabolomics not only offers the possibility to analyse the metabolites in body fluids or tissue biopsies, but also knowledge of tumor associated metabolites that would allow highly sensitive and specific imaging of small tumor nodules based on magnetic resonance imaging (MRI) or Positron Emission Tomography combined with computer tomography (PET/CT).

So far, the applications of metabolomics are mainly concentrated with pharmaceutical evaluations aspects and toxicity studies of new compounds. Moreover, the conceptual possibilities of using metabolomics to predict a patient's responsiveness to treatment and to monitor therapeutic tolerance and success are under intense investigation [25].

In oncology, metabolomics is still in the research and evaluation phase. The first promising results have been reported for the diagnosis of ovarian cancer. The NMR based metabolic spectra of patient's serum have allowed the diagnosis of ovarian cancer with high fidelity [26]. Moreover, analysis of the metabolome in fine needle ovarian biopsies by mass spectrometry has allowed the distinction between borderline tumors and cancer [27]. As mentioned above, metabolite analysis can also be restricted to metabolites specific for defined signalling pathways (metabolite target analysis). This approach may have an important potential in the assessment of breast cancer risk and breast cancer diagnosis. It is generally accepted that the exposure to estrogen is a main risk factor for breast cancer and that oxidative metabolites of estrogen may be causally involved in the development of the disease. Crooke et al. recently presented a mathematical model of the normal mammary gland estrogen metabolism, which was confirmed by in vivo studies. This in silico model was then applied to a breast cancer case-control study and identified a patient population with increased risk of breast cancer based on their enzyme haplotype and the calculation of E(2)-3,4-quinone production, a transient metabolite which so far has not been amenable to chemical quantification [28].

Nano-Particles in Diagnosis and Therapy

Nano-particles are very small particles of 1–1,000 nm diameter comprising a core element used for their detection and a shell allowing the interaction with biological systems. The shells of nano-particles are composed of an organic layer made of a variety of components such as polyethyleneglycols, silicon, or albumin (Fig. 3). Tissue-specific ligands such as tumor specific antibodies can be linked to these organic molecules, enabling targeting of the particles to the desired tissue. The core consists of either fluorescent crystals (quantum dots), metals which are magnetically active (super-magneitic nano-particles) or gold (Raman probes) [29].

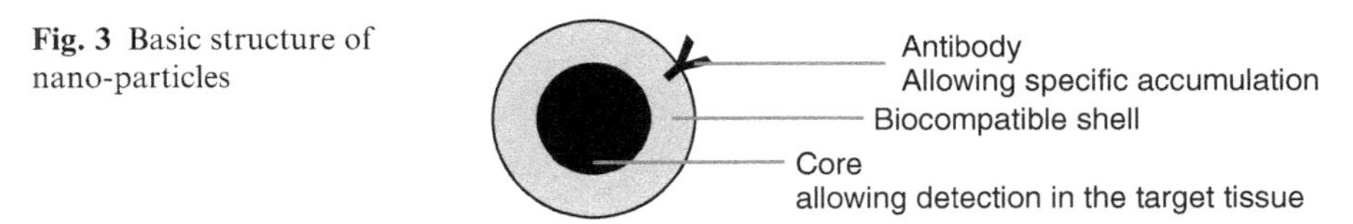

Fig. 3 Basic structure of nano-particles

The fluorescent quantum dots allow the detection and quantification of the target proteins in tumor sections. Since quantum dots can be tuned by changing their size and core composition to emit light with a variety of different wavelengths (450–850 nm), they can be specifically visualized with one light source. Thus, the use of differently fluorescing quantum dots, coated with different antibodies, allows the simultaneous detection of multiple molecular targets in one tumor section or, theoretically, also intra-corporally. The considerable toxicity of quantum dots, however, presently limits their use for diagnostic purposes in vivo [30]. For diagnostic purposes of tumor biopsies, quantum dots are superior to classical immunohistochemistry: (1) they allow the detection of multiple target molecules in one tumor section, (2) they posses a long photostability, and (3) due to their bright fluorescence they allow the accurate detection of low abundant proteins. This technique is not yet widely applied in clinical diagnostics; nevertheless, the recent convincing simultaneous demonstration of c-ErbB2, estrogen receptor, and progesterone receptor in breast cancer cell lines and biopsies suggests their use in clinical practice in the near future [29, 31].

Super-magnetic nano-particles are a powerful means to enhance the sensitivity of MRI and are already widely used in clinical practice and in experimental studies of tumor-associated gene expression, angiogenesis and cellular trafficking. The key advantages of magnetic nano-particles are their low toxicity, high biocompatibility, and efficient accumulation in the target tissue, thereby enabling the imaging of small tumor nodules by safe and non-invasive methods [32, 33].

Gold based nano-particles are very attractive, since they can not only serve diagnostic purposes but also enable therapeutic applications. The concept involves antibody coated gold nano-particles which specifically accumulate in the target tissue. They can be excited by lowest-dose laser energy which in turn can be converted into images by opto-acoustic tomography. By increasing the laser energy to levels still far below the dosage leading to damage of untreated cells, the excited nano-particles convert photo-energy into thermal energy and lead to heat-induced killing of the targeted cells [34]. Ito et al. could show that gold nano-particles bio-conjugated with c-ErbB2 antibodies specifically accumulated in the c-ErbB2 over-expressing SKBR-3 cells and that laser irradiation caused irreversible heat-induced damage leading to cell death [32]. Thus, targeted gold nano-particles may be a potent mean to achieve not only improved imaging of tumor nodules but also their systemic photo-thermal ablation.

Taken together, nano-particles represent a powerful new method of tumor imaging and targeting which promises to improve detection sensitivity and safety and tumor irradiation efficacy. It is to be hoped that the encouraging results of the experimental studies will soon be confirmed by pre-clinical and clinical trials.

Perspectives

Undoubtedly, tumor profiling and nano-technology are powerful means to achieve revolutionary progress in the clinical management of breast cancer. For example, tumor profiling has led to the understanding that estrogen receptor positive and negative breast tumors are different biological diseases which can be further sub-grouped with respect to prognosis and treatment response [35]. Ideally, profiling of an individual tumor by one or a combination of the "omics" approaches will allow the administration of an effective tailored treatment regimen. In the case of recurrence, further profiling of the relapsed tumor cells could reveal their biological changes and treatment could be adapted accordingly. The consequence of this development, however, is that patient groups sharing similar characteristics will get smaller and smaller. Thus, it will be difficult to include enough patients into a clinical study to obtain statistically meaningful data. There is an urgent need to adapt prospective clinical study design to the overwhelming information which can potentially be gained from an individual patient [35, 36]. Primarily, a standardized methodology for tumor profiling has to be established to prevent the presently existing variability and inconsistencies due to technical variations. Moreover, the predictive value and therapeutic suitability has to be proven for every molecule suspected of contributing to the tumor's characteristics. Finally, the benefit of the tailored therapy has to be analysed not only in terms of individual success but also in terms of cost effectiveness. The translation of the technical possibilities into clinical practice will be a major challenge in oncology and will require a comprehensive international collaboration between study groups, clinical centres and research laboratories.

Acknowledgments In thankful memory of Dr. Andrew Ziemiecki. The financial support of the Foundation for Clinical-Experimental Tumour Research is gratefully acknowledged.

References

1. Nicoletta MO, Donach M, De Nicolo A, et al. BRCA-1 and BRCA-2 mutations as prognostic factors in clinical practice and genetic counseling. *Cancer Res Treat Rev.* 2001;27:295–304.
2. Badache A, Goncalves A. The ErbB2 signaling network as target for breast cancer therapy. *J Mammary Gland Biol Neoplasia.* 2006;11:13–25.
3. Consortium IHGS. Finishing the euchromatic sequence of the human genome. *Nature.* 2004;431:931–45.
4. Sorlie T, Tibshirani R, Parker J, et al. Repeated observation of breast tumour subtypes in independent gene expression data sets. *Proc Natl Acad Sci U S A.* 2003;100:8418–23.
5. Farmer P, Bonnefoi H, Becette V, et al. Identification of molecular apocrine breast tumours by microarray analysis. *Oncogene.* 2005;24:4660–71.
6. Sorlie T, Wang Y, Xiao C, et al. Distinct molecular mechanisms underlying clinically relevant subtypes of breast cancer: Gene expression analyses across three different platforms. *BMC Genomics.* 2006;7:127.
7. Van 't Veer VI, Dai H, van de Vijer MJ, et al. Gene expression profiling predicts clinical outcome of breast cancer. *Nature.* 2002;415:530–6.
8. Van de Vijer MJ, He YD, van 't Veer VI, et al. A gene expression signature as a predictor of survival in breast cancer. *N Engl J Med.* 2002;347:1999–2009.
9. Wang Y, Klijn, JG, Zhang Y, et al. Gene expression profiles to predict distant metastases of lymph-node-negative primary breast cancer. *Lancet.* 2005;365:671–9.
10. Sotiriou C, Wirapati P, Loi S, et al. Gene expression profiling in breast cancer: Understanding the molecular basis of histology grade to improve prognosis. *J Natl Cancer Inst.* 2006;98:262–72.
11. Chang JC, Wooten EC, Tsimelzon A, et al. Gene expression profiling for the prediction of therapeutic response to docetaxel in patients with breast cancer. *Lancet.* 2003;362: 362–9
12. Cleator S, Tsimelzon A, Ashworth A, et al. Gene expression patterns for doxorubicin (Adriamycin) and cyclophosphamid (Cytoxan) (AC) response and resistance. *Breast Cancer Res Treat.* 2006;95:229–33.

13. Jansen MP, Foekens JA, van Staveren IL, et al. Molecular classification of tamoxifen-resistant breast carcinomas by gene profiling. *J Clin Oncol.* 2005;23:732–40.
14. Qiu TH, Chandramouli GV, Hunter KW, et al. Global expression profiling identifies signatures of tumor virulence in MMTV-PyMT-transgenic mice: Correlation to human disease. *Cancer Res.* 2004;64:5973–81.
15. Sims A, Ong KR, Clarke RB, et al. Exploiting the potential of gene expression profiling: Is it ready for the clinic? *Breast Cancer Res.* 2006;8:214–20.
16. Miller JC, Zhou H, Kwekel J, et al. Antibody microarray profiling of human prostate cancer sera: antibody screening and identification of potential biomarkers. *Proteomics.* 2003;3:56–63.
17. Knecevic V, Leethanakul C, Bichsel VE, et al. Proteomic profiling of the cancer micro-environment by antibody arrays. *Proteomics* 2001;1:1271–8.
18. Psodas EM, Simpkins F, Liotta AL, et al. Proteomic analysis for the early detection and rational treatment of cancer-realistic hope? *Ann Oncol.* 2005;16:16–22.
19. Merchant M, Weinberger S. Recent advancements in surface enhanced laser desorption/ionisation-time of flight-mass spectrometry. *Electrophoresis.* 2000;21:1164–77.
20. Petricoin EF, Zoon KC, Kohn EC, et al. Clinical proteomics: Translating benchside promise into bedside reality. *Nat Rev Drug Discov.* 2002;1:683–95.
21. Li J, Zhang Z, Rosenzweig J, et al. Proteomics and bioinformatics approaches for identification of serum biomarkers to detect breast cancer. *Clin Chem.* 2002;48:1296–304.
22. Rui Z, Jian-Guo J, Yuan-Peng T, et al. Use of serological proteomic methods to find biomarkers associated with breast cancer. *Proteomics.* 2003;3:433–9.
23. Carter D, Douglas JF, Cornellison CD, et al. Purification and characterization of the mammoglobin/lipophilin B complex, a promising diagnostic marker for breast cancer. *Biochemistry.* 2002;41:6714–22.
24. Hollywood K, Brison DR, Goodacre R. Metabolomics: Current technologies and future trends. *Proteomics.* 2006;6:4716–23.
25. Lindon JC, Holmes E, Nicholson JK. Metabonomics in pharmaceutical R & D. *FEBS J.* 2007;274:1140–51.
26. Odunsi K, Wollmann RM, Ambrosone CB, et al. Detection of epithelial ovarian cancer using H-1-NMR based metabonomics. *Int J Cancer.* 2005;113:782–88.
27. Denkert C, Budczies J, Kind T, et al. Mass-spectometry-based metabolic profiling reveals different metabolite patterns in invasive ovarian carcinomas and borderline tumors. *Cancer Res.* 2006;66:10795–804.
28. Crooke PS, Ritchie MD, Hachey DL, et al. Estrogens, enzyme variants and breast cancer: A risk model. *Cancer Epidemiol Biomarkers Prev.* 2006;1620–9.
29. Yezhelyev MV, Gao X, Al-Hajj A, et al. Emerging use of nanoparticles in diagnosis and treatment of breast cancer. *Lancet Oncol.* 2006;7:657–67.
30. Hardmann R. A toxicologic review of quantum dots: toxicity depends on physiochemical and environmental factors. *Environ Health Perspect.* 2006;114:165–72.
31. Yezhelyev MV, Morris C, Gao X, et al. Simultaneous and quantitative detection of multiple biomarkers in human breast cancer using semiconductor multicolour quantum dots. *Breast Cancer Res Treat.* 2005;94:S48.
32. Ito A, Shinkai M, Honda H, et al. Medical application of functionalized magnetic nanoparticles. *J Biosci Bioeng* 2005;100:1–11.
33. Ackermann ME, Chan WC, Laakkonen P, et al. Nanocrystal targeting in vivo. *Proc Natl Acad Sci U S A.* 2002;99:12617–21.
34. Hirsch LR, Stafford RJ, Blankson J, et al. Nanoshell-mediated infrared thermal therapy of tumors under magnetic resonance guidance. *Proc Natl Acad Sci USA* 2003;100:13549–54.
35. Loi S, Buyse M, Sotiriou C, et al. Challenges in breast cancer clinical trial design in the postgenomic era. *Curr Opin Oncol* 2004;16:536–41.
36. Andre F, Mazouni C, Hortobagyi GN, et al. DNA arrays as predictors of ajuvant/neoadjuvant chemotherapy in breast cancer patients: Current data and issues on study design. *Biochem Biophys Acta.* 2006;1766:197–204.

Pathology Role in Adjuvant Setting

Angelika Reiner-Concin

Introduction

Histopathology provides relevant information on tumors and is generally considered to be the gold standard for diagnostics in oncology. In the last few decades much information on oncology has been gained and tumor characterization has been achieved by histology, including many more details than in former times. In association with this the classification and characterization of tumors have become more complex and therefore communication between clinicians and pathologists needs to be intensified. This becomes evident by the increased implementation of interdisciplinary tumor boards where pathologists take part as important players in a multidisciplinary team.

In this chapter, basic information on histology of breast cancer and conventional histoprognostic factors is given. In addition, the current knowledge on critical questions like observer variability is addressed. Some clinically relevant questions regarding technical aspects are discussed and finally a look is taken at future aspects.

Examination of Pathology Specimens

Core Needle Biopsy – Preoperative Diagnosis

Core needle biopsies (CNB) are widely accepted for preoperative diagnosis in breast lesions. Their diagnostic reliability is very high. The lesion miss rate and the false negative rate are reported in several studies and clinical follow up, being 1.1% and 1% respectively [1]. Taking five or six cores, the diagnostic rate for breast masses is increased up to 97% and for microcalcifications to over 90% [2]. Due to increased mammography screening, preoperative diagnosis on

A. Reiner-Concin (✉)
Department of Pathology, Danube Hospital, Vienna, Austria
e-mail: angelika.reiner@wienkav.at

M. Castiglione, M.J. Piccart (eds.), *Adjuvant Therapy for Breast Cancer*, Cancer Treatment and Research 151, DOI 10.1007/978-0-387-75115-3_4,

CNB is recommended as a quality criterion with respect to preoperative planning of therapy for breast cancer and should be performed at a very high frequency. Also, with respect to neoadjuvant therapy, CNB is a valuable tool for pretherapeutic diagnosis. In CNB, histologic diagnosis can be performed reliably and additional information on prognostic and predictive markers can be obtained by applying immunohistochemistry (IHC) and fluorescent in situ hybridization (FISH). By these methods, steroid hormone receptors and HER-2/neu can be determined very reliably [3–6]. Preoperative profiling with respect to tumor typing and grading is less reliable and reaches only 60–70%. The major problem is of undersampling informative areas in the CNB due to heterogeneity within the tumor. This is especially true for examination of the number of mitoses which is a major factor contributing to tumor grade [7, 8].

To achieve diagnostic accuracy, proper specimen handling is obligatory. This includes that CNB specimens of masses are placed in fixative immediately and that CNB performed due to microcalcifications are X-rayed and also fixed properly. Frozen sections on CNB are not recommended because tissue artefacts due to the freezing procedure may interfere seriously with microscopic interpretation.

Surgical Specimens

In all cases, careful specimen handling and optimal fixation are mandatory. The specimen must not be incised before arriving in the histologic laboratory. For palpable tumors, in case of proven malignant lesions, the surgeon removes the tumor together with an additional rim of surrounding parenchyma in order to achieve clear margins. To guarantee histological orientation, clear marking of the specimen by the surgeon is obligatory. He should preferably attach sutures at the external surface of the specimen. At least three stitches are needed for proper orientation, one to the lateral, one to the medial and one to the superior part of the specimen. For each breast unit it is advisable to establish a code for the orientation of the sutures to avoid misinterpretation. The pathologist should ink the entire surface of the specimen with proper dyes resistant to histologic work up and thus evaluate the margin status exactly. The distance from the tumor to the margins needs to be measured histologically and carefully documented. In case of tumor involved margins at the first excision, the reexcision specimen needs to be oriented again and marked following a standardized protocol. For these specimens, special care needs to be taken on the peripheral margins and they should be sampled exhaustively in histology. The original tumor cavity should be sampled as well in order to detect residual tumor tissue.

In impalpable tumors, which are frequently detected by screening, the lesion is usually localized by wire. Also, for these specimens, orientation using sutures as described above is mandatory. The specimens need to be X-rayed without incision prior to histologic work up. A correlation between the X-ray and the result of histology is necessary to determine whether the relevant lesion has been removed.

Specimens from axillary dissection need to be sliced thinly and palpated. For all identified lymph nodes, histologic examination is necessary. Lymph nodes smaller than 5 mm should be paraffin embedded entirely. Larger lymph nodes need to be cut in half or sliced and then paraffin embedded. To increase diagnostic accuracy, all paraffin blocks from lymph nodes should be step sectioned at three levels.

For sentinel lymph nodes, special standardized work up protocols need to be followed. Sentinel lymph nodes need to be embedded completely and step sectioned till extinction of tissue. Steps should be taken at defined intervals and conventional hematoxylin eosin (H&E) stained sections should be followed by immunhistochemically stained sections using an anticytokeratin antibody. Immunohistochemistry (IHC) should be performed in all sentinel lymph nodes presenting free of tumor on H&E sections.

Frozen Sections

Frozen sections for palpable breast tumors are widely used intraoperatively. With the invention of preoperative diagnosis on CNB their use is limited mainly to assess margin status and sentinel lymph nodes. It is a reliable method for palpable lesions and especially for those larger than 1 cm in diameter [9]. Some authors were able to show that it was also reliable for non-palpable lesions [10]. However, it is not recommended for impalpable lesions and lesions smaller than 1 cm. In most cases with discrepant results between frozen sections and following paraffin histology, the discrepancies are false negative results with a frequency of approximately 1–2% [9]. False positives with frozen sections are very rare events of fewer than 0.1% or do not even occur [11]. However, in some cases (approximately 5%) definitive diagnosis in frozen sections has to be deferred to paraffin sections. Thus sensitivity is over 90% and specificity is around 97%. The main reasons for failure are due to sampling errors, histologic misinterpretation, ignorance of macroscopic features, and poor technical quality of the frozen sections [12].

Frozen sections for margin assessment are described as having a lower diagnostic accuracy. A sensitivity and specificity of 86% and 83% respectively are described [13]. This is mainly due to intraductal tumor components not included in frozen sections but detected only by examination in paraffin sections. The third field of application of frozen sections is intraoperative examination of sentinel lymph node biopsies for the purpose of sparing patients with a positive sentinel lymph node a two step surgery.

Tissue Banks

With growing interest in proteomic and molecular genetic profiling of tumors the interest in establishing multiinstitutional tissue banks for research and its translational application for patients is growing [14].The conventional role of pathologists is professional management of tissue for diagnosis. With this new interest in mind, and the need for high quality removal of representative tumor areas and storage of frozen and paraffin embedded tumor tissue, pathologists need to be involved in these projects. The pathologist can guarantee that tissue is removed from representative areas within a tumor since he recognizes necrotic or fibrotic areas macroscopically which are not applicable to laborious and expensive analysis. In a second step he can prove areas of tissue removal by histologic analysis of corresponding tumor areas. In any event, for high quality biological specimens it has to be guaranteed that tissue removal and freezing is performed immediately after biopsy and tissue fixation has to be performed properly.

Tumor Classification

Malignant breast tumors are divided into epithelial and mesenchymal tumors. Epithelial tumors are far more common and are discussed in this chapter. They are designated as carcinomas and subdivided into invasive and in situ carcinomas. Classification should be performed according to WHO [15]. The classification is based only on the morphological picture of presentation and does not reflect a cell of origin. It distinguishes invasive ductal carcinomas NOS (not otherwise specified) as the major tumor type at a frequency of 75%. Beside this, there occur invasive lobular carcinomas in 10–15%. They almost consistently lack E-cadherin expression [16]. Invasive ductal and lobular carcinomas do not differ in their prognostic significance. More important because of their more favorable prognosis are several rare types of cancers. These include special types as invasive tubular, mucinous, or cribriform carcinomas. These rare tumor types occur at frequencies between 1% and at the most up to 3% (for an overview see [17]). Rather frequently, mixed patterns also occur. Ductal carcinomas in situ are detected at increasing frequencies due to increased use of screening mammography and their increased detection of up to 20% is agreed upon to be a quality parameter for screening mammography. They present with different architectures as solid, comedo, cribriform, and papillary type. Their biological potential is mainly influenced by nuclear grade. They should be carefully sampled for possible microinvasion (invasive focus smaller than 1 mm) which occurs with increasing frequency at higher nuclear grades [18, 19]. Any intraductal carcinoma with an invasive focus larger than 1 mm is classified according to the rules concerning invasive carcinomas.

Histopathologic Prognostic Factors

Tumor and Axillary Lymph Node Staging

Staging of breast cancer applies to the definitions of UICC [20]. Thus, according to tumor size, several tumor stages are discriminated. Traditionally, tumors are staged from category T1 to T4. Due to the increased use of screening mammography, most tumors detected meanwhile are in the T1 category. This made a subdivision into T1a (<5 mm), T1b (5–10 mm) and T1c (10–20 mm) necessary. Today most tumors occur in the T1c category. In addition, axillary lymph node staging is performed. Ipsilateral axillary lymph node status is the most important prognostic indicator. It is well known that the number of axillary lymph node metastasis is associated with increasing probability of recurrences and mortality [21]. According to the TNM staging, the main groups are negative axillary lymph nodes, one to three positive and more than three positive lymph nodes. Additionally, in the most recent edition of the TNM classification, patients with minor lymph node involvement are classified. These are isolated tumor cells (ITC) in the category pN0(i+). ITC are defined as single tumor cells or small clusters of tumor cells measuring not more than 0.2 mm without evidence of a stroma reaction or invasion through vascular channels or lymph node sinuses. A second category of minor lymph node involvement consists of micrometastasis defined as lymph node involvement smaller than 2 mm and larger than 0.2 mm (pN1mi).

Accurate axillary lymph node staging depends critically on the accuracy of pathohistological work up. This is true for conventional axillary lymph node dissection and for sentinel lymph node biopsy. For a correct lymph node staging of conventional axillary lymph node dissection a critical number of lymph nodes needs to be examined. This is usually given when at least ten axillary lymph nodes are examined [22]. If only the low axillary level is removed at least six lymph nodes need to examined for a reliable staging. But several other factors also contribute to accurate lymph node staging. These include the surgeońs skills, as well as hospital and patient factors [23]. However, the main factor seems to be the ability of the pathologist to retrieve the nodes from the axillary fat [24]. The number of axillary lymph nodes removed has an impact on local control of the disease even if it is negative. Regional relapse is significantly increased with smaller numbers of nodes removed when patients do not receive systemic therapy [25]. This means that recovery of only small numbers of negative lymph nodes at axillary dissection likely understages patients and leads to undertreatment.

Besides conventional axillary lymph node dissection, a routinely applied lymph node staging procedure is sentinel lymph node biopsy (SLN). It is accepted as an alternative to routine staging axillary lymph node dissection for patients with early-stage breast cancer with clinically negative axillary nodes [26] and also for intraductal carcinomas with microinvasion [27].

The very high predictive value of SLN biopsy in staging allows avoiding of conventional axillary dissection in approximately 65–70% of patients. This results in a significant reduction in morbidity, especially lymph edema. In cases of positive SLN biopsy the standard therapy is completion of axillary dissection for a complete lymph node staging. The critical question remaining is patient selection after SLN biopsy for conventional lymph node dissection to avoid understaging of axillary lymph nodes. Because the existing criterion is negative histology of SNL, avoiding false negative diagnosis of sentinel lymph nodes is an important issue. Therefore the histopathologic examination of each SLN must be particularly accurate. Unfortunately there still exists considerable heterogeneity of pathological examination of SLN biopsies. Furthermore, no standardized guidelines or protocols for SLN examination exist. Substantial differences exist in work up regarding the number of sections cut and the cutting intervals ranging from 50 μm or less to more than 250 μm or even more. In addition, for detection of micrometastasis IHC is used, more or less, and with the application of various antibodies [28, 29]. Moreover, there exist considerable differences in reported histological findings in SLN. Especially regarding minimal lymph node involvement, various terms like submicrometastases and varying definitions of ITC exist [28]. Therefore, despite existing national or regional guidelines, effort needs to be undertaken in formulating widely accepted international guidelines which focus on standardizing histological work up and microscopic examination. The guidelines should recommend techniques that identify macro- and micrometastases as a minimum standard. Very importantly, they also need to focus on a commonly used terminology to lead to uniform histological reporting. This is necessary to be able to compare patients included in different clinical studies. Such work has already been undertaken but still needs further attention [30]. With respect to ITC, it is important to define strictly the criteria for histological detection, including application of IHC or even molecular methods to clarify the biological potential of such minor lymph node involvement. At the moment it seems likely that ITC are indeed clinically relevant as could be demonstrated from a recent study [31].

Lymph and Blood Vessel Invasion

Tumor cell invasion into both lymphatic and blood vessels are defined by the UICC and specified as L1 and V1 respectively. In routine histology using H&E sections, differentiation between lymphatic and small blood vessels may be difficult due to the lack of a muscular wall in both of them. This is of practical importance because tumor emboli mostly affect small vessels without a muscular wall. In addition, cleft artifacts which occur quite frequently around the tumors may pose diagnostic problems. It is currently believed that they are retraction artifacts due to tissue fixation and processing. For discrimination of lymph and blood vessels from cleft artifacts, special techniques like IHC using antibodies for endothelial markers such as, for example, CD 31 or CD 34 may be used. However, in routine diagnostic pathology this cannot be performed on a regular basis. This point is reflected further by studies which found rather low consistency levels of reproducibility of identification vascular invasion [32]. With respect to patient outcome, it is known that lymphatic invasion correlates with axillary lymph node involvement and with survival and local recurrence [33]. Moreover, lymphovascular invasion was proven to be an independent prognostic factor in node-negative breast cancer and could be considered in decisions about adjuvant treatment in these patients [34]. Not much is known about the significance of tumor cells in cleft artifacts. In a recent study a significant correlation between cleft artifacts and unfavorable tumor parameters such as tumor grade could be demonstrated. In addition, tumors with significant amounts of cleft artifacts were associated significantly with lymphatic invasion and axillary lymph node metastasis. In a multivariate analysis, prominent cleft artifacts were associated with overall and disease-free survival even in lymph node negative patients [35]. Due to this data it was speculated that the cleft artifacts were not due to an artifactual phenomenon explained by fixation and tissue processing. However, it could well be that this phenomenon was due to abnormalities in the basement membrane and to altered tumor stroma interactions. For this hypothesis further investigation is needed.

Tumor Size

Tumor size is critical for tumor staging and is also used as a quality assurance parameter in breast cancer screening programs with respect to judging the ability of the radiologist in the detection of small impalpable cancers. There exist no strict rules how measurement of tumor size should be performed. Preferably the tumor should be measured on the fresh tissue before fixation. Dimensions should be taken in three planes and the biggest is recorded as the maximal tumor diameter and thus is the basis for the T stage. If the specimens arrive in the laboratory fixed in formalin one has to keep in mind that fixation results in insignificant shrinkage of the tissue and thus the tumor diameter may be underestimated insignificantly. Problems may arise in cases where multiple CNB have been taken from a small tumor and only small parts of residual tumor are left in the surgical specimen. In these cases, one has to estimate tumor size by adding together the size of the residual tumor in the excision specimen and the tumor in the CNB and correlate it with tumor size in the mammogram. This may help to avoid significant underestimation of tumor size. If there exists any doubt on tumor size of the fresh tissue, it is recommended to measure tumor diameter on the histologic sections. For the tumor stage the invasive component only should be taken into account. It is important that intraductal parts of the tumor must not be considered. Questions still difficult to answer are posed by cases with multiple tumor nodules. The question of how far apart tumor nodules have to be to be considered as two separate tumors will in most cases be answered subjectively. In such cases the diameter of the larger tumor is taken into account for T staging. Summarizing tumor size is reported as one of the problematic areas of interpretation for staging [36]. There also exist some data on variability of measurement of tumor size [37]. Overall, in this study size determination was generally acceptable. Size was more consistent for invasive breast cancers than for in situ cancers and it was related to tumor subtypes. This was also confirmed by measuring tumor size on histologic slides [32]. This finding is probably due to clearer circumscription of invasive than of intraductal cancers and to clearer circumscription in certain invasive tumor types.

Tumor Grading

For many years a large number of publications has confirmed a powerful prognostic value of histologic tumor grade in terms of overall and recurrence free survival. Tumor grading was proposed first in the 1920s and in a simplified modification suggested by Bloom and Richardson in 1957 [38]. It uses three variables: tubule formation, nuclear pleomorphism (variability in size and shape of nuclei), and mitotic counts. The basic principle of tumor grading is summation of scores of the three variables. For each variable one to three points are given according to the degree of deviation. A total score of 5 or less defines grade 1, a score 6 to 7 grade 2, and a score of 8 and 9 grade 3. Tubule formation and nuclear pleomorphism are determined throughout the whole tumor. Tubule formation is defined by the area containing tubules compared to the whole tumor. Thus if more than 75% of the tumor is composed of tubules, score 1 is allocated. Two points are given if the tumor contains between 10% and 75% tubules and score 3 contains less than 10% tubules. Nuclear pleomorphism is the least defined variable in tumor grading. In the Nottingham modification [39] it was suggested to use the size and shape of normal epithelial cells present in the breast tissue adjacent to the tumor as a reference. If normal epithelial cells are not present, lymphocytes could be used. If tumor cell nuclei are small and show little variation in shape compared with normal nuclei, score 1 should be given. Score 2 should be allocated when tumor cell nuclei are larger than normal and show little variation and small nucleoli. Marked variation and large size of tumor cell nuclei with vesicular appearance and prominent nucleoli is designated as score 3. Most importantly, the Nottingham modification of tumor grading also suggested a standardized semiquantitative evaluation of mitotic counts. It was suggested to use a defined field area in the microscope for determination of the number of mitoses. It is known that the high power fields which are used for counting of mitoses vary in size depending on the type of the microscope. Therefore one has to adapt the mitotic numbers to the field diameter of the microscope used. Mitotic counting should be performed in ten high power fields containing the highest numbers of mitotis in the tumor. This is usually given at the periphery of the tumor. Only mitotic figures which clearly fulfill the morphologic criteria for mitoses should be included for counting. Hyperchromatic nuclei which could well represent apoptotic figures should not be taken into account. This modification of the histologic tumor grading is now recommended by the WHO for all invasive carcinomas [15]. This includes invasive lobular and mucinous carcinomas. Only medullary carcinomas which are by definition grade 3 are not to be graded.

A major concern regarding histologic tumor grading in patient management is interobserver variability. The existence of a wide variation in the proportion of each grade is well known. Grade 1 carcinomas are described in the literature at frequencies between approximately 10 and 30%. For grade

2 carcinomas frequencies are reported between 25 and 55% and for grade 3 carcinomas between 25 and 65% (for an overview see [40]). These differences are affected by several factors. Criteria not fully defined or agreed upon or difficulties in the application of these criteria are a main source of variability. The variability in interpretation is also partly due to tumor heterogeneity and the borderline nature of the presentation of the single factors used for grading. Several studies from the 1980s and even before have shown acceptable levels of agreement between 70 and even 90% between observers. It has to be mentioned that in these studies extremely subjective methods were used. In addition it can be assumed that at that time not so much care was taken on tissue fixation. Immediate tissue fixation is also critical for tumor grading because it is known that the number of mitoses is reduced significantly with delay of fixation. This may result in an underestimation of tumor grade. In the 1990s it became evident that tumor grading is possible with a good interobserver agreement if applied criteria are defined relatively strictly and followed strictly and if training of pathologists is carried out. Thus in several studies, interobserver agreement of almost 90% could be achieved. This corresponds in statistical terms in kappa-statistics to very good overall agreement of 0.7 [41, 42]. Further detailed analysis demonstrated that major differences in grading are attributed by grade 2 cancers. The accuracy for grade 1 and 3 is substantially higher. Thus for grade 1 an agreement with a mean of 83% and for grade 3 a mean of 92% could be achieved when 13 pathologists reviewed breast cancer cases. In contrast, the mean for grade 2 cancers was only 64% [43]. Similar results were found by the European Working Group of Breast Cancer Screening Pathology. Kappa-statistics demonstrated only poor consistency for grade 2 cancers while it showed higher consistency for grades 1 and 3 [32]. Regarding the three factors contributing to tumor grading, it was demonstrated that tubularity and mitotic index were associated with good kappa-statistics and are thus rather robust factors while nuclear pleomorphism showed only poor kappa-statistics [44]. In conclusion, and bearing these difficulties of tumor grading in mind, one can conclude that for selection of patients for therapy it would be wise to put more weight on grade 1 and 3 cancers and to use combinations of different prognostic factors, especially for grade 2 cancers. Further, one should pay attention to the "gray zones" of grading. A grade 1 carcinoma with a score 5 may behave more like a grade 2 cancer score 6 in contrast to a grade 1 carcinoma score 3 [45].

Immunhistochemical Assays

Immunohistochemical analyses (IHC) of biomarkers in breast cancer is extensively used for tumor characterization and to predict prognosis and response or resistance to therapy, respectively. Markers examined on a regular routinely basis are steroid hormone receptors and HER-2/neu.

Steroid Hormone Receptors

Steroid hormone receptors determined in breast cancer are estrogen (ER) and progesterone (PR) receptors. ER in primary breast cancer occurs at a frequency of approximately 75–80% and PR at approximately 60%. ER should be determined on every primary breast cancer prior to decision regarding systemic adjuvant therapy. ER is able to identify patients who are likely to benefit or fail to respond to endocrine therapy. The prognostic value of ER with respect to overall survival is difficult to interpret. There exist many reports in the literature finding positive correlations for ER positive tumors with overall and disease free survival [46–48]. However, one has to keep in mind that there exist strong correlations between steroid hormone receptor positivity and high tumor differentiation. Thus, regarding current opinion, the importance of steroid hormone receptors is mainly given by its predictive value for therapy. Additional PR assays should be performed to characterize patients whose tumors are ER low or negative. The subset of patients with ER low/negative and PR positive tumors may also respond to endocrine therapy [49].

The preferred method for steroid hormone receptor determination is IHC. This is now applied on paraffin sections of formalin fixed tissue. The success of using paraffin sections is founded on the fact that it can be performed on routinely prepared diagnostic sections and that by this method the receptors can be localized to the specific tissue compartment, thus avoiding false assay interpretation. Therefore it is thought that IHC is more reliable and reproducible compared to the formerly used ligand binding assays which used cytosolic preparations of the tissue. Moreover, it could be demonstrated that immunohistochemical detection of ER is superior compared to ligand binding assay [50]. These authors suggested that IHC is easier, safer, and less expensive, and has an equivalent or better ability to predict response to adjuvant endocrine therapy.

However, despite these advantages, there still exist some problems with immunohistochemical assays. One reason for discrepancies in results is the fact that the robustness of IHC is susceptible to differences in tissue fixation and processing. In histopathology, morphology and thus preservation of antigens to be detected in IHC is influenced for example by the type of fixative, delay of fixation after tumor removal, duration of fixation, and the paraffin wax processing schedule. Several studies were performed on these topics. It is recommended that fixation takes place immediately after tumor removal. Therefore it is also recommended that tumor specimens be sent to the pathology laboratory immediately after surgical removal. As fixative, ideally 10% buffered formalin should be used. Fixation time should be at least 6 h and should not be extended to more than 48 h. Too short or prolonged fixation times cause decreasing positivity of ER [51]. For IHC there exist many clones of antibodies against ER and PR and to date by comparison none seems to be superior to another. This is also true for the secondary detection systems. Most of the modern antibodies for paraffin sections need antigen retrieval. Antigen retrieval is needed to overcome some of the problems caused by suboptimal tissue fixation. The method superior to others for ER and PR is heat mediated either using microwave or pressure cooker techniques. In fact, antigen retrieval seems to be a crucial point for obtaining reliable receptor IHC [52, 53]. These studies demonstrated that participating laboratories adequately detected tumors with high levels of receptor expression but a significant number of laboratories failed to detect receptors in low or medium ER expressing carcinomas and this was mainly due to non-exhaustive antigen retrieval. To avoid underestimation of steroid hormone receptor IHC and thus prevent patients with low levels of ER in their cancers from not receiving needed endocrine therapy, much care needs to be taken in raising assay sensitivity. Some improvement regarding variability could be achieved by using automated staining systems for ER and PR IHC which were shown to give better consistency compared to manual staining methods [54].

Another as yet unanswered question concerns scoring of ER and PR IHC and definition of a threshold for discrimination between receptor positive and negative breast cancers. Most laboratories and clinical studies use the 10% receptor positive threshold. This was validated in many clinical studies but it has to be mentioned that this cut off is selected arbitrarily. Other thresholds, like any positive cell or 1–20% receptor positive cells are also used [49, 50]. From the standpoint of laboratory procedure, the problem for setting a cut-off to distinguish between receptor negative and positive carcinomas is critically associated with achieving a balance between assay sensitivity and specificity. This question was discussed nicely by Barnes and coworkers and these authors suggest that rather high cut-offs with respect to response to endocrine therapy may be reasonable [55]. There also exist different systems for scoring. Practically all of them use percentage of positively stained cells and staining intensity as the basis. It was shown that simple scoring systems are most effective. Therefore a "quick score" has been recommended [56]. This awards points for nuclear staining and staining intensity and results in a score from zero to eight points

To overcome the problems with IHC, at least partly technical guidelines for steroid hormone receptor assays and for interpretation and scoring should be formulated urgently. To improve consistency of steroid hormone receptor IHC participation of laboratories in quality assurance programs with slide circulations and bench marking between laboratories on a regularly basis is recommended. These have been set up successfully for many years, for instance by UK NEQAS-ICC or College of American Pathologists. EUSOMA suggests that ER and PR IHC must only be performed in laboratories working with internal and external quality assessment schemes to assure the major goal for the patients in guaranteeing consistency and quality of receptor measurements [49].

HER-2/neu

For several years there has existed a major interest in HER-2/neu (HER-2) for breast cancer patients. The development of Trastuzumab (Herceptin) therapy made testing necessary to consider a patients eligibility in the metastatic disease and adjuvant setting. Accurate assessment of HER-2 status is essential to ensure that patients who may benefit from Trastuzumab are correctly identified. Because of considerable and particularly cardiovascular side effects and high costs of this therapy, it is necessary that patients with HER-2 negative tumors are identified correctly. As revealed in recent extensive and critical studies, approximately 20% of HER-2 positive cancers can be expected [57].

HER-2 status is assessed routinely by IHC at the level of protein expression and by fluorescent in situ hybridization (FISH) assays at the DNA level of gene amplification. It is recommended that it is determined in all primary breast cancers.

HER-2 Immunohistochemistry

In contrast to steroid hormone receptor IHC, many guidelines exist for HER-2 assessment [58, 59]. These focus on technical questions as well as interpretation. As was described above for steroid hormone receptor IHC, the quality of the assays are also influenced by the type of fixative, delay of fixation after tumor removal, duration of fixation, and the paraffin wax processing schedule. The American Society for Clinical Oncology and the College of American Pathologists recommend optimal tissue handling and fixation in a recent publication of their guidelines. As suggested for steroid hormone receptors, fixation should be performed using 10% buffered formalin and last between minimally 6 and maximally 48 h. Time from tissue acquisition to fixation should be as short as possible. In a recent paper, acceleration of fixation by applying high frequency, high intensity ultrasound is suggested, which is proven to preserve uniform tissue morphology and less altered protein antigenicity [60]. This approach may be useful in the future. As for other IHC assays, HER-2 IHC is also influenced by various other factors like the antibodies used, the methodology – especially with respect to antigen retrieval, and the experience of the personnel. Many HER-2 polyclonal and monoclonal antibodies and test kits are commercially available. Some of them are approved by the FDA. Many studies demonstrated broad variations in staining results depending on the antibody. Press and collaborators demonstrated these differences convincingly and the variation affected the FDA approved antibodies as well [61]. It was suggested to use cell lines with differing but constant levels of HER-2 expression as standard material against which assay sensitivity could be checked. In these studies, HercepTest™ had the highest level of reproducibility in sensitivity and evaluation [62, 63]. Laboratories using other individually set up assays were able to improve their sensitivities over several runs of a quality assessment scheme but did not reach results obtained with the HercepTest™. Further it was suggested that IHC can be performed at a higher level and thus more reliably when a large enough number of specimens is examined in a laboratory. For HER-2 IHC it could be demonstrated that in a central reference laboratory there was less discrepancy with HercepTest™ compared to small volume community based laboratories. A substantial proportion of assays (18%) of these small laboratories could not be confirmed by the reference laboratory [64].

HER-2 FISH

The other routinely applied assay method is fluorescent in situ hybridization (FISH). The product identified by this method is gene amplification determined by assessment of copy numbers of the HER-2 gene. Tissue requirements are similar to IHC and the method can be performed on formalin fixed paraffin embedded tissue. Basically, two tests are available. One determines the copy number of the HER-2 gene only. The other test determines the gene copy level as the ratio of the copies of chromosome 17 centromere and the HER-2 gene. By this test aneuploidy of chromosome 17 can be excluded because the HER-2 gene is located on chromosome 17 and its centromeric probe is used as an internal control for aneuploidy of chromosome 17. The specific test product is labeled by fluorescent dyes and can be visualized using a fluorescent microscope. The slides are not permanent and fade rather rapidly. Both tests are approved by the FDA. Several studies compare results of FISH and IHC assays. All of them prove that FISH based tests resulted in more accurate determination of HER-2 expression levels [61, 65]. This higher accuracy of FISH assays may partly be due to microscopic interpretation which is described below. In the future an alternative to FISH testing could become chromogenic in situ hybridization (CISH) or the rather new concept of SISH (silver in situ hybridization). These are modifications of the FISH technique for detection of amplification of genes in paraffin embedded material. The methods are based on the same principle but detection of the oncogene probe is based on a peroxidase or silver reaction which allows the use of a conventional light microscope rather than a fluorescent microscope. Another advantage lies in the fact that permanent slides are produced. Recent studies revealed concordant results between FISH and CISH in more than 90%. Just a few tumors were amplified only in either FISH or CISH respectively [66]. Thus this method may become a reasonable alternative.

Interpretation and Scoring

Immunohistochemistry

For IHC, scoring is performed by determination of the proportion of cells with positive and complete membrane staining and evaluation of the staining intensity. Only membrane staining is to be evaluated. Cytoplasmic staining may occur and sometimes be intense but should be omitted from evaluation. This may result in difficulties in interpretation because discrimination between these closely adjacent regions may be difficult, especially when stained in the same color. The scoring system was published by DAKO Corporation and is part of the FDA approved HercepTest™Kit. Negative IHC results are achieved by score 0 and 1 + . A positive result is given at score 3 + . IHC scores 0, 1 + and 3 + are accepted as reliable and need no further testing. An equivocal result is represented by IHC score 2 + . Guidelines recommend retesting all cases with IHC score 2 + by FISH. In IHC score 2 + some cases may turn out to be HER-2 positive on retesting by FISH and are then eligible for Herceptin treatment. However, the majority of IHC score 2 + cancers are not accompanied by gene amplification and represent "false positive" IHC. Only a small proportion of IHC score 2 + represent true 2 + IHC positivity accompanied by gene amplification [67]. One has to stress that interpretation in IHC is subjective in any case and thus includes observer bias. Interpretation of staining intensity and estimation of membrane staining in a percentage of cells compared to the total of cells within a tumor is variable. Regarding this topic, it was demonstrated that overall discrimination between HER-2 negativity and positivity in IHC (score 0, 1 + vs score 2 + , 3 +) was very high, kappa statistics being 0.96. The main difficulty derives from distinguishing weakly from highly positive cases (score 2 + vs 3 +), their kappa statistics being only 0.38 [68]. Therefore, in these cases, retesting by FISH is very important. In addition, with respect to minimize subjectivity in microscopic evaluation there exist efforts in application of automated image analysis systems for scoring. Applying such systems which are able to evaluate membrane staining only and exclude cytoplasmic staining from evaluation and evaluate percentage of stained cells, these biases may be overcome in the future.

FISH

Scoring FISH affords determination of the copy number of the gene and chromosome 17. This simply requires counting of two colored signals and therefore is easier to perform compared to immunohistochemical evaluation. For such analysis, interscorer errors are reported below 10% [64] and therefore FISH scoring seems to be rather robust against observer bias. According to the guidelines at least 20 nonoverlapping cells in two separate areas of the invasive cancer need to be counted [58]. Based on the counting test interpretation is performed as follows. For HER-2 gene copy number, more than six copies are scored as amplified which means HER-2 positivity, four to six copies are scored equivocal and less than four copies are regarded nonamplified or HER-2 negative. For the HER-2 gene/chromosome 17 ratio a positive result is given by HER2/CEP17 ratio >2.2. A ratio of 1.8–2.2 represents an equivocal result and a ratio of <1.8 is a HER-2 negative result.

Which Score to Be Used?

In conclusion, and taking the recommendations of the guidelines into account, every primary breast cancer should be tested for HER-2. The best method with respect to type of assay and optimal performance remains controversial. The most reasonable way is screening breast cancers for HER-2 using IHC for the purpose of identification of HER-2 negative cases or exclude them. HER-2 positive cancers and especially equivocal score 2+ cases need validating by further testing by FISH prior to therapy. For quality assurance it is strongly recommended that performing laboratories participate in an appropriate external quality assurance program such as the UK NEQAS. On a regularl basis, unstained slides are circulated to the laboratories and are requested to be stained by the routine laboratory method. In addition, their own in house control needs to be returned to the organizing center. All sections will be reviewed by an expert panel. In case of inappropriate results, advice for improvement should be given.

Future Aspects

Microarray Technology

Microarrays can be described as large numbers of samples in an ordered arrangement on a grid. Depending on the specimens to be analyzed, several arrays can be distinguished. Tissue arrays contain patients specimens. Using this technology, a bioprobe can be analyzed for hundreds of patients at a time in a very economic way. The second approach uses hundreds to thousands of biomarker probes upon which a single patient biospecimen can be examined. Most of these arrays use nucleic acid – preferably DNA but also RNA. In these microarrays the nucleic acid is hybridized against the patient specimen and quantified. This means that thousands of genetic markers can be determined at once. Problems have been identified regarding sensitivity because, due to using such large numbers of genetic markers, each single marker cannot be optimized for its sensitivity. This may be a problem for markers expressed at a low level. Another limiting factor is tissue quality. High quality of the samples is required and immediately snap frozen tissue remains the gold standard for such analysis. However, for patient material this cannot be guaranteed in any case within the routine practice in a hospital. Another problem arising with this high complexity technology is the creation of huge data sets which need to be analyzed and interpreted. For this purpose specialized algorithms and IT programs have been developed to convert the raw data into numerical values ready for interpretation. To date this technology can only be applied in very specialized laboratories. Therefore microarray technology today still remains a research tool.

Nevertheless, several interesting and intriguing studies have been performed. Many studies have used gene expression profiles for creating predictive signatures of prognosis such as local recurrences and metastasis. Breast cancer gene signatures have been identified that predicted absolute survival [69]. Patients with cancers with a good prognosis signature have an overall survival of approximately 95% at 10 years compared to only approximately 55% in patients with tumors with poor prognosis signature. The difference remained significant even after stratification into lymph node negative and positive patients respectively. The usedprognostic marker gene profile consisted of 70 genes and the poor prognosis signature included genes regulating the cell cycle, angiogenesis, invasion and metastatis [70]. This suggests that it should be possible to identify patients who are at very low risk of metastasis and therefore adjuvant chemotherapy could safely be omitted. This concept is intriguing because a large number of patients with breast cancer are candidates for adjuvant therapy and as many as up to 80% do not develop metastasis and therefore probably do not need adjuvant chemotherapy. The advantage for these patients is avoiding unnecessary side effects. Other studies demonstrated that microarray analysis is able to identify subgroups of patients for prediction of treatment response. A set of genes identified patients who show significant differences with respect to response to endocrine therapy [71]. Other studies identified patients by their gene signature who are likely to respond at a high probability to neoadjuvant chemotherapy or their gene profile correlated to response to certain chemotherapeutic agents like docetaxel [72, 73]. A step further this leads to the possibility of tailored adjuvant chemotherapy for individual patients [74].

Another field of application of microarray technology regards reclassification of present tumor types. Conventional morphologically based tumor classification relies on anatomic site and tissue of origin. Of special clinical interest – keeping this in mind – is subclassification of histologically nondistinguishable tumor entities with respect to differences in prognosis and treatment. Thus the new technology may be used as a “microarray microscope”. Microarray technology can clearly demonstrate different tumor types among breast cancers. Amongst others, basal cell and luminal cell type cancers were first characterized differently by gene profiling [75]. Meanwhile, it is known that among invasive ductal carcinomas grade 3 approximately 20% and among invasive ductal carcinomas in general 10% are of basal cell type. They are usually triple negative which means they are negative for estrogen and progesterone receptors and for HER-2. In addition, they frequently present with negative axillary lymph nodes. They tend to develop less bone and liver metastasis but more frequently brain metastasis, and they are reported to be associated with a poor clinical outcome [76]. Furthermore, there exists an association between basal cell carcinoma and medullary breast carcinoma. In a large study on medullary breast carcinomas, many showed a basal phenotype [77]. This finding is interesting with respect to the fact that medullary breast carcinomas have an excess of BRCA1 germ-line mutations and, therefore, an association even with hereditary breast cancer may exist. There exists currently no internationally agreed consensus for diagnostic criteria of basal cell carcinomas, nor are they searched for in routine histology. In many studies they are identified by positivity for cytokeratin 14, cytokeratin 5/6 or P-cadherin in IHC. Within the basal cell carcinomas different patterns of cytokeratin 14 expression are associated with differences in prognosis and response to chemotherapy [78]. These findings suggest that in this field new clinically relevant tumor identities may be recognized in the future. It may also be speculated that a combination of conventional histoprognostic factors and the molecular signatures of tumors may be used for determination of prognosis and prediction of therapy in individual patients. If this indeed happens, it will be a real advantage in comparison to our present knowledge.

Summarizing the present possibilities for microarray technology for breast cancer, there remains much to be clarified and optimized. One has to keep in mind that transferring this currently scientifically applied method into widely applied clinical diagnostic assays may have a long way to go. Scientific data have to be reproduced, compared to each other, and clinically proved. Currently results in the literature are often not comparable to each other. Agreements have to be established on the relevant gene profiles for answering specific questions. For a successful application of microarray technology to therapeutic decision-making, high sample quality is required and thus the sample collection under routine hospital conditions has to be optimized. Finally, much more clinical correlative data need to be validated.

References

1. Riedl CC, Pfarl G, Memarsadeghi M, et al. Lesion miss rates and false-negative rates for 1115 consecutive cases of stereotactically guided needle-localized open breast biopsy with long-term follow-up. *Radiology*. 2005;237:847–53.
2. Liberman L, Dershaw DD, Rosen PP, et al. Stereotaxic 14-gauge breast biopsy: how many core biopsy specimens are needed? *Radiology*. 1994;192:793–95.
3. Jacobs TW, Siziopikou KP, Prioleau JE, et al. Do prognostic marker studies on core needle biopsy specimens of breast carcinoma accurately reflect the marker status of the tumor? *Mod Pathol*. 1998;11:259–64.
4. Taucher S, Rudas M, Mader RM, et al. Prognostic markers in breast cancer: the reliability of HER2/neu status in core needle biopsy of 325 patients with primary breast cancer. *Wien Klin Wochenschr*. 2004;116:26–31.
5. Al Sarakbi W, Salhab M, Thomas V, et al. Is preoperative core biopsy accurate in determining the hormone receptor status in women with invasive breast cancer? *Int Semin Surg Oncol*. 2005;2:15.
6. Cahill RA, Walsh D, Landers RJ, et al. Preoperative profiling of symptomatic breast cancer by diagnostic core biopsy. *Ann Surg Oncol*. 2006;13:45–51.
7. Harris GC, Denley HE, Pinder SE, et al. Correlation of histologic prognostic factors in core biopsies and therapeutic excisions of invasive breast carcinoma. *Am J Surg Pathol*. 2003;27:11–15.
8. Andrade VP, Gobbi H. Accuracy of typing and grading invasive mammary carcinomas on core needle biopsy compared with the excisional specimen. *Virchows Arch*. 2004;445:597–602.

9. Niemann TH, Lucas JG, Marsh WL Jr. To freeze or not to freeze. A comparison of methods for the handling of breast biopsies with no palpable abnormality. *Am J Clin Pathol.* 1996;106:225–8.
10. Bianchi S, Palli D, Ciatto S, et al. Accuracy and reliability of frozen section diagnosis in a series of 672 nonpalpable breast lesions. *Am J Clin Pathol.* 1995;103:199–205.
11. Fessia L, Ghiringhello B, Arisio R, et al. Accuracy of frozen section diagnosis in breast cancer detection. A review of 4436 biopsies and comparison with cytodiagnosis. *Pathol Res Pract.* 1984;179:61–6.
12. Cserni G. Pitfalls in frozen section interpretation: a retrospective study of palpable breast tumors. *Tumori.* 1999;85:15–18.
13. Noguchi M, Minami M, Earashi M, et al. Pathologic assessment of surgical margins on frozen and permanent sections in breast conserving surgery. *Breast Cancer.* 1995;2:27–33.
14. Riegman PH, Dinjens WN, Oomen MH, et al. TuBaFrost 1: Uniting local frozen tumour banks into a European network: an overview. *Eur J Cancer.* 2006;42:2678–83.
15. Tavassoli FA, Devilee P. World Health Organization Classification of Tumors: Tumors of the breast and female genital organs. IARC Press, International Agency for Research on Cancer: Lyon, 2003.
16. Acs G, Lawton TJ, Rebbeck TR, et al. Differential expression of E-cadherin in lobular and ductal neoplasms of the breast and its biologic and diagnostic implications. *Am J Clin Pathol.* 2001;115:85–98.
17. Elston CW, Ellis IO. Classification of malignant breast disease. In: Elston CW, Ellis IO, eds. *The Breast. Systemic Pathology.* Vol. 13, Oxford, UK Churchill Livingstone; 1998:243.
18. Prasad ML, Osborne MP, Giri DD, et al. Microinvasive breast carcinoma: clinicopathologic analysis of a single institution experience. *Cancer.* 2000;88:1403–9.
19. de Mascarel I, MacGrogan G, Mathoulin-Pelissier S, et al. Breast ductal carcinoma in situ with microinvasion: a definition supported by a long-term study of 1248 serially sectioned ductal carcinomas. *Cancer.* 2002;94:2134–42.
20. Sobin LH, Wittekind C. TNM classification of malignant tumors. *UICC.* 6th ed. New York, NY: Wiley; 2002.
21. Fisher B, Bauer M, Wickerham L, et al. Relation of number of positive axillary nodes to the prognosis of patients with primary breast cancer: An NSABP update. *Cancer.* 1983;52:1551–57.
22. Wilking N, Rutquist LE, Carstensen J, et al. Prognostic significance of axillary nodal status in primary breast cancer in relation to the number of resected nodes. *Acta Oncol.* 1992;31:29–35.
23. Petrik DW, McCready DR, Sawka CA, et al. Association between extent of axillary lymph node dissection and patient, tumor, surgeon, and hospital factors in patients with early breast cancer. *J Surg Oncol.* 2003;82:84–90.
24. Reynolds JV, Mercer P, McDermot EWM, et al. Audit of complete axillary dissection in early breast cancer. *Eur J Cancer.* 1994;30A:148–49.
25. Weir L, Speers C, D'yachkova Y, et al. Prognostic significance of the number of axillary lymph nodes removed in patients with node-negative breast cancer. *J Clin Oncol.* 2002;20:1793–9.
26. Lyman GH, Giuliano AE, Somerfield MR, et al. American Society of Clinical Oncology guideline recommendations for sentinel lymph node biopsy in early-stage breast cancer. *J Clin Oncol.* 2005;23:7703–20.
27. Intra M, Zurrida S, Maffini F, et al. Sentinel lymph node metastasis in microinvasive breast cancer. *Ann Surg Oncol.* 2003;10:1160–5.
28. Cserni G, Amendoeira I, Apostolikas N, et al. Discrepancies in current practice of pathological evaluation of sentinel lymph nodes in breast cancer. Results of a questionnaire based survey by the European Working Group for Breast Screening Pathology. *J Clin Pathol.* 2004;57:695–701.
29. Viale G, Sonzogni A, Pruneri G, et al. Histopathologic examination of axillary sentinel lymph nodes in breast carcinoma patients. *J Surg Oncol.* 2004;85:123–8.

30. Cserni G, Amendoeira I, Apostolikas N, et al. Pathological work-up of sentinel lymph nodes in breast cancer. Review of current data to be considered for the formulation of guidelines. *Eur J Cancer*. 2003;39:1654–67.
31. Colleoni M, Rotmensz N, Peruzzotti G, et al. Size of breast cancer metastases in axillary lymph nodes: clinical relevance of minimal lymph node involvement. *J Clin Oncol*. 2005;23:1379–89.
32. Sloane JP, Amendoeira I, Apostolikas N, et al. Consistency achieved by 23 European pathologists from 12 countries in diagnosing breast disease and reporting prognostic features of carcinomas. European Commission Working Group on Breast Screening Pathology. *Virchows Arch*. 1999;434:3–10.
33. Pinder SE, Ellis IO, Galea M, et al. Pathological prognostic factors in breast cancer. III. Vascular invasion: relationship with recurrence and survival in a large study with long-term follow-up. *Histopathology*. 1994;24:41–7.
34. Lee AH, Pinder SE, Macmillan RD, et al. Prognostic value of lymphovascular invasion in women with lymph node negative invasive breast carcinoma. *Eur J Cancer*. 2006;42:357–62.
35. Acs G, Dumoff KL, Solin LJ, et al. Extensive retraction artifact correlates with lymphatic invasion and nodal metastasis and predicts poor outcome in early stage breast carcinoma. *Am J Surg Pathol*. 2007;31:129–40.
36. Connolly JL. Changes and problematic areas in interpretation of the AJCC cancer staging manual, 6th ed. for breast cancer. *Arch Pathol Lab Med*. 2006;130:287–91.
37. Ellis IO, Coleman D, Wells C, et al. Impact of a national external quality assessment scheme for breast pathology in the UK. *J Clin Pathol*. 2006;59:138–45.
38. Bloom HJG, Richardson WW. Histological grading and prognosis in breast cancer. *Br J Cancer*.1957;11:359–77.
39. Elston CW, Ellis IO. Pathological prognostic factors in breast cancer. I. The value of histological grade in breast cancer: experience from a large study with long-term follow-up. *Histopathology*. 1991;19:403–10.
40. Elston CW, Ellis IO. Assessment of histological grade. In: Elston CW, Ellis IO, eds. *The Breast. Systemic Pathology*, 3rd ed. Vol. 13. Edinburgh, London, New York, Philadelphia, San Francisco, Sydney, Toronto: Churchill Livingstone. 1998: 365–84.
41. Dalton LW, Page DL, Dupont WD. Histologic grading of breast carcinoma. A reproducibility study. *Cancer*. 1994;73:2765–70.
42. Page DL, Ellis IO, Elston CW. Histologic grading of breast cancer. Let's do it. *Am J Clin Pathol*. 1995;103:123–4.
43. Longacre TA, Ennis M, Quenneville LA, et al. Interobserver agreement and reproducibility in classification of invasive breast carcinoma: an NCI breast cancer family registry study. *Mod Pathol*. 2006;19:195–207.
44. Meyer JS, Alvarez C, Milikowski C, et al. Breast carcinoma malignancy grading by Bloom-Richardson system vs proliferation index: reproducibility of grade and advantages of proliferation index. *Mod Pathol*. 2005;18:1067–78.
45. Dalton LW, Pinder SE, Elston CE, et al. Histologic grading of breast cancer: linkage of patient outcome with level of pathologist agreement. *Mod Pathol*. 2000;13:730–35.
46. Kinsel LB, Szabo E, Greene GL, et al. Immunocytochemical analysis of estrogen receptors as a predictor of prognosis in breast cancer patients: comparison with quantitative biochemical methods. *Cancer Res*. 1989;49:1052–6.
47. Pertschuk LP, Kim DS, Nayer K, et al. Immunocytochemical estrogen and progestin receptor assays in breast cancer with monoclonal antibodies. Histopathologic, demographic, and biochemical correlations and relationship to endocrine response and survival. *Cancer* 1990;66:1663–70.
48. Reiner A, Neumeister B, Spona J, et al. Immunocytochemical localization of estrogen and progesterone receptor and prognosis in human primary breast cancer. *Cancer Res*. 1990;50:7057–61.

49. Blamey RW; EUSOMA. Guidelines on endocrine therapy of breast cancer EUSOMA. *Eur J Cancer*. 2002;38:615–34.
50. Harvey JM, Clark GM, Osborne CK, et al. Estrogen receptor status by immunohistochemistry is superior to the ligand-binding assay for predicting response to adjuvant endocrine therapy in breast cancer. *J Clin Oncol*. 1999;17:1474–81.
51. Goldstein NS, Ferkowicz M, Odish E, et al. Minimum formalin fixation time for consistent estrogen receptor immunohistochemical staining of invasive breast carcinoma. Am *J Clin Pathol*. 2003;120:86–92.
52. Rhodes A, Jasani B, Balaton AJ, et al. Immunohistochemical demonstration of oestrogen and progesterone receptors: correlation of standards achieved on in house tumours with that achieved on external quality assessment material in over 150 laboratories from 26 countries. *J Clin Pathol*. 2000;53:292–301.
53. Rhodes A, Jasani B, Balaton AJ, et al. Study of interlaboratory reliability and reproducibility of estrogen and progesterone receptor assays in Europe. Documentation of poor reliability and identification of insufficient microwave antigen retrieval time as a major contributory element of unreliable assays. *Am J Clin Pathol*. 2001;115:44–58.
54. Regitnig P, Reiner A, Dinges HP, et al. Quality assurance for detection of estrogen and progesterone receptors by immunohistochemistry in Austrian pathology laboratories. *Virchows Arch*. 2002;441:328–34.
55. Barnes DM, Millis RR, Beex LV, et al. Increased use of immunohistochemistry for oestrogen receptor measurement in mammary carcinoma: the need for quality assurance. *Eur J Cancer*. 1998;34:1677–82.
56. Leake R, Barnes D, Pinder S, et al. Immunohistochemical detection of steroid receptors in breast cancer: a working protocol. UK Receptor Group, UK NEQAS, The Scottish Breast Cancer Pathology Group, and The Receptor and Biomarker Study Group of the EORTC. *J Clin Pathol*. 2000;53:634–5.
57. Owens MA, Horten BC, Da Silva MM. HER2 amplification ratios by fluorescence in situ hybridization and correlation with immunohistochemistry in a cohort of 6556 breast cancer tissues. *Clin Breast Cancer*. 2004;5:63–9.
58. Wolff AC, Hammond ME, Schwartz JN, et al. American Society of Clinical Oncology/College of American Pathologists guideline recommendations for human epidermal growth factor receptor 2 testing in breast cancer. *J Clin Oncol*. 2007;25:118–45.
59. Ellis IO, Bartlett J, Dowsett M, et al. Best Practice No 176: Updated recommendations for HER2 testing in the UK. *J Clin Pathol*. 2004;57:233–7.
60. Chu WS, Furusato B, Wong K, et al. Ultrasound-accelerated formalin fixation of tissue improves morphology, antigen and mRNA preservation. *Mod Pathol*. 2005;18:850–63.
61. Press MF, Slamon DJ, Flom KJ, et al. Evaluation of HER-2/neu gene amplification and overexpression: comparison of frequently used assay methods in a molecularly characterized cohort of breast cancer specimens. *J Clin Oncol*. 2002;20:3095–105.
62. Rhodes A, Jasani B, Anderson E, et al. Evaluation of HER-2/neu immunohistochemical assay sensitivity and scoring on formalin-fixed and paraffin-processed cell lines and breast tumors: a comparative study involving results from laboratories in 21 countries. *Am J Clin Pathol* 2002;118:408–17.
63. Rhodes A, Borthwick D, Sykes R, et al. The use of cell line standards to reduce HER-2/neu assay variation in multiple European cancer centers and the potential of automated image analysis to provide for more accurate cut points for predicting clinical response to trastuzumab. *Am J Clin Pathol*. 2004;122:51–60.
64. Paik S, Bryant J, Tan-Chiu E, et al. Real-world performance of HER2 testing – National Surgical Adjuvant Breast and Bowel Project experience. *J Natl Cancer Inst*. 2002;94:852–4.
65. Bartlett JM, Going JJ, Mallon EA, et al. Evaluating HER2 amplification and overexpression in breast cancer. *J Pathol*. 2001;195:422–8.

66. Isola J, Tanner M, Forsyth A, et al. Interlaboratory comparison of HER-2 oncogene amplification as detected by chromogenic and fluorescence in situ hybridization. *Clin Cancer Res*.2004;10:4793–8.
67. Barrett C, Magee H, O'Toole D, et al. Amplification of the HER-2 gene in breast cancers testing 2 + weak positive by HercepTestTM immunohistochemistry: false positive or false negative IHC? *J Clin Pathol*. 2006 Jul 5 [Epub ahead of print].
68. Hsu CY, Ho DM, Yang CF, et al. Interobserver reproducibility of Her-2/neu protein overexpression in invasive breast carcinoma using the DAKO HercepTest. *Am J Clin Pathol*. 2002;118:693–8.
69. van de Vijver MJ, He YD, van't Veer LJ, et al. A gene-expression signature as a predictor of survival in breast cancer. *N Engl J Med*. 2002;347:1999–2009.
70. van't Veer LJ, Dai H, van de Vijver MJ, et al. Gene expression profiling predicts clinical outcome of breast cancer. *Nature*. January 31, 2002;415:530–6.
71. Glinsky GV, Higashiyama T, Glinskii AB. Classification of human breast cancer using gene expression profiling as a component of the survival predictor algorithm. *Clin Cancer Res*. 2004;10:2272–83.
72. Ayers M, Symmans WF, Stec J, et al. Gene expression profiles predict complete pathologic response to neoadjuvant paclitaxel and fluorouracil, doxorubicin, and cyclophosphamide chemotherapy in breast cancer. *J Clin Oncol*. 2004;22:2284–93.
73. Chang JC, Wooten EC, Tsimelzon A, et al. Gene expression profiling for the prediction of therapeutic response to docetaxel in patients with breast cancer. *Lancet*. 2003;362:362–9.
74. Cleator S, Tsimelzon A, Ashworth A, et al. Gene expression patterns for doxorubicin (Adriamycin) and cyclophosphamide (cytoxan) (AC) response and resistance. *Breast Cancer Res Treat*. 2006;95:229–33.
75. Sorlie T, Perou CM, Tibshirani R, et al. Gene expression patterns of breast carcinomas distinguish tumor subclasses with clinical implications. *Proc Natl Acad Sci U S A*. 2001;98:10869–74.
76. Banerjee S, Reis-Filho JS, Ashley S, et al. Basal-like breast carcinomas: clinical outcome and response to chemotherapy. *J Clin Pathol*. 2006;59:729–35.
77. Jacquemier J, Padovani L, Rabayrol L, et al. Typical medullary breast carcinomas have a basal/myoepithelial phenotype. *J Pathol*. 2005;207:260–8.
78. Fulford LG, Reis-Filho JS, Ryder K, et al. Basal-like grade III invasive ductal carcinoma of the breast: patterns of metastasis and long-term survival. *Breast Cancer Res*. 2007;9:R4.

Guidelines, Consensus Conferences and Overviews (Meta-analysis)

Kathleen I. Pritchard

Introduction

In the practice of oncology, and even in sub-specialties such as the care of women with breast cancer, it can be challenging and sometimes overwhelming to keep up to date with the latest discoveries and publications. In past years, the review article [1, 2] was the standard vehicle for keeping up to date for most clinicians. Review articles of this type, while often excellent summations of the available data, did not use explicit criteria for the inclusion or weighting of evidence from articles which often had wide variability in methodologic quality. Furthermore, today's methods of rapid computer-based formalized literature retrieval were not available at that time. In spite of that limitation, however, published articles were usually accessible using hand searching methods which are still an important part of all literature reviews and guideline production [3–5]. More problematic in such reviews was the lack of access to unpublished material, since review articles and indeed even consensus documents, guidelines and meta-analyses of published data do not usually attempt to retrieve such data.

In 1984, the first formal meeting of investigators and statisticians devoted to the conduct of a meta-analysis of all data concerning the treatment of early breast cancer took place. Although meta-analysis was actually an older technique, used mainly in the social sciences literature, it had not been widely appreciated in medical circles until around this time. The first meeting of the Early Breast Cancer Trials Collaborative Group (EBCTCG) Overview, or meta-analysis, colloquially referred to as the Oxford Overview, actually took place in Heathrow Airport. Here for the first time clinicians from all over the world involved in studies of treatment of early breast cancer gave 1-min summaries of their data and Richard Peto and others described the techniques for meta-analysis and the

K.I. Pritchard (✉)
Senior Scientist, Sunnybrook Research Institute Medical Oncologist, Sunnybrook Odette Cancer Centre, Professor, Department of Medicine, Faculty of Medicine, University of Toronto, Toronto, Canada

M. Castiglione, M.J. Piccart (eds.), *Adjuvant Therapy for Breast Cancer*, Cancer Treatment and Research 151, DOI 10.1007/978-0-387-75115-3_5,

then startling results of the application of this technique to adjuvant systemic therapy with tamoxifen and chemotherapy.

Consensus meetings are held and documents written in many venues but the prototype consensus conferences and documents for adjuvant therapy of breast cancer as well as for many other medical topics are those of the National Institutes of Health in the United States (NIH US). Subsequently a wide variety of consensus meetings have been held by other organizations such as the National Comprehensive Cancer Network (NCCN), the European Organization for Research and Treatment of Cancer (EORTC), and many other national and international groups. In particular, the biannual St. Gallen Primary Therapy of Breast Cancer Meeting traditionally holds a consensus panel which is then written up as a consensus guideline. The American Society for Clinical Oncology (ASCO) also publish guidelines in particular areas such as the role of sentinel node biopsy, the role of bisphosphonates in breast cancer, the role of aromatase inhibitors in breast cancer and others. Guidelines such as those put forward by NCCN and the St. Gallen Group tend to be less evidence driven and more consensus based then those of ASCO or other organizations. Particularly evidence based guidelines include those written by the Practice in Evidence Based Care (PEBC) Program of Cancer Care Ontario (CCO).

The advantage of Consensus Meetings held by organizations such as NIH is that they frequently find and present unpublished and preliminary data from a variety of groups. This can only occur in so far as these data are known to exist because they are funded through NIH or other major agencies or are registered as part of the current required world wide trials registration mechanisms [6].

All of these newer processes, like those associated with the traditional review article, suffer from the problems of rapid data accumulation and hence a requirement for frequent updating. Often literature searches are out of date and evidence based guidelines can require last minute additions of data before publishing. Decisions as to whether to include only fully published and peer reviewed articles or also abstracts from meetings plague these processes, as they did the production of up-to-date review articles in the 1970s and earlier. Computer access to on-line publications which presage printed material is a help in this process, as is the availability of slides from major meetings such as the ASCO meetings and the San Antonio Breast Cancer Symposiums (SABCS). The fact that such materials do represent preliminary data is sometimes problematic however, since data may change when final analyses are made [7].

Meta-analysis or Overviews

The concept of pooling or summing of clinical trials results, the meta-analysis or overview technique was originally developed by T.C. Chalmers and others and was initially used in the medical field to examine the role of anticoagulants following myocardial infarction [8]. The first so-called “Oxford” Overview

Group meetings were in fact held in Heathrow Airport in London in 1984 and in Bethesda, Maryland in 1985. Prior to each of these meetings, Sir Richard Peto of Oxford and his team requested raw data from all investigators who had carried out randomized trials of adjuvant therapy of any type. By literature searches and communication with individual investigators, the Oxford group eventually obtained raw data from virtually every randomized trial of (1) tamoxifen as adjuvant therapy, (2) radiation as adjuvant treatment, (3) chemotherapy of any type as adjuvant treatment and (4) ovarian ablation ± prednisone as adjuvant treatment. The Overview was subsequently expanded to include randomized trials of immunotherapy (never much of a rewarding exercise) and more modern endocrine and targeted treatments such as the aromatase inhibitors (AIs) and trastuzumab (Herceptin). Initially in 1984 only crude mortality data were requested as outcome endpoints but by the time of the Bethesda meeting more detailed data including time of first recurrence, nodal and receptor status were being collected. Since these initial meetings, quinquenial data collections and meetings have been held. More recently the EBCTCG exercise has taken on an ongoing nature in which data is continuously retrieved and updated from all known randomized studies.

A number of mathematical techniques are available [9] for conducting an overview or meta-analysis. The use of correct methodology in assembling the data to be included is much more crucial than the mathematical techniques to be used however. The basic principle of overview or meta-analysis is that treated patients from one study are compared only to controls from the same study and never directly to patients in other studies. The results of each individual comparison from each trial are then pooled to obtain an overall estimate of treatment effect. One excellent discussion of overview methodology is entitled "The problems of pooling, drowning and floating" by Goldman and Feinstein [10]. Some of the issues of meta analysis are briefly discussed below:

1. Patients from various studies being pooled must have the same diagnosis. This may seem obvious and in the case of adjuvant treatment of breast cancer it is probably a fairly simple matter but it is crucial to the technique.
2. Patients from various studies being pooled may have mixes of clinical severity of disease. Meta-analysis can use stratification to select groups of patients from each study who have similar characteristics, for example positive axillary nodes versus negative axillary nodes, estrogen receptor positivity versus negativity, etc.
3. If data are to be pooled each study must use the same therapeutic maneuver. This sounds obvious but may not always be so simple. For example, some studies of adjuvant tamoxifen gave tamoxifen for 1 year, others 2 years and 5 years. Doses varied. Should all of these studies be pooled or separated? More complex difficulties arise when looking at studies of combination chemotherapy. The cyclophosphamide, methotrexate, and five fluorouracil (CMF) regimens were generally grouped together and single agent regimens were grouped. However, amongst different studies, regimens of CMF

known to be differentially effective are used. Single agents were different in both types of drug and scheduling. More recently the issues of how to group "dose dense" therapies and various "intense" and less intense anthracycline-containing regimens have added complexity. For example, regimens such as AC are not the same as regimens such as CEF or FEC 100 but have been generally grouped as anthracycline-containing regimens in the EBCTCG meta-analyses.

4. Studies to be pooled will need the same outcome measures. Mortality should be specified as cause specific or crude mortality and disease free survival or event free survival differentiated. Any of these outcomes are valid but different ones should not be mixed.
5. When a number of studies are pooled, the results are weighted so that studies containing more patients have more weight than studies containing fewer patients. Each trial is analyzed separately producing one log rank statistic per trial. Trials can be stratified by age, nodal status, receptor status and then combined to give an overall estimate of the effect of different treatments overall and in different subgroups.
6. One must be careful in applying the results of pooled "old" data to current medical practice. For example, the pooling of data from radiation therapy techniques of 20 and 30 years ago may not give the same results as one might achieve with more sophisticated techniques today.
7. Only data from strictly randomized studies should be included in meta-analysis. The results of any meta-analysis are only as valid as the data from the original studies pooled. If individual studies did not have strictly blinded randomization, they may be biased and such bias will be reflected in the meta analysis.
8. Pooled results must include the results of all patients randomized in each trial, at risk of creating bias.
9. Any overview of a given therapeutic maneuver must include all of the randomized studies which exist of that maneuver. If only the published studies of a given maneuver are included in an overview, a bias toward positive results might occur. This publication may occur because investigators are more likely to submit positive studies for publication and journals more likely to accept them.
10. Above all, it must be remembered that an overview is only as good as the individual trials included in it. Some of the data included in overviews such as the EBCTCG are unpublished. These data may not have been peer-reviewed and therefore must be carefully and accurately scrutinized within the overview process. Breaks in randomization may have occurred in individual trials which could be unknown to the overview investigators. Therefore the input of the investigators responsible for each study in the overview is essential at all stages of the overview process. The EBCTCG Group have had considerable strength concerning these matters since, as part of the EBCTCG Process, collaboration amongst statisticians, methodologists and clinicians has been sought, built, and sustained.

Over the history of the EBCTCG Overview, the first data from 1984 showed that tamoxifen [4] CMF chemotherapy [4] and ovarian ablation [11–13] each improved survival. While this seems obvious in retrospect, at that time North Americans were very skeptical about the efficacy of tamoxifen while the British and Europeans were more skeptical about the efficacy of CMF. Everyone was dubious that ovarian ablation was effective because such small trials had been done and few had shown any statistically significant benefits. The meta-analytic summing however showed clear benefit for all three approaches.

By 1990 the Overview showed that longer tamoxifen treatment seemed better and that tamoxifen effects were clearly greater in ER positive women. It was also shown that tamoxifen reduced the rate of contralateral breast cancer and that chemotherapy was effective in both older and younger women [14].

By 1995 the huge magnitude of effect of 5 years of tamoxifen had been seen and it was very clear from direct and indirect comparisons that tamoxifen given for 5 years was better than 1 or 2 years. It also became clear, somewhat unexpectedly, that tamoxifen prevented contralateral breast cancer only in women with ER positive disease. The 1995 Overview also showed that anthracycline-containing regimens in general were better than CMF although it seemed that some anthracycline containing regimens were better than others [15].

The 2000 Overview was able to demonstrate clearly the persisting benefits of both polychemotherapy and of tamoxifen at 15 years. (Figs. 1 and 2). Ovarian oblation or suppression was also shown to be effective at 15 years of follow up (Fig. 3). It remained clear that while ovarian suppression or ablation was effective when given alone, it was not significantly so when added to chemotherapy. Because of the availability of early data from the Adjvuant Tamoxifen Longer versus Shorter (ATLAS) and Adjuvant Tamoxifen or More (ATOM) trials the door was opened to the suggestion that more than 5 years of tamoxifen might be even better than 5 years of such therapy [5].

In 2005, the main comparisons included (1) chemotherapy subdivided by (i) high dose therapy (transplant-type therapy), (ii) taxanes, (iii) anthracyclines and (iv) CMF-type chemotherapy, (2) ovarian ablation/suppression, (3) tamoxifen, (4) aromatase inhibitors, (5) neoadjuvant therapy, and (6) local therapy. New baseline data requested included sentinel node biopsy and HER2 data. By September 2006, 37 more groups and 182 more trials had been added to the EBCTCG database and processed. The 2006 Overview included 76 groups and 389 trials of which 112 were new and 277 updated, and 264,000 women, 70,000 in new and 194,000 in updated trials [16]. About 80,000 women had been studied in chemotherapy trials of whom 4,000 were in trials of single agents versus nil, more than 30,000 were in trials of prolonged chemotherapy versus nil, more than 30,000 were in trials of anthracycline versus non-anthracycline based chemotherapy, more than 10,000 were in trials of taxane versus non-taxane containing therapy, and more than 6,000 were on trials of bone marrow (BMT) or stem cell transplant (SCT) associated with high dose chemotherapy. More than 80,000 women had been studied in tamoxifen trials, more than 50,000 of whom were in trials of tamoxifen versus none and about 30,000 in

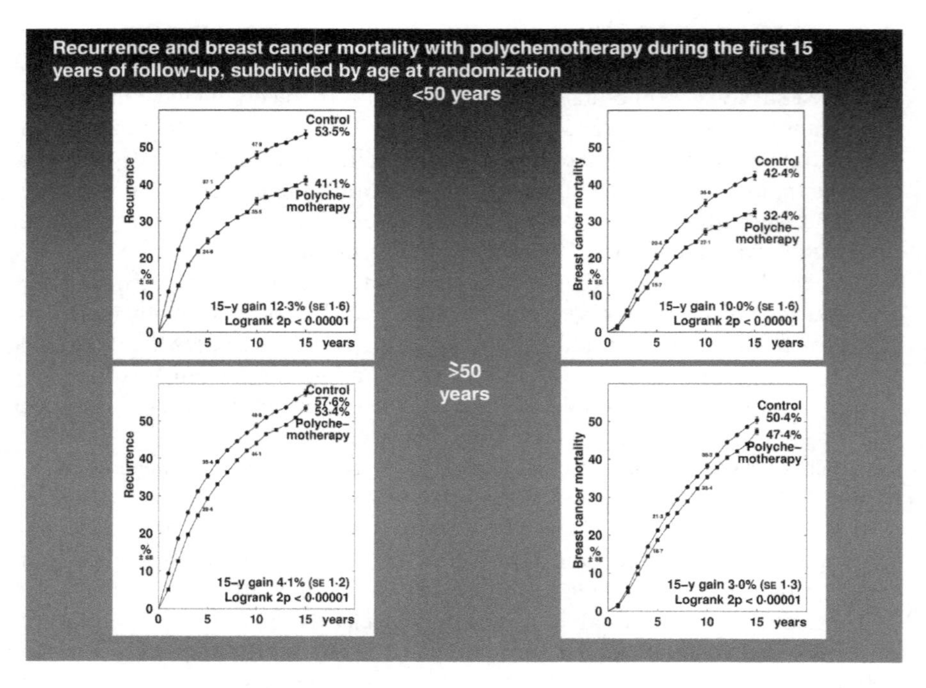

Fig. 1 Early breast cancer trialists collaborative group 2005/2006

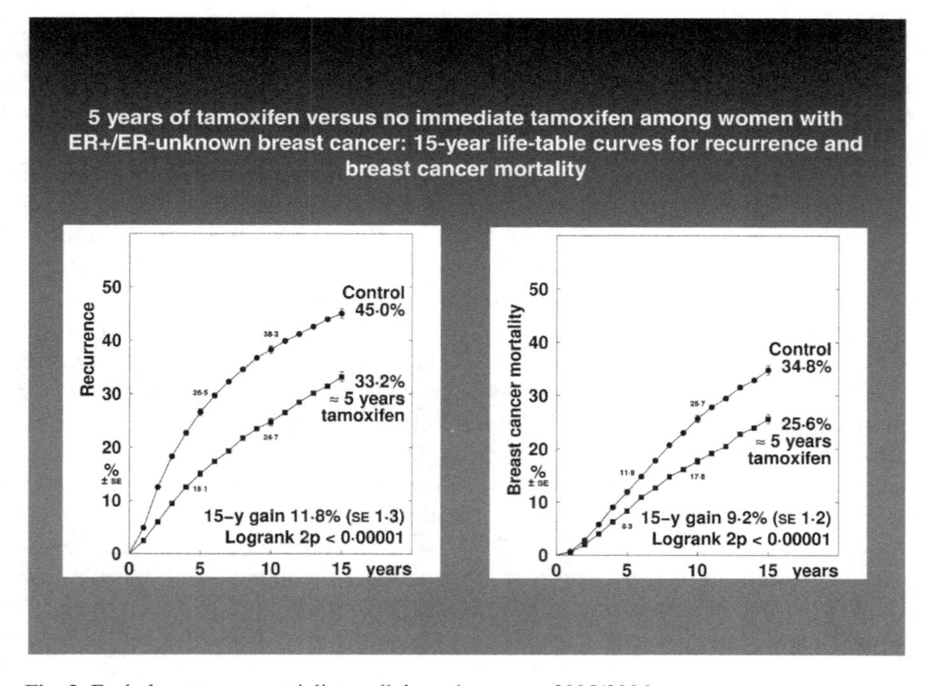

Fig. 2 Early breast cancer trialists collaborative group 2005/2006

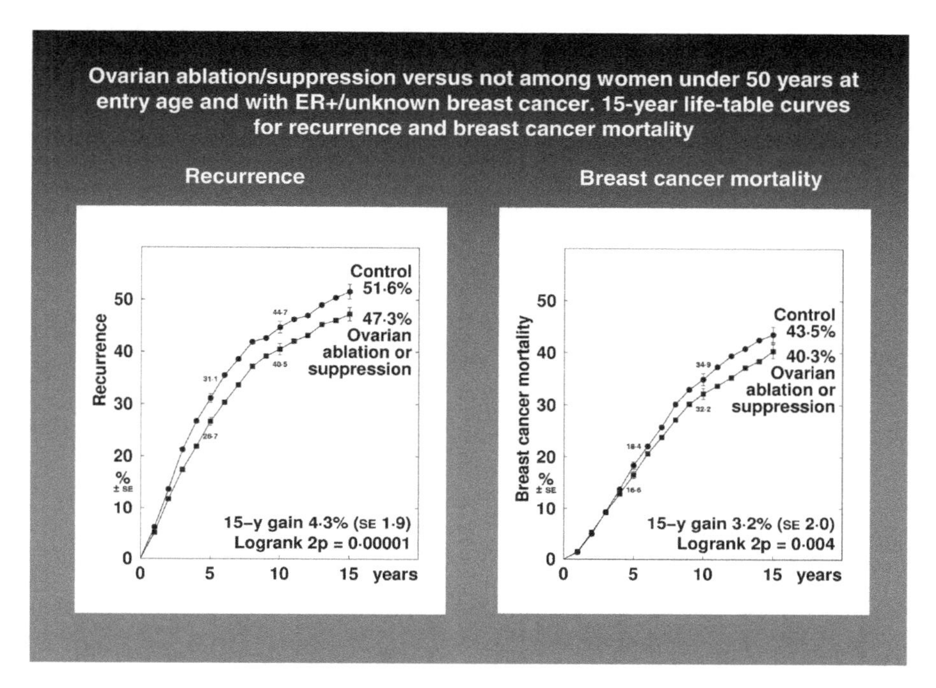

Fig. 3 Early breast cancer trialists collaborative group 2005/2006

direct comparisons of a longer versus shorter tamoxifen treatment. In addition about 12,000 women were in trials of ovarian ablation or suppression versus none and 30,000 women in trials of aromatase inhibitors (AIs).

An AI meta analysis process has been carried forward by a subgroup of the Oxford Overview acting independantly as the AI Overview Group but collaborating with the EBCTCG trialists. This group presented data at the San Antonio Breast Cancer 2008 Symposium (SABCS) [17] which will be published shortly. In summary, the 2006 ASCO Overview shows that AIs reduce recurrence and appear to add to survival overall although the early termination and cross-over seen in many of these trials makes overall survival difficult to assess. These trials however require separation by control group (tamoxifen versus placebo/control), sequenced versus primary after 2–3 or 5 years and possibly by type of AI.

Meta-analysis of the newer chemotherapy trials is now ongoing. This meta-analysis will include for the first time a specific meta-analysis of BMT/SCT supported high dose therapies. This meta-analysis is plagued however by the problems of differing control arms, some of which are less than standard treatment. Similarly, the taxane trials will be separated into trials of taxane versus no taxane and taxane versus taxane trials including a grouping for concurrent versus sequential trials of taxanes. Once again the grouping of taxane trials is problematic since all taxane regimens are not the same and control arms also differ. A subcommittee of Oxford investigators are working together to classify these trials and hence most appropriately structure their meta-analysis which is currently ongoing. The EBCTCG 2005 Overview will also attempt to look at "dose dense" versus "non-dose dense" regimens and dose intense versus non-dose intense regimens. Table 1 lists a general grouping of the types of trials and the numbers of patients in them.

Table 1 Early breast cancer trialists collaborative group 2005/2006 overview

Trials exploring dose or schedule questions (except BMT/SCT trials)		
Type of question	No. of trials	No. of pts.
• DI(dose level)	3	±4,000
• CD (treatment duration)	16	±10,000
• DI + CD	10	±10,000
• DD (dose interval)	3	±3,500
• Weekly vs q 3 wks (different dose levels)	2	±5,000
• Sequential vs Combo (same agents)	5	±14,000

BMT = Bone marrow transplant
SCT = Stem cell transplant
DI = Dose intensity
CD = Chemotherapy duration
DD = Dose density
q = every

In the 2005 Overview of tamoxifen trials the protracted advantages of tamoxifen at 15 years follow up are seen. It seems clear that ER poor PR poor patients show no benefit and similarly that ER poor PR positive show no benefit either. ER positive PR negative and ER positive PR positive patients showed similar and impressive benefits (see Figs. 4 and 5). The Overview of 5 years versus longer tamoxifen also appeared to show significant improvement in recurrence free survival for longer therapy. These results together with those of both ATLAS [18] and ATOM [19] as individual trials have been shown.

The strengths of the Oxford Overview remain the power of the technique and the processes that assure that the data are correct and comprehensive. The meta-analysis technique gives the ability to assess both the magnitude and length of effects and improves understanding of the long term natural history of breast cancer. The collaboration between methodologists, statisticians, and investigators is extremely strong.

The EBCTC Overview has however been plagued by weaknesses and frustrations that include long timelines because of the data collection and verification required. In addition, there are genuine intellectual disagreements about how much one can split or one should split or lump the data. For example, although we lose quite large amounts of the data when we try to assess treatment effects within clinically relevant subgroups that include grade, nodes, and ER and PgR we must nonetheless look at these subgroups since the largest such subgroups are available within the EBCTCG Overview. Some involved in the EBCTCG Overview continue to be frustrated by the reluctance of others to

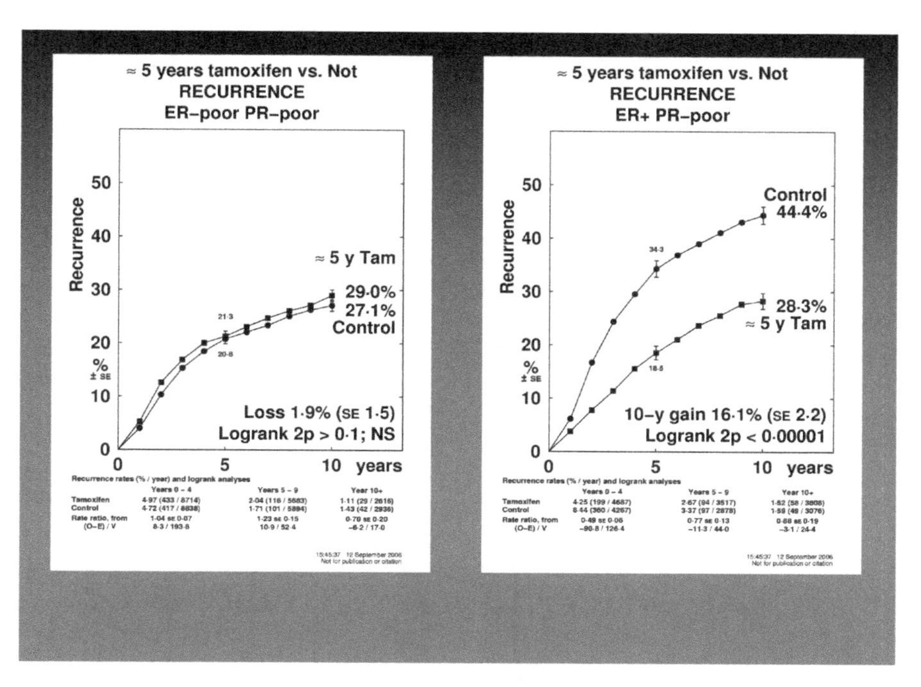

Fig. 4 Early breast cancer trialists collaborative group 2005/2006

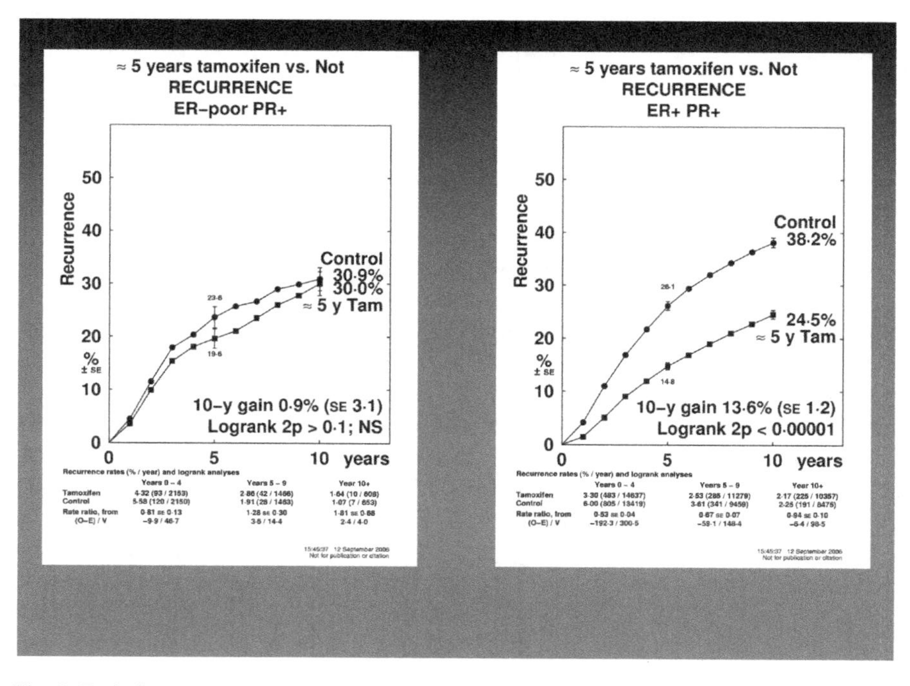

Fig. 5 Early breast cancer trialists collaborative group 2005/2006

explore subsets while some remain concerned about over-interpretation of subset analyses and attempting to take the data far beyond what the subset sizes can carry. These differing scientific points of view will continue to be explored in vigorous debate in the EBCTCG process.

In addition, all involved in the Overview process fear the loss of long term follow up in the individual trials that make up the Overview. Currently many groups are no longer following their breast cancer trial patients beyond 10 years because of lack of funding. However, it seems very clear from the most interesting results seen after 15 and 20 years of follow up in the EBCTCG Overview that such follow up is crucial and should be continued at all costs.

The future potentials of the EBCTCG Overview include further elucidation of long term recurrence and mortality patterns, examination of the long term efficacy of tamoxifen, the AIs and chemotherapy as well as the potential to describe long term side effects of these therapies. Regardless of the limits associated with subgroup analysis there will clearly be the potential for more analyses concerning predictive factors such as HER2. In summary, the EBCTCG Overview exercise is still extremely valuable. The potential remains enormous, collaboration remains crucial and flexibility amongst investigators will be key.

Consensus Meetings and Documents

While a broad variety of consensus exercises and documents are held and published, the prototype probably remains the NIH US consensus process [20]. The number of NIH Consensus Development Conferences covering the area of adjuvant therapy of breast cancer have been held as part of the overall NIH program. The NIH, the lead government agency for federally sponsored research in the United States, beginning in 1977, organized Consensus Development Conferences to review controversial areas of medical research [21]. Several hundred such conferences were subsequently held on a wide variety of diseases and medical disciplines. Adjuvant therapy of breast cancer has been one of the most popular topics for consensus development conferences with meetings held in 1980, 1985, 1990 and 2000 [22–25].

NIH Consensus Development Conferences are structured to emphasize a balanced critical review of the scientific evidence. A planning committee develops key questions and selects experts in the field who then present pertinent research results to an independent non-governmental panel consisting of academic and community-based physicians, biostatisticans, nurses, basic researchers and members of other appropriate disciplines along with lay patient advocates. The panelists are selected for their general expertise in their chosen field but they can not have published extensively or be considered opinion leaders on the topic selected for Consensus Development. The most recent Consensus Conference on the adjuvant therapy of breast cancer held November 1–3, 2000 was open to the public and admission was free. The Panelists had reviewed the existing literature prior to the conference and their review was then supplemented by presentations from 33 expert speakers, most of whom contributed original articles to the subsequently published monograph. The Consensus meeting reviewed a series of questions which included (1) which factors should be used to select systemic adjuvant therapy? (2) for which patients should adjuvant hormonal therapy be recommended? (3) for which patients should adjuvant chemotherapy be recommended, which agents should be used and at what dose and schedule? (4) for which patients should postmastectomy radiotherapy be recommended? (5) how do side effects and quality of life issues factor into individual decision making about adjuvant therapy? and (6) what are promising new research directions for adjuvant therapy? Discussion sections were interspersed through the formal presentations. At the conclusion of the expert presentations the panel met in closed sessions and developed a draft consensus statement. The panel chair person read the entire draft to all meeting participants who offered suggestions before the panelists finalized the statement. At the close of the conference the Consensus Statement was presented to the National Press, made available on the NIH website, http://consensus.nih.gov, and was subsequently published [26]. The entire statement was reproduced in a monograph [26] and provided a useful summary recommendation to professionals and the public.

The advantage of a Consensus Conference such as this is that invited expert speakers presented data that had not previously been published or presented. For example, Bryant, Fisher and Dignam published data on optimal duration of tamoxifen therapy [27]. Similarly data from investigators on topics such as ovarian ablation with or without chemotherapy, that had not previously been published, were presented for the first time [28].

Such Consensus meetings certainly provide a focus pulling together data that has emerged over the preceeding number of years. The lack of systemic searching for data in specific areas such as occurs in an exercise like the EBCTCG Overview, however, sometimes leads to problems. For example, the early presentations and publication of data on length of tamoxifen suggested that longer tamoxifen might be worse than 5 years of tamoxifen. This has turned out with further follow up and results of other studies probably not to be the case. Thus, a more systematic process that collects data from all of available sources over a more protracted period of time is likely more useful.

Clinical Practice Guidelines

Clinical practice guidelines have gained increasing visibility and importance in clinical practice. They are also used for health policy formulation and reimbursement. Such guidelines may be based on expert consensus or highly evidence based. The translation of clinical research results into practice guidelines can be slow but methods are evolving to improve the timeliness of guideline creation and maximize their impact on the quality of cancer patient care.

The guidelines created by ASCO have been viewed as among the most influential. ASCO began publishing guidelines in 1994 and has since published 25 guidelines. They subsequently began producing clinical guideline tools and resources and are currently developing 9 new and 11 updated guidelines. ASCO now conducts full updates of guidelines every 3 years and conducts an annual surveillance for literature focusing on evidence which could potentially affect previous recommendations. The ASCO Health Services Committee also publishes Provisional Clinical Opinions (PCOs) which are based on the expedited review of potentially practiced containing changing evidence. Nonetheless, the ASCO guidelines are limited by their small number and by difficulty of implementation into daily practice. A number of new initiatives by ASCO and others in partnership with a variety of commited professional organizations such as Cancer Care Ontario have resulted in improvements to the timely development, dissemination and implementation of Clinical Practice Guidelines. These initiatives include the development of rapid updating options, a guideline endorsement policy, and the development of mutiple derivative products including an executive summary, a patient guide, or powerpoint slides with each guideline in order to enhance dissemination [29].

The ASCO and the Program in Evidence Based Care (PEBC) group of Cancer Care Ontario Guidelines are both based on systematic reviews of evidence defined by critically developed criteria. The PEBC of Cancer Care Ontario is a guidelines program of the cancer system in Ontario, Canada. It is a key initiative of Cancer Care Ontario (CCO), the advisory body of the Ontario government in matters related to cancer. The Evidence Advice Cycle (formerly called the Guideline Development Cycle) [3] serves as the map to guide the development of all PEBC Guidelines. Systematic review has been the methological foundation of all PEBC produced clinical guidelines. Formally structured reviews address explicitly framed questions formulated to be answered by analysis and interpretation of the synthesized evidence. The PEBC process, while strongly evidence driven, has recently also expanded to look beyond the published literature in order to consider the environmental scan, an explicit and transparent search and review of the "gray" literature that features descriptions of or data related to solving an organizational or system problem that could be applied locally – and formalized consensus methods. The Provincial Disease Site Groups of the PEBC as part of their overall portfolio have developed 143 practice guidelines related to chemotherapy and a number of others related to a variety of other aspects of care. There are 25 breast cancer guidelines [29].

Many organizations such as the NCCN, EORTC and a wide variety of others have developed guideline programs which are not perhaps as strongly evidence based as those of ASCO or the PEBC of CCO. As the practice environment changes, every organization involved in composing and administering clinical guidelines will need to remain alert and willing to adapt to that change in order to achieve more effective guideline implementation. Well done practice guidelines such as those of ASCO or the PEBC of CCO reflect the evidence-based approach of meta analysis at one end and the less formalized consensus conference approach at the other. While largely evidence driven, practice guidelines may also take into account practice activities through environmental scans or practitioner feedback that are not based on such hard evidence. The need for constant updating remains problematic. Barriers to the incorporation of clinical guidelines can exist at physician, patient, technical, and economically based levels. However, the role of clinical practice guidelines will continue to evolve and such guidelines will prove useful in day to day care of women with breast cancer. Collaboration amongst various groups such as that between ASCO and the PEBC will help to conserve resources, not reinvent the wheel, and generally provide better quality guidelines available to all [29].

Summary

In summary, traditional reviews, consensus conferences, practice guidelines, and meta-analyses can each provide relevant data that is useful in patient care. It is clear that the traditional review has to some degree fallen out of favor but may in fact still be extremely useful. Meta-analysis is dependent on collaboration amongst investigators, together with vigorous data cleaning, processing and analysis by expert statistical and methodologic groups. The interactions between clinicians, methologists and statisticans in this area are clearly pivotal. The EBCTCG meta-analysis in particular has clearly provided new insights into adjuvant therapy. The extension of this process to look in more detail at predictive factors, while controversial, may prove useful over the coming decades.In the meantime, rigorously conducted consensus processes and well done guidelines developed according to rigorous approaches and meeting quality standards will continue to prove useful.

References

1. Henderson IC, Canellos GP. Cancer of the breast: The past decade (first of two parts). *N Engl J Med.* 1980;302:17–30.
2. Henderson IC, Canellos GP. Cancer of the breast: The past decade (second of two parts). *N Engl J Med.* 1980;302:78–90.
3. Browman GP, Levine MN, Mohide EA, et al. The practice guidelines development cycle: A conceptual tool for practice guidelines development and implementation. *J Clin Oncol.* 1995;13:502–12.
4. Early Breast Cancer Trialists' Collaborative Group. Effects of adjuvant tamoxifen and of cytotoxic therapy on mortality in early breast cancer: An overview of 61 randomized trials among 28,896 women. *N Engl J Med.* 1988;319:1681–92.
5. Early Breast Cancer Trialists' Collaborative Group. Effects of chemotherapy and hormonal therapy for early breast cancer on recurrence and 15-year survival: An overview of the randomised trials. *Lancet.* 2005;365:1687–717.
6. De Angelis C, Drazen JM, Frizelle F, et al. Clinical trial registration: A statement from the International Committee of Medical Journal Editors. *Ann Intern Med.* 2004;141:477–8.
7. Tam VC, Hotte SJ. Consistency of phase III clinical trials abstracts presented at an annual meeting of the American Society of Clinical Oncology compared with their subsequent full-text publications. *J Clin Oncol.* 2008;26:2205–11.

8. Chalmers TC, Matta R.J., Smith H Jr, Kunzler AM. Evidence favouring the use of anticoagulants in the hospital phase of acute myocardial infarction. *N Eng J Med.* 1977;297:1097.
9. Rosenthal R. Combining results of independent studies. *Psych Bulletin.* 1978;85:185–93.
10. Goldman L, Feinstein AR. Angicoagulants and myocardial infarction: The problems of pooling, drowning and floating. *Ann Inter Med.* 1979;90:92–4.
11. Delozier T, Juret P, Couette JE, Mace-Lesech J. Ovarian irradiation in postmenopausal women with breast cancer and positive axillary nodes. In: Early Breast Cancer Trialists' Collaborative Group, ed. Treatment of Early Breast Cancer. Worldwide Evidence 1985–1990. *A Systematic Overview of all Available Randomized Trials of Adjuvant Endocrine and Cytoxic Therapy.* Oxford: Oxford University Press; 1990:114.
12. Pritchard KI. Ovarian ablation as adjuvant therapy for premenopausal women with early breast cancer: Phoenix arisen? (Editorial). *Lancet.* 1992;339:95–6.
13. Early Breast Cancer Trialists' Collaborative Group. Ovarian ablation in early breast cancer: An overview of the randomized trials. *Lancet.* 1996;348:1189–96.
14. Early Breast Cancer Trialists' Collaborative Group. Tamoxifen for early breast cancer: An overview of the randomized trials. *Lancet.* 1998;351:1451–67.
15. Early Breast Cancer Trialists' Collaborative Group. Polychemotherapy for early breast cancer: An overview of the randomized trials. *Lancet.* 1998;352:930–42.
16. Personal communication with Sir Richard Peto. 2008.
17. Ingle JN, Dowsett AG, Cuzick J, Davies C, Early Breast Cancer Trialists' Collaborative Group. Aromatase inhibitors versus tamoxifen as adjuvant therapy for postmenopausal women with estrogen receptor positive breast cancer: Meta-analysis of randomized trials of monotherapy and switching strategies. *Br Cancer Res Treat.* 2008;106. Abstract 107.
18. Peto R, Davies C. ATLAS (Adjuvant Tamoxifen, Longer Against Shorter): international randomized trial of 10 versus 5 years of adjuvant tamoxifen among 11 500 women preliminary results [abstract]. *Br Cancer Res Treat.* 2007;106.Abstract 48.
19. Earl H, Gray R, Kerr D, Lee M. The optimal duration of adjuvant tamoxifen treatment for breast cancer remains uncertain: Randomize into ATom. *Clin Oncol (R Coll Radiol).* 1997;9:141–43.
20. Abrams JS, Eifel P. Monograph Overview. *Monogr Natl Cancer Inst.* 2001;30:1–4.
21. Office the Director NIH. Guidelines for the planning and management of NIH Consensus Development Conferences. NIH. 1993. Report http://consensus.nih.gov
22. Moxley JH, Allegra JC, Henney J, Muggia FM. Treatment of primary breast cancer: Summary of the National Institutes of Health Consensus Development Conference. *JAMA.* 1980;244:797–803.
23. Consensus Conference. Adjuvant chemotherapy for breast cancer. *JAMA.* 1985; 254:3461–3.
24. NIH Consensus Conference. Treatment of early stage breast cancer. *JAMA.* 1991;265:391–5.
25. National Institutes of Health Consensus Development Panel. The National Institutes of Health Consensus Development Conference: Adjuvant therapy for breast cancer. *J Natl Cancer Inst.* 2001;30:1–152.
26. National Institutes of Health Consensus Panel. National Institiutes of Health Consensus Development Conference statement: Adjuvant therapy for breast cancer, November 1–3, 2000. *J Natl Cancer Inst.* 2001;93:979–89.
27. Bryant J., Fisher B, Dignam J. Duration of Adjuvant Tamoxifen Therapy. *J Natl Cancer Inst.* 2001;30:56–61.
28. Davidson N.E. Ovarian ablation as adjuvant therapy for breast cancer. *J Natl Cancer Inst.* 2001;30:67–71.
29. Balaban EP, Brouwers M, Temin SB, Lyman GH. Issues in clinical practice guideline implementation and utilization. *ASCO Educational Book.* In press 2009.

Statistical Issues and Challenges

Meredith M. Regan

Adjuvant therapy clinical trials for early breast cancer have historically been treatment focused—for example assessing the role of chemotherapy, tamoxifen, ovarian ablation—rather than patient-population focused. Therapeutic effects of adjuvant therapies for early breast cancer have been assessed "across the board" and implemented using the principle that if a treatment is effective "on average" then it is effective "for all patients." There is new effort to tailor early breast cancer clinical trials to populations of patients who might have the best chance to benefit from the therapies being studied. For example, estrogen receptor (ER) and progesterone receptor (PgR) are the most important factors used today to tailor adjuvant therapies [1, 2], and recent pivotal trials of adjuvant trastuzumab (Herceptin) demonstrated its benefit among patients whose tumors overexpressed HER2/*neu* [3–5]. Exploration and improved understanding of the biological basis for predicting response to available adjuvant therapies is essential to enhance patient care.

Completed clinical trials, initiated and matured as biological knowledge developed inparallel, present an opportunity to learn from the past. The novel STEPP (Subpopulation Treatment Effect Pattern Plots) method was motivated by the inadequacy of statistical approaches for presenting results of clinical trials to tailor treatments properly. The future looks forward to using molecular profiling or gene expression of a tumor to tailor treatments for early breast cancer. Two landmark clinical trials, MINDACT and TAILORx, were launched in 2006 with the objective to validate the utility of a signature of molecular profiling or gene expression in clinical practice.

M.M. Regan (✉)
IBCSG Statistical Center, Department of Biostatistics and Computational, Biology, Dana-Farber Cancer Institute and Harvard School of Public Health, Boston, MA, USA
e-mail: meredith_regan@dfci.harvard.edu

M. Castiglione, M.J. Piccart (eds.), *Adjuvant Therapy for Breast Cancer*, Cancer Treatment and Research 151, DOI 10.1007/978-0-387-75115-3_6,

Learning from the Past

The setting. Adjuvant therapy trials for early breast cancer are often designed as blinded or unblinded, randomized controlled trials in which patients are randomly assigned to receive one of two therapies. The primary analysis tests the null hypothesis (H_0) of treatment equality vs an alternative hypothesis (H_A) of a difference in treatment efficacy. The primary outcome measure is usually a time-to-event variable (e.g., disease-free survival; DFS), defined as the duration of time from the date of randomization to the date of an event of interest (e.g., breast cancer recurrence or death from any cause) or to the date of last follow-up when the patient was known to be free from the event of interest (censored observation). The survival distributions for patients randomized to each therapy arm are calculated and displayed using the method of Kaplan and Meier [6]. The hazard ratio (HR) and 95% confidence interval (CI) for the treatment comparison (the "treatment effect") are estimated from a Cox proportional hazards (PH) model and a log-rank test [6] is used for the hypothesis test (H_0: $HR = 1$ vs H_A: $HR \neq 1$). If the hypothesis test indicates rejecting the null in favor of the alternative hypothesis (i.e., a statistically significant p-value is obtained and one treatment is declared superior to the other treatment), then a secondary analysis may re-evaluate the treatment effect after "adjusting" or "controlling" for other known prognostic factors, e.g., nodal status and tumor grade and size, using Cox PH modeling. If the hypothesis test for the treatment comparison in this model reaches the same result, then one concludes that, in patients who have the same nodal status, tumor grade and tumor size, the one treatment is superior to the other treatment. These analyses address the average treatment effect in the population of patients who were eligible for the trial. These analyses do not help to discover in which patients the treatment might be most beneficial.

The subgroup controversy. To address this issue, the subsequent analyses in most clinical trials will estimate the treatment effect (i.e., HR and 95% CI) within different subgroups of patients, e.g., groupings of age at randomization (e.g., <35, 35–49, 50–59, ≥ 60 years), nodal status (negative, positive). An appropriate hypothesis test would be to test for a treatment-by-covariate interaction in a Cox PH model, e.g., testing whether the magnitude of the treatment effect is different for patients with node-positive than for those with node-negative disease.

Subgroup analyses are controversial because of concerns of spurious results and incorrect conclusions [7, 8]. There are concerns of inflating alpha (type I error) levels because of repeated hypothesis testing (i.e., false-positive results wherein statistically significant results emerge by chance alone). On the other hand, when the trial is statistically powered only for the primary treatment comparison in the entire trial population and not for a smaller subgroup of the trial population, then false-negative results are likely. Similarly tests for treatment-by-covariate interactions may produce false-negative or false-positive results [7, 9] when in fact the magnitude of the treatment effect is not different between subgroups. Thus recommending treatments based only on the overall results from a clinical trial and avoiding recommendations based on subgroup analyses is advocated by many. However, this approach again applies an average treatment effect "across the board."

Some argue that limited, pre-specified, hypothesis-based subgroup analyses can be useful in the appropriate context, with recognition that results of subgroup analyses must always be presented and interpreted cautiously [10, 11]. Coates et al. [11] argued that the primary question is whether the treatment works; but if it does work, then the emergent secondary question concerns the magnitude of the therapeutic benefit, and that the analytical approach and use of subgroup analyses for these two questions differ. That is, the primary analytical hypothesis test is to be undertaken in the entire trial population (log-rank test of H_0: $HR = 1$ vs H_A: $HR \neq 1$; estimating HR and 95% CI) and if this result is statistically significant then estimating the treatment effect in clinically-relevant subgroups is valuable.

Recently Lagakos [12], who has been widely referenced as opposed to subgroup analyses, restated the need for cautious interpretation of subgroup analyses writing "When subgroup analyses are properly conducted, presentation of their results can be informative, especially when the treatments being compared are used in practice. . .avoiding any presentation of subgroup analyses because of their history of being over-interpreted is a steep price to pay for a problem that can be remedied by more responsible analysis and reporting. Ultimately, medical research and patients are best served when subgroup analyses are well planned and appropriately analyzed and when conclusions and recommendations about clinical practice are guided by the strength of the evidence."

Forest plots. Borrowed from meta-analysis, forest plots [13] now abound in the adjuvant therapy literature to summarize subgroup analyses; Fig. 1 provides an example from the *HER*ceptin *A*djuvant (HERA) trial [3]. The horizontal axis is the value of the HR, displayed as a box with the size proportional to the information for the subgroup (the larger the box the more information available for the subgroup, which is based on the number of patients in the subgroup who experiencing events), and the 95% CI is indicated by "whiskers" which extend from the box. A vertical line is indicated at $HR = 1.0$, the null value for the primary analysis of treatment equality, and a second vertical line is indicated at the overall HR of treatment effect among all trial patients. Traditionally the vertical line at 1.0 is solid, and the line indicating the overall treatment effect is dashed. However Cuzick [14] recommended using the solid line to indicate the overall treatment effect which provides a visual reminder that the focal question of subgroup analyses is of heterogeneity in the magnitude of the treatment effect among subgroups relative to the overall treatment effect. This approach was implemented in the HERA trial report [3] with the solid vertical line at $HR = 0.54$, the treatment effect among all patients, and the dashed vertical line at $HR = 1.0$. The authors concluded that there was no evidence of heterogeneity in the relative treatment effect among the selected subgroups [3].

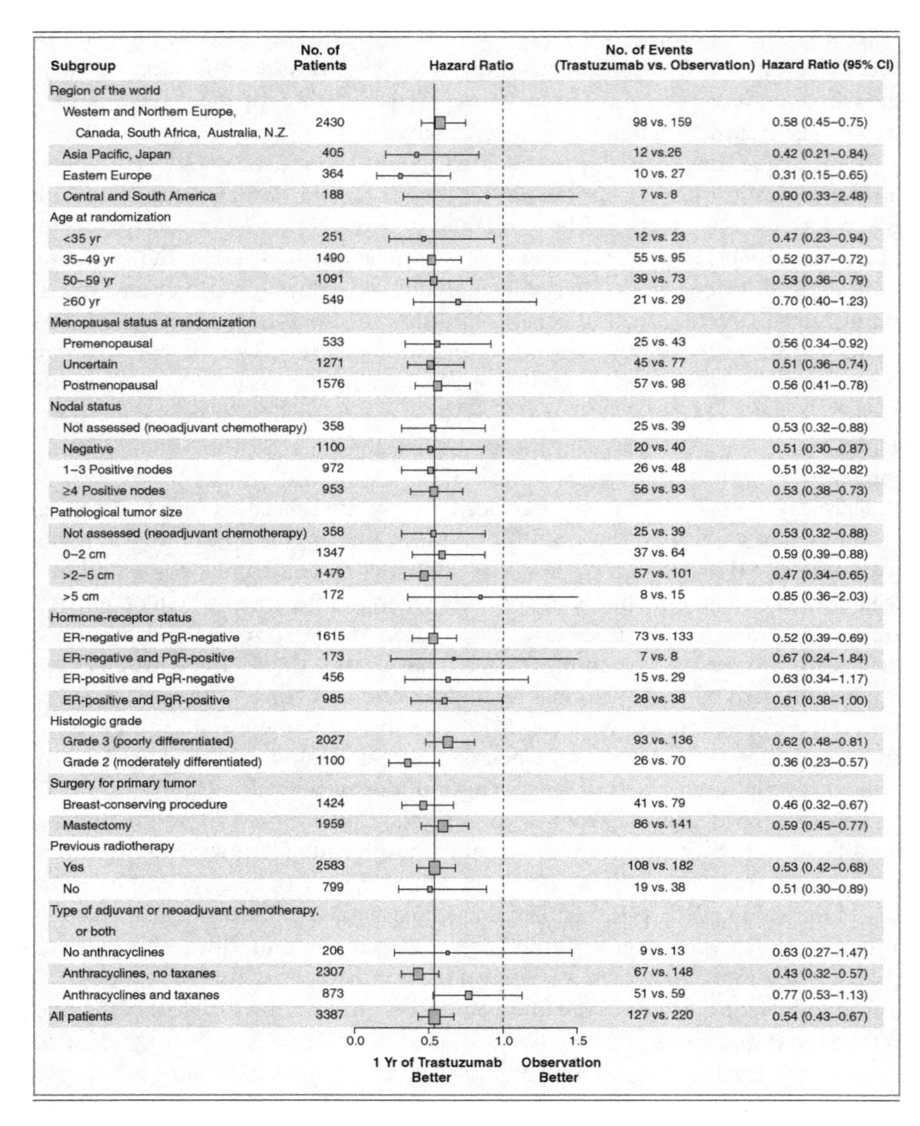

Fig. 1 Analyses of disease-free survival according to subgroup in the HERA trial (from Piccart-Gebhart et al. [3]. by permission). The hazard ratios (with 95% confidence intervals) are for the patients assigned to trastuzumab for 1 year, as compared with those assigned to observation, and were obtained from an unadjusted Cox model. The *solid vertical line* indicates a hazard ratio of 0.54, which is the value for all patients, and the *dashed vertical line* indicates the hazard ratio of 1.00, which is the null-hypothesis value. The size of the squares is proportional to the number of events in the subgroup. CI denotes confidence interval, N.Z. New Zealand, ER estrogen receptor, and PgR progesterone receptor

Cut-points for defining subgroups. The subgroups in subgroup analyses are sometimes formed by dividing a continuously-measured variable of interest into two or more categories; for example, age at randomization and pathological tumor size were divided into categories in the HERA trial report [3]. Laboratory values or biomarkers such as ER expression level are frequently categorized. The cut-points may be based on those previously proposed or established in prior research, based on observed quantiles of the distribution, or may be derived by using a statistical method of finding an "optimal" cutpoint. Clinical decision-making is facilitated by considering prognostic/predictive factors in categories rather than along a continuum. However, for statistical analysis categorization is unnecessary, results in loss of information and power, may lead to bias by using data-derived optimal cutpoints and incorrect conclusions, and is not recommended [15–16].

STEPP. The novel STEPP (*S*ubpopulation *T*reatment *E*ffect *P*attern *P*lots) method was motivated by the inadequacy of statistical approaches for presenting results of clinical trials to tailor treatments properly [17–19]. STEPP is a nonparametric methodology developed to explore the pattern of treatment effects across subpopulations defined by a continuously-measured variable, e.g., degree of ER expression or patient age. Its aim is to identify features that predict responsiveness to the treatments under study in a randomized clinical trial and generate biologically-plausible hypotheses to be tested further using other clinical trial datasets. The STEPP method avoids arbitrary division of a continuously-measured variable into categories and, by focusing on the continuum rather than on categories, it reduces the risk that individual subgroup analyses might be over-interpreted.

STEPP involves defining several overlapping subpopulations of patients on the basis of a variable of interest and studying the resulting pattern of the treatment effects estimated within each subpopulation. The subpopulations contain a fixed number of patients; the patients are ordered according to the value of the variable of interest and each subpopulation is formed starting with the fixed number patients with the lowest variable values and then dropping approximately 10–20 patients with the lowest variable value and adding approximately 10–20 patients with the next highest variable values. This is the "sliding-window" approach. The fixed number of patients and the number dropped and added with each subsequent population are chosen in consideration of the sample size. The plot's x-axis indicates the median variable value of patients in each subpopulation; the y-axis indicates the measure of treatment effect in each subpopulation, either t-year time-to-event percentage (e.g., 5-year DFS) estimated in each therapy arm using the Kaplan-Meier method, or the HR estimated from a Cox PH model.

Figures 2,3,4 provide examples from IBCSG Trial IX [20], a randomized trial investigating whether sequential treatment with three 28-day courses of "classical" CMF (cyclophosphamide, methotrexate and 5-fluorouracil) chemotherapy followed by tamoxifen for 57 months significantly improved DFS as compared with tamoxifen alone for 5 years in postmenopausal women with

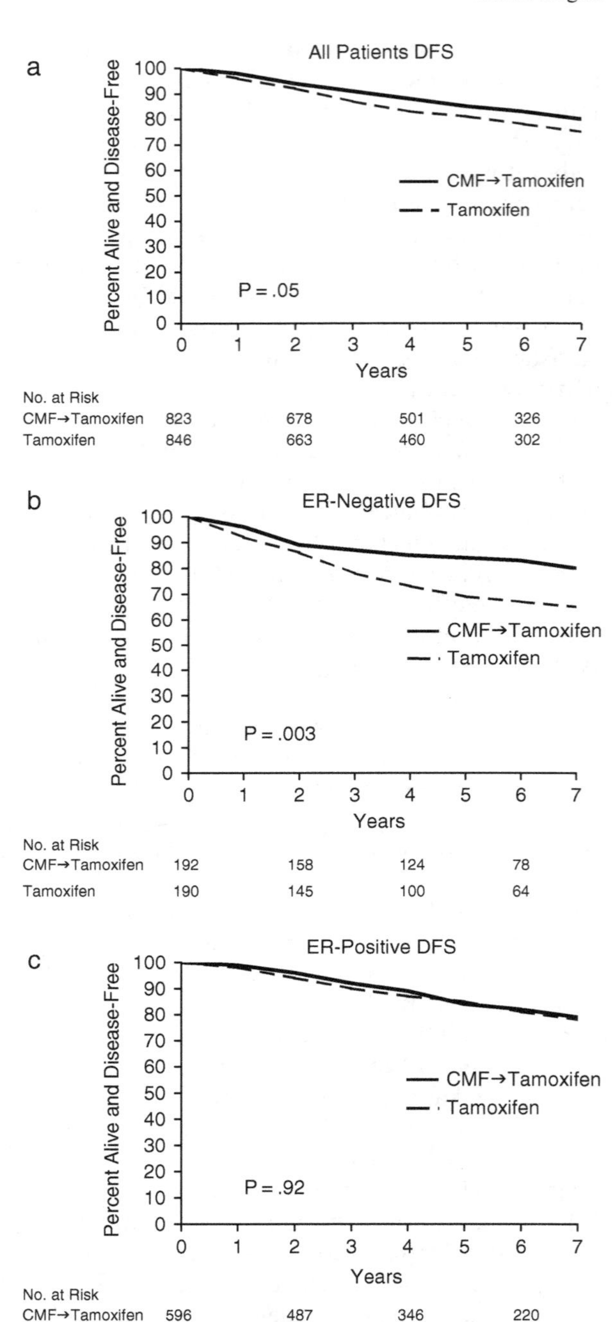

Fig. 2 Kaplan-Meier plots of disease-free survival (DFS) for postmenopausal women with lymph node-negative breast cancer according to randomized treatment group (CMF followed by tamoxifen or tamoxifen alone for 5 years) at a median follow-up time of 6 years in IBCSG Trial IX (adapted from IBCSG [20]). **a** For all 1,669 women. **c** For 382 women with ER-negative breast cancer. **e** For 1,217 women with ER-positive breast cancer.

lymph node-negative breast cancer. IBCSG reported, at a median follow-up of 6 years, that CMF followed by tamoxifen significantly improved DFS as compared with tamoxifen alone (HR = 0.80; 95% CI 0.64–1.00; Fig. 2). ER-status of the primary tumor was determined by the local pathologists prior to randomization and used as a randomization stratification factor. For ER-status, the test of treatment-by-covariate interaction in the Cox PH model was statistically significant (p = 0.01), as the effectiveness of adding CMF to the adjuvant treatment regimen was observed exclusively among women with ER-negative disease (HR = 0.52, 95% CI 0.34–0.79) and no treatment difference was observed for women with ER-positive tumors (HR = 0.99; 95% CI 0.75–1.30).

Figure 3 presents the STEPP analysis according to quantitative ER values measured using biochemical assays. Figure 3a measures the treatment effect as 5-year DFS percent and Fig. 3b measures the treatment effect using the Cox model HR. The two STEPPs highlight the strong treatment effect associated with adding chemotherapy for women with tumors expressing no or low levels of ER compared with virtually no treatment effect on DFS for women with tumors having higher values of ER (those subpopulations with median ER exceeding 10 fmol/mg cytosol protein). Because ER-status was defined for most women based on biochemical assays as ≤ 10 vs >10 fmol/mg cytosol protein to indicate ER-negative vs ER-positive tumors, respectively, the conclusions based on the analysis using categorical or using continuous ER levels are consistent.

Figure 4 presents the STEPP analysis according to the women's age at randomization, using 5-year DFS as the measure of treatment effect; there is no obvious pattern differential treatment response according to age (i.e., of age-by-treatment interaction). Note, however, that if subgroup analysis had been undertaken with age dichotomized as <60 vs ≥ 60 years then the analysis would have concluded that there was no age-by-treatment interaction (p = 0.42) with estimated treatment effect stronger among younger (HR = 0.71, 95% CI 0.50–1.02) than older women (HR = 0.87, 95% CI 0.65–1.16). If instead age had been dichotomized as <65 vs ≥ 65 then the analysis would have concluded no interaction (p = 0.52) but with estimated treatment effect stronger for older (HR = 0.72, 95% CI 0.49–1.06) than for younger women (HR = 0.84, 95% CI 0.64–1.11). Examining the pattern of treatment response across the continuum of age would reduce the risk that a subgroup analysis based on a single selected cut-point might be over-interpreted.

The STEPP method was developed because of the inadequacy of approaches for presenting results of clinical trials to properly tailor treatments. It estimates the treatment effect within each subpopulation by well-known statistical measures, the Kaplan-Meier estimate of *t*-year survival or hazard ratio. The STEPP method focuses on the patterns of treatment response across the continuum, avoiding the need for arbitrary cut-points while generating biologically-plausible hypotheses to be tested further using other clinical trial datasets. The method also investigates an alternative "tail-oriented" pattern, which

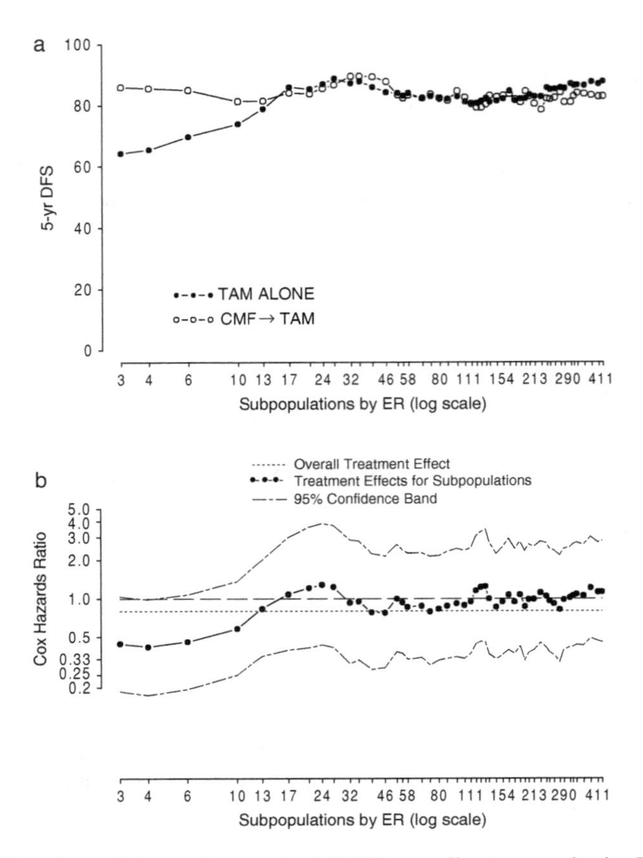

Fig. 3 STEPP analysis of disease-free survival (DFS) according to quantitative ER values for postmenopausal women with lymph node-negative breast cancer according to randomized treatment group (CMF followed by tamoxifen vs tamoxifen alone for 5 years) in IBCSG Trial IX [20]. For these sliding-window STEPP analyses, each subpopulation contained approximately 200 women, and each subsequent subpopulation was formed by moving from left to right by dropping approximately 10 observations with the lowest values for ER and adding approximately 10 observations with the next higher values of ER. The x-axis indicates the median ER value for the women in each subpopulation. **a** STEPP showing 5-year DFS percent. **b** STEPP showing Cox model HR. *Horizontal dashed line* = no difference between treatments (HR = 1.0); *horizontal dotted line* – the observed treatment difference for the overall population (HR = 0.80). *Solid circles* = HRs for each of the sliding-window subpopulations; bands around these points – the simultaneous (across all subgroups) 95% CI for the HRs

concentrates on the influence of extreme values of the covariate on the magnitude of the treatment effect [17, 19]. An S-Plus (Insightful Corp., Seattle, WA) function is available from the original authors or through the IBCSG (http://www.ibcsg.org).

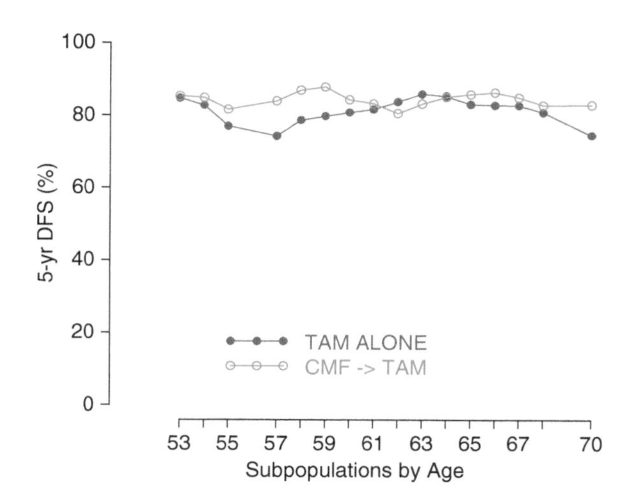

Fig. 4 STEPP analysis of 5-year DFS according to age at randomization for women treated with CMF followed by tamoxifen vs women treated with tamoxifen alone in IBCSG Trial IX. For this sliding-window STEPP analyses, each subpopulation contained approximately 250 patients and each subsequent subpopulation was formed by dropping and adding approximately 20 women.

Planning for the Future

Developing and validating genomic classifiers. The introduction of DNA microarray technology has brought about exciting possibility for tailoring treatments in early breast cancer. With the growing incorporation of this technology into research, guidelines continue to evolve for the design, analysis and reporting of microarray expression profiling studies [21, 22] as well as for the development and validation of an expression signature classifier prior to clinical application [23]. In the meantime two landmark clinical trials, MINDACT and TAILORx, were launched in 2006 for women with early stage breast cancer with the objective of validating the utility of signatures of molecular or gene expression profiles in clinical practice. The trials focus on the question of whether the signature identifies a subset of patients with node-negative early-stage breast cancer who do not need chemotherapy.

As defined by Simon [23], "a multigene expression signature classifier is a function that provides a classification of a tumor based on the expression levels of the component genes." The tumor classes depend on the setting, e.g., low-risk vs high-risk of breast cancer recurrence. A classifier is developed using an archival set of tumor samples for which the relevant, possibly long-term, clinical outcome data are available. Ideally the samples are from a clearly-defined, homogeneously-treated patient population, but the availability of archival material often is limiting, and the clinical data should be uniformly collected with standardized variable and outcome definitions for forming the classes. In the development stage a large set of genes is screened to discover a subset of genes whose expression is strongly correlated with outcome and a classifier function is defined and internally validated—ideally on a subset of the samples that were not used for selecting the genes and defining the classifier—to estimate the error rate of the classifier. The classifier is subsequently externally validated on a different, independent set of clinically-annotated tumor samples, with careful attention paid to differences in the cohort characteristics and variable definition as compared with the original samples. Expression levels of the subset of genes comprising the classifier are determined and the classifier function is applied to these values to assess the performance of the classifier for predicting outcome and the rate of misclassification in the new cohort. As with any novel drug or treatment regimen, the ultimate validation of its clinical application is achieved by conducting a large, prospective clinical trial. The design of such novel trials to validate a biological marker or signature classifier presents challenges.

The MINDACT trial. A 70-gene prognostic gene expression signature for patients with node-negative disease which was developed by researchers at the Netherlands Cancer Institute in Amsterdam [24, 25] and validated by the TRANSBIG Consortium [26] is the basis of the *M*icroarray *I*n *N*ode negative *D*isease may *A*void *C*hemo*T*herapy (MINDACT) trial [27, 28]. MINDACT is an international, prospective, randomized phase III trial to compare the 70-gene expression signature with the *Adjuvant! Online* clinical-pathological prognostic tool [29] (http://www.adjuvantonline.com/) to select patients who should and should not receive chemotherapy for node-negative disease.

Women with operable node-negative breast cancer are eligible. After surgery a frozen tumor sample will be sent for evaluation of the 70-gene expression signature which will classify it as low- or high-risk molecular prognosis. The risk classification will be compared with that determined by *Adjuvant! Online* using the clinical-pathological features as assessed by the local pathologist. Patients for whom the two risk evaluations are discordant will then be randomly assigned to use one risk evaluation or the other to decide whether or not the patient will receive chemotherapy, which is equivalent to randomly assigning these patients to receive chemotherapy or not. The objective is to confirm that patients with "low-risk" molecular prognosis but "high-risk" clinical-pathological prognosis can safely be spared chemotherapy without affecting long-term outcome, defined as distant metastasis-free survival. The planned trial sample size is 6,000 patients, with 672 expected to fall into this discordant group who do not receive chemotherapy based on the low-risk molecular prognosis classification.

The TAILORx Trial. A 21-gene Recurrence Score™, which was developed and validated by Genomic Health Inc. with collaboration from the National Surgical Adjuvant Breast and Bowel Project (NSABP) [30–33] and is marketed under the name Onco*type* DX™ (Genomic Health, Inc., Redwood City, CA), is the basis of the *T*rial *A*ssigning *I*ndividua*L*ized *O*ptions for Treatment (*Rx*), or TAILORx study. TAILORx is a prospective randomized Phase III trial being undertaken in U.S. and Canada to determine whether the 21-gene Recurrence Score™ (RS) can be used to assign patients with endocrine-responsive node-negative disease to the most appropriate and effective adjuvant treatment: hormonal therapy alone or chemotherapy and hormonal therapy [34–36].

Women with ER-positive and/or PgR-positive, HER2-negative, node-negative operable breast cancer are eligible. After surgery a formalin-fixed paraffin-embedded tumor sample will be sent for evaluation of the 21-gene RS, which ranges from 1 to 100 with a higher score associated with increased risk of recurrence, and which will classify patients into three risk categories: low RS<11; intermediate RS = 11–25; high RS>25. The "primary study group" is the intermediate (RS = 11–25) risk category; these patients will be randomly assigned to receive or not receive chemotherapy in addition to hormonal therapy with the objective to demonstrate that long-term outcome, defined as disease-free survival, for patients treated with adjuvant hormonal therapy alone is not inferior to that for patients treated with adjuvant chemotherapy and hormonal therapy. The planned trial sample size is over 10,000 patients, with about 44% (4,390) of the population expected to fall into this "primary study group" whose use of adjuvant chemotherapy is randomly assigned.

Trial design issues. Though the conceptual objective of the trials is clear—demonstrate that patients with node-negative disease for whom it is decided not to administer adjuvant chemotherapy on the basis of a signature of molecular or gene expression profile will not experience poorer than expected long-term outcome—the differences in the designs of the two trials demonstrate that realization of the concept is not straightforward.

Both trials will enroll a very large number of patients and focus the randomization and statistical hypothesis test on a smaller subset of patients for whom decision-making about chemotherapy is deemed less clear. For TAILORx it is those patients with an intermediate RS (11–25), whereas for MINDACT it is those patients with discordant gene signature and clinical-pathological evaluations. Interestingly, the RS cut-off values being used to classify risk groups in the TAILORx trial [34] (low RS<11; intermediate RS = 11–25; high RS>25) are different to those developed [31–33] and proposed for clinical practice (low RS<18; intermediate RS = 18–30; high RS ≥31) [37].

The MINDACT trial did not initially focus on the patients with discordant gene signature and clinical-pathological evaluations; in the original design, patients were randomly assigned to have either the gene signature evaluation or the clinical-pathological evaluation used for chemotherapy decision-making [28]. One concern is evidenced in the revised design: for a large proportion of patients the decision based on the gene signature and clinical-pathological evaluations would be concordant and they would not inform the randomized comparison [28].

Another concern, which remains an issue for both trials, is that of non-adherence to the signature-based decision because the clinical-pathological factors traditionally used in decision-making are known. Non-adherence with the randomized assignment in a clinical trial has the impact of diluting the treatment effect and reducing power for the treatment comparison and hence necessitating an increase in planned sample size. The MINDACT trial includes a pilot phase at 7 centers in 7 countries among the first 800 patients to evaluate adherence with the randomization and also whether there is bias in patient selection for the trial [28]. In the TAILORx trial, the planned sample size was increased in anticipation of non-adherence following a standard methodology [34].

An issue fundamental to the design of both trials is that the conceptual question is fundamentally one of equivalence or non-inferiority: that omitting chemotherapy will not result in poorer outcome. Non-inferiority trials are difficult to conduct, are subject to criticism regarding the choice of "non-inferiority" threshold, and often require larger sample sizes than superiority trials [8]. Each trial avoids a classical statistical non-inferiority design and hypothesis testing. Part of the concern about the original design of the MINDACT trial was the use of a non-inferiority design [28]. The new design resulted in formulation of a one-sample statistical hypothesis test (H_0: 92% 5-year DMFS vs H_A: 95% 5-year DMFS; DMFS = distant metastasis-free survival) among the subset of patients with discordance of low-risk gene signature and high-risk clinical-pathological evaluation who are randomly assigned to use the gene signature for decision-making and thus not receive chemotherapy; the sample size was planned with one-sided type I error $\alpha = 2.5\%$ and type II error $\beta = 20\%$ (i.e., 80% power) [28]. Thus if the lower confidence interval on the observed 5-year DMFS is above 92%, then the trial will conclude that the omission of chemotherapy was not unacceptably detrimental. The TAILORx trial suggests a non-inferiority design, but uses a null hypothesis of no difference between the two groups assigned by randomization, as when testing for superiority, and specifies larger type I error (one-sided $\alpha = 10\%$) and smaller type II error ($\beta = 5\%$) than would be used in planning a superiority trial to detect an unacceptably large decrease in 5-year DFS from 90% with chemotherapy to 87% or lower without chemotherapy [34]. This allows a larger chance of erroneously rejecting the null hypothesis of no treatment difference (i.e., concluding that chemotherapy *is superior* than no chemotherapy) when in fact there is no treatment difference, and a smaller chance of erroneously failing to reject the null hypothesis of no treatment difference (i.e., concluding that chemotherapy *is not better* than no chemotherapy) when in fact there is a treatment difference and chemotherapy is superior to no chemotherapy.

The trials also have other differences between them, and each has differences from their developmental research which underscores the need for the trials. The TAILORx and MINDACT trials both have broader eligibility criteria than were used in their developmental and validation studies, but differ with respect to the eligible patient population; both enroll only patients with node-negative disease, but TAILORx is limited to patients with ER and/or PgR-positive, HER2-negative disease whereas MINDACT is not [28, 34]. The trials use different endpoint definitions, both of which are different to those used in the development and validation of the studies. Both of the trials face the logistical hurdles of submitting material for central laboratory evaluation before the patient is treated; the MINDACT is using the pilot phase to assess logistical problems [28].

MINDACT and TAILORx trials are expected to involve 3 years of accrual to achieve the planned sample sizes plus about 3 to 4 additional years of follow-up until the first reporting of results [28, 34]. Despite the challenges, these two landmark trials offer exciting potential to tailoring treatments for women with early stage breast cancer.

References

1. Goldhirsch A, Glick JH, Gelber RD, et al. Meeting highlights: International expert consensus on the primary therapy of early breast cancer 2005. *Ann Oncol.* 2005;16:1569–83.
2. Goldhirsch A, Coates AS, Gelber RD, et al. First—select the target: Better choice of adjuvant treatments for breast cancer patients. *Ann Oncol.* 2006;17;1772–6.
3. Piccart-Gebhart MJ, Proctor M, Leyland-Jones B, et al. Trastuzumab after adjuvant chemotherapy in HER2-positive breast cancer. *N Engl J Med.* 2005;353;1659–72.
4. Romond EH, Perez EA, Bryant J, et al. Trastuzumab plus adjuvant chemotherapy for operable HER-2 positive breast cancer. *N Engl J Med.* 2005;353:1673–84.
5. Slamon D, Eiermann W, Robert N, et al. BCIRG 006: 2nd interim analysis phase III randomized trial comparing doxorubicin and cyclophosphamide followed by docetaxel (AC→T) with doxorubicin and cyclophosphamide followed by docetaxel and trastuzumab (AC→TH) with docetaxel, carboplatin and trastuzumab (TCH) in Her2neu positive early breast cancer patients. *Breast Cancer Res Treat.* 2006;100(1):52.
6. Collett D. Modelling survival data in medical research, 2nd ed. Boca Raton, FL: Chapman & Hall/CRC; 2003.
7. Peto R. Statistical aspects of cancer trials. In: Halnan, KE, ed. *Treatment of Cancer.* London: Chapman & Hall; 1982:867–71.
8. Green S, Benedetti J, Crowley J. Clinical trials in oncology: Interdisciplinary statistics. Boca Raton: Chapman & Hall/CRC; 1997.
9. Lee KL, McNeer JF, Starmer CF, et al. Clinical judgment and statistics: Lessons from a simulated randomized trial in coronary artery disease. *Circulation* 1980;61:508–15.
10. Friedman LW, Furberg CD, DeMets DL. *Fundamentals of clinical trials.* New York: Springer-Verlag; 1998:304–6.
11. Coates AS, Goldhirsch A, Gelber RD. Overhauling the breast cancer overview: Are subsets subversive? *Lancet Oncol.* 2002;3:525–6.
12. Lagakos SW. The challenge of subgroup analyses—reporting without distorting. *N Engl J Med.* 2006;354:1667–9.
13. Lewis S, Clarke M. Forest plots: Trying to see the wood and the trees. *BMJ.* 2001;322:1479–80.
14. Cuzick J. Forest plots and the interpretation of subgroups. *Lancet.* 2005;365:1308.
15. Royston P, Altman DG, Sauerbrei W. Dichotomizing continuous predictors in multiple regression: A bad idea. *Stat Med.* 2006;25:127–41.
16. McShane LM, Altman DG, Sauerbrei W, et al., for the Statistics Subcommittee of the NCI-EORTC Working Group on Cancer Diagnostics. REporting recommendations for tumor MARKer prognostic studies (REMARK). *J Natl Cancer Inst.* 2005;97:1180–4.
17. Bonetti M, Gelber RD. A graphical method to assess treatment – covariate interactions using the Cox model on subsets of the data. *Stat Med.* 2000;19:2595–609.
18. Bonetti M, Gelber RD, Goldhirsch A, Castiglione-Gertsch M, Coates AS, for the International Breast Cancer Study Group. 8. Innovative strategies of adjuvant treatments. Features that predict responsiveness to chemotherapy and endocrine therapies. *Breast.* 2001;10:147–57.
19. Bonetti M, Gelber RD. Patterns of treatment effects in subsets of patients in clinical trials. *Biostatistics.* 2004; 5:465–81.
20. International Breast Cancer Study Group. Endocrine responsiveness and tailoring adjuvant therapy for postmenopausal lymph node-negative breast cancer: A randomized trial. *J Natl Cancer Inst.* 2002;94:1054–65.
21. Simon RM, Korn EL, McShane LM, et al. Design and analysis of DNA microarray investigations. New York: Springer, 2003.
22. Dupuy A, Simon RM. Critical review of published microarray studies for cancer outcome and guidelines on statistical analysis and reporting. *J Natl Cancer Inst.* 2007;99:147–57.

23. Simon R. Roadmap for developing and validating therapeutically relevant genomic classifiers. *J Clin Oncol.* 2005;23:7332–41.
24. van't Veer LJ, Dai H, van de Vijver MJ, et al. Gene expression profiling predicts clinical outcome of breast cancer. *Nature.* 2002;415:530–6.
25. van de Vijver MJ, He YD, van't Veer LJ, et al. A gene-expression signature as a predictor of survival in breast cancer. *N Engl J Med.* 2002;347:1999–2009.
26. Buyse M, Loi S, van't Veer L, et al. on behalf of the TRANSBIG Consortium. Validation and clinical utility of a 70-gene prognostic signature for women with node-negative breast cancer. *J Natl Cancer Inst.* 2006;98:1183–92.
27. European Organization for Research and Treatment of Cancer (EORTC), TRANSBIG. MINDACT: Microarray In Node negative Disease may Avoid ChemoTherapy (dated 18. 07.06). Available at: http://www.breastinternationalgroup.org/downloads/latestnews/27_07_05/MINDACT_trial_overview.pdf. Accessed March 29, 2007.
28. Bogaerts J, Cardoso F, Buyse M, et al. on behalf of the TRANSBIG consortium. The signature evaluation as a prognostic tool: challenges in the design of the MINDACT trial. *Nature Clin Practice.* 2006;3:540–51.
29. Ravdin PM, Siminoff LA, Davis GJ, et al. Computer program to assist in making decisions about adjuvant therapy for women with early breast cancer. *J Clin Oncol.* 2001;19:980–91.
30. Cronin M, Pho M, Dutta D, et al. Measurement of gene expression in archival paraffin-embedded tissues: Development and performance of a 92-gene reverse transcriptase-polymerase chain reaction assay. *Am J Pathol.* 2004;164:35–42.
31. Paik S, Shak S, Tang G, et al. A multigene assay to predict recurrence of tamoxifen-treated, node-negative breast cancer. *N Engl J Med.* 2004;351:2817–26.
32. Habel LA, Shak S, Jacobs MK, et al. A population-based study of tumor gene expression and risk of breast cancer death among lymph node-negative patients. *Breast Cancer Res.* 2006;8:R25.
33. Paik S, Tang G, Shak S, et al. Gene expression and benefit of chemotherapy in women with node-negative, estrogen receptor-positive breast cancer. *J Clin Oncol.* 2006;24:1–12.
34. Eastern Cooperative Oncology Group (ECOG), The Breast Cancer Intergroup. Program for the Assessment of Clinical Cancer Tests (PACCT-1): Trial Assigning Individualized Options for Treatment: The TAILORx Trial [Trial Protocol]. Version dated April 7, 2006.
35. The National Cancer Institute. The TAILORx breast cancer trial (posted 5/23/06). Available at: http://www.cancer.gov/clinicaltrials/digestpage/TAILORx/. Accessed March 29, 2007.
36. Eastern Cooperative Oncology Group (ECOG). Patient education materials available for TAILORx (revised March 8, 2007). Available at: http://www.ecog.org/general/tailorx.html. Accessed March 29, 2007.
37. Genomic Health, Inc. OncotypeDX.com for healthcare professionals: Onco*type* DX results. Available at: http://www.genomichealth.com/oncotype/about/results.aspx. Accessed March 29, 2007.

Part II
Treatments

Multidisciplinary Care: Optimising Team Performance

Frances M. Boyle

Introduction

The 2006 ASCO-ESMO consensus statement on Quality Cancer Care states that "optimal treatment of cancer should be provided by a team that includes, where appropriate, multidisciplinary medical expertise composed of medical oncologists, surgical oncologists, radiation oncologists, and palliative care experts, as well as oncology nurses and social workers. Patients should also have access to counselling for their psychosocial, nutritional and other needs" [1]. The statement highlights the need for patients to receive adequate information to allow participation as desired in decision making, to have their privacy protected and to be treated with dignity at all times. Access to clinical trials is identified as a hallmark of quality care, adding yet another layer of complexity to patients' experience of a cancer diagnosis.

Multidisciplinary care in breast cancer, in so far as it facilitates access to all therapeutic modalities and is a marker of volume, has been shown to reduce mortality and improve quality of life [2–5]. In addition to those mentioned above, core treatment team members include pathologists and radiologists. Input from other specialties such as geneticists, reconstructive surgeons, gynaecologists and psychiatrists will be needed for some patients [6]. Research staff provides valuable support and information when treatment options include a clinical trial [7]. During a woman's journey with breast cancer, she and her family will meet a multitude of health professionals, and perhaps receive care in more than one institution, as well as in her local community.

So how do we fashion "multidisciplinary teams" (MDTs) which are consistent in their approach across these multiple settings, timely and accurate in their communication both with one another and with the patient and her care-givers, and at the same time conscious of protecting sensitive information? Without the luxury of a team jersey with names and position numbers clearly labelled on the

F.M. Boyle (✉)
Pam McLean Centre, University of Sydney
e-mail: franb@med.usgd.edu.au

M. Castiglione, M.J. Piccart (eds.), *Adjuvant Therapy for Breast Cancer*, Cancer Treatment and Research 151, DOI 10.1007/978-0-387-75115-3_7,

back, and without the defined boundaries and time-keepers of a sporting field [8], how do we clearly identify our roles, and optimise and sustain our performance on our patients' behalf?

Sharing Goals and Strategies

Marshall and Begeman, drawing on their experience with "knowledge teams" in technical industries, highlight the "synergy that is the real 'gold' of teamwork. This involves the producing of an outcome through interaction that could not be achieved by the same individuals working separately, either in series or in parallel" [9]. They highlight the importance of shared goals, shared resources and mutual accountability for outcomes.

A shared understanding of the "rules" is key to any team's function, forming the framework within which individual strategies can be plotted for differing circumstances. Yet in managing breast cancer, emerging evidence results in a complex "rule book" which is constantly changing. The crafting of clinical practice guidelines with a multidisciplinary approach [10, 11] assists teams to share relevant progress, educate new members and identify overlapping concerns. Regular updates such as the biannual St Gallen consensus on adjuvant therapy [12] have been shown, when implemented in MDTs in Canada, to improve survival at a population level [13]. Team meetings provide opportunities for learning around the care of individual patients [14]. More formal educational events for team members, perhaps even an annual "camp" where each discipline presents what is new in their area, may be of benefit in stimulating discussion and updating of local care plans.

A high level of technical expertise is a prerequisite for effective cancer care, but does not in itself ensure effective team functioning in knowledge teams [13] – tacit knowledge or "know how" is often as important as "know what" in fast moving organisations. Developing a creative strategy to implement a newly published recommendation, e.g. routine Her 2 testing, will require an understanding of local processes, identification of key individuals who can champion change, and potential funding opportunities. This tacit knowledge is rarely formally documented and will be unique to each MDT and indeed each patient – it is shared in dialogue rather than in national guidelines, and is the (usually unstated) rationale for Multidisciplinary Meetings (MDMs).

Effective Team Meetings

Regular meetings of the team to develop individual game plans and discuss previous performance are critical to coordinating action on the field, and allow tacit knowledge to be "extracted, explored, developed and shared quickly, efficiently and spontaneously, and often unconsciously" [9]. Ideally meetings to plan patient management should take place when all relevant information to underpin decision making is available, along with key team members. Such meetings may occur face to face, or via video- or teleconference for smaller or remote sites [6]. Hallmarks of effective MDMs include [14, 15]:

1. Facilitation of active participation by all relevant clinicians, with adequate time to discuss contentious or emerging issues of relevance.
2. A climate of trust that allows the asking of "dumb questions" and the contributions of all participants to be recognised and respected, regardless of seniority or status [9].
3. Representation of the woman's perspective and circumstances, either directly or by a clinician with knowledge of her concerns e.g. a breast care nurse or family physician
4. Documentation of attendance and decisions, and mechanisms for rapid communication of these to relevant treating clinicians e.g. fax or email.
5. Educational opportunities for junior clinicians and students.
6. Data collection to assess both process and outcomes of care, including patient satisfaction and waiting times, and to foster research.
7. Appropriate facilities for the meeting, including audio visual equipment for presentation of diagnostic material e.g. data projection, and a set up of the chairs that encourages discussion e.g. a u-shape or around a table rather than rows of seats.
8. Regular involvement of research staff and improved accrual to clinical trials [16].
9. Adequate administrative and logistic support.

Troubleshooting

All too often, however, our experience of MDT meetings is far from this ideal – frustrating, time wasting and conflict ridden. We may be asked to consider too many cases or too few, be dogged by missing results or absent decision makers, or find our input undervalued by others. Time for MDT meetings takes a particularly heavy toll on diagnostic specialists, who may be required to assist multiple cancer teams within the institution, without release from their own clinical workload. A single dominant voice may drown out more reticent opinions. Poor remuneration for meeting time, and scheduling meetings before or after working hours may be barrier to participation by some members [14, 17]. Concerns of some members about medico-legal exposure may inappropriately discourage the recording of a dissenting view [18]. How might we optimise performance when the reality falls short of the theoretical ideal?

Development and Coaching

One would not place 15 elite sportsmen on a field and expect them to win the World Cup that afternoon. Trust, "the extent to which team members feel they can be open, honest and direct with each other, and rely on each other for support... is a characteristic that develops over time as a result of positive experiences and a deepening level of understanding between team members" [9]. Tuckman [19] has identified that effective teams develop through a series of stages, and our experience working with breast cancer teams indicates that several years may be required for this process.

1. Forming – the players are "selected" and make a commitment to the team, they identify their individual roles and begin to train together.
2. Storming – in which conflicts arise due to differences of opinion and style, different levels of skill and fitness, with the emergence of training needs.
3. Norming – in which teams develop "plays" – strategies for dealing with particular challenges, which offer a smoother decision making process. They begin to communicate in "code" allowing economical signalling of intent.
4. Performing – the team has reached a satisfactory level of function and morale rises as success is observed and trust is evident.
5. Reforming – a key player retires, or the rules change, and the process begins again, at least in miniature.

Failure to identify and respond to the challenges of each of these phases will lead to poor functioning. We would not expect a sporting team to achieve success without a coach, yet it is rare for cancer teams to receive external advice and assistance. In Australia, the National Breast Cancer Centre and the Cancer Institute of NSW, in collaboration with the Pam McLean Centre, have undertaken a "coaching" program for MDTs, leading to improvements in satisfaction. Lesley Fallowfield is currently undertaking a training program for MDTs in Wales, aiming to improve communication processes that will facilitate clinical trial accrual (personal communication). Results are awaited with interest, as this process of training may benefit MDTs in other countries.

Inspirational Leadership

Key to the successful transition through each of these phases is leadership – someone who has the big picture in view and a sense of guardianship of the group over an extended period of time. A recent study of breast cancer teams in the United Kingdom [20] identified that the most effective teams were those which utilised a dispersed model of leadership, i.e. more than one discipline led team discussions. Absence of one person thus did not cause the meetings to grind to a halt, and greater participation resulted. Having a single clear leader could result in satisfactory functioning, but was less likely to promote innovation. The most destructive influence on team effectiveness identified in this study was lack of clarity or conflict over leadership.

Transition in leadership will challenge all teams and requires careful succession planning as the next generation are groomed to take on this role. Stepping into the captaincy may also affect a clinicians' performance in their usual role, since they are fulfilling two tasks in the meeting – watching and listening to the whole group as well as considering their own clinical cases. Coaching emerging leaders to better understand and influence team processes may be a particularly effective strategy, although one as yet untested in the cancer arena.

The team leader may not necessarily be the best meeting facilitator – this role can be rotated amongst those the skills necessary to ensure all relevant opinions are expressed and consensus is arrived at and documented.

Strengthening Commitment

Lack of commitment to the process of meetings may be a particular issue for diagnostic specialists, who tended to have the most negative perception of MDTs in the UK study [20]. They are less likely to see the direct benefits to patients of the process of case review, and may instead be looking for satisfaction from the streamlining of their own clinical workload that comes from better understanding of the surgeon's and oncologists' needs. The development of sentinel node biopsy in particular has required closer collaboration between diagnostic specialists. Workforce shortages are likely to be particularly acute in these disciplines in future, particularly in academic settings. Measures to enhance their satisfaction with MDT participation and clinical trial research will need to be considered in many countries if we are not to lose a vital resource, whose involvement underpins all treatment decisions.

The responsibility of MDT members to ensure that decisions made and recorded by the group reflect their views accurately has been highlighted recently in discussions around the medico-legal implications of MDTs [18]. MDMs would be regarded from a legal perspective as a formal referral process constituting a duty of care in most jurisdictions, and as such, all present are considered responsible and potentially liable for decisions made within their area of expertise, regardless of whether they see the patient subsequently in consultation. Such knowledge may assist in focusing attention!

MDTs therefore require mechanisms to document decisions (including dissenting views and patient choices which might be at variance to recommendations) and to remind members of their responsibilities. Since MDTs are increasingly considered best practice [1], their appropriate use should in fact reduce the risk of litigation in the future. A formal process of obtaining consent from patients to have their situation discussed is also considered wise in view of privacy issues and the sensitive nature of information that may be disclosed [17, 18].

Managing Conflict and Poor Performance

Poor performance in an elite sporting team leads to the player being dropped, and disruptive behaviour leads to penalties. In most MDTs the opportunities to remove and replace dysfunctional members are limited unless true misdemeanour occurs. Monitoring the team "climate" is another responsibility of leadership and may be assisted by the use of diagnostic tools [9, 20].

Differences in learning styles [21] might be expected in MDTs – more reflective types such as diagnostic specialists might enjoy dwelling on details of immunohistochemical stains they have lovingly prepared, and the theoretical radiation oncologist might be keen to quote the latest data, whilst the action oriented surgeon might prefer a "25 words or less" approach ("Do I need to go back, or not?"). The pragmatic medical oncologist has already tuned out and is checking e-mails, because the patient is 82 years old and has significant co-morbidity, ruling out adjuvant systemic therapy. Solving any complex problem such as breast cancer will require all to contribute, and gaining an understanding of and respect for each other's approach will reduce annoyances.

Dealing with conflict in MDTs requires acknowledgement of the problem, identification of a champion to take on the issue and get the full story, brainstorming outside of the team meeting to identify contributing factors and potential solutions, and gaining agreement to try out the most feasible options [22]. Active listening and empathy are useful communication tools in this setting, just as they would be in settings where conflict with patients occurs. This process may also benefit from external facilitation if the problem is major, especially if the team leader is one of the protagonists.

Preventing Burnout

Sometimes conflict and poor performance will be caused by burnout in one or more team members [23], manifesting as emotional exhaustion, depersonalisation or a low sense of professional accomplishment. This is not surprising considering workloads and the emotional demands of caring for cancer patients. A well functioning team is potentially protective against burnout – when we notice a team member struggling with a particular patient, taking some time outside the meeting to listen and share the burden, mobilise additional psychosocial support for the patient, and reassure our colleague of understanding will assist in maintaining team members' mental health [20, 24].

Poorly functioning teams however can increase stress, increasing demands on the already overburdened. Depression in team members may manifest as disruptive behaviour and an increased frequency of errors or absenteeism. Institutional and regulatory mechanisms for referral of health care professionals for assistance will vary from country to country, but we who are increasingly willing to consider specialist psychological care for our patients may be reluctant to accept it for ourselves. A team leader who encourages open discussion of the need for management of workload and supports self-care strategies may assist in this regard.

Improving Communication with Patients

There is now open acknowledgement of the adverse impact of insensitive delivery of bad news and prognostic information on patients and families [11], and the importance of providing information in ways that meet varying patient needs [25]. Training in small group settings which allow review of the evidence, opportunity for discussion and practice (with actors as simulated patients) has been demonstrated to improve communication skills of cancer professionals [28]. In the setting of multidisciplinary care, however, the appropriate communication of one team member may be undermined by the less skilful approach of another, leading to confusion and distress for patients when the "story keeps changing". Finding opportunities to undertake communication skills training as a team may assist members to understand the different approach that each member brings to the interaction and increase the repertoire of skills within the group [27].

Developing orientating information for patients, e.g. a brochure which identifies team members and how the team functions, is also suggested by research with Australian consumers [28], who report that the word "multidisciplinary" may not be readily understood by newly diagnosed women. Local circumstances will dictate the most appropriate format for such information, e.g. website, printed material, which will require regular updating and consumer input.

Conclusions

Writing about keys to success in Rugby, former Australian captain John Eales highlights the critical role of communication: "You may have the best moves in the world, but if you don't let others know about them, they will never work."[29]. A multidisciplinary team climate which promotes effective communication with both health professionals and patients will also be one in which patient outcomes will be optimised and team members health will be safeguarded. Improving our understanding of cancer care team processes through further research, meanwhile availing ourselves of opportunities for training, will assist cancer professionals to reach these goals.

Acknowledgments The work of the Pam McLean Centre in multidisciplinary communication has been a team effort, with creative input from Stewart Dunn, Paul Heinrich and Emma Robinson, and Robert Marshall of K-teams International P/L. Breast Cancer MDTs throughout Australia and New Zealand have shared their experience with us and the NHMRC National Breast Cancer Centre has enthusiastically implemented training initiatives. We are also grateful for the support of the Australian and New Zealand Rugby Unions, from whom we have learnt that great teams don't just happen.

References

1. Horning SJ, Mellstedt H. ASCO-ESMO Consensus statement on Quality Cancer Care. *JCO*. 2006;24:3497–98.
2. Chang JH, Vines E, Bertsch H, et al.The impact of a multidisciplinary breast cancer centre on recommendations for patient management. *Cancer*. 2001;91:1231–7.
3. Sainsbury R, Hayward B, Johnston C, et al. Influence of clinician workload and patterns of treatment on survival from breast cancer. *Lancet*. 1995;345:1265–70.
4. Gillis CR, Hole DJ. Survival outcome of care by specialist surgeons in breast cancer. *BMJ*. 1996;312:145–8.
5. Gabel M, Hilton NE, Nathanson SD. Multidisciplinary breast cancer clinics. Do they work? *Cancer*. 1997;79:2380–4.
6. Zorbas H, Barraclough B, Rainbird K, et al. Multidisciplinary care for women with early breast cancer in the Australian Context: What does it mean? *Med J Aust*. 2003;179:528–31.
7. Loh WP, Butow PN, Brown RF, Boyle F. Ethical communication in clinical trials: Issues faced by data managers in obtaining informed consent. *Cancer*. 2002, 95:2414–21.
8. Boyle FM, Robinson E, Heinrich P, Dunn SM. "Cancer: Communicating in the team game" *ANZ J Surg*. 2004,74:477–81.
9. Marshall RJ, Begeman M. Necessary but not sufficient: The role of expertise in technical team success. *Cutter IT J*. 2005;18:1–6.
10. National Breast Cancer Centre (Australia). *Clinical Practice Guidelines for the Management of Early Breast Cancer*. 2nd ed. Canberra: NHMRC; 2001.
11. National Breast Cancer Centre (Australia). *Clinical Practice Guidelines: Providing Information, Support and Counseling for Women with Breast Cancer*. Canberra. NHMRC; 2000.
12. Goldhirsch A, Glick JH, Gelber RD, et al. Meeting highlights: International expert consensus on the primary therapy of early breast cancer. *Ann Oncol*. 2005;16:1569–83.
13. Herbert-Croteau N, Brisson J, Latreille J, Rivard M, Abdelaziz N, Marting G. Compliance with consensus recommendations for systemic therapy is associated with improved survival of women with node-negative breast cancer. *JCO*. 2004;22:3685–93.
14. Fleissig A, Jenkins V, Catt S, Fallowfield L. Multidisciplinary teams in cancer care: are they effective in the UK. *Lancet Oncol*. 2006;7:935–43.
15. National Breast Cancer Centre (Australia). Multidisciplinary meetings for cancer care: A guide for health services providers. National Breast Cancer Centre, Camperdown 2005 (http://www.nbcc.org.au/bestpractice/mdc/resources.html).
16. Magee LR, Laroche CM, Gilligan D. Clinical trials in lung cancer: Evidence that a programmed investigation unit and a multidisciplinary clinic may improve recruitment. *Clin Oncol*. 2001;13:310–11.
17. Boyle FM, Robinson E, Heinrich P, Dunn SM. Barriers to communication in multidisciplinary breast cancer teams. *Proc ASCO*. 2004.
18. Sidhom MA, Poulsen MG. Multidisciplinary care in oncology: Medicolegal implications of group decisions. *Lancet Oncol*. 2006;7:951–4.
19. Tuckman BW, Jensen MA. Developmental sequence in small groups. *Psychol Bulletin* 1965;63:384–99.
20. Haward R, Amir Z, Borrill C, et al. Breast cancer teams: The impact of constitution, new cancer workload and methods of operation on their effectiveness. *BJC*. 2003;89,15–22.
21. Honey P, Mumford A. *Using Your Learning Style*. Maidenhead, UK: Peter Honey Publications; 1986.
22. Back AL, Arnold RM. Dealing with conflict in caring for the seriously ill. *JAMA*. 2005;293:1374–81.
23. Lyckholm L. Dealing with stress, burnout and grief in the practice of oncology. *Lancet Oncol*. 2001;2:750–5.

24. Hall P, Weaver L. Interdisciplinary education and teamwork: A long and winding road. *Med Educ*. 2001;35:867–75.
25. Brown RF, Butow PN, Henman MJ, Dunn SM, Boyle FM, Tattersall MNH. "Responding to the active and passive patient: flexibility is the key." *Health Expectations*. 2002,5:330–40
26. Fallowfield L, Jenkins V, Farewefll V, Saul J, Duffy A, Eves R. Efficacy of a Cancer Research UK communication skills training model for oncologists: A randomized controlled trial. *Lancet*. 2002;359:650–6.
27. Maguire P, Pitceathly C. Key communication skills and how to acquire them. *BMJ*. 2002;325:697–700.
28. Neil S, Scott C, Galetis S, Rodger A. The celluloid version of the multidisciplinary meeting:perceptions of consumers. *ANZJ Surg*. 2003;73:A7.
29. Eales J, Batchelor L. *Rugby Facts for Kids*. Sydney: ABC Books; 2003.

Preoperative Chemo- and Endocrine Therapy

Rosalba Torrisi

Primary Systemic Therapy: Rationale and State of the Art

Primary systemic therapy (PST) or preoperative therapy has been part of the multidisciplinary approach to locally advanced and inflammatory breast cancer since the early 1970s. The administration of chemotherapy allowed surgical resection of inoperable tumours and improved clinical outcome [1]. The chance of downsizing the tumour extended its use to operable large breast tumour candidates for mastectomy in order to reduce the extent of surgery. A series of phase II trials reporting an objective response rate ranging from 60 to 90%, showed the feasibility of this approach in terms of significant activity with no detriment to survival [2]. In addition, the early administration of medical treatment appeared an attractive means to improve clinical outcome. In fact, according to preclinical models, it was suggested that a primary tumour may induce the growth of micro-metastatic foci through the production of growth stimulating factors [3]. Preoperative systemic therapy could lead to less favourable growth kinetics for development of micro-metastasis and decrease the development of drug resistant clones through early exposure to systemic therapy [3]. Other theoretical advantages of preoperative administration of chemotherapy are the possibility to assess the response in vivo and tailor further treatments accordingly.

To exploit this hypothesis, a number of randomised trials comparing PST with postoperative administration of systemic treatment (adjuvant therapy) were designed in the 1990s (Table 1).

Although heterogeneous in the design, the selection of patients and the choice of chemotherapy, all these trials were consistent in showing that, albeit a high objective response rate and a relevant proportion of patients

R. Torrisi (✉)
Research Unit of Medical Senology, Department of Medicine,
European Institute of Oncology, via Ripamonti 435, 20141,
Milan, Italy
e-mail: rosalba.torrisi@ieo.it

M. Castiglione, M.J. Piccart (eds.), *Adjuvant Therapy for Breast Cancer*,
Cancer Treatment and Research 151, DOI 10.1007/978-0-387-75115-3_8,

Table 1 Randomised trials of primary vs adjuvant chemotherapy

Study (year)	No. of patients	Treatment	RR (%)	pCR (%)	DFS %	OS (%)
Mauriac (1991) [4]	272	EVM × 3→MTV × 3	33	NR	79 vs 81	55 vs 55
Semiglazov (1994) [5]	212	TMF × 6 + Radiotherapy	29	NR	81 vs 72*	86 vs 78
Scholl (1994) [6]	414	FAC × 4 + Radiotherapy	65	NR	59 vs 55	86 vs 78*
NSABP-B18 (1997) [7]	1,523	A C × 4	36	13	67 vs 67	80 vs 80
Makris (1998) [8]	309	MMM+ TAM × 4-pre + 4 adj vs MMT × 8	83	10	ND	ND
Jakesz (2001) [9]	423	CMF × 3 pre+ CMF × 3 adj vs CMF × 6 adj	68	6	NR	66 vs 59
EORTC (2001) [10]	698	FEC × 4	49	4	65 vs 70	82 vs 84
NSABPB-27 (2003–2006) [11, 12]	2,411	AC × 4 pre → D × 4 AC × 4+ D × 4 adj	91 85	14 26	71 70	ND
ECTO (2005) [13]	1,355	A T × 4 → CMF × 4	78	23	ND	ND

RR = response rate; pCR = pathological complete remission; DFS = disease-free survival; OS = overall survival; * = $p<0.05$ NR = not reported; ND = no difference; Pre = primary; adj = adjuvant; EORTC = European Organisation for Research and Treatment of Cancer; ECTO = European Cooperative Trial in Operable Breast Cancer; EVM = epirubicin, vincristine, methotrexate; MTV = mytomicin C, thiotepa, vindesine; TMF = thiotepa, methotrexate, fluorouracile; FAC = fluorouracile, doxorubicin, cyclophosphamide; AC = doxorubicin, cyclophosphemide; MMM = mytomicin C, mitoxantrone, methotrexate; TAM = tamoxifen; CMF = cyclophosphamide, methotrexate, fluorouracile; FEC = fluorouracile, epirubicin, cyclophosphamide; D = docetaxel; AT = doxorubicin, paclitaxel.

submitted to breast conserving surgery, the clinical outcome in terms of disease free survival (DFS) and overall survival (OS) was not affected by the timing of systemic therapy [4–13] (Table 1). A meta-analysis of nine randomised studies confirmed the equivalence between preoperative and adjuvant therapy in terms of survival and disease progression, while primary therapy was associated with an increased risk of loco-regional recurrence, especially in patients who received radiotherapy instead of surgery as local treatment [14].

The results of these studies appear to disclaim the use of PST whenever no benefit in terms of more conservative surgery is expected. At the same time, however, these results suggested that the administration of PST is safe and no detriment arises from postponing surgery. In addition, no excess of surgical complications was observed in patients receiving preoperative therapy.

A further analysis of some of these trials led to a new insight into the approach to PST. The NSABP B-18 study, including over 1,500 patients and comparing 4 courses of standard AC administered preoperatively vs the same regimen administered after surgery, showed that, although either DFS and OS were comparable overall, patients who experienced a complete pathological response (pCR) benefited from an improved DFS. This finding suggested that PST may also be useful as a means to identify subsets of patients at different prognosis [15].

The Role pf pCR

After the results of the NSABP B-18, a number of studies have confirmed that the disappearance of neoplastic cells in the primary tumour may be considered as a surrogate of a complete eradication of viable tumour cells either of loco-regional or micro-metastatic systemic disease, as suggested by the improved outcome [12, 16–19] (Table 2). Pathologic complete remission has then been proposed as a surrogate or intermediate marker of clinical outcome and indicated as the principal endpoint for subsequent trials aimed at optimising pre-operative regimens [20, 21].

However, the heterogeneous definition of pCR used across studies renders the comparisons of these results troublesome [20]. Even considering just large randomised trials, the definition of pCR ranges from the disappearance of neoplastic invasive cells in the primary tumour without considering the nodal status [7, 11–13] to the lack of neoplastic cells both in the breast and in the axilla

Table 2 Clinical outcome and pathological complete response (pCR)

Study	No. of patients	Treatment	Definition of pCR	pCR (%)	DFS %	OS %
NSABP B-18 [15]	1,523	AC × 4	Breast	13	75 vs 58	85 vs 73
Royal Marsden [16]	435	EC\CMF	Breast and axilla	23	NS	91 vs 73
EIO [17]	399	Various regimens	Breast	16	NS	NR
NSABP B-27 [12]	2,411	AC × 4 → D × 4	Breast	14	84 vs 67	93 vs 81
MD Anderson [18]	1,731	Anthracylines and/or taxane based CT	Breast and axilla	13	87 vs 61*	91 vs 80
ECTO [13]	1,355	AT × 4 → CMF × 4	Breast	23	89 vs 75 #	NR

pCR = pathological complete response; DFS = disease free survival; OS = overall survival; NS = not significant; NR = not reported; # freedom from progression was reported; EIO = EIO = European Institute of Milan; ECTO = European Cooperative Trial in Operable Breast Cancer; AC = doxorubicin, cyclophosphamide; EC = epirubicin, cyclophosphamide; CMF = cyclophosphamide, methotrexate, fluorouracil; D = docetaxel; AT = doxorubicin, paclitaxel

[18, 22] to the lack of both invasive and in situ neoplastic cells [20]. The more restrictive the definition of pCR, the greater benefit in terms of outcome may be expected. However, while the occurrence of negative pathological nodes has been confirmed as an independent prognostic factor in different series [12, 23], it has been clearly demonstrated that the persistence of residual DCIS does not affect patient outcome in terms of local recurrence or survival [24]. Another important consideration is that the results of the studies have consistently shown an advantage in terms of DFS but not of OS. It may be hypothesised that, since the likelihood of achieving a pCR is diluted by the heterogeneity of study population, the number of pCR observed in most trials is too small to translate in a survival advantage.

However, up to now, pCR represents the best available predictor of clinical outcome after preoperative therapy. The search of early predictors of pCR by identifying the associated clinical and biological factors has been encouraged in order to select patients who may benefit more from PST and to avoid unnecessary toxicity to others.

The studies aimed at identifying early predictors of response, particularly of pCR, have not been fully successful. The early (short term) change of proliferative activity during preoperative treatment rather than baseline value was significantly correlated with clinical and/or pathological response either after preoperative endocrine-, chemo-endocrine- and chemotherapy [25–28]. On the other hand, the absence of a significant reduction of Ki67 did not predict lack of clinical response, rendering this marker useless for the early identification of patients who are more likely to benefit from preoperative treatment.

Hormone receptors represent the most established tumour characteristic associated with increased likelihood to achieve pCR. Estrogen (ER) and progesterone receptor (PgR) negative tumours generally have a two- to sevenfold greater pCR rate than ER and PgR positive tumours and this finding is consistent across studies irrespective of design and schedule used [11, 13, 16–18, 29–31 (Table 3). The low pCR rate obtained in ER and PgR positive tumours conflicts with the improved outcome generally associated with this tumour population which has been confirmed both in large randomised studies such as the European Cooperative Trial in Operable Breast Cancer (ECTO) study and in large retrospective series such as those from MD Anderson, Royal Marsden and the European Institute of Oncology (EIO) [16–19]. It has also been questioned whether pCR rate represents an appropriate endpoint in ER positive tumours, as suggested by the results of the retrospective analysis of the Royal Marsden series showing a correlation of pCR and clinical outcome in ER negative but not in ER positive tumours [16]. This finding was disclaimed by the retrospective analysis of the MD Anderson series showing that patients achieving pCR experienced a better prognosis irrespective of hormone receptor status [18]. However, the limited number of pCR observed in both series among ER positive tumours may account for this inconsistency and the question is still open.

Table 3 Pathological complete remission (pCR) overall and according to hormone receptor status

Study	No. patients	Treatment	pCR %		
			Overall	HR+ve	HR–ve
Royal Marsden [16]	438	EC/CMF	12	8	22
EIO [17]	399	Various regimens	16	7	33
AGO [29]	475	ddE $\times$ 3 $\rightarrow$ T $\times$ 3 ET $\times$ 4	18 10	8	26
GEPAR-DUO [30]	913	AC $\times$ 4 $\rightarrow$ D $\times$4 ddAD $\times$ 4	14.3 7	6	23
ECTO [19]	438	AT $\times$ 4 $\rightarrow$ CMF $\times$ 4	23	12	42
GEPAR-TRIO [31]	285	TAC $\times$ 6 TAC $\times$ 2 $\rightarrow$ NX $\times$ 4	18 3	3*	27
NSABP B-27 [12]	2,411	AC $\times$ 4 AC $\times$ 4 $\rightarrow$ D $\times$ 4	13 26	8	17
MD Anderson [18]	1,731	Anthracycline and taxane based CT	13	8	24

pCR = pathological complete response; HR+ve = hormone receptor positive; HR-ve = hormone receptor negative; EIO = European Institute of Milan; AGO = Arbeitsgemeninschaft Gastroenterologische Onkologie; GEPARDUO = German Preoperative Adriamyicin and Docetaxel Study II; ECTO = European Cooperative Trial in Operable Breast Cancer; GEPAR-TRIO = German Preoperative Adriamyicin and Docetaxel Study III; EC = epirubicin, cyclophosphamide; CMF = cyclophosphamide, methotrexate, fluorouracil; Dd = dose dense; E = epirubicin; T = paclitaxel; D docetaxel; TAC = docetaxel, doxorubicin, cyclophosphamide; NX = vinorelbine, capecitabine.

Tumour histologic type has been also correlated with pathological remission in large retrospective series, showing that patients with a lobular carcinoma obtained a pCR ranging from 1 to 3% as compared to the 9–15% of the ductal histology, although their long term prognosis was better [32, 33].

HER2 status was investigated as a predictive marker of response to different primary chemotherapy regimens but results are not consistent in showing a significant association between pCR rate and HER2 positivity [34, 35] and up to now it should be considered only as a marker of sensitivity to trastuzumab.

Anthracyclines and Taxanes: Which is the Gold Standard?

As mentioned above, although it is generally accepted that regimens containing both anthracyclines and taxanes yield the best results, much debate is ongoing as to whether combined or sequential administration represent the best schedule [20, 21]. Indirect comparisons suggest that concurrent administration of anthracyclines and taxanes is associated with a pCR rate which is generally lower than that obtained with a sequential schedule, except for the study from the ECTO which, however, included four additional courses of a non-cross resistant regimen after the combination of doxorubicin and paclitaxel [20, 21]. Table 4 summarises the results of randomised trials, including an adequate number of patients, investigating different anthracyclines and taxanes containing regimens and addressing the issues of schedule and duration.

Table 4 Randomised trials of primary chemotherapy including different schedules and duration of anthracyclines and taxanes

Study	No. patients	Treatment	cRR(%)	pCR (%)	pN0 %
Anthracyclines vs Taxanes					
Dieras [36]	200	AC × 4 vs AT × 4	89	16	22
			70	10	20
ACCOG [37]	632	AC × 6 vs	61	24	39
		AD × 6	70	21	34
Anthracyclines + Taxanes (concurrent or sequential)					
Aberdeen [38]	162	CVAP × 8	66	16	67
		CVAP × 4 → D × 4	94	34	62
NSABP B-27 [12]	2,411	AC ×4	86	14	51
		AC × 4 → D × 4	91	26	58
GEPARDUO [30]	913	AC × 4 → D × 4	79	14.3	61
		ddAD × 4	69	7	55
AGO [29]	475	ET × 4	NR	10	42
		ddE × 3 → T × 3		18	51
Green [39]	258	T q3 wk × 4 → FAC × 4	85	16	51
		wT × 12 → FAC × 4	86	28	59
Different duration					
Romieu [41]	232	AT × 4 vs	20 *	17	NR
		AT × 6	32 *	11	
EORTC [42]	448	CEF × 6 vs	80	14	NR
		dd EC × 6	88	10	
ABCSG 14 [43]	292	ED × 3 vs	76 #	7.7	43
		ED × 6	89 #	18.6	57

cRR = clinical response rate; pCR = pathological complete response; pN0 pathological negative nodes; ACCOG = Anglo-Celtic Cooperative Group; GEPARDUO = German Preoperative Adriamyicin and Docetaxel Study II; AGO = Arbeitsgemeninschaft Gastroenterologische Onkologie; EORTC = European Organisation for Research and Treatment of Cancer; ABCSG = Austrian Breast Cancer Study Group; AC = doxorubicin, cyclophosphamide; AT = doxorubicin, paclitaxel; AD = doxorubicin, docetaxel; CVAP = cyclophosphamide, vincristine, doxorubicin, prednisone; dd = dose dense; ET = epirubicin, paclitaxel; FAC = fluorouracil, doxorubicin, cyclophosphamide; CEF = cyclphosphamide, epirubicin, fluorouracil.
* only clinical complete responses were reported
# stable disease were included

The two largest studies which compared the concurrent administration of anthracyclines and taxanes vs anthracyclines and cyclophosphamide did not show an advantage for the taxane-containing regimen [36, 37].

The first study randomised 200 patients to either standard doxorubicin plus cyclophosphamide or doxorubicin plus paclitaxel every 3 weeks for four courses. The pCR rate was 10% vs 16% (6% vs 8% in independent review) in the two arms respectively, while clinical response rate was greater in the taxane-containing arm [36]. The Anglo-Celtic Cooperative Group (ACCOG) compared six cycles of either AC or doxorubicin + docetaxel; no difference in pCR, clinical response or long term outcome was observed [37].

The Aberdeen study randomised patients who showed a clinical response after four cycles of CVAP (cyclophosphamide, vincristine, doxorubicin and prednisone) to an additional four cycles of the same regimen or four cycles of docetaxel [38]. Non-responding patients received four cycles of docetaxel. The addition of docetaxel significantly improved either clinical response and pCR rate as compared to eight cycles of the same regimen (94% and 34% vs 66% and 16%, respectively). This study demonstrates the clear advantage of the addition of a taxane comparing regimens of the same duration but the number of patients included (162) was relatively small.

Two pivotal studies showing the benefit of adding taxotere to anthracyclines based regimens, the NSABP B-27 and the German Preoperative Adriamyicin and Docetaxel Study (GEPAR-DUO) have compared schedules with different durations [12, 13, 30]. The GEPARD-DUO study compared standard four courses of AC followed by four courses of docetaxel and dose dense doxorubicin + docetaxel (AD) for four courses [30]. Both response rate and pCR were significantly higher in the sequential arm (pCR = 14.3% vs 7%, p<.001) [30]. The NSABP B-27, the largest published trial of preoperative therapy including more than 2,400 patients, showed that adding four courses of docetaxel to AC × 4 courses doubled pCR rate [12]. We therefore cannot rule out that the advantage may also be due to a longer treatment other than the addition of a new agent.

A direct comparison between concurrent vs sequential administration of anthracyclines and taxanes has been performed other than in the GEPARDUO study also in a trial by the Arbeitsgemeninschaft Gastroenterologische Onkologie (AGO) group who has compared three courses of epirubicin followed by three courses of paclitaxel administered every 2 weeks vs the two drugs administered concurrently every 3 weeks for four courses [29]. The sequential schedule proved to be superior, also in the latter study, where the duration of treatment was similar, although the total dose delivered was different.

These two trials raise also the issue of dose dense schedules, obtaining inconsistent results. The MD Anderson also explored this issue, comparing in a randomised trial the weekly vs standard administration of paclitaxel; similarly to what observed in the advanced disease, weekly paclitaxel was shown to double pCR rate than the standard schedule (29% vs 14%, p<.01) [39]. In a small phase II study including 66 patients with operable breast cancer, weekly administration of cisplatin, paclitaxel and epirubicin for eight courses yielded a pCR rate of 55% [40]. Thus the weekly schedule more than the classical dose dense schedule appears to improve clinical and pathological response rate and merits to be further exploited.

The optimal duration of preoperative therapy also is still unknown. Indirect evidence of a greater activity for the longer duration is provided by the NSABP B-27, the AGO and the GEPAR-DUO studies, although other variables may have concurred to these results. Very few studies have specifically addressed this issue comparing fewer vs more courses of the same chemotherapeutic regimen [41–43]. The largest of these studies, the ABCSG 14, which randomly compared three vs six cycles of epirubicin and docetaxel, showed that longer treatment resulted in a significantly higher pCR rate (18.6% vs 7.7%, p = .0045) and pathological negative nodes at surgery (56.6% vs 42.8%, p = .02) [43]. Four to six courses are currently recommended as primary therapy outside a clinical trial [20].

Another poorly addressed issue is the activity of a second-line therapy in non-responding patients. The Aberdeen study clearly showed the advantage of switching to taxotere in patients responding to CVAP, while in non-responding patients a pCR of only 2% was observed [38]. The GEPAR-TRIO study randomised patients not responding after TAC for two cycles to four additional courses of the same regimen or to a non-cross-resistant therapy including capecitabine + vinorelbine (NX). Clinical response rate was similar between the two groups (22.5% vs 21.9%, respectively) and pCR were fewer in the NX group (3.1% vs 7.3%) [31].

Another piece of evidence derives from a randomised study investigating a non-cross resistant regimen vs five additional cycles of the same preoperative regimen as adjuvant treatment in patients with suboptimal response (>1 cm^3 of residual tumour) to three cycles of an anthracyclines based therapy. No difference in terms of relapse-free survival (RFS) and a trend vs an improved survival (655 vs 47% p = .06) for the non cross resistant regimen was observed [44].

Although a suggestion towards a poor activity of a second line regimen emerged from these randomised studies, the small number of patients included does not allow drawing definitive conclusions on these issues and further trials either in the preoperative or in the adjuvant setting are warranted.

Primary Treatment of Endocrine Responsive Tumours

Preoperative treatment of endocrine responsive tumours represents a challenge for medical oncologists. Although chemotherapy is able to induce a high number of objective responses the chance of obtaining a pCR is from two- to sevenfold lower than in hormone receptor negative tumours [20,21]. In addition, while chemotherapy schedule makes the difference in the likelihood of pCR among ER negative tumours, pCR rate in ER positive tumours ranges consistently from 6 to 10%, regardless of the use of more intensive chemotherapeutic regimens (see Table 3).

It is reasonable to speculate that conversely these tumors may benefit of an endocrine maneuver. Endocrine therapy has been historically limited to patients who were not suitable for chemotherapy and surgery. Earlier phase II studies with tamoxifen focused primarily on elderly and/or frail patients, often unselected for hormone receptor status of the tumour and showed a response rate of 49–68% [45]. The proven superiority of third-generation aromatase inhibitors in the advanced disease prompted the investigation of these agents in the preoperative setting in postmenopausal women with hormone receptor positive tumors. Initially, phase II studies showed a response rate up to 80% for letrozole and comparison studies of aromatase inhibitors with tamoxifen were started [45].

In a phase III study, the P-024 , which included 337 postmenopausal hormone receptor positive breast cancer patients, *letrozole* was shown to increase response rate (55 vs 36%, $p<.001$) and to increase breast conserving surgery rate (45 vs 35%, $p = .022$) as compared with tamoxifen [46] Interestingly, subgroup analyses showed that patients with HER1 and/or HER2 overexpressing tumors benefited of letrozole (RR = 88 vs 21%) while in tumors not overexpressing HER1 and/or HER2 response rate was similar between the two treatments (54 vs 42%) [47].

The second randomised trial, the IMPACT trial, comparing *anastrozole* vs tamoxifen vs the combination of the two agents in 330 postmenopausal women with ER positive tumors failed to show any difference as for response rate among treatments (37 vs 36 vs 39%), although patients receiving anastrozole were significantly more likely to undergo breast conservative surgery (46 vs 22%) [48]. In this study, again, patients with HER2 overexpressing tumors responded better to the aromatase inhibitor than to tamoxifen although the difference was not statistically significant (58 vs 22%) [48].

In the third trial, the PROACT trial, where 451 postmenopausal women with ER positive tumors were allowed to receive chemotherapy in addition to endocrine agents, anastrozole and tamoxifen yielded a similar response rate, except in the subgroup of patients who did not receive concurrent chemotherapy who benefited, although not significantly, from anastrozole (36.2 vs 26.5%, $p = .09$) in terms of response rate while feasible surgery was improved after 3 months in a significantly higher proportion of patients on anastrozole (43% vs 31%, $p = .04$) [49].

Exemestane has been compared with tamoxifen in a randomised study including 151 postmenopausal women with ER and/or PgR positive breast cancer [50]. The aromatase inhibitor significantly increased clinical response rate (76 vs 40%, $p = .05$) and the rate of breast conserving surgery (36.8 vs 20%, $p = .05$) but not the rate of imaging response [50].

The results of these randomised trials together with those of phase II studies have shown that preoperative endocrine therapy is a feasible and safe option in postmenopausal patients with hormone receptor positive tumors. However the pCR rate reported in these studies is very low (1–3%) [20]. Given the time lag to reaching full therapeutic effect for endocrine therapies, the issue of duration of preoperative endocrine therapy is crucial, as demonstrated by an increased response rate observed with prolonged letrozole in studies comparing different durations [51].

Another critical issue is the selection of patients according to the endocrine responsiveness. In a study of the Edinburgh group, 83 postmenopausal women were treated with neoadjuvant letrozole for 3 months. Tumours were subdivided according to their ER ALLRED scores and 60 tumours were scored 8 while 23 were scored as ALLRED 6 or 7. Although response rates were similar in both groups, a significant greater reduction in tumour volume was observed in patients whose tumours had the highest ER level [52].

Thus, an adequately prolonged endocrine therapy may be deemed equally active as chemotherapy in a selected population of exquisite endocrine responsive tumours. The results of a randomised comparison between chemotherapy and endocrine therapy in postmenopausal women with ER positive breast cancer seems to confirm this speculation, in that four courses of doxorubicin and paclitaxel yielded comparable objective responses (64%) and slightly less breast conserving surgery (24% vs 33%) as exemestane and anastrozole, while pCR rate was higher although not significantly after chemotherapy (6% vs 3%) [53].

The experience with endocrine preoperative therapy in premenopausal patients is very limited. A phase II study investigating letrozole in combination with GnRH analogue in a population of ER and PgR positive breast cancer showed a clinical response rate assessed by ultrasound of 50%, a pCR rate of 3%, while breast conserving surgery was feasible in 47% of patients, figures that are comparable with the results observed in postmenopausal patients [54]. Importantly, longer treatment duration appeared to be the major determinant of clinical response.

Another strategy theoretically active, which has not been pursued extensively, is the combination of chemotherapy and endocrine therapy. Both the NSABP B-18 and the B-27 studies allowed the association of tamoxifen 20 mg/day concurrent with chemotherapy in patients older than 50 years old regardless of hormone receptor status. The German group compared in a randomised study (GEPARDO) the addition of tamoxifen to dose-dense doxorubicin and docetaxel [55]. Again the patients were not selected for hormone receptor status and about 40% of patients turned out to have ER negative tumours at surgery. The pCR rate was comparable in the two groups (9% vs 10.3%) and the authors concluded that the effect of endocrine therapy should be exploited in regimens with longer duration [55].

Another phase III randomised study investigated the association of tamoxifen with epirubicin [56]. Both clinical and pathological response rate were comparable, while proliferative activity was significantly down regulated by the addition of tamoxifen [56].

These discouraging results should be blunted by the observation that in no study were patients selected according to hormone receptor status. In addition, results of the SWOG study suggested that sequential administration of tamoxifen and chemotherapy is more advantageous than the concomitant administration [57]. Thus the combination of chemotherapy and different endocrine manipulations in selected population of ER positive tumours may be still pursued. The results of a small non-randomised study suggested that the concurrent administration of GnRH analogue and chemotherapy with ECF improved either clinical and pathological response rate as compared to the chemotherapy alone in a series of premenopausal patients with ER positive breast cancer [58]. Similarly the concurrent administration of exemestane and chemotherapy has been investigated in two small phase I studies, reporting a high activity which warranted the investigation of this combination in phase II studies [45].

A different approach to combination of endocrine therapy with chemotherapy explored the association of letrozole with oral low-dose cyclophosphamide in elderly postmenopausal patients with ER positive locally advanced breast cancer. A not significantly higher response rate and a significantly greater suppression of Ki67 and circulating VEGF were observed in the combination arm [59]. However, at the present time the combination of chemotherapy and endocrine therapy should be considered investigative in the preoperative setting.

Open Issues

Identifying Powerful Predictors of Response

A number of studies have focused on evaluating the predictive value of different gene expression profiles but no conclusive evidence has been achieved .The largest study on 133 patients treated with preoperative anthracyclines and taxane based chemotherapy showed that a set of 30 genes were able to predict the occurrence of pCR, with an higher sensitivity than the combination of conventional parameters as age, ER status and grade (92 vs 61%). However, to what extent this set of genes is a generic predictor for chemotherapy sensitivity or specific for the chemotherapeutic regimen is not determined [60].

The Oncotype DX, a RT-PCR based assay including a 16 genes mostly related to proliferation, invasion, ER and HER2 plus five references genes yielding a recurrence score (RS), has been shown as a powerful prognostic indicator within large randomised trials [61]. In addition, it has been shown to indicate patients who benefit from the addition of chemotherapy to tamoxifen [62]. The RS was also shown to correlate significantly with the likelihood of pCR in a series of 89 patients treated with preoperative doxorubicin + paclitaxel, confirming that patients who benefit more from chemotherapy are more likely to obtain a pCR [63]. In the same series of patients a set of 86 genes, selected among 386 genes, and including proliferation related, immune-related and oestrogen receptor related genes, were associated with the likelihood of achieving a pCR [63].

Gene expression profiles were also used to identify five different molecular breast cancer subtypes bearing substantially different prognosis [64]. Molecular subtypes were also shown to respond differently to preoperative chemotherapy since basal-like (hormone receptor and HER2 negative tumours) and HER2 positive subtypes achieved 45% of pCR while luminal A and B tumours (ER positive tumours) obtained only a 2% of pCR rate [65].

Beyond pCR

Although pCR represents the most sensitive available predictor of clinical outcome, it has also been shown that residual tumor either in the breast or in the axilla correlates with prognosis [12, 20, 21, 30]. It can be speculated that varying degrees of residual tumor other than the dichotomization presence/absence may be useful to identify a continuum of subsets of patients at different prognosis, improving the prognostic value of pathologic response. This hypothesis has been recently supported by the recognition of residual cancer burden (RCB) calculated as a continuous index combining pathologic measurements of size and cellularity of the primary tumor with number and size of nodal metastasis [66]. Four different scores of RCB were identified which were independently associated with clinical outcome in a multivariate analysis. Importantly, patients with RCB score I carried the same prognosis than patients with no residual cancer burden (corresponding to the conventional definition of pCR) [66]. A validation of this index in larger series may help in the future to allow a better prediction of clinical outcome after response to primary therapy.

Integrating Targeted Agents

The evidence of a synergistic activity between chemotherapy and *trastuzumab* in the treatment of HER2 overexpressing advanced and early breast cancer has prompted a number of phase II studies investigating the association of trastuzumab and various agents, particularly platinum salt derived agents and spindle poison agents (taxanes and vinorelbine). These studies showed a high response rate and an appreciable pCR rate ranging from 18% to 47% [20]. The first phase III randomised study, which compared the addition of trastuzumab to paclitaxel followed by FEC vs chemotherapy alone was closed prematurely including only 42 patients, due to the dramatic difference between the trastuzumab and no-trastuzumab arms [67]. Interestingly, in this study there was a similar pCR rate both in HR+ve and HR–ve tumors (70 vs 61.5%), differently from what is generally observed in studies of preoperative chemotherapy. More recently preliminary results of a larger phase III trial NOAH (NeOAdjuvant Herceptin) comparing three cycles of doxorubicin in combination with paclitaxel, followed by four cycles of paclitaxel and four cycles of intravenous CMF with or without trastuzumab in locally advanced HER2 positive breast cancer showed a significantly improved pCR rate (43 vs 23%, $p = .002$) also when considering inflammatory breast cancer [68]. The results of this trial together with those of phase II trials are going to change in the near future the recommendations of the international panel consensus of 2006 leading to the inclusion of trastuzumab in the standard preoperative treatment of HER2 positive breast cancer.

Other targeted agents have been less investigated. The activity of *gefitinib*, a small EGFR tyrosine kinase inhibitor, has been investigated in combination with anastrozole in a phase II randomised study in postmenopausal patients with ER and EGFR positive breast cancer. The combination of gefitinib and anastrozole induced a significantly greater decrease of ki67 as compared to gefitinib alone, while clinical response rate was similar in the two arms [69]. On the other hand, the addition of gefitinib to anastrozole did not change proliferative activity and overall response rate in ER positive breast cancer unselected for EGFR positivity [70]. The biological activity of gefitinib has been investigated in combination with chemotherapy in a phase II randomised study. No increased effect on biomarkers of EGFR pathway and on proliferation rate was observed as compared with chemotherapy alone [71].

The dual EGFR and HER2 tyrosine kinase inhibitor *lapatinib* has been investigated as single agent in locally advanced and inflammatory breast cancer. A clinical response rate was observed in 62% of patients with refractory and recurrent inflammatory HER2 positive breast cancer [72]. The overexpression of HER2 and of its phosphorylated form was the most powerful predictor of response, while the loss of PTEN was not predictive of treatment failure.

The activity of lapatinib in the preoperative setting will be explored in a phase III multicentric trial comparing lapatinib and trastuzumab as single agents and in combination for 6 weeks followed by the same biological treatment in association with weekly paclitaxel for 12 weeks (neo-Adjuvant Lapatinib Trastuzumab Trial Optimization, neo-ALTTO).

As for the monoclonal antibody anti VEGF *bevacizumab*, the biological effects other than the clinical activity have been investigated in inflammatory breast cancer. After the administration of bevacizumab as single agent a decrease of VEGFR2 and of vascular permeability (assessed by MRI parameters), correlated with clinical response were observed [73].

The results of these studies, although heterogeneous and conflicting, all together underscore the relevance of the appropriate selection of patients when considering targeted therapies.

Conclusions

At the present time the only established benefit of primary systemic therapy is to render suitable to surgery inoperable tumours and to enable breast conserving surgery for large operable tumours candidate to mastectomy. No general benefit in terms of improved outcome has been demonstrated, except for patients achieving a complete pathological disappearance of viable tumour cells.

However, administration of primary therapy has other theoretical advantages:

1. The chance of assessing response in vivo may avoid the large number of patients and longer time of observation required to estimate the activity of new treatment strategies in the adjuvant setting although the lack of a clear improvement in OS may reduce this benefit
2. Primary systemic therapy represents an unique opportunity to get invaluable insights into the biology of the tumour and to identify biological and molecular markers associated with response and resistance to treatments

As stated in the 2006 recommendations of an international expert consensus panel, preoperative therapy may be considered for all patient candidates for receiving a systemic therapy after surgery. However, except in cases when a benefit in terms of improved surgery is expected, preoperative treatment should be offered within controlled clinical trials. A set of randomised trials designed to investigate not only new drug combinations but also early biomarkers of benefit are currently ongoing. The results of these trials will allow in the near future to optimise tailored preoperative strategies for selected subsets of breast cancer.

References

1. Giordano SH. Update on locally advanced breast cancer. *The Oncologist*. 2003;8:521–530.
2. Wolff AC and Davidson NE. Primary systemic therapy in operable breast cancer. *J Clin Oncol*. 2000;18:1558–69.
3. Fisher B, Gunduz N, Saffer EA. Influence of the interval between primary tumour removal and chemotherapy on kinetics and growth of metastasis. *Cancer Res*. 1983;43:1488–92.
4. Mauriac L, Mc Grogan G, Avril A, et al. Neoadjuvant chemotherapy for operable breast carcinoma larger than 3 cm : A unicentre randomized trial with a 124-month median follow-up. Institute Bergonie Bordeaux Group Seine (IBBGS). *Ann Oncol*. 1999;10:47–52.
5. Semiglazov VF, TopuzovEE, Bavli JL, et al. Primary (neoadjuvant) chemotherapy and radiotherapy compared with primay radiotherapy alone in stage IIb–IIIa breast cancer. *Ann Oncol*. 1994;5:591–95.
6. Scholl SM, Fourquet A, Asselain B, et al. Neoadjuvant vs adjuvant chemotherapy in premnopausal patients with tumours considered too large for breast conserving surgery: Preliminary results of a randomized trial. *Eur J Cancer*. 1994;30A:645–52.
7. Fisher B, Bryant J, Wolmark N, et al. Effect of preoperative chemotherapy on the outcome of women with operable breast cancer. *J Clin Oncol*. 1998;16:2672–85.

8. Makris A, Powles TJ, Ashley SE, et al. A reduction in the requirements for mastectomy in a randomized trial of neoadjuvant chemoendocrine therapy in primary breast cancer. *An Oncol.* 1998;9:1179–84.
9. Jakesz R, for the ABCSG. Comparison of pre- of postoperative chemotherapy in breast cancer patients. Four-year results of Austrian Breast & Colorectal Cancer Study Group (ABCSG) trial 7. *Proc Am Soc Clin Oncol.* 2001;20:125
10. Van der Hage JA, van der Velde CJ, Julien JP, et al. Preoperative chemotherapy in primary operable breast cancer: Results from the European Organization for Research and Treatment of Cancer trial 10902. *J Clin Oncol.* 2001;19:4224–37.
11. Bear HD, Anderson S, Brown A, et al. The effect on tumour response of adding sequential preoperative docetaxel to preoperative doxorubicin and cyclophosphamide: Preliminary results from National Surgical adjuvant Breast and Bowel Project Protocol B-27. *J Clin Oncol.* 2003;21:4165–74.
12. Bear HD, Anderson S, Smith RE, et al. Sequential preoperative or postoperative docetaxel added to preoperative doxorubicin plus cyclophosphamide for operable breast cancer: National Surgical Adjuvant Breast and Bowel Project Protocol B-27. *J Clin Oncol.* 2006;24:2019–27.
13. Gianni L, Baselga J, Eiermann V, et al. European Cooperative Trial in Operable Breast Cancer (ECTO): Improved freedom from progression (FFP) from adding paclitaxel (T) to doxorubicin (A) followed by cyclophosphamide, methotrexate and fluorouracile (CMF). *Proc Am Soc Clin Oncol.* 2005;24:513.
14. Mauri D, Pavlidis N, Ioannidis JP. Neoadjuvant versus adjuvant systemic treatment in breast cancer: A meta-analysis. *J Natl Cancer Inst.* 2005;97(3)188–94.
15. Wolmark N, Wang J, Mamounas E, et al. Preoperative chemotherapy in patients with operable breast cancer. Nine-year results from National Surgical adjuvant Breast and Bowel Project B-18. *J Natl Cancer Inst Monogr.* 2001;30:96–102.
16. Ring AE, Smith IE, Ashley S, Fulford LG, Lakhani SR. Oestrogen receptor status, pathological complete response and prognosis in patients receiving neoadjuvant chemotherapy for early breast cancer. *Br J Cancer.* 2004;91:2012–17.
17. Colleoni M, Viale G, Zahrieh D, et al. Chemotherapy is more effective in patients with breast cancer not expressing steroid hormone receptors: A study of preoperative treatment. *Clin Cancer Res.* 2004;10:6622–8.
18. Guarneri V, Broglio K, Kau SW, et al. Prognostic value of pathologic complete response after primary chemotherapy in relation to hormone receptor status and other factors. *J Clin Oncol.* 2006;24:1037–44.
19. Gianni L, Baselga J, Eiermann W, et al. Feasibility and tolerability of sequential doxorubicin/paclitaxel followed by cyclophosphamide, methotrexate, and fluorouracil and its effects on tumour response as preoperative therapy. *Clin Cancer Res.* 2005;11:8715–8721.
20. Kaufmann M, Hortobagyi GN, Goldhirsch A, et al. Recommendations from an international expert panel on the use of neoadjuvant (primary) systemic treatment of operable breast cancer: An update. *J Clin Oncol.* 2006;24:1940–9.
21. Sachelarie I, GRossband ML, Chadha M, et al. Primary systemic therapy of breast cancer. *The Oncologist.* 2006;11:574–89.
22. Kuerer HM, Newman LA, Smith TL, et al. Clinical course of breast cancer patients with complete pathologic primary tumour and axillary lymph node response to doxorubicin-based neoadjuvant chemotherapy. *J Clin Oncol.* 1999;17:460–69.
23. Hennessy BT, Hortobagyi GN, et al. Outcome after pathologic complete eradication of cytologically proven breast cancer axillary node metastases following primary chemotherapy. *J Clin Oncol.* 2005;23:9304–11.
24. Mazouni CX, Peintinger F, Wan-Kau S, et al. Residual ductal carcinoma in situ in patients with complete eradication of invasive breast cancer after neoadjuvant chemotherapy does not adverse patient outcome. *J Clin Oncol.* 2007;25:2650–5.

25. Beresford MJ, Wilson GD, Makris A. Measuring proliferation in breast cancer: Practicalities and applications. *Breast Cancer Res*. 2006;8:216 (doid:10.1186/bcr1618).
26. Chang J, Powles T, Allred D, et al. Biologic markers as predictors of clinical outcome from systemic therapy for primary operable breast cancer. *J Clin Oncol*. 1999;17:3058–63.
27. Burcombe RJ, Makris A, Richman PI, et al. Evaluation of ER, PgR, HER2 and Ki-67 as predictors of response to neoadjuvant anthracycline chemotherapy for operable breast cancer. *Br J Cancer*. 2005;92:147–55.
28. Dowsett M, Ebbs SR, Dixon M, et al. Biomarker changes during neoadjuvant anastrozole, tamoxifen, or the combination: influence of hormonal status and HER2 in breast cancer – a study from the IMPACT trialists. *J Clin Oncol*. 2005;23:2477–92.
29. Untch M, Konecny G, Ditsch N, et al. Dose-dense sequential epirubicin-paclitaxel as preoperative treatment of breast cancer: Results of a randomized AGO study. *Proc Am Soc Clin Oncol*. 2002;21:133a.
30. Von Minckwitz G, Raab G, Caputo A, et al. Doxorubicin with cyclophosphamide followed by docetaxel every 21 days compared with doxorubicin and docetaxel every 14 days as preoperative treatment in operable breast cancer: The GEPARDUO study of the German Breast Group. *J Clin Oncol*. 2005;23:2676–85.
31. Von Minckwitz G, Blohmer J-U, Raab G et al. *In vivo* chemosensitivity – adapted preoperative chemotherapy in patients with early-stage breast cancer: The GEPARTRIO pilot study. *Ann Oncol* 2005;16:56–63.
32. Cristofanilli M, Gonzalez-Angulo A, Sneige N, et al. Invasive lobular carcinoma classic type: Response to primary chemotherapy and survival outcomes. *J Clin Oncol*. 2007;23:41–48.
33. Tubiana-Hulin M, Stevens D, Lasry S, et al. Response to neoadjuvant chemotherapy in lobular and ductal breast carcinomas: A retrospective study on 860 patients from one institution. *Ann Oncol*. 2007;17:1228–33.
34. Andre F, Mazouni C, Liedtke C, et al. HER2 expression and efficacy of preoperative paclitaxel/FAC chemotherapy in breast cancer. *Breast Cancer Res Treat*. 2007; DOI 10.1007/s10549-007-9594-8.
35. Colleoni M, Viale G, Zahrieh D, et al. Expression of ER, PgR, HER1, HER2 and response: A study of preoperative chemotherapy. *Ann Oncol*. 2007, Epub 6 Nov.
36. Dieras V, Fumoleau P, Romieu G, et al. Randomized parallel study of doxorubicin plus paclitaxel and doxorubicin plus cyclophosphamide as neoadjuvant treatment of patients with breast cancer. *J Clin Oncol*. 2004;22:4958–65.
37. Evans TR, Yellowlees A, Foster E, Earl H et al. Phase III randomized trial of doxorubicin and cyclophosphamide as primary medical therapy in women with breast cancer: An anglo-celtic cooperative oncology group study. *J Clin Oncol*. 2005;23:2988–95.
38. Smith IC, Heys SD, Hutcheon AW, et al. Neoadjuvant chemotherapy in breast cancer: Significant enhanced response with docetaxel. *J Clin Oncol*. 2002;20:1456–66
39. Green MC, Buzdar AU, Smith T, et al. Weekly paclitaxel improves pathological complete remission in operable breast cancer when compared with paclitaxel one every 3 weeks. *J Clin Oncol*. 2005;23:5983–92.
40. Frasci G, D'Aiuto G, Comella P, et al. A 2-month cisplatin-epirubicin-paclitaxel (PET) weekly combination as primary systemic therapy for large operable breast cancer: A phase II study. *Ann Oncol*. 2005;16:1268–75.
41. Romieu G, Tubiana-Hulin M, Fumoleau P, et al. A multicenter randomized phase II study of 4 or 6 cycles of Adriamycin/taxol (paclitaxel) AT as neoadjuvant treatment of breast cancer. *Ann Oncol*. 2002;13(suppl):33–34.
42. Therasse P, Mauriac L, Welnicka-Jaskiewicz M, et al. Final results of a randomized phase III trial comparing cyclophosphamide, epirubicin and fluorouracil with a dose-intensified epirubicin and cyclophosphamide + filgrastim as neoasduvant treatment in locally advanced breast cancer: An EORTC-NCIC-SAKK multicenter study. *J Clin Oncol*. 2003;21:843–50.

43. Steger GG, Galid A, Gnant M, et al. Pathologic complete response with six compared with three cycles of neoadjuvant epirubicin plus docetaxel and granulocyte colony-stimulating factor in operable breast cancer: Results of ABCSG-14. *J Clin Oncol.* 2007;25:2012–18.
44. Thomas E, Holmes FA, Smith TL, et al. The use of alternate, non-cross resistant adjuvant chemotherapy on the basis of pathologic response to a neoadjuvant doxorubicin-based regimen in women with operable breast cancer: Long term results from a prospective randomized trial. *J Clin Oncol.* 2004;22:2294–302.
45. Abrial C, Mouret-Reynier M-A, Curé H, et al. Neoadjuvant endocrine therapy in breast cancer. *Breast.* 2006;15:9–19.
46. Eiermann W, Paepke S, Appfelstaedt J, et al. Preoperative treatment of postmenopausal breast cancer patients with letrozole: A randomized double-blind multicenter study. *Ann Oncol.* 2001;12:1527–32.
47. Ellis MJ, Coop A, Singh B, et al. Letrozole is more effective neoadjuvant endocrine therapy than tamoxifen for ErbB-1- and/or ErbB-2-positive, estrogen receptor-positive primary breast cancer: evidence from a phase III randomized trial. *J Clin Oncol.* 2001;19:3808–16.
48. Smith IE, Dowsett M, Ebbs SR, et al. Neoadjuvant treatment of postmenopausal breast cancer with anastrozole, tamoxifen, or both in combination: The immediate preoperative anastrozole, tamoxifen, or combined with tamoxifen (IMPACT) multicenter double-blind randomized trial. *J Clin Oncol.* 2005;23:5108–16.
49. Cataliotti L, Buzdar A, Noguchi S, et al. Comparison of anastrozole versus tamoxifen as preoperative therapy in postmenopausal women with hormone receptor-positive breast cancer. The pre-operative "Arimidex" compared to tamoxifen (PROACT) trial. *Cancer.* 2006;106:2095–103.
50. Semiglazov V, Kletsel A, Semiglazov V, et al. Exemestane versus tamoxifen as neoadjuvant endocrine therapy for postmenopausal women with ER+ breast cancer (T2N1-2, T3N0-1 T4N0M0). *Proc ASCO.* 2005;23 abs 530.
51. Paepke S, Jacobs VR, Paepke D, et al. Critical appraisal of primary systemic endocrine therapy in receptor-positive postmenopausal breast cancer: An update. *Onkologie.* 2006;29:210–17.
52. Dixon JM, Jackson J, Renshaw L, Miller WR. Neoadjuvant tamoxifen and aromatase inhibitors: Comparisons and clinical outcomes. *J Steroid Biochem Mol Biol.* 2003;86:295–9.
53. Semiglazov VF, Semiglazov VV, Dashyan GA, et al. Phase 2 randomized trial of primary endocrine therapy versus chemotherapy in postmenopausal patients with estrogen-receptor positive breast cancer. *Cancer.* 2007;110:244–54.
54. Torrisi R, Bagnardi V, Pruneri G, et al. Antitumour and biological effects of letrozole and GnRH analogue as primary therapy in premenopausal women with ER and PgR positive locally advanced operable breast cancer. *Br J Cancer.* 2007;97:802–8.
55. Von Minckwitz G, Costa SD, Raab G, et al. Dose-dense doxorubicin, docetaxel and granulocyte colony-stimulating factor support with or without tamoxifen as preoperative therapy in patients with operable carcinoma of the breast: A randomized, controlled open phase IIb study. *J Clin Oncol.* 2001;19:3506–15.
56. Bottini A, Berruti A, Brizzi MP, et al. Cytotoxic and antiproliferative activity of the single agent epirubicin versus epirubicin plus tamoxifen as primary chemotherapy in human breast cancer: A single-institution phase III trial. *Endocrine Related Cancer.* 2005;12:383–92.
57. Albain KS. Adjuvant chemo-endocrine therapy for breast cancer: Combined or sequential? *Breast.* 2003;12:12.
58. Torrisi R, Colleoni M, Veronesi P, et al. Primary therapy with ECF in combination with a GnRH analogue in premenopausal women with hormone receptor positive T2-T4 breast cancer. *Breast.* 2007;16:73–80.

59. Bottini A, Generali D, Brizzi MP, et al. Randomized phase II trial of letrozole and letrozole plus low-dose metronomic oral cyclophosphamide as primary systemic treatment in elderly breast cancer patients. *J Clin Oncol.* 2006;24:3623–8.
60. Hess KR, Anderson K, Symmans WF, et al. Pharmacogenomic predictor of sensitivity to preoperative chemotherapy with paclitaxel and fluorouracile, doxorubicin and cyclophosphamide in breast cancer. *J Clin Oncol.* 2007;24:4236–44.
61. Paik S, Shak S, Tang G, et al. A multigene assay to predict recurrence of tamoxifen-treated, node-negative breast cancer. N Engl J Med. 2004;351:2817–26.
62. Paik S, Tang G, Shak S, et al. Gene expression and benefit of chemotherapy in women with node-negative, estrogen receptor positive breast cancer. *J Clin Oncol.* 2006;24:3726–34.
63. Gianni L, Zambetti M, Clark K, et al. Gene expression profiles in paraffin-embedded core biopsy tissue predict response to chemotherapy in women with locally advanced breast cancer. *J Clin Oncol.* 2005;23:7266–77.
64. Sorlie T, Perou CM, Fan C, et al. Gene expression profiles do not consistently predict the clinical treatment response in locally advanced breast cancer. *Mol Cancer Ther.* 2006;5:2914–8.
65. Rouzier R, Perou CM, Symmans WF, et al. Breast cancer molecular subtypes respond differently to preoperative chemotherapy. *Clin Cancer Res.* 2005;11:5678–85.
66. Symmans WF, Peintinger F, Hatzis C, et al. Measurement of residual cancer burden to predict survival after neoadjuvant chemotherapy. *J Clin Oncol.* 2007;25:4414–22.
67. Buzdar AU, Ibrahim NK, Francis D, et al. Significantly higher pathologic complete remission rate after neoadjuvant therapy with trastuzumab, paclitaxel and epirubicin chemotherapy: Results of a randomized trial in human epidermal growth factor receptor 2-positive operable breast cancer. *J Clin Oncol.* 2005;23:3676–85.
68. Gianni L, Semiglazov V, Manikhas GM, et al. Neoadjuvant trastuzumab in locally advanced breast cancer (NOAH): Antitumour and safety analysis. 2007 ASCO Annual Meeting Proceedings Part I. Vol 25, No. 18S (June 20 Suppl), 2007:532.
69. Polychronis A, Sinnett HD, Hadjiminas D, et al. Preoperative gefitinib versus gefitinib and anastrozole in postmenopausal patients with oestrogen-receptor positive and epidermal-growth-factor-receptor-positive primary breast cancer: A double-blind placebo-controlled phase II randomised trial. *Lancet Oncol.* 2005;6:383–91.
70. Smith IE, Walsh GW, Skene A, et al. A phase II placebo-controlled trial of neoadjuvant anastrozole alone or with gefitinib in early breast cancer. *J Clin Oncol.* 2007;25:3816–22.
71. Guarneri V, Frassoldati A, Ficarra, et al. Phase II randomized trial of preoperative epirubicin-paclitaxel ± gefitinib with biomarker evaluation in operable breast cancer. *Breast Cancer Res Treat.* 2007; DOI 10.1007/s10549-007-9688-3.
72. Spector NL, Blackwell K, Hurley J, et al. EGF 103009, a phase II trial of lapatinib monotherapy in patients with relapsed/refractorty inflammatory breast cancer (IBC): Clinical activity and biologic predictors of response. *J Clin Oncol.* 2006;24 (suppl):3S (abs 502).
73. Wedam SB, Low JA, Yang SX, et al. Antiangiogenic and antitumour effects of bevacizumab in patients with inflammatory and locally advanced breast cancer. *J Clin Oncol.* 2006;24:769–77.

Adjuvant Chemotherapy

M. Tubiana-Hulin and M. Gardner

Apparently localized breast cancer which has been treated with optimal locoregional therapy can recur months or years later, ultimately resulting in death. This is generally believed to be due to the development of occult micrometastases disseminated in the body and already present at the time of the initial surgery. Destruction of these micrometastases is the aim of adjuvant and neoadjuvant therapy. Adjuvant therapies have been widely used since the 1970s and, although the absolute survival benefit they confer is modest (10%), they have been credited, together with screening and improvement of loco-regional treatment, for the reduction in breast cancer mortality observed in recent decades.

Over the past few decades, several generations of adjuvant chemotherapy randomized trials have been conducted specially for patients with positive axillary nodes that have demonstrated increasing efficacy: monochemotherapy, CMF (cyclophosphamide-methotrexate-fluorouracil) based polychemotherapy, anthracyclines based combinations, anthracyclines and taxanes-based combinations and recently, for patients with HER 2 oncoprotein overexpression) trastuzumab combined with anthracyclines-taxanes regimens that represented a very important advance. Concurrently, adjuvant hormonal treatments either alone or combined with chemotherapy have been developed: ovarian suppression, tamoxifen and more recently, aromatase inhibitors for postmenopausal patients. At 15 year of follow-up, on the whole, reduction of risk of mortality from adjuvant therapies is about 50% [1].

The interest of adjuvant chemotherapy for breast cancer was demonstrated in the early 1980s by data from two large randomized trials begun in 1972 and 1973, which had a considerable impact on the management of operable breast cancer. Patients with positive axillary lymph nodes who received 2 years of treatment with melphalan by mouth in the NSABP B-05 trial [2] or 1 year of CMF (cyclophosphamide, methotrexate, 5-fluorouracil) in the Milan Cancer Institute study [3] were found to have benefited in terms of disease-free survival

M. Tubiana-Hulin (✉)
Centre René Huguenin St Cloud France

M. Castiglione, M.J. Piccart (eds.), *Adjuvant Therapy for Breast Cancer*,
Cancer Treatment and Research 151, DOI 10.1007/978-0-387-75115-3_9,

in comparison with the placebo group. Subgroup analysis showed that this benefit concerned mainly patients who were under the age of 50 years with moderate nodal involvement.

A great many comparative studies of different chemotherapy protocols have subsequently been conducted to evaluate the efficacy of chemotherapy in different patient populations.

The Oxford international meta-analysis of adjuvant trials [1, 4, 5] has been carried out every 5 years since 1985. This analysis comprises 80% of randomized adjuvant trials published or conducted worldwide, in which individual patient data are taken into account. The 2005 update reports 10- and 15-year disease-free survival and overall survival rates. It concerns 4,000 patients in monochemotherapy trials and 29,000 in polychemotherapy trials, the latter mainly involving CMF for 6 or 12 months, or a combination with anthracyclines for 6 months. In several studies vincristine or prednisone were associated with the above drugs. Very few of the patients were over 70 years of age. Globally, monochemotherapy lowered the annual event rate (hazard ratio 0.86, SE 0.04 $2p<0.001$) but did not affect mortality. Polychemotherapy lowered both the annual event rate (HR 0.77, 0.02 $2p<0.00001$) and the mortality rate (HR 0.83, 0.02 $2p<0.00001$). In this case, the efficacy of chemotherapy was demonstrated regardless of age ($p<0.00001$), with a greater benefit before age 50. The relative reduction in the recurrence rate took place in the first 5 years, while overall survival improved throughout the 10 and 15 years of follow-up.

The relative risk reduction was independent of menopausal status, hormone receptor status, and use or not of tamoxifen. Furthermore, the relative benefit was identical for node-positive and node-negative disease.

Because of wide variation between chemotherapy regimens (drugs, doses, methods of administration, duration) that partly explain the variable outcomes reported in these trials, the meta-analysis can establish the minimum effect achieved with adjuvant chemotherapy, but does not allow any conclusions as to specific treatment modalities: dose density or dose intensity, alternating or sequential protocols.

Anthracyclines in Adjuvant Therapy

The anthracyclines are topoisomerase II inhibitors. Doxorubicin and epirubicin appear similar in efficacy, but at larger cumulative doses epirubicin may be less cardiotoxic. Anthracyclines are among the most active drugs in metastatic breast cancer. Used as early as 1974 by the M.D. Anderson group in Texas [6] in non-randomized trials, the FAC protocols (5-fluorouracil, doxorubicin, cyclophosphamide) already appeared to demonstrate a survival benefit in node-positive patients (particularly with more than three positive nodes), irrespective of age. In France, anthracyclines, especially epirubicin, have been included in the majority of adjuvant chemotherapy protocols used over the past 15 years [7, 8]. The Oxford meta-analysis published in 2005 [1] combined data from 14,000 women (two-thirds of whom were under the age of 50 years) and directly compared anthracyclines' protocols and CMF-based protocols for 6 months. The superiority of the anthracyclines protocols was established: risk of recurrence with a hazard ratio of 0.89 ($2p = 0.001$) and risk of death (HR 0.84, $2p = 0.001$). The absolute difference in survival was 3% at 5 years and 4% at 10 years regardless of age or estrogen receptor status.

A review of trials conducted by the major cooperative groups provides additional data. The NSABP B-11 [9] trial compared melphalan + 5-fluorouracil (PF) with melphalan + 5-fluorouracil + doxorubicin (PAF) in patients aged 50–59 years with progesterone receptor-negative tumors. Here, the addition of doxorubicin conferred a benefit in terms of disease-free survival and overall survival at 6 years. On the other hand, the same combination to which concomitant tamoxifen was added (NSABP B-12), or PFT vs PAFT in patients with progesterone receptor-positive tumors did not show any significant difference in disease-free survival or overall survival [9].

It should be noted that the doxorubicin doses used in these trials (30 mg/m^2 per cycle for six cycles) can be considered suboptimal. The Bonadonna group from the Milan Cancer Institute also evaluated the effect of doxorubicin in patient populations with one to three positive nodes. Doxorubicin given after six cycles of CMF vs CMF alone did not provide any significant benefit [10].

The NSABP trial (B-15) [11] is noteworthy in that it compared the combination doxorubicin/cyclophosphamide with classical CMF. More than 2,000 patients with positive axillary nodes were randomized to receive either four cycles of AC (doxorubicin 60 mg/m^2, cyclophosphamide 600 mg/m^2) over 2 months vs six cycles of classical CMF over 6 months. A third arm evaluated the sequence AC → CMF with a 6-month interval between the last cycle of AC and the first cycle of CMF. This study did not find any reduction in the recurrence risk or overall survival, but quality of life and toxicities were improved with AC as compared to CMF.

The Onco-France trial [12] compared AVCF (doxorubicin, vincristine, cyclophosphamide, 5-fluorouracil) vs CMF. After a long (10-year) follow-up, the anthracyclines arm was superior in terms of disease-free survival and overall survival in premenopausal patients.

The International Breast Cancer Cooperative Group [13] compared classical CMF (six cycles) vs eight cycles of EC 60 mg/m^2 and 500 mg/m^2 or HEC (epirubicin 100 mg/m^2 + cyclophosphamide 830 mg/m^2). At 4 years there was no significant difference as compared with the CMF protocol, although a dose effect was observed with epirubicin and the HEC protocol was superior to EC. There were about 250 pre- and post-menopausal patients in each arm and the follow-up was fairly short, which makes the results difficult to interpret.

The National Cancer Institute of Canada trial, updated by Levine in 2005 [14], compared six cycles of CMF (cyclophosphamide 100 mg/m^2, methotrexate 40 mg/m^2, 5-fluorouracil 600 mg/m^2) vs six cycles of CEF (cyclophosphamide

75 mg/m^2, epirubicin 60 mg/m^2 days 1 and 8, and 5-fluorouracil 500 mg/m^2) in pre- and peri-menopausal women with axillary node-positive breast cancer. The epirubicin dose intensity had to be reduced due to hematologic toxicity. The 10-year results were in favor of CEF, with 52% relapse-free survival vs 45% (p = 0.007) and 62% overall survival vs 58% (p = 0.08). Long-term cardiotoxicity was slightly higher with CEF (1.1%) than with CMF (0.3%).

A publication by Poole [15] combining data from two English studies recently confirmed the superiority of anthracyclines-containing protocols, with a benefit on disease-free survival (79 vs 69%, p<0.001) and overall survival (82 vs 75%, p<0.001) at 5 years. Altogether, four trials comparing anthracyclines-containing chemotherapy with classical CMF showed a significant reduction in the risk of relapse and death. The use of suboptimal doses of anthracyclines (per cycle or cumulative dose), concomitant tamoxifen, late introduction of anthracyclines, might explain certain "negative" studies. The NSABP B-15 trial was the landmark trial in establishing the four-cycle AC regimen as the American standard and the basis of a sequence from which, today, most adjuvant trials are still designed by the major cooperative groups like (cancer and leukemia group B) CALBG, Southwest oncology group SWOG, etc.

Duration of treatment

Many randomized trials have addressed the question of the duration of adjuvant chemotherapy which, in the oldest studies, was 1–2 years. The report from Milano [16] comparing six vs twelve cycles of CMF continues to have an influence on most current protocols. With 5 years of follow-up in 460 patients, no significant differences were found in either disease-free survival (65.6 vs 59%, p = 0.17) or overall survival (77 vs 72%, six cycles, p = 0.20). The same was true in all the subgroups analyzed. A single perioperative cycle or an early postoperative cycle [25] gave significantly worse outcomes than 6 months of CMF (Ludwig Breast Cancer Study Group, [17].

The 1998 Oxford meta-analysis [5] looked at outcomes of short or long treatment durations in 6,000 patients and found similar results between 3–6 months of chemotherapy vs longer treatment durations. However, the treatment duration differed according to the drugs used: 2.5 months of AC appeared to be equivalent to six cycles of CMF(NSABP B15), but three cycles of FEC 50 or 75 mg were inferior to six cycles of FEC 50 mg [18]. The French trial PACS 05, which recently completed patient recruitment, is comparing four cycles of FEC 100 mg with six cycles of FEC 100 mg in high-risk node-negative patients.

While the minimum duration of treatment appears to be 3 months (four cycles) with anthracyclines or taxanes-based regimens, it is possible that sequential regimens will demonstrate the superiority of longer treatment durations of 4–6 months [19].

Dose Intensity

Hryniuk [20] defines dose intensity as the quantity of drug in milligrams per square meter of body surface area per week. This enables a comparison of protocols in terms of administered and theoretical dose and makes it possible to define potential modulations, such as dose escalation (increasing the unit dose of the drug(s) each cycle without changing the interval between cycles or maintaining the doses but reducing the interval between cycles). Two trials in favor of high doses [CALGB 8541 (FAC 30, 40 or 60 mg/m^2) [21] and FAGS 05(FEC 50 vs 100 mg/m^2) [22] used anthracyclines doses which are currently considered to be suboptimal and therefore merely demonstrated the deleterious effect of a dose reduction.

NSABP trials [23, 24] as well as CALBG 9344 [19] used the same standard treatment comprising four sequences of doxorubicin 60 mg/m^2 plus cyclophosphamide 600 mg/m^2. The NSABP B 25 [23] evaluated the effect of increasing the cyclophosphamide dose (same dose in two instead of four cycles or total dose multiplied two- or fourfold), while the CALBG trial investigated the effect of increasing the anthracyclines dose by 50% [19]. Disease-free and overall survival were unchanged. On the other hand, acute toxicities were substantially higher, with a tenfold increase in the complication rate in the high-dose arm of trial B-25 relative to the standard treatment, despite systematic support with hematopoietic factors.

In conclusion, increasing the doses of adjuvant chemotherapy by a factor of four at the most has not been shown to have superior efficacy. However, reducing the doses to suboptimal levels has been shown to have a deleterious effect.

Randomized Studies of High-Dose Adjuvant Chemotherapy with Hematopoietic Stem Cell Transplantation

The patients in these trials were at high risk of recurrence and in most cases had more than ten positive nodes. Prospective randomized trials involving a large patient cohort were presented at the plenary seminar of the ASCO congress in 1999. The trials reported by Peters [25] and Bergh [26] consisted of four induction cycles with FAC or FEC and an intensified consolidation cycle in the experimental arm. A total of 874 and 525 patients were randomized, respectively. After a median follow-up of 3 and 2 years, no significant differences were found. These data agree with those of Hortobagyi [27] and Rodenhuis [28] in a smaller series of patients who received pre- and post-operative induction with anthracyclines and cyclophosphamide.

Sequential Regimens

The Milan Cancer Institute study [29] has been a decisive factor. In patients with three or more positive nodes (405 randomized patients), this was the first study to also test alternating or sequential schedules: four cycles of doxorubicin followed by eight cycles of CMF vs two cycles of CMF followed by one cycle of doxorubicin in four successive cycles. At 10 years disease-free survival and overall survival were significantly better in the alternating regimen (42 vs 28%, $p = 0.002$ and 58 vs 44%, $p = 0.002$, respectively).

The two treatment arms differed only in terms of the method of administration; the doses of doxorubicin (75 mg/m^2) and CMF were identical. The sequential regimen proved to be significantly superior in terms of relapse-free survival (42 vs 28%, $p = 0.002$) and overall survival (58 vs 44%, $p = 0.002$). The median time to disease progression was doubled in the sequential arm (86 vs 47 months).

These benefits were observed in all subgroups of the study population. In particular, relapse-free survival in patients with the worst prognosis (>10 positive nodes and tumor >2 cm) was 85% in the sequential arm, which is similar to that seen in patients with a better prognosis (4–10 positive nodes and tumor $\leq$2 cm) on an alternating regimen. The dose intensity of the cytotoxic drugs was similar in both arms of the study: 0.92 and 0.94 for the sequential and alternating regimens, respectively. However, by definition, the doxorubicin dose intensity was higher in the sequential arm (four cycles of doxorubicin over 27 weeks). This is believed to explain the advantage of a sequential regimen: the shorter time interval between two doxorubicin cycles would decrease the repopulation of the chemosensitive cell fraction. Later studies of sequential regimens have abandoned CMF in favor of anthracyclines plus taxanes combinations.

Taxanes in the Adjuvant Setting

Of the new drugs developed over the last 15 years, only the taxanes have been found to provide a tangible benefit in terms of breast cancer outcomes [30]. The first studies of these drugs in the neoadjuvant and adjuvant setting began in 1995. Paclitaxel and docetaxel act by stabilizing microtubules, thereby preventing the disassembly of microtubules required for mitosis. Important differences exist between these two drugs. First, the optimal dose and schedule of paclitaxel (175–250 mg/m^2 over 3 h or 24 h or 80 mg/m^2 over 1 h every week) is still controversial whereas the optimal taxotere dose of 100 mg/m^2 given over 1 h as monotherapy every 3 weeks has been established since this drug went into development. In addition, a pharmacokinetic interaction has been found to occur between paclitaxel delivered in a short, 3-h infusion and doxorubicin, which increases the AUC of doxorubicinol [31–33] and is responsible for cardiotoxicity. Paclitaxel plus doxorubicin combinations given at a 16- to 24-h interval circumvent this problem but this schedule is more difficult to administer and also less effective [34]. This is why this drug is only used in sequential regimens in the adjuvant setting.

Paclitaxel

1. The CALBG 9344 [19] trial tested two hypotheses: the effect of increasing the doxorubicin dose in the AC regimen, and the benefit of adding four cycles of paclitaxel after four cycles of AC. The 3,170 patients were randomized according to a bifactorial design: patients were first randomized to AC 60, 75, or 90 mg combined with cyclophosphamide 600 mg/m^2, then secondly randomized to receive or not four additional cycles of paclitaxel (175 mg/m^2 over 3 h). Receptor-positive patients then systematically received hormonal therapy with tamoxifen for 5 years. The results of the interim analysis at 18 and 30 months showed that increasing the doxorubicin dose above 60 mg/m^2 conferred no added benefit, whereas sequential addition of paclitaxel significantly improved survival, with a 22% reduction in the relapse rate and a 26% reduction in mortality. However the main benefit was seen in HR-negative patients. These findings are difficult to interpret, since it is not known if the observed benefit was due to the paclitaxel or to the longer duration of chemotherapy.
2. The NSABP B-28 trial [35] was similar to the above study (3,060 node-positive patients, four cycles of AC vs four AC followed by four cycles of paclitaxel), but there were some notable differences in terms of the paclitaxel dose (225 mg/m^2), the cohort (70% with one to three positive nodes) and especially tamoxifen, which was concomitant to chemotherapy, after menopause and even in HR-negative patients over the age of 50 years. After a median follow-up of 64 months, the relative risk of recurrence decreased by 17% ($p = 0.008$) but there was no impact on overall survival. Concomitant administration of CT and tamoxifen appears to be less effective than CT followed by tamoxifen for positive hormonal status patients.
3. The CALBG 9741 trial [36] tested the concept of dose density as described by L. Norton, which states, briefly, that an identical fraction of exponentially growing tumor cells is destroyed by a given dose of a drug. Breast cancer usually grows according to non-exponential Gompertzian kinetics. Repopulation of tumor cells after cytoreduction is faster in Gompertzian models than in experimental models of exponential growth. Thus, the test hypothesis is that there would be a greater reduction in tumor volume by more frequent administration of cytotoxic drugs than by an increase in dose. Then 2,500 patients were randomized to a sequential schedule (four cycles of each of the three drugs doxorubicin, paclitaxel, cyclophosphamide) or a concomitant regimen (four cycles of AC followed by four cycles of paclitaxel). In each arm, patients were randomized a second time to test dose density: one cycle every 2 weeks with hematopoietic growth factor support vs the usual 3-week interval between cycles. After a median follow-up of 36 months, there was no significant difference between the sequential or concomitant arms, but a significant difference was found in favor of the dose densified arm (2-week interval), with 26 and 31% relative reduction in the risk of recurrence and death, respectively. No density-sequence interaction was found.

4. The M.D. Anderson study involving a smaller cohort is of interest in terms of the equivalence of treatment duration [36]. Here 524 patients were randomized to either eight cycles of FAC or four cycles of paclitaxel (250 mg/m^2 by 24-h infusion every 3 weeks) followed by four cycles of FAC in an adjuvant or neoadjuvant setting and possibly followed by irradiation and by tamoxifen for patients over the age of 50 years or with receptor-positive disease. The classical prognostic factors differed in the two groups in terms of presurgery clinical stage and postsurgery surgical stage as well as ER status, which was more often positive in the paclitaxel group. At 48 months, there was no significant difference in overall survival and a small difference in favor of the paclitaxel arm for relapse-free survival in receptor-negative patients. There was a 30% reduction in the risk of recurrence in the paclitaxel arm (results validated at 3 years) but the modalities are still open to discussion.

Docetaxel was more effective than doxorubicin and paclitaxel in a direct comparison in metastatic setting [37]. This drug has been evaluated in several concomitant or sequential regimens.

The BCIRG 001 trial which began in 1997 [38] compared FAC and TAC regimens (A 50 mg/m^2, C 500 mg/m^2 and 5-fluorouracil 500 mg/m^2 or T docetaxel 75 mg/m^2). Here 1,491 patients under the age of 70 years with node-positive disease were randomized in this study. Patients received six cycles of chemotherapy beginning 2 months after surgery. Irradiation was given following surgery and hormonal therapy was given in receptor-positive patients after completion of chemotherapy. Median dose intensity was equivalent in the two protocols (98 vs 99%). At 55 months, relapse-free survival was significantly higher in the TAC arm ($p = 0.001$), irrespective of subgroup and in particular of receptor or HER2 status. The risk reduction was 39% for one to three positive axillary nodes and 17% for more than three positive nodes. Survival was 87% with TAC and 81% with FAC ($p = 0.008$). Hematologic and other toxicities were more frequent with TAC. In particular, neutropenic fever occurred in 24.7% of patients vs 2.5% in the FAC group, but nonfatal grade 3 or 4 infections were only seen in 3.9% of cases (ciprofloxacin prophylaxis was routinely administered). Amenorrhea was more frequent with TAC (61 vs 52.4%) but no data are yet available concerning the frequency of permanent amenorrhea. Quality of life scores did not differ in the two groups.

The PACS 01 trial [39] randomized 1,999 patients to either six cycles of FEC (epirubicin 100 mg/m^2) or three cycles of FEC followed by three cycles of docetaxel 100 mg/m^2. Chemotherapy began before the 42nd postsurgical day, followed by radiation therapy and then tamoxifen for 5 years in receptor-positive patients. The groups were well balanced for the conventional prognostic factors. The data were in favor of the sequential regimen with a ratio of 0.83 ($p<0.01$) for relapse-free survival and 0.73 ($p<0.05$) for overall survival.

The US oncology [40] compared four cycles of standard AC with four cycles of TC (without anthracyclines: docetaxel 75 mg/m^2 + cyclophosphamide 600 mg/m^2). Radiation therapy, when indicated, was given on completion of chemotherapy followed by hormonal therapy in receptor-positive patients. Here 1,016 patients under 75 years of age were randomized. Patient characteristics were similar in the two arms: 48% node negative, only 11% with >3 positive axillary nodes, 29% receptor-negative. At 5 years, relapse-free survival was significantly higher in the TC group with a hazard ratio of 0.67 ($p = 0.015$) and a favorable but not yet significant effect on overall survival. Muscle and joint pain, edema and febrile neutropenia were more frequent in the TC arm. Digestive disorders and one case of congestive heart failure were observed in the AC arm. There were two deaths in the TC arm including one due to sepsis in a neutropenic patient.

The results of trial E 2197 [41] comparing four cycles of AC vs four cycles of AT (with docetaxel 60 mg/m^2) in 2,952 patients were not significant at 4 years, probably because the docetaxel doses were insufficient. Also, fever, neutropenia and death were more frequent in the AT arm.

Other Drugs in Adjuvant Setting

Other drugs alone or combination of drugs that demonstrated activity in metastatic breast cancer are candidates to be tested in the adjuvant setting. The goal is to find possibly more active (especially in subgroups as basal type (triple negative)) and/or less toxic regimen avoiding cardiac toxicity of anthracyclines-based chemotherapy, more fitted for patients more than 70 year old and/or candidates for trastuzumab chemotherapy that has its specific cardio-toxicity. Amongst these candidate drugs are gemcitabine with moderate toxicity, synergistic to paclitaxel and docetaxel [37, 42], that is incorporated in a number of on going trials, following three or four anthracyclines-based cycles. For example, the TanGo trial [43] will randomize patients to EC (90/600 mg/m^2) followed by paclitaxel (175 mg/m^2) or paclitaxel combined to gemcitabine (1,250 mg/m^2 day 1 and 8) or NSABP B38,a randomized comparison between TAC and dose-dense AC followed by paclitaxel and gemcitabine.

Capecitabine is a well tolerated oral drug with no myelosuppression or alopecia, active in metastatic trial and synergistic to taxanes, that could be specially fitted for older patients: one CALBG trial (49907) will compare capecitabine alone to standard CMF or AC.

Numerous on-going trials will incorporate capecitabine with taxanes, anthracyclines, or vinorelbine [44]. Several biologic agents will very soon be incorporated in adjuvant setting. Lapatinib, an oral inhibitor of epidermal growth factor and HER2 tyrosine kinase appears to be the next candidate in HER2 overexpressing tumors (see dedicated chapter).

Late Adverse Effects of Breast Cancer Adjuvant Chemotherapy

Effectiveness of adjuvant chemotherapy designed to improve cure rates and to extend survival time is tempered by side effects that may impair in some cases seriously quality of life (QOL) or become exceptionally even life-threatening. Acute toxicities differ among chemotherapy regimens and may include nausea, vomiting, mucositis, myelosuppression, neurotoxicity, weight modifications, alopecia and muscle pain. Management of these toxicities has been previously extensively reviewed [45]. Cardiac and hematological toxicities are potentially lethal complications. Lethal outcome due to acute complications is rare, however, particularly since the appropriate use of growth factors [40].

Cardiac Toxicity

The delayed dilated cardiomyopathy may occur as late as several years after completion of anthracyclines therapy and is irreversible [46, 47]. There are several well conducted studies demonstrating increase of incidence of cardiac failure with increasing cumulative dose of doxorubicin, and epirubicin [48, 49]. A 5% risk is seen at 450 mg/m^2 for doxorubicin, 900 mg/m^2 for epirubicin, doses that are not reached in adjuvant setting [50]. Accordingly, the risk of developing a left ventricular dysfunction in early breast cancer patients receiving epirubicin-based adjuvant chemotherapy seems acceptable: at 7 years, 1.36 vs 0.21% without epirubicin [51]. Cofactors for cardiotoxic risk are mediastinal irradiation which includes the heart, age (older than 70 or younger than 15 years), coronary artery disease, valvular or myocardial abnormalities, and hypertension. Transtuzumab and paclitaxel enhance cardiac toxicity [52].

Hematological Complications – Acute Myeloid Leukemia and Myelodysplastic Syndrome

Acute myeloid leukemia (AML) appears relatively early (3 years) after the end of the adjuvant chemotherapy without previous myelodysplastic phase, particularly if anthracyclines and more generally topoisomerase II inhibitors were used. Myelodysplastic syndrome (MS), often associated with abnormalities involving chromosome 5 and/or 7, appears 5–10 years after adjuvant chemotherapy and is more particularly associated with use of alkylating agents and radiotherapy.

The general risk of AML is multiplied by five if standard dose adjuvant chemotherapy without anthracyclines was used (to reach 0.2–0.4% at 10 years). Introduction of anthracyclines at standard dose (single doxorubicine dose <60 mg/m^2; cumulative dose <360 mg/m^2) multiplies this risk by 1.2–1.5.

Higher dose intensity and cumulative dose of epirubicin or cyclophosphamide multiplied the risk for the development of treatment-related AML/MDS by 10 [53–56]. Other agents like mitoxanthrone seem to be associated more strongly with AML and for that reason they are not used any more in adjuvant treatment [57, 58]. Finally, the use of growth factors seems to be associated with an increased risk of AML [59, 60]. Nevertheless, this data was not confirmed by some studies [61].

Pulmonary Toxicity

The late toxicity of cyclophosphamide may appear up to 8 years after initiation of therapy. However, the incidence of cyclophosphamide related lung fibrosis is very low, only isolated case reports of patients in whom cyclophosphamide was the only identifiable etiologic factor for lung toxicity were published. There is no direct dose dependence [62, 63].

Gonadal Dysfunction

Cytotoxic therapy may induce premature menopause or at least temporary amenorrhea as a result of direct ovarian damage causing loss of maturing follicles or failure of follicular recruitment. The incidence of permanent treatment-induced amenorrhea dramatically and continuously increases with age at treatment. The menopause may begin during chemotherapy or subsequently after several years of oligomenorrhea. Although some patients with treatment-induced temporary amenorrhea do display menopausal symptoms, these symptoms are usually indicative or permanent ovarian failure.

Alkylating agents seem to be more particularly responsible for the permanent gonadal failure. The cumulative dose of cyclophosphamide in adjuvant breast cancer chemotherapy appears to be more important than the dose rate. [62, 64]. The addition of taxanes to adjuvant chemotherapy increases the risk of the premature menopause [65].

Quality of Life

Long-term, disease-free breast cancer survivors with no past adjuvant chemotherapy had a better quality of life (QOL) than those who had received adjuvant chemotherapy [66]. Twenty years after adjuvant chemotherapy, 5% of survivors had clinical levels of distress, 15% reported two or more posttraumatic stress disorder symptoms that were moderately to extremely bothersome, 1–6% reported conditioned nausea, emesis, and distress as a consequence of sights, smells, and tastes triggered by reminders of their treatment, and 29%

reported sexual problems attributed to having had cancer. Survivors with persistent physical symptoms long after treatment completion (lymphedema and numbness) that interfered with functioning had significantly more psychologic sequelae compared with survivors with no physical complaints [67].

"Off-treatment" fatigue, weakness, and less vitality are common and distressing symptoms following cancer treatment. No relationship was found between fatigue and extent of treatment or time since treatment completion [68–72]. Cognitive deficits (e.g., problems with memory and concentration) were observed in breast cancer patients receiving adjuvant chemotherapy compared with healthy controls [73, 74]. High-dose chemotherapy appears to impair cognitive functioning more than standard-dose chemotherapy. Central nervous system toxicity may be a dose-limiting factor in high-dose chemotherapy regimens [75].

Recommendations for the Use of Adjuvant Chemotherapy

As adjuvant therapies, prognostic and predictive factors knowledge is a work in progress (dedicated chapters). Nowadays, in clinical practice, recommendations for adjuvant therapies are based on consensus conferences, especially St Gallen experts conferences [76, 77] that take into account two predictive factors: hormonosensitivity and HER 2 status and menopausal status that influences the type of endocrine treatment. Four prognostic factors – tumor size, axillary nodal status, hormonal status, and vascular tumor emboli – determined three groups of risk – low, intermediate. and high.

The St Gallen expert consensus recommends adjuvant systemic treatment for all node-negative premenopausal patients except those at low risk, defined as having pathologic size less or equal to 2 cm, grade 1, ER positive and/or progesterone positive status and age older than 35. Those patients treated with optimal loco-regional therapy have a very good prognosis with overall survival at 8 years equal to 94% [24]. In this low-risk group, no adjuvant treatment or hormonal adjuvant treatment for postmenopausal treatment is required. For the intermediate and high risk node negative group (85% of patients in this classification), adjuvant chemotherapy should be administered to fitted patients, followed by hormonal adjuvant treatment (in case of hormonal status positivity) and trastuzumab in case of HER-2 overexpression: duration of chemotherapy is still debated. However, six cycles of classical CMF is preferred in many countries for HER-2 negative patients (HER 2 positive patients gaining a benefit from anthracyclines-based combinations [78]) as special consideration should be made for late toxicities as absolute overall survival benefit doesn't exceed 5%. In high risk group, six cycles of anthracyclines-based chemotherapy are usually administered. For node positive patients, less than 70 year old, adjuvant chemotherapy is usually administered: sequential regimens three cycles of FEC and three cycles of docetaxel 100 mg/m^2 or four cycles of AC followed by four cycles of paclitaxel (175 mg/m^2), especially in case of negative hormonal status, or combined treatment six cycles of TAC (docetaxel, doxorubicin, cyclophosphamide). For very high risk group, with more than three involved nodes, or basal type (triple negative), other strategies are discussed [79]. New cisplatin-based regimen, or new taxoid (ixabepothilone) tailored a high dose or dose-dense epirubicin-based regimen.

Conclusions

Even if adjuvant chemotherapy for early breast cancer has clearly improved outcome, numerous questions are still unanswered. Little is known on adjuvant chemotherapy for patients more than 70 years old; very young patients probably need tailored treatments [80]. Classical prognostic groups could probably be refined using new molecularly based tools (important on-going trials as MINDACT test this hypothesis) and, moreover, determination of profile of sensitivity to various chemotherapeutic agents should permit one to enhance efficacy and not to overtreat non-responding patients, still the most numerous group.

References

1. Effects of chemotherapy and hormonal therapy for early breast cancer on recurrence and 15-year survival: An overview of the randomised trials. *Lancet*. 2005;365(9472):1687–717.
2. Fisher B, Fisher ER, Redmond C. Ten-year results from the National Surgical Adjuvant Breast and Bowel Project (NSABP) clinical trial evaluating the use of L-phenylalanine mustard (L-PAM) in the management of primary breast cancer. *J Clin Oncol*. 1986;4:929–41.
3. Bonadonna G, Valagussa P, Tancini G, et al. Current status of Milan adjuvant chemotherapy trials for node-positive and node-negative breast cancer. *NCI Monogr*. 1986;4:45–9.
4. Systemic treatment of early breast cancer by hormonal, cytotoxic, or immune therapy. 133 randomised trials involving 31,000 recurrences and 24,000 deaths among 75,000 women. Early Breast Cancer Trialists' Collaborative Group. *Lancet*. 1992;339:1–15.
5. Polychemotherapy for early breast cancer: An overview of the randomised trials. Early Breast Cancer Trialists' Collaborative Group. *Lancet*. 1998;352:930–42.
6. Buzdar AU, Kau SW, Smith TL, et al. Ten-year results of FAC adjuvant chemotherapy trial in breast cancer. *Am J Clin Oncol*. 1989;12:123–8.
7. Bonneterre J, Roche H, Kerbrat P, et al. Epirubicin increases long-term survival in adjuvant chemotherapy of patients with poor-prognosis, node-positive, early breast cancer: 10-year follow-up results of the French Adjuvant Study Group 05 randomized trial. *J Clin Oncol*. 2005;23:2686–93.
8. Hery M, Bonneterre J, Roche H, et al. Epirubicin-based chemotherapy as adjuvant treatment for poor prognosis, node-negative breast cancer: 10-year follow-up results of the French Adjuvant Study Group 03 trial. *Bull Cancer*. 2006;93:E109–E114.
9. Fisher B, Redmond C, Wickerham DL, et al. Doxorubicin-containing regimens for the treatment of stage II breast cancer: The National Surgical Adjuvant Breast and Bowel Project experience. *J Clin Oncol*. 1989;7(5):572–82.

10. Moliterni A, Bonadonna G, Valagussa P, et al. Cyclophosphamide, methotrexate, and fluorouracil with and without doxorubicin in the adjuvant treatment of resectable breast cancer with one to three positive axillary nodes. *J Clin Oncol.* 1991;9:1124–30.
11. Fisher B, Brown AM, Dimitrov NV, et al. Two months of doxorubicin-cyclophosphamide with and without interval reinduction therapy compared with 6 months of cyclophosphamide, methotrexate, and fluorouracil in positive-node breast cancer patients with tamoxifen-nonresponsive tumors: Results from the National Surgical Adjuvant Breast and Bowel Project B-15. *J Clin Oncol.* 1990;8:1483–96.
12. Misset JL, di Palma M, Delgado M. Adjuvant treatment of node-positive breast cancer with cyclophosphamide, doxorubicin, fluorouracil, and vincristine versus cyclophosphamide, methotrexate, and fluorouracil: Final report after a 16-year median follow-up duration. *J Clin Oncol.* 1996;14:1136–1145.
13. Piccart MJ, Di Leo A, Beauduin M, et al. Phase III trial comparing two dose levels of epirubicin combined with cyclophosphamide with cyclophosphamide, methotrexate, and fluorouracil in node-positive breast cancer. *J Clin Oncol.* 2001;19:3103–10.
14. Levine MN, Pritchard KI, Bramwell VH, et al. Randomized trial comparing cyclophosphamide, epirubicin, and fluorouracil with cyclophosphamide, methotrexate, and fluorouracil in premenopausal women with node-positive breast cancer: Update of National Cancer Institute of Canada Clinical Trials Group Trial MA5. *J Clin Oncol.* 2005;23:5166–70.
15. Poole CJ, Earl HM, Hiller L, et al. Epirubicin and cyclophosphamide, methotrexate, and fluorouracil as adjuvant therapy for early breast cancer. N Engl J Med. 2006;355:1851–62.
16. Tancini G, Bonadonna G, Valagussa P, et al. Adjuvant CMF in breast cancer: Comparative 5-year results of 12 versus 6 cycles. *J Clin Oncol.* 1983;1:2–10.
17. Combination adjuvant chemotherapy for node-positive breast cancer. Inadequacy of a single perioperative cycle. The Ludwig Breast Cancer Study Group. *N Engl J Med.* 1988;319:677–83.
18. Fumoleau P, Kerbrat P, Romestaing P, et al. Randomized trial comparing six versus three cycles of epirubicin-based adjuvant chemotherapy in premenopausal, node-positive breast cancer patients: 10-year follow-up results of the French Adjuvant Study Group 01 trial. *J Clin Oncol.* 2003;21:298–305.
19. Henderson IC, Berry DA, Demetri GD, et al. Improved outcomes from adding sequential Paclitaxel but not from escalating Doxorubicin dose in an adjuvant chemotherapy regimen for patients with node-positive primary breast cancer. J Clin Oncol. 2003;21:976–83.
20. Hryniuk WM, Goodyear M. The calculation of received dose intensity. *J Clin Oncol.* 1990;8:1935–37.
21. Wood WC, Budman DR, Korzun AH, et al. Dose and dose intensity of adjuvant chemotherapy for stage II, node-positive breast carcinoma. *N Engl J Med.* 1994;330:1253–59.
22. Bonneterre J, Roche H, Bremond A. Results of a randomized trial of adjuvant therapy with FEC 50 versus FEC 100 in high risk node positive breast cancer patients. *Proc ASCO* 1998;17:473.
23. Fisher B, Anderson S, DeCillis A, et al. Further evaluation of intensified and increased total dose of cyclophosphamide for the treatment of primary breast cancer: Findings from National Surgical Adjuvant Breast and Bowel Project B-25. *J Clin Oncol.* 1999;17:3374–88.
24. Fisher B, Jeong JH, Dignam J, et al. Findings from recent National Surgical Adjuvant Breast and Bowel Project adjuvant studies in stage I breast cancer. *J Natl Cancer Inst Monogr.* 2001;30:62–66.
25. Peters WP, Dansey RD, Klein JL, et al. High-dose chemotherapy and peripheral blood progenitor cell transplantation in the treatment of breast cancer. *Oncologist.* 2000;5:1–13.
26. The Scandinavian breast cancer study group 9401. Results of a randomized adjuvant breast breast cancer study with high dose chemotherapy with CTC [subcript b] supported by autologous bone marrow stem cells versus dose escalated and tailored FEC therapy. *Proc ASCO.* 1999;18,A3.

27. Hortobagyi GN, Buzdar AU. RESPONSE: re: randomized trial of high-dose chemotherapy and blood cell autografts for high-risk primary breast carcinoma. *J Natl Cancer Inst.* 2000;92:1273.
28. Rodenhuis S, Bontenbal M, Beex LV, et al. High-dose chemotherapy with hematopoietic stem-cell rescue for high-risk breast cancer. *N Engl J Med.* 2003;349:7–16.
29. Bonadonna G, Zambetti M, Valagussa P. Sequential or alternating doxorubicin and CMF regimens in breast cancer with more than three positive nodes. Ten-year results. *JAMA.* 1995;273:542–7.
30. Ferguson T, Wilcken N, Vagg R, et al. Taxanes for adjuvant treatment of early breast cancer. *Cochrane Database Syst Rev.* 2007;(4):CD004421.
31. Gehl J, Boesgaard M, Paaske T, et al. Combined doxorubicin and paclitaxel in advanced breast cancer: Effective and cardiotoxic. *Ann Oncol.* 1996;7:687–93.
32. Gianni I, Baselga J, Eiermann W, et al. ECTO Study Group European Cooperative Trial in Operable Breast Cancer: Improved freedom from progression from adding paclitaxel to doxorubicin followed by cyclosphamide methotrexate and fluorouracil. *Proc ASCO.* 2005;23,A513.
33. Gianni L, Munzone E, Capri G, et al. Paclitaxel by 3-hour infusion in combination with bolus doxorubicin in women with untreated metastatic breast cancer: High antitumor efficacy and cardiac effects in a dose-finding and sequence-finding study. *J Clin Oncol.* 1995;13:2688–99.
34. Amadori D, Fabbri M. [Doxorubicin and paclitaxel versus 5-fluorouracil, doxorubicin and cyclophosphamide as first-line treatment in women with metastatic breast carcinoma: final results of a phase III multicenter randomized trial]. *Tumori.* 2001;87:A18–A19.
35. Mamounas EP, Bryant J, Lembersky B, et al. Paclitaxel after doxorubicin plus cyclophosphamide as adjuvant chemotherapy for node-positive breast cancer: Results from NSABP B-28. *J Clin Oncol* 2005;23:3686–96.
36. Citron ML, Berry DA, Cirrincione C, et al. Randomized trial of dose-dense versus conventionally scheduled and sequential versus concurrent combination chemotherapy as postoperative adjuvant treatment of node-positive primary breast cancer: First report of Intergroup Trial C9741/Cancer and Leukemia Group B Trial 9741. *J Clin Oncol.* 2003;21:1431–39.
37. Chan S, Friedrichs K, Noel D, et al. Prospective randomized trial of docetaxel versus doxorubicin in patients with metastatic breast cancer. J Clin Oncol. 1999;17:2341–2354.
38. Martin M, Pienkowski T, Mackey J, et al. Adjuvant docetaxel for node-positive breast cancer. *N Engl J Med.* 2005;352:2302–2313.
39. Roche H, Fumoleau P, Spielmann M, et al. Sequential adjuvant epirubicin-based and docetaxel chemotherapy for node-positive breast cancer patients: The FNCLCC PACS 01 Trial. *J Clin Oncol.* 2006;24:5664–5671.
40. Jones SE, Savin MA, Holmes FA, et al. Phase III trial comparing doxorubicin plus cyclophosphamide with docetaxel plus cyclophosphamide as adjuvant therapy for operable breast cancer. *J Clin Oncol.* 2006;24:5381–87.
41. Goldstein LJ, O'Neill J, Sparano J, et al. E2197:Phase III AT (doxorubicin/docetaxel) vs. AC (doxorubicin/cyclophosphamide) in the adjuvant treatment of node positive and high risk node positive breast cancer. *Proc ASCO.* 2005;23:A512.
42. O'Shaughnessy J. Gemcitabine combination chemotherapy in metastatic breast cancer: Phase II experience. *Oncology* (Williston Park). 2003;17:15–21.
43. Poole C. Adjuvant chemotherapy for early-stage breast cancer: the tAnGo trial. *Oncology* (Williston Park). 2004;18:23–26.
44. Perez E, Muss HB. Optimizing adjuvant chemotherapy in early-stage breast cancer. *Oncology* (Williston Park). 2005;19:1759–67.
45. Shapiro CL, Recht A. Side effects of adjuvant treatment of breast cancer. *N Engl J Med.* 2001;344:1997–2008.

46. Steinherz LJ, Steinherz PG, Tan CT, et al. Cardiac toxicity 4 to 20 years after completing anthracycline therapy. *JAMA*. 1991;266:1672–7.
47. Steinherz LJ. Anthracycline-induced cardiotoxicity. Ann Intern Med. 1997;126:827–828.
48. Von Hoff DD, Rozencweig M, Layard M, et al. Daunomycin-induced cardiotoxicity in children and adults. A review of 110 cases. *Am J Med*. 1977;62:200–8.
49. Von Hoff DD, Layard MW, Basa P, et al. Risk factors for doxorubicin-induced congestive heart failure. *Ann Intern Med*. 1979;91:710–17.
50. Keefe DL. Anthracycline-induced cardiomyopathy. *Semin Oncol*. 2001;28:2–7.
51. Fumoleau P, Roche H, Kerbrat P, et al. Long-term cardiac toxicity after adjuvant epirubicin-based chemotherapy in early breast cancer: French Adjuvant Study Group results. *Ann Oncol*. 2006;17:85–92.
52. Gianni L, Dombernowsky P, Sledge G, et al. Cardiac function following combination therapy with paclitaxel and doxorubicin: an analysis of 657 women with advanced breast cancer. *Ann Oncol*. 2001;12:1067–1073.
53. Praga C, Bergh J, Bliss J, et al. Risk of acute myeloid leukemia and myelodysplastic syndrome in trials of adjuvant epirubicin for early breast cancer: Correlation with doses of epirubicin and cyclophosphamide. *J Clin Oncol*. 2005;23:4179–91.
54. Smith RE, Bryant J, DeCillis A, et al. Acute myeloid leukemia and myelodysplastic syndrome after doxorubicin-cyclophosphamide adjuvant therapy for operable breast cancer: The National Surgical Adjuvant Breast and Bowel Project Experience. *J Clin Oncol*. 2003;21:1195–204.
55. Smith RE. Risk for the development of treatment-related acute myelocytic leukemia and myelodysplastic syndrome among patients with breast cancer: Review of the literature and the National Surgical Adjuvant Breast and Bowel Project experience. *Clin Breast Cancer*. 2003;4:273–9.
56. Smith SM, Le Beau MM, Huo D, et al. Clinical-cytogenetic associations in 306 patients with therapy-related myelodysplasia and myeloid leukemia: The University of Chicago series. *Blood*. 2003;102:43–52.
57. Le Deley MC, Suzan F, Cutuli B, et al. Anthracyclines, mitoxantrone, radiotherapy, and granulocyte colony-stimulating factor: Risk factors for leukemia and myelodysplastic syndrome after breast cancer. *J Clin Oncol*. 2007;25:292–300.
58. Linassier C, Barin C, Calais G, et al. Early secondary acute myelogenous leukemia in breast cancer patients after treatment with mitoxantrone, cyclophosphamide, fluorouracil and radiation therapy. *Ann Oncol*. 2000;11:1289–94.
59. Hershman D, Neugut AI, Jacobson JS, et al. Acute myeloid leukemia or myelodysplastic syndrome following use of granulocyte colony-stimulating factors during breast cancer adjuvant chemotherapy. *J Natl Cancer Inst*. 2007;99:196–205.
60. Muss HB, Berry DA, Cirrincione C, et al. Toxicity of older and younger patients treated with adjuvant chemotherapy for node-positive breast cancer: The Cancer and Leukemia Group B Experience. *J Clin Oncol*. 2007;25:3699–3704.
61. Hudis C, Citron ML, Berry D, et al. Five year follow-up of INT C9741: Dose-dense (DD) chemotherapy (CRx) is safe and effective. *Breast Cancer Res Treat*. 2005;94:A41.
62. Cooper JA, White DA, Matthay RA. Drug-induced pulmonary disease. Part 1: Cytotoxic drugs. *Am Rev Respir Dis*. 1986;133:321–40.
63. Malik SW, Myers JL, DeRemee RA, et al. Lung toxicity associated with cyclophosphamide use. Two distinct patterns. *Am J Respir Crit Care Med*. 1996;154:1851–56.
64. Koyama H, Wada T, Nishizawa Y, et al. Cyclophosphamide-induced ovarian failure and its therapeutic significance in patients with breast cancer. *Cancer*. 1977;39:1403–9.
65. Tham YL, Sexton K, Weiss H, et al. The rates of chemotherapy-induced amenorrhea in patients treated with adjuvant doxorubicin and cyclophosphamide followed by a taxane. *Am J Clin Oncol*. 2007;30:126–132.
66. Ganz PA, Desmond KA, Leedham B, et al. Quality of life in long-term, disease-free survivors of breast cancer: A follow-up study. *J Natl Cancer Inst*. 2002;94:39–49.

67. Kornblith AB, Herndon JE, Weiss RB, et al. Long-term adjustment of survivors of early-stage breast carcinoma, 20 years after adjuvant chemotherapy. *Cancer*. 2003;98:679–89.
68. Andrykowski MA, Curran SL, Lightner R. Off-treatment fatigue in breast cancer survivors: a controlled comparison. *J Behav Med*. 1998;21:1–18.
69. Bower JE, Ganz PA, Desmond KA, et al. Fatigue in long-term breast carcinoma survivors: A longitudinal investigation. *Cancer*. 2006;106:751–758.
70. Broeckel JA, Jacobsen PB, Horton J, et al. Characteristics and correlates of fatigue after adjuvant chemotherapy for breast cancer. *J Clin Oncol*. 1998;16:1689–1696.
71. Goldstein D, Bennett B, Friedlander M, et al. Fatigue states after cancer treatment occur both in association with, and independent of, mood disorder: A longitudinal study. *BMC Cancer*. 2006;6:240.
72. Nieboer P, Buijs C, Rodenhuis S, et al. Fatigue and relating factors in high-risk breast cancer patients treated with adjuvant standard or high-dose chemotherapy: A longitudinal study. *J Clin Oncol*. 2005;23:8296–304.
73. Brezden CB, Phillips KA, Abdolell M, et al. Cognitive function in breast cancer patients receiving adjuvant chemotherapy. *J Clin Oncol*. 2000;18:2695–2701.
74. Wefel JS, Lenzi R, Theriault RL, et al. The cognitive sequelae of standard-dose adjuvant chemotherapy in women with breast carcinoma: Results of a prospective, randomized, longitudinal trial. *Cancer*. 2004;100:2292–99.
75. Van Dam FS, Schagen SB, Muller MJ, et al. Impairment of cognitive function in women receiving adjuvant treatment for high-risk breast cancer: High-dose versus standard-dose chemotherapy. *J Natl Cancer Inst*. 1998;90:210–18.
76. Cinieri S, Orlando L, Fedele P, et al. Adjuvant strategies in breast cancer: New prospectives, questions and reflections at the end of 2007 St Gallen International Expert Consensus Conference. *Ann Oncol*. 2007;18:vi63–vi65.
77. Goldhirsch A, Wood WC, Gelber RD, et al. Progress and promise: highlights of the international expert consensus on the primary therapy of early breast cancer 2007. *Ann Oncol*. 2007;18:1133–44.
78. Gennari A, Sormani MP, Pronzato P, et al. HER2 status and efficacy of adjuvant anthracyclines in early breast cancer: A pooled analysis of randomized trials. *J Natl Cancer Inst*. 2008;100:14–20.
79. Torrisi R, Balduzzi A, Ghisini R, et al. Tailored preoperative treatment of locally advanced triple negative (hormone receptor negative and HER2 negative) breast cancer with epirubicin, cisplatin, and infusional fluorouracil followed by weekly paclitaxel. *Cancer Chemother Pharmacol*. 2008;62(4)667–72.
80. Goldhirsch A, Gelber RD, Yothers G, et al. Adjuvant therapy for very young women with breast cancer: Need for tailored treatments. *J Natl Cancer Inst Monogr*. 2001;93:44–51.

Postoperative Endocrine Therapy for Invasive Breast Cancer

Leisha A. Emens and Nancy E. Davidson

Introduction

Estrogen plays a key role in mammary carcinogenesis, identifying the pathways that regulate estrogen function as major targets for breast cancer therapy. Expression of the estrogen receptor α (ERα) or the progesterone receptor (PR) is a widely recognized predictor of response to hormonal therapy [1]. Studies of endocrine manipulation conducted in advanced breast cancer have revealed response rates of 80% for ER+/PR+ tumors, 40–45% for ER–/PR+ tumors, 25–30% for ER+/PR– tumors, and less than 10% for ER–/PR– tumors. More recently, data have demonstrated that over-expression of ER or PR in at least 1% of breast tumor cells indicates potential responsiveness to endocrine therapy [2, 3]. In the absence of ER or PR expression, endocrine therapy is not indicated. These observations highlight the importance of an accurate measurement of ER and PR expression in the primary tumor in therapeutic decision-making. Currently, quality-controlled quantitative immunohistochemistry is the method of choice [4, 5].

The estrogen pathway can be manipulated by several distinct strategies. Estrogen production itself can be decreased by ovarian ablation/suppression [6] or aromatase inhibitors [7]. Alternatively, ERα activity can be modulated using Tamoxifen or other selective estrogen receptor modulators (SERMs) like Raloxifene [8]. Furthermore, the ERα can be downregulated by Fulvestrant, a selective estrogen receptor destroyer (SERD) [9]. Ovarian function has a major impact on circulating levels of estrogen, and menopausal status drives decision-making when choosing endocrine therapies for women with invasive breast cancer. In premenopausal women, the ovary is the major source of estrogen

L.A. Emens (✉)
Breast Cancer and Tumor Immunology Programs, Department of Oncology, The Johns Hopkins University School of Medicine and the Sidney Kimmel Comprehensive Cancer Center at Johns Hopkins, 1650 Orleans Street, Room 409, Bunting Blaustein Cancer Research Building, Baltimore, MD 21231-1000, USA
e-mail: emensle@jhmi.edu

M. Castiglione, M.J. Piccart (eds.), *Adjuvant Therapy for Breast Cancer*, Cancer Treatment and Research 151, DOI 10.1007/978-0-387-75115-3_10,

production. A smaller amount of estrogen is produced by extragonadal aromatase, which catalyzes the conversion of androstenedione and testosterone to estrone and estradiol respectively. In postmenopausal women, peripheral aromatization is the primary source of estrogen. Therefore, ablating ovarian function by surgical removal, targeted medical suppression, or the indirect effects of chemotherapy is most effective for decreasing estrogen levels in women with intact ovarian function. In contrast, the prevention of extragonadal estrogen production by inhibiting aromatase is the most effective means of decreasing estrogen levels in postmenopausal women. Importantly, the most recent Early Breast Cancer Trialists' Collaborative Group (EBCTCG) overview analysis demonstrated that 5 years of adjuvant Tamoxifen reduced the annual rate of death by 31% among women with ER+ breast cancer, regardless of age [10]. However, recent advances in breast cancer biology have highlighted the heterogeneity of the disease, with gene expression profiles classifying luminal A and luminal B as two distinct biological subtypes of ER+ breast cancer with very different natural histories [11–13]. Further, multiple mechanisms of resistance to endocrine therapy can account for Tamoxifen failure. These include de novo resistance pre-determined by tumor cell biology [14], acquired resistance that develops over time with treatment [15], genetic resistance related to inherited differences in drug metabolism [16], or unresponsive estrogen/progesterone receptor variants [17]. These findings, together with both the emergence of new drugs and the resurgence of old therapies, highlight the complexity of treatment decision-making for women with ER+ disease. Here, we present an overview of the current data guiding the use of endocrine manipulation for early breast cancer treatment, and highlight emerging opportunities for further refinement.

Adjuvant Endocrine Therapy for Premenopausal Women with Early Breast Cancer

About one quarter of newly diagnosed breast cancers occur in women under 50 years of age, a commonly used surrogate for premenopausal status [18]. About 60% of these young women have hormone-responsive tumors [19], and have typically been offered adjuvant Tamoxifen therapy with or without ovarian suppression [20]. Historically, many of these premenopausal women with disease that is potentially hormone-sensitive have also received adjuvant chemotherapy, particularly if there is a high risk of relapse (large tumors or positive lymph nodes) [4]. The use of chemotherapy in women with lymph node-negative ER+ disease has been more controversial. Much of the benefit of chemotherapy may be due to chemotherapy-induced ovarian suppression rather than to the direct cytotoxic effects of chemotherapy in this patient population. These uncertainties have led to two major research initiatives. First, defining the role of ovarian ablation in the management of premenopausal women with early breast cancer is the goal of several ongoing international clinical trials [21]. Second, the development of techniques to define better the relative responsiveness of breast cancers to endocrine manipulation and/or chemotherapy has recently led to a shift in assessing recurrence risk based on tumor biology in addition to tumor size and lymph node status [22–24].

Tamoxifen Alone

The 1995 EBCTCG overview showed that 5 years of Tamoxifen given to women younger than 50 years old resulted in proportional risk reductions in recurrence and mortality of 45 and 32% respectively [25]. A number of randomized trials have defined the role of Tamoxifen in this patient population. The Nolvadex Adjuvant Trial Organization (NATO) [26], the National Surgical Adjuvant Breast and Bowel Project (NSABP) B-14 [27, 28], and the Scottish trials [29–31] tested Tamoxifen therapy alone against observation or placebo. The NSABP and Scottish studies re-randomized patients who remained disease-free after 5 years of Tamoxifen to either stop Tamoxifen or continue it for 5 additional years. All of these clinical trials revealed a substantial benefit for 5 years of Tamoxifen therapy (Table 1). Longer therapy was associated with an increased risk of endometrial cancer in one trial [31], but no additional clinical benefit in any trial. Therefore, 5 years of adjuvant Tamoxifen therapy is currently the standard of care for premenopausal women with hormone receptor-positive early breast cancer.

Tamoxifen plus Chemotherapy

The EBCTCG overview revealed proportional risk reductions of the annual mortality rate for premenopausal women with ER+ breast cancer treated with anthracycline-based chemotherapy plus tamoxifen compared to anthracycline-based chemotherapy alone of 57 and 38% respectively [10]. Tamoxifen has been compared with chemotherapy by the Italian Breast Cancer Adjuvant Study Group (GROCTA) [32] and by the Gynecological Adjuvant Breast Group (GABG) [33]. Although there was no statistically significant difference in outcome in the GROCTA study, those in the GABG study treated with chemotherapy (CMF) had more favorable outcomes (disease free survival (DFS) and overall survival (OS)) than those treated with Tamoxifen alone [33] (Table 1). The Eastern Cooperative Oncology Group ECOG conducted a clinical study testing the efficacy of a doxorubicin-based regimen and 5 or more years of tamoxifen in 533 premenopausal women with lymph node-positive disease; 335 women expressed ERα and 198 women did not. This study demonstrated improved 5 year DFS with the addition of at least 5 years of tamoxifen to chemotherapy for the patients with ER+ disease (78%) compared to those with

Table 1 Trials of adjuvant tamoxifen alone, and tamoxifen with chemotherapy

Study	Patient population	Treatment	Results	Ref
NATO (N = 605)	LN+, premenopausal LN+ or LN-, postmenopausal	Tam 20 mg 2 yr (N = 300) vs No treatment (N = 305)	Better PFS and OS with Tam	[26]
NSABP B-14 (N = 2,644)	LN-, ER+ ≤49 yr and ≥50 yr	Tam 20 mg 5 yr vs Placebo	Tam > placebo DFS 83 vs 77% ; Tam decr RR 44%; No OS difference	[27]
NSABP B-14 Tam > 5 years (N = 1,172)	LN-, ER+ ≤49 yr and ≥50 yr (after 5 yr Tam)	Tam 20 mg 5 more yr (N = 593) vs Placebo (N = 579)	No DFS/OS difference at 4 yr; Tam < placebo at 7 yr	[28]
Scottish trial (N = 1,323)	LN-, premenopausal LN-, postmenopausal	Tam 20 mg 5 yr adjuvant (N = 667) vs Tam 20 mg after relapse (N = 656)	Tam > no treatment DFS/RFS No impact on OS	[29]
Scottish trial Tam beyond 5 yr (N = 342)	LN- (after 5 yr Tam)	Tam 20 mg (N = 173) vs No further therapy (N = 169)	No difference except increase in endometrial cancer with Tam > 5 yr	[30, 31]
GROCTA trial (N = 504)	LN+, ER+ Premenopausal (N = 237)	Tam ×5 yr vs CMF × 6, E × 4 vs CMF × 6, E × 4, Tam × 5 yr	No difference in DFS/OS between Tam and chemo in premenopausal women, except an excess of loco-regional recurrences with Tam	[32]
GABG study (N = 331)	LN+, ER+, <50 yr	CMF × 6 vs Tam × 5 yr	CMF>Tam for DFS/OS	[33]
ECOG study (N = 533)	LN+, ER+ and ER-	chemotherapy vs chemotherapy, Tam X 5–10 yr	Tam no treatment after chemotherapy	[34]
IBCSG 13-93 (N = 1,246)	LN+, pre- and peri-menopausal	AC × 4, CMF × 3, Tam × 5 yr vs AC × 4, CMF × 3, no treatment	Tam>no treatment for DFS	[35]

NATO = Nolvadex Adjuvant Trial Organization; NSABP = National Surgical Adjuvant Breast and Bowel Project; Tam = Tamoxifen; LN = lymph node; ER = estrogen receptor; yr = years; vs = versus; N = number; PFS = progression free survival; OS = overall survival; DFS = disease free survival; decr = decrease; RR = relapse rate; RFS = relapse free survival; GROCTA = Gynecological Adjuvant Breast Group; CMF = cyclophosphamide/metho-trexate/5-fluorouracil; E = epirubicin; DFS = disease-free survival; GABG = Gynecological Adjuvant Breast Group; ECOG = Eastern Cooperative Oncology Group; IBCSG = International Breast Cancer Study Group; AC = Doxorubicin/Cyclophosphamide

ER-negative disease (58%) ($p=0.03$ vs $p=0.63$) [34]. The International Breast Cancer Study Group (IBCSG) Trial 13–93 enrolled 1,246 pre- and perimenopausal patients with lymph node-positive disease, randomizing them to receive chemotherapy alone, or chemotherapy followed by 5 years of Tamoxifen [35]. In this study the addition of Tamoxifen to chemotherapy improved DFS compared to chemotherapy alone in patients with ER+ breast cancers, with a hazard ratio of 0.59 ($p<0.0001$). Tamoxifen was ineffective in those breast cancers classified as ER–, with a hazard ratio of 1.02 ($p=0.89$). An unplanned exploratory analysis revealed that patients with tumors completely devoid of ER expression had a seemingly detrimental effect with the addition of Tamoxifen to chemotherapy, with a hazard ratio of 2.10 ($p=0.04$). Interestingly, those patients with ER+ tumors who experienced chemotherapy-induced amenorrhea had a significantly improved outcome compared to those without chemotherapy-induced amenorrhea (HR = 0.61 for amenorrhea compared to no amenorrhea, $p=0.004$), regardless of whether Tamoxifen therapy was used. This finding highlights the potential importance of directly modulating ovarian estrogen production as primary breast cancer therapy.

Ovarian Ablation/Suppression Alone

The ovaries are the major source of estrogen production in premenopausal women, with a smaller amount of estrogen derived from the peripheral aromatization of androgens. Thus, oophorectomy or ovarian irradiation has been used to ablate ovarian function as breast cancer therapy for over 100 years. Beatson first reported the use of ovarian ablation in the palliation of young women with breast cancer in 1896 [36]. More recently, luteinizing hormone releasing hormone (LHRH) analogues have been used to manipulate ovarian function. These drugs impinge on the hypothalamic-pituitary-ovarian axis to suppress circulating levels of estrogen to post-menopausal levels. Medical suppression has the advantage of lower morbidity, with the potential for restoration of ovarian function upon drug withdrawal to maintain fertility in young premenopausal women. Generally, ovarian ablation and medical ovarian suppression (OA/OS) are considered to have equivalent activity in reducing ovarian function.

Randomized trials of adjuvant ovarian ablation/suppression began in 1948 [6]. The combined analysis of these trials by the EBCTCG conclusively demonstrated that ovarian ablation alone decreases breast cancer recurrence and increases survival in women less than 50 years old [10]. Ovarian ablation/suppression vs not in ER+ breast cancer resulted in an absolute decrease in the 15-year recurrence and mortality rates of 4.3% ($p=0.00001$) and 3.2% ($p=0.004$) respectively. Notably, the efficacy of adjuvant ovarian ablation appeared to be similar to that of adjuvant chemotherapy or Tamoxifen in women less than 50 years old in the early EBCTCG analyses [37]. Ovarian ablation had less impact in women who also received chemotherapy, perhaps due either to the influence of chemotherapy-induced amenorrhea, or due to detrimental interactions between concurrent endocrine therapy and chemotherapy. These are not firm conclusions since they are based on indirect comparisons; incomplete data on ER and PR status were available, and age was used as a surrogate determinant of ovarian function. Moreover, these studies generally did not include Tamoxifen in the chemotherapy arms, nor did they utilize newer chemotherapy regimens containing anthracyclines and taxanes.

Ovarian Ablation/Ovarian Suppression Compared to Chemotherapy

The activity of ovarian ablation suggested by the meta-analyses of the EBCTCG led to multiple clinical trials directly comparing the efficacy of ovarian ablation or ovarian suppression to chemotherapy. Eligibility for these trials was determined by actual menopausal status rather than age; for some of these trials, the hormone receptor status of the tumor was also available. These studies are summarized in Table 2.

The Scottish/Imperial Cancer Research Fund trial randomized women to ovarian ablation or CMF, each with or without 5 years of prednisolone [38]. Follow up at 12 years revealed no difference in event-free survival or OS. Subgroup analysis showed that ovarian ablation improved survival for the 270 women whose tumors expressed ER, whereas CMF improved survival for those women whose tumors did not. A Scandinavian trial compared radiation-induced ovarian failure with nine cycles of intravenous CMF [39]. There was no difference between these treatments, with a hazard ratio of ovarian ablation compared to CMF for DFS of 0.99 at 8.5 years median follow up, and for OS of 1.11 at 10.5 years median follow up. The Takeda Adjuvant Breast Cancer Study with Leuprorelin Acetate (TABLE) study randomized 589 patients with lymph node-positive, ER+ breast cancer to receive six cycles of CMF or 2 years of monthly depot Leuprorelin acetate [40]. No differences in recurrence-free survival or OS emerged. The Zoladex Early Breast Cancer Research Association (ZEBRA) study randomized 1,640 premenopausal women with lymph node-positive breast cancer (80% with ER+ tumors) to six cycles of oral CMF or 2 years of monthly ovarian suppression with goserelin [41]. DFS and OS were equivalent at 6 years median follow up in patients with ER+ disease. Women who developed CMF-related ovarian failure had longer DFS than those who did not; moreover, women with ER- tumors who were treated with CMF had longer DFS than similar women treated with goserelin. Importantly, 76.9% of women treated with CMF remained amenorrheic at 3 years, where as only 22.6% of women treated with goserelin remained amenorrheic at this same time point. Together, these trials support the use of goserelin as a reasonable treatment option for young women with ER+, lymph node-positive breast cancer, particularly those who wish to preserve fertility.

Table 2 Trials assessing the role of adjuvant ovarian ablation/suppression

Study	Patient population	Treatment	Results	Reference
Ovarian ablation vs *chemotherapy*				
Scottish trial (N = 332)	LN+	CMF × 6–8 cycles vs Goserelin x 2 yr	No difference in event-free or OS Goserelin better in HR+ CMF better in HR-	[38]
Scandinavian study (N = 732)	LN+ or T>5 cm HR+	CMF × 9 cycles vs Ovarian irradiation	No difference	[39]
TABLE study (N = 589)	LN+ ER+	CMF × 6 cycles vs Leuprorelin × 2 yr	No difference	[40]
ZEBRA study (N = 1,640)	LN+	CMF × 6 cycles vs Goserelin × 2 yr	No difference for HR+ CMF better for HR-	[41]
Ovarian ablation + chemotherapy				
INT0101 study (N = 1,503)	LN+, ER+	CAF × 6 vs CAF × 6 + Z × 5 yr vs CAF 6 + ZT × 5 yr	Better TTR/DFS with CAFZT No diff OS CAFZ better for <40 yrs?	[44]
ZIPP trial (N = 2,648)* *43% of enrolled patients also received chemotherapy	Stage 1/11	T × 2 yr vs Z × 2 yr vs TZ x 2 yr vs No hormonal Rx	Z better for DFS/OS	[45]
IBCSG 11-93 (N = 174)	LN+, ER+	AC x 4 + OA/OS + T × 5 yr vs OA/OS + T x 5 yr	No difference	[46]
IBCSG VIII (N = 1,063)	Stage 1/11, LN-	Z × 2 yr vs CMF × 6 vs CMF × 6, Z × 1.5 yr	CMF>Z in HR- patients CMF = Z in ER+ patients	[47]

Table 2 (continued)

Study	Patient population	Treatment	Results	Reference
Arriagada et al. (N = 926)*	LN+, high grade *63% HR+ 77% received anthracycline-based chemo	Chemo vs Chemo + OA/OS	No difference overall Lower recurrence <40, ER+	[48]
Ovarian ablation + tamoxifen				
INT0142 (N = 350)* *closed early due to poor accrual	LN-, HR+	T × 5 yr vs OA + T × 5 yr	No difference	[49]
Vietnamese (N = 709)	Stage 1/11	OA + T vs Observation	Better DFS/OS with OA + T	[50]
GROCTA (N = 244)	LN+, HR+	Z + T vs CMF × 6	No difference	[51]
FASG06 (N = 333)	LN+, ER+	Triptorelin × 3 yr + T vs FEC × 6	No difference	[52]
French (N = 162)	LN+, ER+	OA + T vs FAC	No difference	[53]
ABC (OAS) (N = 2,144)	Stage 1/11/III	T +/–chemo + OA/OS vs T +/– chemo	No difference	[54]
ABCSG-5 (N = 1,045)	Stage 1/11, HR+	Z × 3 yr + T × 5 yr vs CMF × 6	Better DFS with Z + T No difference in OS	[55]

N = number; LN = lymph node; CMF = Cyclophosphamide/Methotrexate/5-Fluorouracil; vs = versus; OS = overall; survival; HR = Hormone receptor; Tu = tumor; cm = centimeter; TABLE = Takeda Adjuvant Breast Cancer Study with Leuprorelin; Acetate; ER = Estrogen receptor; ZEBRA = Zoladex Early Breast Cancer Research Association; CAF = Cyclophosphamide/ Doxorubicin/5-Fluororacil; Z = Goserelin; T = Tamoxifen; TTR = time to recurrence; ZIPP = Zoladex in Premenopausal Patients; AC = Doxorubicin/Cyclophosphamide; IBCSG = International Breast Cancer Study Group; OA/OS = ovarian ablation/ovarian suppression; GROCTA = Gruppo di Ricerca in Oncologia Clinica e Terapie Associate; FASG = French Adjuvant Study Group; FEC = 5-Fluorouracil/Epirubicin/Cyclophosphamide; FAC = 5-Fluorouracil/Doxorubicin/Cyclophosphamide; ABC (OAS) = Adjuvant Breast Cancer (Ovarian Ablation Suppression); ABCSG = Adjuvant Breast Cancer Study Group

Ovarian Suppression Combined with Chemotherapy

Younger women are less likely to develop permanent amenorrhea as the result of adjuvant chemotherapy [42]. It has been suggested that these women may be at higher risk of relapse than older premenopausal patients with a higher likelihood of chemotherapy-induced amenorrhea, arguing that ovarian ablation/suppression could be an effective adjuvant therapy for them [43]. At least four studies have examined whether the addition of ovarian ablation to standard adjuvant chemotherapy improves outcomes in young women with early breast cancer (Table 2). The Intergroup study INT0101 enrolled 1,503 eligible premenopausal women with lymph node-positive, ER+ breast cancer, randomizing them to six cycles of oral CAF alone (CAF), six cycles of CAF followed by goserelin (CAF-Z), or six cycles of CAF followed by goserelin and tamoxifen (CAF-ZT) [44]. At a median follow up of 9.6 years, treatment with CAF-ZT improved time to recurrence (TTR) and DFS, but not OS (hazard ratios of 0.73, 0.74, and 0.91 with p values of <0.01, <0.01, and 0.23 respectively). There was no advantage for the addition of goserelin to CAF (CAF-Z). These data are limited by the lack of a treatment arm evaluating the efficacy of CAF and tamoxifen alone, as tamoxifen was not regarded as an active agent for premenopausal women when INT0101 was launched. An unplanned subset analysis suggested that any benefit associated with CAF-Z was limited to patients younger than 40 years old. The Zoladex in Premenopausal Patients (ZIPP) trial used a two by two factorial design in a four arm study comparing 2 years of treatment with tamoxifen, goserelin, tamoxifen and goserelin, or no hormonal therapy [45]. This patient population was heterogeneous: 42% had positive lymph nodes, 56% had ER+ breast cancer, and 43% received adjuvant chemotherapy. At a median follow-up of 5.5 years, goserelin treatment was associated with a 20% decrease in first events ($p=0.002$), and a 19% improvement in OS ($p=0.038$). The clinical benefit was greatest in patients with ER+ tumors, and was less pronounced in those who also received tamoxifen or chemotherapy. The IBCSG Trial 11–93 treated 174 patients, comparing the efficacy of ovarian ablation/suppression combined with tamoxifen and four cycles of anthracycline-based chemotherapy to that of ovarian ablation/suppression combined with tamoxifen alone in premenopausal women with lymph node-positive, ER+ breast cancer [46]. Although the power of the study is small, no differences emerged. The IBCSG VIII trial compared oral CMF followed by 1.5 years of goserelin to either six cycles of oral CMF alone or 2 years of goserelin alone in 1,063 pre- and perimenopausal women with lymph node-negative breast cancer [47]. The majority of these women had ER+ breast cancers. At a median follow up of 5.7 years, CMF was superior to goserelin in patients with ER- disease, but equivalent to goserelin in ER+ patients. Another trial randomized 926 premenopausal patients with positive lymph nodes or high grade breast cancers to adjuvant chemotherapy alone, or adjuvant chemotherapy plus ovarian ablation/suppression (radiation or triptorelin for 3 years) [48]. In this study, 63% of enrolled patients had HR+ tumors, and 77% received anthracycline-based chemotherapy. There was no difference between the treatments arms with regard to 10 year DFS or OS. However, patients younger than 40 years old had a lower rate of recurrence with the addition of ovarian ablation/suppression.

In the aggregate, these trials do not establish a clear benefit for combined ovarian suppression and chemotherapy. However, the subgroup of young premenopausal women less than 40 years of age with ER+ breast cancers who do not become postmenopausal with chemotherapy may benefit from the addition of ovarian ablation. Adequately powered, randomized, prospective clinical trials are essential to define the role of ovarian ablation/suppression in this patient population.

Ovarian Ablation Combined with Tamoxifen

Tamoxifen was not routinely used for the management of premenopausal women with hormone-sensitive breast cancer until after the results of the EBCTCG were released in 1995. These data showed that tamoxifen resulted in a proportional reduction in the risk of recurrence and death of 42% and 32% respectively, regardless of chemotherapy administration [25]. Two trials have examined the addition of tamoxifen to ovarian ablation in the absence of chemotherapy. An Intergroup trial (INT0142) enrolled 350 premenopausal women with lymph node-negative, hormone receptor-positive breast cancer less than 3 cm in size, randomizing them to 5 years of tamoxifen or 5 years of tamoxifen plus ovarian ablation. This trial was closed early due to poor accrual, so the data lack statistical power. Nevertheless, there was no difference between treatment with tamoxifen alone or tamoxifen plus ovarian ablation [49]. The second trial conducted in Southeast Asia enrolled 709 women with early breast cancer, randomizing them to receive oophorectomy plus tamoxifen at the time of primary breast surgery or at first relapse [50]. At a mean follow up of 3.6 years, the 5 year DFS rates were 75% and 58% respectively ($p=0.0075$, adjusted). Corresponding OS rates were 78% and 70% ($p=0.41$, unadjusted). The cost efficacy analysis showed a cost per year of life gained of $351, compared to $11,300 for chemotherapy in the setting of negative lymph nodes, and $5,000 in the setting of positive lymph nodes. These data support oophorectomy and tamoxifen as active and cost-effective first-line adjuvant therapy for premenopausal women with operable hormone-sensitive breast cancer.

Several clinical trials have tested the combination of tamoxifen and ovarian ablation/suppression compared to chemotherapy. The Gruppo di Ricerca in Oncologia Clinica e Terapie Associate (GROCTA) trial compared six cycles of oral CMF to tamoxifen combined with ovarian ablation (surgery, radiation, or 2 years of goserelin) [51]. At a median follow up of 76 months, there was no difference between the treatments. The French Adjuvant Study Group (FASG) 06 trial compared 3 years of tamoxifen plus the LHRH agonist triptoreline to six cycles of FEC in 333 premenopausal women with lymph node-positive,

HR+ breast cancer. At a median follow up of 54 months, there were no significant differences [52]. A small French study compared FAC to ovarian ablation and tamoxifen in women with lymph node-positive, hormone receptor-positive disease [53]. This study similarly showed no difference, although it was underpowered. The Adjuvant Breast Cancer Trialists' Collaborative Group conducted the Ovarian Ablation/Suppression Trial (ABC OAS Trial), enrolling 2,144 pre- and perimenopausal patients receiving 5 years of tamoxifen with or without chemotherapy to receive ovarian ablation/suppression, or no additional therapy. Of these patients, 942 (88%) received ovarian ablation/suppression. Relapse-free survival (RFS) and OS were similar between the two groups, arguing against the addition of ovarian manipulation to standard adjuvant therapy [54]. Finally, the ABCSG conducted a trial of therapy with 3 years of goserelin plus 5 years of tamoxifen to six cycles of intravenous CMF in 1,045 women with Stage I or II hormone receptor-positive breast cancer [55]. At a mean follow up of 42 months, combination endocrine therapy resulted in a statistically significant improvement in DFS compared to CMF ($p=0.02$), with no difference in OS. Notably, the women in the CMF group who developed ovarian failure had significantly longer DFS and OS compared to those who did not. A limitation of all of these trials is that they failed to incorporate tamoxifen into the chemotherapy arms.

Emerging Data Regarding Endocrine Therapy for Premenopausal Women

The role of ovarian ablation in the management of premenopausal women with early breast cancer remains uncertain. Recently, the EBCTCG reported a meta-analysis of 11,906 premenopausal women with early breast cancer randomized in 16 trials of LHRH agonists [56]. While the use of LHRH agonists alone was ineffective therapy for hormone receptor-positive tumors, the addition of LHRH agonists to tamoxifen, chemotherapy, or both reduced recurrence by 12.7% ($p=0.02$), and death after recurrence by 15.1% ($p=0.03$). LHRH agonists showed a similar efficacy to chemotherapy, but no trials assessed an LHRH agonist compared to chemotherapy, each followed by tamoxifen. LHRH agonists were ineffective in hormone receptor-negative tumors. Several randomized Phase III clinical trials are prospectively evaluating the role of ovarian ablation/suppression with tamoxifen or an aromatase inhibitor as a component of primary therapy for ER+ breast cancer (Table 3). Additionally, the Oncotype Dx test, a 21-gene risk stratification tool, has recently emerged as a means of determining recurrence risk and guiding therapeutic decision-making [23, 24]. In retrospective studies, women with ER+, lymph node-negative tumors and a high recurrence score appear to benefit from the addition of chemotherapy to endocrine therapy to decrease the risk of relapse, whereas those with low to intermediate recurrence scores benefit primarily from endocrine therapy. A large, prospective trial (TAILORx) has been launched in the United States to validate

Table 3 Ongoing clinical trials of ovarian ablation/suppression

Trial	Patient population	Intervention
ABCSG-12	Premenopausal Stage I/II/III HR+	G + A vs G + A + Z vs G + T vs G + T + Z
IBSCG 24-02/BIG 2-02: SOFT	Premenopausal HR+ No adjuvant chemotherapy or premenopausal after adjuvant chemotherapy	T vs OS + T vs OS + AI
IBSCG 25-02/BIG 3-02: TEXT	Premenopausal women with HR+ tumors who require OS with or without chemotherapy from the start of adjuvant therapy	OS + T vs OS + AI

ABCSG = Adjuvant Breast Cancer Study Group; BIG = Breast International Group; HR = hormone receptor; G = Goserelin; A = anastrozole; Z = Zolendronate; T = Tamoxifen; IBSCG = International Breast Cancer Study Group; SOFT = Suppression of Ovarian Function Trial; AI = aromatase inhibitor; TEXT = Tamoxifen and Exemestane Trial

Oncotype Dx as a tool that can be used to tailor adjuvant therapy to the biology of the primary breast tumor [57]. Finally, for hormone receptor-positive tumors, it is clear that over 50% of recurrences and over 66% of breast cancer deaths occur more than 5 years after diagnosis [10, 25, 58]. This observation, along with the results of the MA.17 trial discussed below, supports the concept of extending endocrine treatment beyond 5 years, which is the current standard. Currently, the Adjuvant Tamoxifen: Longer Against Shorter (ATLAS) trial, and the Adjuvant Tamoxifen Treatment, Offer More? (ATTOM) trials are following women treated with Tamoxifen for up to 10 years [59]. The ATLAS study is comparing 5–10 years of adjuvant Tamoxifen therapy, and the ATTOM trial is randomizing women who discontinue Tamoxifen treatment after at least 2 years to receive an additional 5 years of Tamoxifen or no additional therapy. In the interim, 5 years of tamoxifen is standard for premenopausal women with hormone receptor-positive breast cancer.

Adjuvant Endocrine Therapy in Postmenopausal Women

As discussed above, for the last 30 years tamoxifen was the drug of choice for postmenopausal women with hormone receptor positive-breast cancer. It cuts the risk of both disease recurrence and new contralateral breast cancers by about 50%, and reduces mortality by about 31% [10, 25]. However, tamoxifen therapy is discontinued by 23–40% of patients who take it because of issues related to quality of life. Risks of tamoxifen therapy include hot flashes, vaginal bleeding and discharge, endometrial cancer, hysterectomy, ischemic cerebrovascular events, and venous thromboembolic events. Multiple third generation aromatase inhibitors have been developed as an alternative to tamoxifen for postmenopausal women. Of these drugs, anastrozole, letrozole, and exemestane are currently available in the United States.

Aromatase Inhibitors Instead of Tamoxifen

Several studies have examined the activity of initial adjuvant treatment with aromatase inhibitors (Table 4). The Arimidex, Tamoxifen, Alone or in Combination (ATAC) trial compared 5 years of therapy with anastrozole alone, tamoxifen alone, or the combination of anastrozole and tamoxifen in 9,366 postmenopausal women with hormone receptor-positive early breast cancer [60]. The primary endpoints of this study were DFS and safety/tolerability. At first analysis, with a median follow-up of 33 months, treatment with anastrozole resulted in a better DFS than treatment with tamoxifen (89.4 vs 87.4% respectively; p=0.13). Results for the combination arm were not significantly better than the tamoxifen alone arm, so it was closed. Notably, treatment with anastrozole also reduced the incidence of contralateral breast cancers and distant metastases by 42 and 14% respectively as compared to tamoxifen. Anastrozole

Table 4 Trials comparing initial tamoxifen with aromatase inhibition

Study	Patient population	Intervention	Results	Ref
ATAC (N = 9,366)	Postmenopausal	A × 5 yr vs T × 5 yr vs A + T × 5 yr	A>T for DFS A+T = T	[60, 61]
BIG I-98 (N = 8,028)	Postmenopausal ER+ and/or PR+	T × 5 yr vs L × 5 yr vs T × 2 yr, L × 3 yr vs L × 2 yr, T × 3 yr	L>T for DFS* L>T for distant recurrence *T compared to L upfront only	[62, 63]
TEAM	Postmenopausal	T × 5 yr vs E × 5 yr vs T × 2 yr, E × 3 yr vs E × 2 yr, T × 3 yr	NR, ongoing	–

ATAC = Arimidex, Tamoxifen, Alone or in Combination; A = Arimidex; T = Tamoxifen; DFS = disease-free survival; BIG = Breast International Group; ER = estrogen receptor; PR = progesterone receptor; L = Letrozole; TEAM = Tamoxifen and Exemestane Adjuvant Multicenter; E = Exemestane; NR = not reported was better tolerated with regard to hot flashes, thromboembolic events, endometrial cancer, vaginal bleeding, and cerebrovascular events, but resulted in a higher rate of musculoskeletal symptoms, bone density loss, and bone fractures. The ATAC trial was recently updated at 68 months of follow up; at this time only 8% of patients remained on therapy [61]. The DFS for anastrozole compared with tamoxifen was superior, with a hazard ratio of 0.87 (p=0.002), and an absolute difference of 3.7% between the two arms. There is no statistically significant OS difference between the two arms. Based on these data, the U.S. Food and Drug Administration (FDA) approved anastrozole as initial adjuvant endocrine therapy for postmenopausal women with ER+ early breast cancer.

The Breast International Group (BIG) 1-98 trial randomized 8,028 postmenopausal women with hormone receptor-positive breast cancer to 5 years of tamoxifen alone, 5 years of letrozole alone, 2 years of tamoxifen followed by 3 years of letrozole, or 2 years of letrozole followed by 3 years of tamoxifen. The first analysis of this study compared the two groups assigned to initial tamoxifen therapy (4,007 patients) to the two groups assigned to initial letrozole therapy (4,003 patients). At a median follow up of 25.8 months, letrozole significantly improved DFS compared to tamoxifen, with a hazard ratio of 0.81 (p=0.003) [62]. Five-year DFS estimates were 84% for the letrozole group and 81.4% for the tamoxifen group, for an absolute difference of 2.6% between the two groups. Letrozole therapy was associated with decreased rates of distant recurrence, with a hazard ratio of 0.73 (p=0.001). A subsequent update at a median follow up of 51 months revealed an 18% reduction in the risk of recurrence, with a hazard ratio of 0.82 (p=0.007) [63]. These results are similar to the results of the ATAC study; the spectrum of side effects for aromatase inhibition and tamoxifen were also similar to those observed in the ATAC trial. There is currently no significant difference in OS between these two groups. Based on these data, letrozole was approved by the U.S. FDA for the adjuvant treatment of postmenopausal women with early ER+ breast cancer. Data from the sequential arms are not yet available.

The Tamoxifen and Exemestane Adjuvant Multicenter (TEAM) trial was designed to randomize 4,400 postmenopausal patients with early breast cancer to exemestane or tamoxifen for 5 years [64]. Based on the results of the Intergroup Exemestane Study (IES) showing that Exemestane given after 2–3 years of Tamoxifen improves DFS compared to tamoxifen alone (discussed below), the TEAM trial has been amended to permit those initially randomized to receive tamoxifen to cross over to exemestane.

Aromatase Inhibitors After Tamoxifen

Several randomized trials have further analyzed the sequential use of tamoxifen and aromatase inhibitors (Table 5). The Italian ITA study randomized 426 postmenopausal women with hormone receptor-positive breast cancer who had

Table 5 Trials testing aromatase inhibitors in sequence with tamoxifen

Study	Patient population	Intervention	Result	Ref
Italian ITA (N=426)	Postmenopausal, HR+	T × 2 yr, T × 3 yr vs T × 2 yr, A × 3 yr	T+A>T for RFS	[65]
ABCSG-8/ ARNO (N=3,224)	Postmenopausal, HR+	T × 2 yr, T × 3 yr vs T × 2 yr, A × 3 yr	T+A>T for DFS, OS	[66, 67]
IES (N=4,742)	Postmenopausal, ER+ and/or PR+	T × 2–3 yr, T × 2–3 yr vs T × 2–3 yr, E × 2–3 yr	T+E>T for DFS, OS	[68, 69]
NCIC-CTG MA.17 (N=5,187)	Postmenopausal ER+ and/or PR+	T × 5 yr, P × 5 yr vs T × 5 yr, L × 5 yr	T+L>T for DFS T+L>T for OS if LN+	[70, 71]

HR = hormone receptor; T = Tamoxifen; A = Anastrozole; RFS = relapse-free survival; ABCSG = Austrian Breast and Colorectal Cancer Study Group; ARNO = German Adjuvant Breast Cancer Group; DFS = disease-free survival; OS = overall survival; IES = Intergroup Exemestane Study Group; ER = estrogen receptor; PR = progesterone receptor; E = exemestane; NCIC-CTG MA.17 = National Cancer Institute of Cancer Clinical Trials Group MA.17 Trial; P = placebo; L = Letrozole; LN = lymph node

already completed 2 years of tamoxifen to continue tamoxifen to complete a total of 5 years, or to switch to anastrozole for 3 years to complete a total of 5 years of endocrine therapy [65]. At a median follow up of 64 months, sequential therapy with tamoxifen and anastrozole resulted in improved event-free and RFS, with hazard ratios of 0.57 (p=0.005) and 0.56 (p=0.01) respectively. There was a trend toward fewer deaths in the anastrozole group, although this did not reach statistical significance. The Austrian Breast and Colorectal Cancer Study Group (ABSCG)-8 and the Arimidex-Nolvadex (ARNO) trials randomized a combined total of 3,224 postmenopausal women who had been on tamoxifen for 2 years to continue tamoxifen to complete a total of 5 years of treatment, or to switch to anastrozole for 3 years to complete a total of 5 years of endocrine therapy [66]. At a median follow up of 28 months, sequential therapy with tamoxifen and anastrozole resulted in a 41% proportional improvement in DFS (p=0.0009). At this time, there was a 3.1% absolute improvement in event-free survival. An updated analysis revealed that, at a median follow up of 30.1 months, there was a 39% reduction in the relative risk of disease recurrence or death, with a hazard ratio of 0.61 (p=0.01) [67]. It also revealed a survival benefit for sequential therapy, with 15 deaths in the group treated with tamoxifen followed by anastrozole compared to 28 deaths in the group treated with tamoxifen alone (p=0.045). The International Exemestane Study (IES) randomized 4,742 postmenopausal women with hormone receptor-positive breast cancer who had already received 2–3 years of adjuvant tamoxifen to complete 5 years total of tamoxifen, or switch to exemestane to complete a total of 5 years of endocrine therapy [68]. At a median follow up of 36 months, sequential treatment with tamoxifen and exemestane resulted in proportional and absolute reductions in the risk of recurrence of 32 and 4.7% respectively ($p=0.0005$). Subsequent analysis of these data showed that the DFS benefit was maintained, with a hazard ratio of 0.76 ($p=0.0001$), and a statistically significant survival benefit was associated with sequential therapy in the ER+/ER unknown subgroup of patients. At the most recent report of these results with a median follow up of 55.7 months, there was a 24% improvement in DFS with exemestane therapy, with a hazard ratio of 0.76 ($p=0.0001$), and an absolute benefit of 3.3% [69]. Further, there was a 15% improvement in OS in this group, with a hazard ratio of 0.85 ($p=0.08$). It is important to remember that only those patients who had completed 2–3 years of tamoxifen without early recurrence were included in this study, so it is a highly selected patient population compared to those populations treated initially with endocrine therapy in the ATAC or BIG 1-98 studies.

Finally, the MA.17 trial randomized 5,187 women to 5 years of letrozole or placebo after completing 5 years of adjuvant tamoxifen therapy [70, 71]. At a median follow up of 30 months, letrozole was associated with a statistically significantly better DFS and distant DFS than placebo, with HRs of 0.58 ($p<0.001$) and 0.60 ($p=0.002$) respectively. There was no difference between the arms for OS. However, the OS of lymph node-positive patients was significantly improved with letrozole, with a HR of 0.61 ($p=0.04$).

The data were unblinded in October 2003, and all patients were offered open-label letrozole. Among the 2,594 women initially randomized to placebo, 1,655 chose to receive open-label letrozole. As a group, these women were younger, had disease at higher risk for relapse, and were more likely to have been treated with chemotherapy than those who did not choose to take letrozole. At 54 months of follow up, there was a statistically significant improvement in DFS in women who chose to take letrozole, with a hazard ratio of 0.31 ($p<0.0001$) [72]. Thus, women with hormone-sensitive breast cancer may benefit from letrozole therapy even after a significant period of time off tamoxifen therapy. Based on the results of the MA.17 study, the U.S. FDA approved letrozole as extended adjuvant endocrine therapy after 5 years of tamoxifen.

A retrospective analysis of this study demonstrated that the impact of letrozole compared to placebo may be greatest in women with ER+/PR+ tumors [73]. Furthermore, data from cohorts of patients defined by randomization date (12, 24, 36, and 48 months) revealed a significant decrease in the risk of recurrence with letrozole treatment regardless of time from randomization [74]. The hazard ratios for DFS continued to decrease over time, from 0.52 at 12 months to 0.19 at 48 months. This observation suggests that longer letrozole exposure affords greater clinical benefit, at least out to 48 months. The MA.17R trial is an extension of the MA.17 trial that randomly assigns patients to either five more years of letrozole, or to observation. This study will provide data guiding the optimal duration of treatment for efficacy in addition to long-term toxicity for patients treated over 10 years from initial diagnosis.

No direct comparisons of the aromatase inhibitors in the adjuvant setting have been reported. MA.27 is a randomized, Phase III trial comparing 5 years of anastrozole to 5 years of exemestane as initial therapy for patients with early hormone receptor-positive breast cancer. The Femara vs Anastrozole Clinical Evaluation (FACE) trial is a randomized Phase III study comparing the efficacy and safety of letrozole and anastrozole in postmenopausal patients with lymph node-positive early breast cancer.

A small trial conducted by the Austrian Breast and Colorectal Cancer Study Group (ABCSG), trial ABCSG 6a, examined the addition of 3 years of adjuvant anastrozole therapy after the completion of 5 years of adjuvant tamoxifen therapy [75]. There was longer event-free survival in women who received sequential therapy compared to 5 years of tamoxifen alone with or without aminoglutethimide. Finally, a meta-analysis of the "switching trials", with 4,006 patients and a median follow up of 30 months, confirmed an improvement in DFS, with a hazard ratio of 0.59 ($p=0.0001$) [76]. The hazard ratio for OS was 0.71 ($p=0.038$).

All of the clinical trials examining the efficacy of adjuvant aromatase inhibitors have demonstrated an adverse effect on bone mineral density. A subprotocol of the ATAC trial studied 308 patients from the study, and a control group of 46 nonrandomized postmenopausal patients with invasive, early breast cancer who did not receive endocrine therapy [77]. Anastrozole was associated with a decrease in bone mineral density in the spine and hip at both 1 and 2 years, whereas tamoxifen was associated with an increase. The rate of bone loss with anastrozole occurred at a constant rate over the 2-year period. The analysis of bone mineral density at 5 years showed that bone loss continued unabated in the hip, but that the rate of bone loss decreased in the lumbar spine ($p=0.0002$). Importantly, no patient with a normal baseline bone density developed osteoporosis by 5 years. A similar analysis was performed on the IES study [78]. Within 6 months of switching to exemestane, baseline bone mineral density was lowered by 2.7% ($p<0.0001$) at the lumbar spine and 1.4% ($p<0.0001$) at the hip. Bone mineral density decreases were only 1.0% ($p=0.002$) and 0.8% ($p=0.003$) in year 2 at the lumbar spine and hip, respectively. No patient with normal bone mineral density at trial entry developed osteoporosis. The NCIC CTC MA.17 study also reported similar findings [79]; 226 patients (122 letrozole, 104 placebo) were enrolled. At 24 months, patients receiving letrozole had a significant decrease in total hip and lumbar spine bone mineral density compared to those receiving placebo, with a loss of 3.6% compared to 0.71% ($p=0.044$) and 5.35% compared to 0.70% ($p=0.008$) respectively. No patient developed osteoporosis in the hip, whereas at the L2-L4 (posteroanterior view), more women developed osteoporosis while receiving letrozole compared to those receiving placebo, at 4.1 and 0% respectively ($p=0.064$). Other side effects commonly reported with the use of aromatase inhibitors are hot flashes and arthralgias. Aromatase inhibitors may also adversely impact the lipid profile, potentially resulting in a slight increase in cardiovascular disease; this is under active investigation.

Recommendations for Adjuvant Endocrine Therapy from Consensus Meetings

Several consensus statements about the use of adjuvant endocrine therapy have been released. In 2000, the United States NIH Consensus Development Conference on the Adjuvant Therapy for Breast Cancer concluded that standard adjuvant chemotherapy should be recommended for the majority of premenopausal women with early stage breast cancer. Women with ER+ breast cancer should be given tamoxifen for 5 years, with consideration of ovarian ablation/suppression as an alternative to tamoxifen for selected women. The panel concluded that there was insufficient evidence to support the addition of ovarian ablation/suppression to standard adjuvant chemotherapy combined with tamoxifen [80]. The American Society of Clinical Oncology convened a Technology Assessment Panel in 2002, 2003, and 2004 to review data on the use of aromatase inhibitors in the adjuvant setting. The panel concluded that the optimal adjuvant endocrine therapy for postmenopausal women with hormone sensitive breast cancer should include an aromatase inhibitor as initial therapy, or after a period of tamoxifen therapy [81].

The 2005 International Consensus Conference on the Adjuvant Therapy of Primary Breast Cancer emphasized that the first consideration for adjuvant breast cancer therapy should be the endocrine responsiveness of the tumor [22]. The Conference defined breast cancers as endocrine-responsive, endocrine-nonresponsive, and tumors of uncertain endocrine responsiveness, with each category further divided by menopausal status. Importantly, axillary lymph node involvement itself did not define high risk. Intermediate risk tumors included lymph node-negative disease if the primary tumor presented high risk features, and lymph node-positive disease (one to three positive lymph nodes) if the tumor did not present high risk features. The panel recommended chemotherapy for endocrine-nonresponsive disease, endocrine therapy for endocrine-responsive disease, and the combination of endocrine therapy and chemotherapy for some intermediate and all high risk disease. Both endocrine therapy and chemotherapy were recommended for tumors of uncertain endocrine responsiveness, except for those tumors in the low risk category (small, lymph node-negative tumors).

Lingering Questions, Emerging Considerations and Future Directions for Research

Despite its longstanding use as the mainstay of therapy for hormone-responsive breast cancer, many issues remain unresolved regarding distinct aspects of endocrine manipulation. For premenopausal women, the benefit of adding ovarian ablation/suppression to those premenopausal women who do not become amenorrheic as the result of adjuvant chemotherapy remains unknown, and ongoing clinical trials are addressing this issue. These trials are also testing the use of combined endocrine therapy with ovarian ablation/suppression and aromatase inhibition in this setting. The appropriate duration of the use of medical ovarian suppression also remains unknown—most clinical trials have continued LHRH analogues for 2–3 years. For postmenopausal women, the optimal use of aromatase inhibition remains to be defined. The most appropriate sequencing strategy with tamoxifen, the optimal duration of therapy, and the optimal aromatase inhibitor remain unknown. It is critical to remember that aromatase inhibitors are contraindicated in women who are premenopausal, and should be used with extreme caution in women with chemotherapy-induced amenorrhea [82]. For both premenopausal and postmenopausal women, the long-term sequelae of estrogen deprivation with ovarian ablation/suppression and/or aromatase inhibition are also unknown. Finally, host and tumor biology are becoming increasingly important in therapeutic decision-making. Pharmacogenomic variables impacting the efficacy of endocrine therapy have emerged as important considerations in choosing tamoxifen therapy, and molecular determinants of tumor biology distinct from the endocrine signaling pathways have been suggested as potential predictors of improved response to therapy with aromatase inhibitors as compared to tamoxifen.

References

1. Osborne CK, Yochmowitz MG, Knight WA III, McGuire WL. The value of estrogen and progesterone receptors in the treatment of breast cancer. *Cancer*. 1980;46(12 Suppl):2884–8.
2. Harvey J, Clark G, Osborne C, Allred D. Estrogen receptor status by immunohistochemistry is superior to the ligand-binding assay for predicting response to adjuvant endocrine therapy in breast cancer. *J Clin Oncol*. 1999;17:1474–81.
3. Mohsin S, Wiess H, Gutierrez M, et al. Neoadjuvant Trastuzumab induces apoptosis in primary breast cancers. *J Clin Oncol*. 2005;23:2460–8.
4. Goldhirsch A, Wood W, Gelber R, et al. Meeting highlights: Updated international expert consensus on the primary therapy of early breast cancer. *J Clin Oncol*. 2003; 21:3357–65.
5. Zafrani B, Aubriot H, Mouret E, et al. High sensitivity and specificity of immunohistochemistry for the detection of hormone receptors in breast carcinoma: Comparison with biochemical determination in a prospective study of 793 cases. *Histopathol*. 2000; 37:536–45.
6. Clarke M. Ovarian ablation in breast cancer, 1896–1998: Milestones along hierarchy of evidence from case report to Cochrane review. *BM J*. 1998;317:1246–8.
7. Smith IE, Dowsett M. Aromatase inhibitors in breast cancer. *N Engl J Med*. 2003; 348:2431–42.
8. Osborne CK, Zhao H, Fuqua SA. Selective estrogen receptor modulators: Structure, function, and clinical use. *J Clin Oncol*. 2000;18(17):3172–86.
9. Dauvois S, Danielian PS, White R, Parker MG. Antiestrogen ICI 164,384 reduces cellular estrogen receptor content by increasing its turnover. *Proc Natl Acad Sci U S A*. 1992; 89(9):4037–41.
10. Early Breast Cancer Trialists' Collaborative Group (EBCTCG). Effects of chemotherapy and hormonal therapy for early breast cancer on recurrence and 15-year survival: An overview of the randomized trials. *Lancet*. 2005;365:1687–717.

11. Perou C, Sorlie T, Eisen M, et al. Molecular portraits of human breast tumors. *Nature*. 2000; 406:747–52.
12. Sorlie T, Perou C, Tibshirani R, et al. Gene expression patterns of breast carcinomas distinguish tumor subclasses with clinical implications. *Proc Natl Acad Sci U S A*. 2001; 98(19):10869–74.
13. Sorlie T, Tibshirani R, Parker J, et al. Repeated observation of breast tumor subtypes in independent gene expression data sets. *Proc Natl Acad Sci U S A*. 2003;100(14):8418–23.
14. Dowsett M, Harper-Wynne C, Beoddinghaus I, et al. HER-2 amplification impedes the antiproliferative effects of hormone therapy in estrogen receptor-positive primary breast cancer. *Cancer Res*. 2001;61:8452–8.
15. Moy B, Goss P. Estrogen receptor pathways: resistance to endocrine therapy and new therapeutic approaches. *Clin Cancer Res*. 2006;15:4790–3.
16. Choi J, Nowell S, Blanco J, Ambrosone C. The role of genetic variability in drug metabolism pathways in breast cancer prognosis. *Pharmacogenomics* 2006;7:613–24.
17. Wiebe V, Osborne C, Fuqua S, DeGregorio M. Tamoxifen resistance in breast cancer. *Crit Rev Oncol Hematol*. 1993;14:173–88.
18. Smigal C, Jemal A, Ward E, et al. Trends in breast cancer by race and ethnicity: Update 2006. *CA Cancer J for Clinicians*. 2006;56:168–83.
19. Pujol P, Daures J, Thezenas S, et al. Changing estrogen and progesterone receptor patterns in breast carcinoma during the menstrual cycle and menopause. *Cancer*. 1998; 83:698–705.
20. Goldhirsch A, Glick J, Gelber R, et al. Meeting highlights: International consensus panel on the treatment of primary breast cancer. Seventh international conference on adjuvant therapy of primary breast cancer. *J Clin Oncol*. 2001;19(18):3817–27.
21. Prowell T, Davidson N. What is the role of ovarian ablation in the management of primary and metastatic breast cancer today? *Oncologist*. 2004;9:507–17.
22. Goldhirsch A, Glick J, Gelber R, et al. Meeting highlights: International expert consensus on the primary therapy of early breast cancer 2005. *Annals Oncol*. 2005;16:1569–83.
23. Paik S, Shak S, Tang G, et al. A multigene assay to predict recurrence of tamoxifen-related, node-negative breast cancer. *N Engl J Med*. 2004;351:2817–26.
24. Paik S, Tang G, Shak S, et al. Gene expression and benefit of chemotherapy in women with node-negative, estrogen-receptor-positive breast cancer. *J Clin Oncol*. 2006; 24:3726–34.
25. Early Breast Cancer Clinical Trialists' Collaborative Group (EBCTCG). Tamoxifen for early breast cancer: Overview of the randomized trials. *Lancet*. 1998;351:1451–67.
26. Nolvadex Adjuvant Trial Organization (NATO). Controlled trial of tamoxifen as a single adjuvant agent in the management of early breast cancer. *Br J Cancer*. 1988;57:608–11.
27. Fisher B, Costantino J, Redmond C, et al. A randomized clinical trial evaluating tamoxifen in the treatment of patients with node-negative breast cancer who have estrogen-receptor-positive tumors. *N Engl J Med*. 1989;320:479–84.
28. Fisher B, Dignam J, Bryant J, Wolmark N. Five versus more than five years of tamoxifen for lymph node-negative breast cancer: Updated findings from the National Surgical Adjuvant Breast and Bowel Project B-14 randomized trial. *J Natl Cancer Inst*. 2001;93:684–90.
29. Stewart H. The Scottish trial of adjuvant tamoxifen in node-negative breast cancer. *J Natl Cancer Inst*. 1992;11:117–20.
30. Stewart H, Forrest A, Everington D, et al. Randomised controlled trial of conservation therapy for breast cancer: 6-year analysis of the Scottish trial. Scottish Cancer Trials Breast Group. *Lancet*. 1996;348:708–13.
31. Stewart H, Prescott R, Forrest A. Scottish adjuvant tamoxifen trial: A randomized study updated to 15 years. *J Natl Cancer Inst*. 2001;93:456–62.
32. Boccardo F, Amoroso D, Rubagotti A, et al. Endocrine therapy of breast cancer: The experience of the Italian cooperative group for chemohormonal therapy of early breast cancer. *Annals New York Acad Sci*. 1993;698:318–29.

33. Kaufmann M, Jonat W, Abel U, et al. Adjuvant randomized trials of doxorubicin/cyclophosphamide versus doxorubicin/cyclophosphamide/tamoxifen and CMF chemotherapy versus tamoxifen in women with node-positive breast cancer. *J Clin Oncol.* 1993;11:454–60.
34. Tormey DC, Gray R, Abeloff MD, et al. Adjuvant therapy with a doxorubicin regimen and long-term tamoxifen in premenopausal breast cancer patients: An Eastern Cooperative Oncology Group trial. *J Clin Oncol.* 1992;10:1848–56.
35. Colleoni M, Gelber S, Goldhirsch A, et al. Tamoxifen after adjuvant chemotherapy for premenopausal women with lymph node-positive breast cancer: International Breast Cancer Study Group Trial 13-93. *J Clin Oncol.* 2006;24:1332–41.
36. Beatson G. On the treatment of inoperable cases of carcinoma of the mamm: Suggestions for new method of treatment. *Lancet.* 1896;2:104–7.
37. Early Breast Cancer Trialists' Collaborative Group (EBCTCG). Ovarian ablation in early breast cancer: overview of the randomized trials. *Lancet.* 1996;348:1189–96.
38. Scottish Cancer Trials Breast Group and ICRF, Breast Unit, Guy's Hospital, London. Adjuvant ovarian ablation versus CMF chemotherapy in premenopausal women with pathological stage II breast carcinoma: the Scottish trial. *Lancet.* 1993;341:1293–8.
39. Ejlertsen B, Mouridsen H, Jensen M, et al. Similar efficacy for ovarian ablation compared with cylcophosphamide, methotrexate, and fluorouracil: From a randomized comparison of premenopausal patients with node-positive, hormone receptor-positive breast cancer. *J Clin Oncol.* 2006;24:4956–62.
40. Schmid P, Untch M, Wallwiener D, et al. Cyclophosphamide, methotrexate and fluorouracil (CMF) versus hormonal ablation with leuprorelin acetate as adjuvant treatment of node-positive, premenopausal breast cancer patients: preliminary results of the TABLE-study (Takeda Adjuvant Breast cancer study with Leuprorelin Acetate). *Anticancer Res.* 2002;22:2325–32.
41. Jonat W, Kaufmann M, Sauerbrei W, et al. Goserelin versus cyclophosphamide, methotrexate, and fluorouracil as adjuvant therapy in premenopausal patients with node-positive breast cancer: The Zoladex Early Breast Cancer Research Association study. *J Clin Oncol.* 2002;20:4628–35.
42. Petrek J, Naughton M, Case L, et al. Incidence, time course, and determinants of menstrual bleeding after breast cancer treatment: A prospective study. *J Clin Oncol.* 2006;24:1045–51.
43. Goldhirsch A, Gelber R, Yothers G, et al. Adjuvant therapy for very young women with breast cancer: need for tailored treatments. *J Natl Cancer Inst Monogr.* 2001;30:44–51.
44. Davidson N, O'Neill A, Vukov A, et al. Chemoendocrine therapy for premenopausal women with axillary lymph node-positive, steroid hormone receptor-positive breast cancer: Results from INT0101 (E5188). *J Clin Oncol.* 2005;23:5973–82.
45. Baum M, Hackshaw A, Houghton J, et al. Adjuvant goserelin in pre-menopausal patients with early breast cancer: Results from the ZIPP study. *Eur J Cancer.* 2006;42:895–904.
46. International Breast Cancer Research Study Group. Randomized controlled trial of ovarian function suppression plus tamoxifen versus the same endocrine therapy plus chemotherapy: Is chemotherapy necessary for premenopausal women with node-positive, endocrine-responsive breast cancer? First results of International Breast Cancer Study Group Trial 11–93. *Breast.* 2001;10:130–8.
47. Castiglione-Gertsch M, O'Neill A, Price K, et al. Adjuvant chemotherapy followed by goserelin versus either modality alone for premenopausal lymph node-negative breast cancer: A randomized trial. *J Natl Cancer Inst.* 2003;95:1833–46.
48. Arriagada R, Le M, Spielmann M, et al. Randomized trial of adjuvant ovarian suppression in 926 premenopausal patients with early breast cancer treated with adjvuant chemotherapy. *Annals Oncol.* 2005;16:389–96.
49. Robert N, Wang M, Wood W. Phase III comparison of tamoxifen with ovarian ablation in premenopausal women with axillary node-negative, receptor-positive breast cancer <3 cm. *Proc Am Soc Clin Oncol.* 2003;22:16a.

50. Love R, Duc N, Allred D, et al. Oophorectomy and tamoxifen adjuvant therapy in premenopausal Vietnamese and Chinese women with operable breast cancer. *J Clin Oncol* 2002;20:2559–66.
51. Boccardo F, Rubagotti A, Amoroso D, et al. Cyclophosphamide, methotrexate, and fluorouracil versus tamoxifen plus ovarian suppression as adjuvant treatment of estrogen receptor-positive pre-/perimenopausal breast cancer patients: results of the Italian Breast Cancer Adjuvant Study Group 02 randomized trial. *J Clin Oncol*. 2000;18:2718–27.
52. Roche H, Kerbrat P, Bonneterre J, et al. Complete hormonal blockade versus epirubicin-based chemotherapy in premenopausal, one to three node-positive, and hormone-receptor positive, early breast cancer patients: 7-year follow-up results of French Adjuvant Study Group 06 randomised trial. *Annals Oncol*. 2006;17:1221–7.
53. Roche H, Mihura J, de Lafontan B, et al. Castration and tamoxifen versus chemotherapy (FAC) for premenopausal, node- and receptor-positive breast cancer patients: A randomized trial with a 7 years median follow up. *Proc Am Soc Clin Oncol*. 1996;15:117.
54. The Adjuvant Breast Cancer Trials Collaborative Group. Ovarian ablation or suppression in premenopausal early breast cancer: Results from the International Adjuvant Breast Cancer Ovarian Ablation or Suppression Randomized Trial. *J Natl Cancer Inst*. 2007;99:516–25.
55. Jakesz R, Hausmaninger H, Kubista E, et al. Randomized adjuvant trial of tamoxifen and goserelin versus cyclophosphamide, methotrexate, and fluorouracil: Evidence for the superiority of treatment with endocrine blockade in premenopausal patients with hormone-responsive breast cancer–Austrian Breast and Colorectal Cancer Study Group Trial 5. *J Clin Oncol*. 2002;20:4621–7.
56. Early Breast Cancer Trialists' Collaborative Group (EBCTCG). Use of luteinising-hormone-releasing hormone agonists as adjuvant treatment in premenopausal patients with hormone-receptor-positive breast cancer: a meta-analysis of individual patient data from randomized adjuvant trials. *Lancet*. 2007;369:1711–23.
57. Paik S. Molecular profiling of breast cancer. *Curr Opin Obst Gynecol*. 2006;18:59–62.
58. Kennecke H, Olivotto I, Speers C, et al. Late risk of relapse and mortality among postmenopausal women with estrogen responsive early breast cancer after 5 years of tamoxifen. *Annals Oncol*. 2007;18:45–51.
59. Bryant J, Fisher B, Dignam J. Duration of adjuvant tamoxifen therapy. *J Natl Cancer Inst Monogr*. 2001;30:56–61.
60. Baum M, Budzar A, Cuzick J, et al. Anastrozole alone or in combination with tamoxifen versus tamoxifen alone for adjuvant treatment of postmenopausal women with early breast cancer: First results of the ATAC randomised trial. *Lancet*. 2002;359:2131–9.
61. Howell A, Cuzick J, Baum M, et al. Results of the ATAC (Arimidex, Tamoxifen, Alone or in Combination) trial after completion of 5 years' adjuvant treatment for breast cancer. *Lancet* 2005;365:60–2.
62. Thurlimann B, Keshaviah A, Coates AS, et al. Breast International Group (BIG) 1-98 Collaborative Group: A comparison of letrozole and tamoxifen in postmenopausal women with early breast cancer. *N Engl J Med*. 2005;353:2747–57.
63. Coates A, Keshaviah A, Thurlimann B, et al. Five years of letrozole compared with tamoxifen as initial adjuvant therapy for postmenopausal women with endocrine-responsive early breast cancer: Update of study BIG 1-98. *J Clin Oncol*. 2007;25:486–92.
64. Ryan P, Goss P. Adjuvant hormonal therapy in peri- and postmenopausal breast cancer. *The Oncologist*. 2006;11: 718–31.
65. Boccardo F, Rubagotti A, Puntoni M, et al. Switching to anastrozole versus continued tamoxifen treatment of early breast cancer: preliminary results of the Italian Tamoxifen Anastrozole *Trial. J Clin Oncol*. 2005;23:5138–47.
66. Jakesz R, Jonat W, Gnant M, et al. Switching of postmenopausal women with endocrine-responsive early breast cancer to anastrozole after 2 years' adjuvant tamoxifen: combined results of ABCSG trial 8 and ARNO 95 trial. *Lancet*. 2005;366:455–62.

67. Kaufmann M, Jonat W, Hilfrich H, et al. Survival benefit of switching to anastrozole after 2 years of treatment with tamoxifen versus continued tamoxifen therapy: The ARNO 95 study (abstract 547). *J Clin Oncol.* 2006;24(18S):14s.
68. Coombes R, Hall E, Gibson L, et al. A randomized trial of exemestane after two to three years of tamoxifen therapy in postmenopausal women with primary breast cancer. *N Engl J Med* 2004;350:1081–92.
69. Coombes R, Kilburn L, Snowdon C, et al. Survival and safety of exemestane versus tamoxifen after 2–3 years' tamoxifen treatment (Intergroup Exemestane Study): A randomised controlled trial. *Lancet.* 2007;369:559–70.
70. Goss P, Ingle J, Martino S, et al. A randomized trial of letrozole in postmenopausal women after five years of tamoxifen therapy for early-stage breast cancer. *N Engl J Med.* 2003;349:1793–802.
71. Goss P, Ingle J, Martino S, et al. Randomized trial of letrozole following tamoxifen as extended adjuvant therapy in receptor-positive breast cancer: updated findings from NCIC CTG MA.17. *J Natl Cancer Inst.* 2005;97:1262–71.
72. Robert N, Goss P, Ingle J, et al.. Updated analysis of NCIC CTG MA.17 (letrozole vs placebo to letrozole vs placebo) post unblinding (abstract 550). *Proc Am Soc Clin Oncol.* 2006;24(18s):5s.
73. Goss P, Ingle J, Martino S, et al. Efficacy of letrozole extended adjuvant therapy according to estrogen receptor and progesterone receptor status of the primary tumor: National Cancer Institute of Canada Clinical Trials Group MA.17. *J Clin Oncol.* 2007;25:2006–11.
74. Ingle J, Tu D, Pater J, et al. Duration of letrozole treatment and outcomes in the placebo-controlled NCIC CTG MA.17 extended adjuvant therapy trial. *Breast Cancer Res Treat.* 2006;99:295–300.
75. Jakesz R, Samonigg R, Greil M, et al. Extended adjuvant treatment with anastrozole: Results from the Austrian Breast and Colorectal Cancer Study Group Trial 6a (ABCSG-6a). *Proc Am Soc Clin Oncol.* 2005;23(16s):10s.
76. Jonat W, Gnant M, Boccardo F, et al. Effectiveness of switching from adjuvant tamoxifen to anastrozole in postmenopausal women with hormone-sensitive early-stage breast cancer: A meta-analysis. *Lancet Oncol.* 2006;7:991–6.
77. Eastell R, Hannon RA, Cuzick J, et al. Effect of an aromatase inhibitor on bone mineral density and bone turnover markers: 2-year results of the Anastrozole, Tamoxifen, Alone or in Combination (ATAC) trial (18233230). *J Bone Mineral Res.* 2006;21:1215–23.
78. Coleman R, Banks L, Girgis S, et al. Skeletal effects of exemestane on bone-mineral density, bone biomarkers, and fracture incidence in postmenopausal women with early breast cancer participating in the Intergroup Exemestane Study (IES): A randomised controlled study. *Lancet Oncol.* 2007;8:119–27.
79. Perez EA, Josse RG, Pritchard KI, et al. Effect of letrozole versus placebo on bone mineral density in women with primary breast cancer completing 5 or more years of adjuvant tamoxifen: A companion study to NCIC CTG MA.17. *J Clin Oncol.* 2006;24:3629–35.
80. National Institutes of Health Consensus Development Panel. National Institutes of Health Consensus Development Conference Statement: adjuvant therapy for breast cancer, November 1–3, 2000. *J Natl Cancer Inst Monogr.* 2001;30:5–15.
81. Winer E, Hudis C, Burstein H, et al. American Society of Clinical Oncology technology assessment on the use of aromatase inhibitors as adjuvant therapy for postmenopausal women with hormone receptor-positive breast cancer: Status report 2004. *J Clin Oncol.* 2005;23:619–29.
82. Smith I, Dowsett M, Yap Y, et al. Adjuvant aromatase inhibitors for early breast cancer after chemotherapy-induced amenorrhoea: Caution and suggested guidelines. *J Clin Oncol.* 2006;24:2444–7.

Adjuvant Therapy of Breast Cancer – Bisphosphonates

Tiina Saarto

The skeleton is a first site of recurrence in every third relapse in breast cancer. Approximately 70% (50–80%) of metastatic breast cancer patients have bone metastases [1]. Bisphosphonates have been used successfully in the treatment of malignant hypercalcaemia and skeletal metastases [2]. The use of bisphosphonates in addition to hormone therapy or chemotherapy reduces the risk of developing skeletal events (new skeletal lesions, progression of existing bone lesions, hypercalcaemia, pathological fractures, palliative radiotherapy or surgery) and the skeletal event rate, as well as increases the time to skeletal event in women with advanced breast cancer and clinically evident bone metastases. Bisphosphonates also reduce bone pain but did not appear to affect survival. During the last 15 years bisphosphonates have been investigated in treatment of primary breast cancer either in prevention of breast cancer recurrences or treatment related bone loss.

Bisphosphonates are synthetic analogues of natural pyrophosphates, characterized by two carbon-phosphate bonds (P-C-P) instead of an oxygen atom [3]. In contrast to the natural pyrophosphate, bisphosphonates are resistant to breakdown by enzymatic hydrolysis. Bisphosphonates act specifically on bone, because of their strong affinity for calcium phosphate. According to the structure of side chain, the bisphosphonates can be divided into those resembling the natural bisphosphonate or non-aminobisphosphonates (clodronate and etidronate) and those with a nitrogen-containing side chain, aminobisphosphonates (pamidronate, alendronate, zoledronic acid, risedronate, ibandronate). Bisphosphonates inhibit bone resorption by a variety of mechanisms. When osteoclasts ingest bisphosphonate-containing bone, their cytoskeleton becomes disrupted and the apoptosis of the osteoclasts is activated. The non-aminobisphosphonates act as analogues of ATP and inhibit ATP dependent intracellular enzymes leading to apoptosis and death of the osteoclasts. The aminobisphosphonates, on the other hand, inhibit enzymes of the mevalonate pathway by disrupting the signalling functions of key regulatory proteins and lead to osteoclast apoptosis. Bisphosphonates also inhibit development of osteoclast from monocyte-precursors by diminishing the recruitment and

T. Saarto (✉)
Department of Oncology, Helsinki University Central Hospital, Helsinki, Finland
e-mail: tiina.saarto@hus.fi

M. Castiglione, M.J. Piccart (eds.), *Adjuvant Therapy for Breast Cancer*,
Cancer Treatment and Research 151, DOI 10.1007/978-0-387-75115-3_11,

activity of osteoclasts. Bisphosphonates have demonstrated direct antitumour activity against neoplastic cells especially in the bone [4]. Bisphosphonates inhibit the adhesion of tumour cells to the bone and induce tumour cell apoptosis in vitro [4, 5]. In an animal model, bisphosphonates not only halted osteolysis but also reduced skeletal tumour burden mainly in bone but in some models also in visceral organs [4]. However, no effect has been demonstrated on the apoptosis of breast cancer cells at extraskeletal metastases, suggesting that local concentration of bisphosphonates is sufficient to induce apoptosis of tumour cells only in the bone [4].

Adjuvant Bisphosphonate Therapy

There are three controlled prospective trials published on adjuvant bisphosphonate treatment in early stage breast cancer. These trials all with oral clodronate provide conflicting data on the potential role of adjuvant bisphosphonates among patients with no evidence of distant metastases after definitive local surgery. The first trial conducted by Diel et al. [6] randomly assigned 302 women with node-positive and node-negative primary breast cancer and positive bone marrow aspirate for tumour cells to receive either clodronate 1,600 mg/day orally for 2 years or no bisphosphonate. The type of adjuvant systemic therapy was selected in accordance with specific guidelines (hormonal therapy, chemotherapy, or both, or no systemic therapy). In the initial report, with a median follow-up of 36 months, the incidence of bony metastasis (8 vs 17%, $p = 0.003$), and visceral metastasis (8 vs 19%, $p = 0.003$) were significantly lower in the clodronate arm than in the control arm. There was also a significant overall survival advantage with clodronate: six clodronate treated patients (4%) vs 22 control patients (15%) died ($p = 0.001$). Later, after 8.5 years of follow-up, the difference in incidence of bone or visceral metastases, as well as in DFS, disappeared. However, OS still remained somewhat superior in the clodronate group than in the controls [7].

Saarto et al. [8] reported results of an open trial of 299 women with node-positive breast cancer who were randomly assigned to receive clodronate 1,600 mg/day or to the control group for 3 years. All patients received adjuvant therapy; premenopausal women received CMF chemotherapy and postmenopausal women were treated with antiestrogens. After a follow-up of 5 years, there was no significant difference in the frequency of bone metastases between the clodronate and control arms (21 vs 17%), even though bone as a first site of relapse was significantly less frequent in the clodronate group than in the controls (14 vs 30%). In contrast to the Diel study, the incidence of nonosseous metastases was significantly higher in the clodronate arm (43 vs 25%, $p = 0007$). Both DFS (56 vs 71%, $p = 0.0007$) and OS (70 vs 83%, $p = 0.009$), were significantly worse in the clodronate arm than in the controls. However, the baseline characteristics were unbalanced in favour of the controls with more progesterone receptor negative tumours in the clodronate group.

Thus, in multivariate analyses of OS treatment effect remained only borderline significant. In updated 10-year follow-up data the results have remained stable, except that clodronate treatment no longer compromised overall survival [9].

In the largest and only double-blind placebo controlled trial by Powles et al. [10], 1,069 women with node-negative or node-positive breast cancer were randomly assigned to receive either clodronate 1,600 mg/day or placebo for the duration of 2 years. During the 2 years of clodronate use, skeletal metastases were significantly less frequent in the treatment group as compared to the placebo group (2.3 vs 5.2%, $p = 0.016$). However, at 5 years of follow-up, the incidence of bone metastases was no longer significantly different between the clodronate and control arms (9.6 vs 9.7%). No difference in the frequency of nonosseous metastases was observed at any time. Overall survival was significantly improved in the clodronate arm during the total follow-up period (81.5 vs 76%, $p = 0.047$), but no difference was seen in DFS. In a later reanalyses of this study, however, the incidence of bone metastases turned out to be significantly lower in the clodronate treated patients than in the controls (9.6 vs 13.5%, $p = 0.043$), while overall survival benefit lost its significance [11].

According to the Cochrane meta-analyses of bisphosphonates for breast cancer [2], adjuvant oral clodronate does not significantly reduce the risk of developing skeletal metastases (RR 0.82, 95% CI 0.66–1.10; $p = 0.07$), or visceral metastases (RR 0.95, 95% CI 0.80–1.12; $p = 0.53$), but may improve survival (RR 0.82, 95% CI 0.69–0.97). However, there is a significant heterogeneity among these three studies emphasizing the uncertainty of these findings. The major difference between these studies is that the Diel study included only women who had tumour cells in bone marrow, whereas Saarto included only nodal positive breast cancer patients. Also the Saarto study was unbalanced, having significantly more women with hormone receptor negative tumours in the clodronate arm than in the control arm, but the sensitivity analyses indicated that the results remain robust in spite of this. Nevertheless, the most likely explanation for the heterogeneity is the small number of events in these trials [2].

In summary, given that the three adjuvant trials are inconsistent without any long term disease free or breast cancer specific survival benefit, it remains uncertain whether bisphosphonates are beneficial as adjuvant treatment. Five adjuvant bisphosphonate studies are ongoing: the AZURE trial with 3,360 women with early stage breast cancer randomized to receive standard chemotherapy and zoledronic acid for 5 years or standard chemotherapy only, the NSABP trial B-34 with 3,200 early stage breast cancer patients randomly assigned to adjuvant clodronate or placebo for 3 years, the North American Intergroup trial (SWOG 0307), which compare adjuvant oral clodronate to oral ibandronate and intravenous zoledronic acid and two oral ibandronate studies (GAIN and ICE). Hopefully these trials could give a conclusive answer of the role of bisphosphonates in adjuvant setting.

Bisphosphonates and Treatment Related Bone Loss

Bone Health and Risk of Osteoporosis

Osteoporosis is defined as a systemic skeletal disease characterised by low bone mass and micro-architectural deterioration of bone tissue, with a consequent increase in bone fragility and susceptibility to fractures with minimal or no trauma. Based on the World Health Organisation (WHO) criteria, osteoporosis is defined to exist when DXA-measured bone mineral density (BMD) values fall more than 2.5 standard deviation (SD) below the population average in young healthy adults. Osteopenia, by comparison, is defined as a loss in T-score between –1 and –2.5 SD below the mean by WHO criteria.

Bone health tends to deteriorate with age: peak bone mass is attained in the third decade of life and age related bone loss starts around the age of 40. The role of oestrogen deficiency in menopausal and age related bone loss in women is well documented. Oestrogen inhibits bone resorption. The withdrawal of sex steroids leads to accelerated bone loss because bone formation is unable to keep pace with osteoclastic bone resorption. During the menopause women lose excessive amounts of cancellous bone and frequently develop "crush type" vertebral fractures. In senile osteoporosis bone loss is proportional for both cortical and cancellous bone, and is manifested by hip and radius fractures as well as vertebral fractures. The main contributory factors in the development of osteoporosis are too little peak bone mass formed during adolescence and the total amount of continuous bone loss thereafter. The risk of fractures increases steeply with age and most of those affected are over 75 years. It has been estimated that fractures caused by osteoporosis affect one in two women and one in five men over the age of 50 [12].

Epidemiologic studies show that the risk of breast cancer is greater in postmenopausal women with higher BMD [13, 14]. Paradoxically, however, breast cancer survivors are at increased risk of osteoporosis and fracture as compared with women in general [14]. Recently, Chen et al. reported a 15% (HR 1.15 95% CI 1.05–1.25) increased rate of fractures in breast cancer survivors in the observational component of the Women Health Initiative Study (WHI) [14]. Interestingly, the increased risk was seen only among survivors who had a breast cancer diagnosis before 55 years (HR 1.78 95% CI 1.28–2.46). It is likely that this paradox is explained by oestrogen deficiency that develops in women treated for breast cancer, particularly chemotherapy, which induces early menopause and accelerated bone loss in most of the premenopausal women. Thus, women who develop breast cancer may well have normal or high BMD at the time of diagnosis, but, due to oestrogen deficiency induced by, e.g., chemotherapy or aromatase inhibitors, they have an increase in bone turnover, accelerated bone loss, and increased risk of fracture later in life.

Chemotherapy Induced Bone Loss and Bisphosphonates

Adjuvant chemotherapy causes ovarian failure in a majority of premenopausal women with early breast cancer. The average rate of chemotherapy-induced amenorrhoea varies from 50 to 70% [15–17]. However, the rate of amenorrhoea associated with different therapies shows significant variation among studies. The risk of chemotherapy-induced amenorrhoea is age related [15]. Women most prone to develop ovarian failure are those in their 40s, while women under 40 years of age have better preservation of menstruation after combination chemotherapy. The onset of amenorrhea after initiation of chemotherapy is also longer in women younger than 40 years. Even though ovarian function is persisted shortly after chemotherapy, chemotherapy causes some degree of ovarian dysfunction in most of the premenopausal women leading to early menopause.

In premenopausal women treated with adjuvant chemotherapy, the changes in BMD are strongly associated with menstrual function after chemotherapy [18] (see Fig. 1). Chemotherapy induced ovarian suppression induces rapid bone loss in premenopausal women with breast cancer. In a study by Saarto et al. [18], the decrease in BMD at 12 months in patients with chemotherapy-induced permanent amenorrhoea was –6.8% in the lumbar spine and –1.9% in the femoral neck, as compared to women with menstrual cycle irregularities (–1.8 and –1.2%) and women with regular menstruating cycles (–1.05 and –0.3%), respectively. As expected, women with permanent amenorrhoea were significantly older (mean age 49 years) than women who perceived either regular menstruation cycles (37 years) or with irregular menses (43 years). Similarly, in a study by Shapiro et al. [19] the first annual BMD decrease in patients with chemotherapy-induced amenorrhoea was –7.7% in the lumbar spine and –4.6% in the femoral neck. The annual bone losses rate at spine of 6.8–7.7% for women with chemotherapy-induced early menopause appeared to

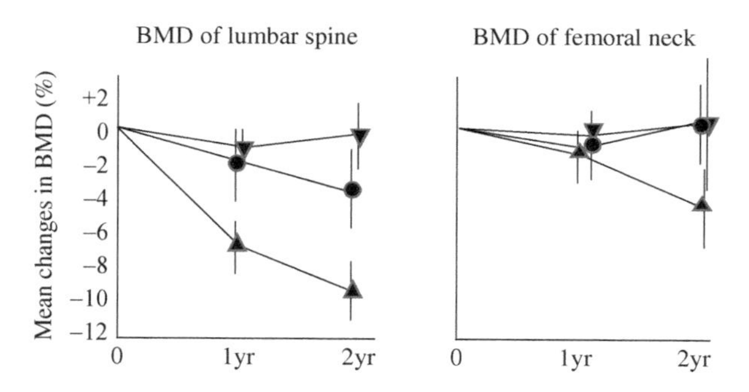

Fig. 1 Changes from baseline and 95% confidence intervals in BMD of lumbar spine and femoral neck at 1 and 2 years in 81 premenopausal women who experienced permanent amenorrhoea, menstrual irregularities or persisted regular menstrual cycles after CMF chemotherapy.
Courtesy of Dr. Tiina Saarto

be significantly larger than those found in longitudinal studies of natural menopause. According to longitudinal study of Pouilles, the mean annual bone loss rate of lumbar spine during the premenopause is –0.79 ± 1.5%, perimenopause –2.35 ± 1.5% and for postmenopause –1.24 ± 1.5% [20]. Following the first year after the chemotherapy, however, the annual bone loss rate slowed down being approximately –1.5% during the next few years, which is in line with the average annual bone lose rate in postmenopause [21]. Women with imminent amenorrhoea after chemotherapy are not the only ones in risk of accelerated bone loss. During the 5-year follow-up period every second women who were still menstruating 12 months after initiation of chemotherapy experienced menopause and accelerated bone loss. Hence, no difference was seen in total amount of bone loss after 5 years in women who experienced amenorrhoea shortly after chemotherapy or later during the 5-year follow-up period [21]. Therefore, not only premenopausal women who experience permanent amenorrhoea shortly after chemotherapy, but also women who continue to menstruate for some years after chemotherapy seem to be in increased risk of early menopause and osteoporosis. No clinical data exist of chemotherapy and bone loss in postmenopausal women. However, as the detrimental effect of chemotherapy on bone seems to be predominantly due to effect of chemotherapy on ovarian function, it seems that chemotherapy does not have significant effect on bone health in postmenopausal women with ovarian function suppressed already.

The efficacy of oral bisphosphonates in prevention of chemotherapy related bone loss has been studied with 148 premenopausal women, who were randomized to start 3-year oral clodronate (1,600 mg daily) treatment simultaneously with adjuvant CMF chemotherapy or no additional therapy [18] (see Fig. 2). Three-year oral clodronate treatment reduced spinal bone loss almost 60% as compared to the control group (3-year spinal bone loss –7.4% in the control and –3.0% in the clodronate group, p = 0.003) [21]. Even a rapid bone loss related to chemotherapy induced amenorrhea was significantly reduced by clodronate

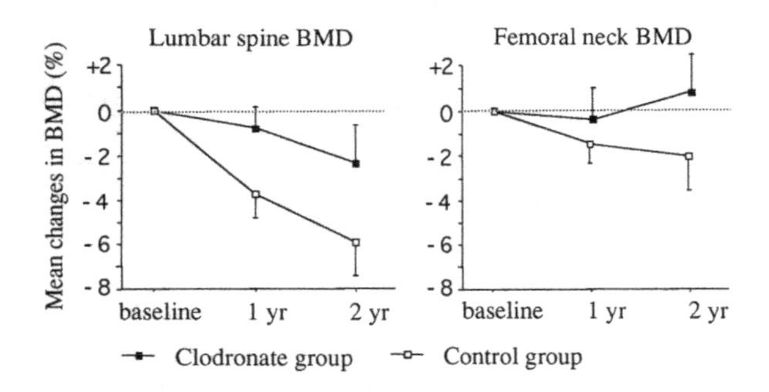

Fig. 2 Changes from baseline and 95% confidence intervals in BMD of lumbar spine and femoral neck at 1 and 2 years in 148 premenopausal women treated with adjuvant clodronate treatment alongside with chemotherapy or with chemotherapy alone.
From Saarto et al. [18], by permission of *J Clin Oncol*

(–9.0 and –5.1%). The effect of clodronate persisted at least 2 years after treatment termination (5-year lumbar spine bone loss –9.7% in the controls and –5.8% in the clodronate group, p = 0.008). The changes in femoral neck were in line with spinal BND changes, but less significant (at 3 years –2.8 and –1.7%, at 5 years –5.1 and –3.5%, respectively) [21].

In line with previous study with oral clodronate, intermittent intravenous pamidronate 60 mg every 3 months simultaneously with chemotherapy effectively prevented chemotherapy induced bone loss in 40 premenopausal breast cancer patients [22]. Bone loss in lumbar spine was totally prevented by pamidronate (+1.9%) as compared to placebo group (–3.2%) at 12 months (p = 0.002). The similar effect was also seen in femur, but the difference did not reached statistically significant level (–0.3 vs – 2.8%). This was also true in women with chemotherapy-induced amenorrhoea (lumbar spine +0.9 vs –4.0%, $p<0.03$), and femoral neck +1.2 vs –4.0%, $p<0.03$). However, in a small study of intermittent intravenous clodronate infusions of 1,500 mg alongside with adjuvant chemotherapy, it was shown that this failed to prevent or reduce chemotherapy related bone loss in 48 premenopausal women [23].

In summary, chemotherapy induced ovarian failure causes rapid bone loss especially from the lumbar spine. Women who perceived menstrual cycles experienced a moderate if any bone loss shortly after chemotherapy, but the bone loss rate accelerates during the following years, as many of them develop early menopause later in life. Consequently, chemotherapy in premenopausal women expose them to early menopause and rapid bone loss, both of which are strong predictors of osteoporosis. Bisphosphonates, either orally or intravenously, significantly reduce or even prevent chemotherapy induced rapid bone loss. The effect persisted at least some years after treatment termination. However, no fracture data exist.

Ovarian Suppression Induced Bone Loss and Bisphosphonates

Ovarian ablation (surgical, radiation or chemical) causes a sudden decline in oestrogen levels and leads to a rapid decrease in BMD [24, 25]. Adjuvant treatment with LHRH analogue induces bone loss comparable to bone loss related to chemotherapy-induced amenorrhea [25]. After 2-year goserelin treatment, BMD decreased in lumbar spine and hip by –10.5 and –6.4% compared to –6.5 and –4.5% after CMF chemotherapy. However, 1 year after cessation of goserelin, BMD showed a partial recovery, and no difference was found between goserelin and chemotherapy thereafter.

Zoledronic acid every 6 months for 3 years was studied in combinations of goserelin and tamoxifen or goserelin and anastrozole in 401 premenopausal women (ABCSG-12 trial) [26]. Endocrine treatment without zoledronic acid led to significant overall bone loss. The bone loss rate was significantly more severe in patients receiving goserelin and anastrozole (3-year BMD decrease from lumbar spine –17.3% and trochanter –11.3%) compared with goserelin and tamoxifen (–11.6 and –5.1%, respectively) ($p<0.0001$). In contrast, BMD remained stabile in zoledronic acid-treated patients; 25% of the patients treated with goserelin and anastrozole developed spinal osteoporosis, while no osteoporosis was seen in tamoxifen or zoledronic acid groups. In summary, ovarian suppression induces a rapid bone loss. The risk of spinal osteoporosis is significantly increased with the combination of aromatase inhibitor and ovarian suppression, which can be prevented by bisphosphonates.

Antiestrogens and Bisphosphonates

Antiestrogen tamoxifen has oestrogen agonistic or antagonistic effect depending on the target organ and endogenous oestrogen levels [14]. In postmenopausal women tamoxifen has oestrogen agonistic effects on bone and therefore prevents bone loss in postmenopausal women [27]. In premenopausal women tamoxifen induces a modest bone loss. A –3.3% decline in lumbar spine and –1.6% in hip bone density was demonstrated with 3-year tamoxifen treatment in premenopausal women who remained premenopausal throughout the study period as compared to a small gain per annum for women on placebo ($p<0.001$ and <0.05) [28]. Likewise, the effect of tamoxifen on bone after chemotherapy depends on ovarian function in premenopausal women ($p<0.0001$) [29]. Women who perceived menstruation cycles experienced a modest bone loss in lumbar spine if tamoxifen was used after chemotherapy (3-year BMD changes in lumbar spine –4.6% and femoral neck –1.8%, respectively), but no bone loss was seen without tamoxifen (+0.6 and –1.4%, respectively). On the contrary, tamoxifen reduced bone loss in premenopausal women who developed amenorrhoea after chemotherapy. Three-year bone loss rate in lumbar spine was –9.5% in amenorrhoeic women without tamoxifen and –6.8% with tamoxifen treatment. In femoral neck 3-year bone loss rate was –4.9% without tamoxifen and –3.6% with tamoxifen. In addition, tamoxifen seems partially to counteract the demineralising effects of LHRH analogues in premenopausal women. A Swedish study randomized 89 premenopausal women with early breast cancer to receive goserelin alone, goserelin plus tamoxifen or tamoxifen alone for 2 years [30]. The loss in total body BMD within 2 years was greatest in women receiving goserelin alone (–5.0%), while tamoxifen plus goserelin (–1.4%) and tamoxifen alone (–1.5%) resulted in smaller declines in BMD. However, 1 year after cessation of the treatment, the goserelin group showed a partial recovery from bone loss (+1.5%).

Even though antiestrogens prevent bone loss in postmenopausal women, bone mineral density can even be augmented by combining bisphosphonate to the antiestrogen treatment [31]. Two-year oral clodronate (1,600 mg daily) treatment markedly increased BMD in lumbar spine and femoral neck by 2.9 and 3.7%, while there was no significant changes in BMD with single antiestrogen (tamoxifen 20 mg or toremifene 60 mg) therapy in 121 postmenopausal women (difference between the groups in spine and femoral neck p = 0.001 and 0.006). In another study of Powles et al. [32], 311 both pre- and postmenopausal women were randomly allocated to the clodronate 1,600 mg /day or to the placebo group along with various adjuvant therapies, either chemotherapy, tamoxifen or both. The treatment effect of clodronate on spine was 2.38% after 1 and 1.72% after 2 years, which was in line with menopausal status and treatments.

In summary, tamoxifen prevents bone loss in postmenopausal women, which can be augmented by combining bisphosphonate to the antiestrogen therapy. In the presence of premenopausal oestrogen level, however, the net effect of tamoxifen is antiestrogenic with respect to skeletal metabolism.

Aromatase Inhibitors Induced Fracture Risk and Bisphosphonates

In postmenopausal women, aromatase inhibitors lower circulating oestrogen levels by preventing the conversion of androgen substrates into oestrogen and therefore accelerate bone loss and increase the risk of bone fractures. There are six controlled prospective trials where third-generation aromatase inhibitor is compared to tamoxifen [33–37] and one study to placebo [38]. In two studies, 5-year primary aromatase inhibitor therapy were compared to tamoxifen treatment [33, 34], and in four studies sequential therapy of tamoxifen and aromatase inhibitors was compared to 5-year tamoxifen therapy (ABCSG trial 8, ARNO 95 trial, ITA trial, and the Intergroup Exemestane study) [35–37]. MA17 is the only large placebo controlled study of aromatase inhibitors in adjuvant setting, where letrozole or placebo was introduced after 5 years of tamoxifen [38]. Fracture data is available from all these trials (see Table 1). In all but ITA trial fractures were more frequent in the aromatase inhibitor group than in the tamoxifen group. In MA17 study no significant difference in fracture rate was seen between extended letrozole and placebo [38], but in the letrozole group there was a higher frequency of newly diagnosed osteoporosis 8.1% as compared to the placebo group 6.0% ($p = 0.003$). Likewise, in the primary report of sequential exemestane trial with median follow up time of 30.6 months osteoporosis was reported significantly more frequently in the exemestane 7.4% than in the tamoxifen group 5.7% ($p = 0.023$) [37]. In four studies BMD data is available (see Table 2) [39–42]. In all studies except one the bone loss rate was accelerated [39–41]; however, the bone loss rate, at least in the spine, seemed to slow down after the first year [39, 40]. In ATAC trial, 5 out of 162 patients (3%) treated with anastrozole become osteoporotic during the 5-year follow-up [39]. In MA.17 trial 4.1% of women became osteoporotic detected by BMD measurement while receiving letrozole as compared to no osteoporosis in the placebo group ($p = 0.064$) [40]. Of note, no patient with BMD in the normal range at trial entry developed osteoporosis in neither of the studies.

As aromatase inhibitors increase the risk of fractures in postmenopausal breast cancer patients, adjuvant bisphosphonate treatment along with

Table 1 Aromatase inhibitors and fracture rate

Studies	Aromatase inhibitor	Follow-up time	Fracture rate in aromatase inhibitor group	Fracture rate in tamoxifen group	
Primary aromatase inhibitor vs tamoxifen treatment					
ATAC (33)	Anastrozole	68 months	11%	7.7%	OR 1.49, 95% CI 1.25–1.77, p<0.0001
BIG-1-98 (34)	Letrozole	25.8 months	5.7%	4.0%	p<0.001
Sequential tamoxifen and aromatase inhibitor vs tamoxifen treatment					
ABCSG8/ ARNO95 (35)	Anastrozole	28 months	2%	1%	OR 2.14 95% CI 1.14–4.17, p = 0.015
ITA (36)	Anastrozole	36 months	2 patients	2 patients	NS
IES (37)	Exemestane	58 months	7%	5%	OR 1.45 95% CI 1.13–1.87 p = 0.003
Extended aromatase inhibitor therapy after 5-year tamoxifen vs placebo					
MA.17 (38)	Letrozole	30 months	5.3%	4.6%[a]	NS

[a]Placebo

Data from Howell et al. [33], Breast International Group (BIG) 1–98 Collaborative Group [34], Jakesz et al. [35], Boccardo et al. [36], Coombes et al. [37] and Goss et al. [38]

aromatase inhibitors are under intensive investigation. In one study zoledronic acid 4 mg every 6 months was given for 602 postmenopausal women treated with letrozole either upfront (starting at the same time with letrozole treatment) or delayed-start (starting if T-score decreases below 2.0 SD or in the case of fracture) [43]. After 12 months of letrozole treatment, BMD of lumbar spine and hip were increased in the upfront arm by 1.9 and 1.3%, while BMD was decreased in the delayed group by 2.4 and 2.0%, respectively (p<0.0001 for both). Of patients in the delayed group, 8.3% required zoledronic acid by the protocol. No patients developed osteoporosis. Low-trauma fractures occurred in 1% of the patients in both groups. In line with the previous study, a preliminary report of oral ibandronate 150 mg per month vs placebo in postmenopausal women with osteopenia before anastrozole treatment showed that oral ibandronate once a month even increased BMD both in spine and hip as compared to bone loss without ibandronate [44].

In summary, aromatase inhibitors increase bone resorption leading to accelerated bone loss, especially during the first few years. The decline progressively slowed down thereafter, but continued to decline. Aromatase inhibitors increase frequency of osteoporosis and osteoporotic fractures as compared to

Table 2 Aromatase inhibitors and BMD changes

	No. of patients treatments	Follow-up time	BMD changein AI group	BMD change in control group	
Lumbar spine					
ATAC (39)	167	1 year	−2.2%	+1.4%	p<0.0001
	Anastrozole vs tamoxifen	2 years	−4.0%	+2.1%	
		5 years	−6.1%	+2.8%	
MA17 (40)	226 Letrozole vs placebo	2 years	−5.4%	−0.7%	0.008
IES (41)	206 Exemestane vs tamoxifen	6 months	−2.7%		p<0.0001[a]
Lonning (42)	147 Exemestane vs placebo	2 years	−4.3%	−3.7%	NS
Hip					
ATAC (39)		1 years	−1.5%	+0.9%	p<0.0001
		2 years	−3.9%	+1.2%	
		5 years	−7.2%	+0.7%	
MA 17 (40)		2 years	−3.6%	−0.7%	p = 0.44
IES (41)		6 months	−1.4%		p<0.0001[a]
Lonning (42)		2 years	−5.4%	−3.0%	NS

[a]Compared to baseline BMD within the aromatase inhibitor group
Data from Coleman et al. [39], Coleman [40], Perez et al. [41] and Lonning et al. [42]

tamoxifen. Patients at risk of osteoporosis are those with osteopenia before the therapy [39, 40, 42]. Initial dual-energy X-ray absorptiometry (DEXA) bone scan is therefore recommended for all patients before the treatment with aromatase inhibitors to select risk patients for closer follow-up. Bisphosphonates significantly prevent aromatase inhibitors inducing bone loss, but no data exist, so far, as to whether fractures related to aromatase inhibitors can be prevented by adjuvant bisphosphonate treatment.

Bisphosphonates in Prevention of Treatment Related Osteoporosis

There is solid evidence that bisphosphonates prevent cancer treatment related bone loss (chemotherapy, LHRH analogue, aromatase inhibitors). However, very few data exist of prevention of treatment related osteoporosis: in one study zoledronic acid every 6 months prevented spinal osteoporosis induced by goserelin and anastrozole treatment (25% vs no osteoporosis) [26], and in another preliminary report 3-year oral clodronate treatment prevented spinal osteoporosis in breast cancer patients treated with chemotherapy or antiestrogen (23 vs 5%) [45]. No data exist of prevention of hip osteoporosis or fracture prevention in cancer survivors.

To select breast cancer patients at risk of osteoporosis, an initial dual-energy X-ray absorptiometry (DEXA) bone scan is recommended. According to several reports, breast cancer patients with normal BMD before the initiation of adjuvant cancer treatments have a minimal risk of osteoporosis at least within the next 5 years [40, 45]. However, patients at risk of osteoporosis are those with osteopenia before the therapy [39, 40, 42, 45]. Even though bisphosphonates successfully prevent treatment related bone loss, so far evidence is lacking of fracture prevention in non-osteoporotic patients. The need for therapy in non-osteoporotic patients should therefore be considered individually, taking into account other risk factors for fracture like advanced age, previous fracture, family history of hip fracture, premature menopause, propensity to fall, smoking, corticosteroid therapy and other disorders associated with increased bone resorption. Patients with osteoporosis, in contrast, should be treated according to guidelines for treatment of osteoporosis including physical exercise, vitamin D and calcium intake and bisphosphonates.

Safety of Bisphosphonates

Bisphosphonate therapy is generally well tolerated [46]. Intravenous administration of the aminobisphophonates can induce transient flu-like symptoms with fever, myalgia and arthralgia. Oral administration of bisphosphonates in turn may be accompanied by gastrointestinal discomfort, nausea, dyspepsia, vomiting, diarrhoea and even oesophageal ulceration [46]. Some deterioration of renal function is reported in patients treated with bisphosphonates [46]. Though the renal complications during bisphosphonate therapy are often mild and apparent only occur as transient increases in serum creatinine, serum electrolyte and creatinine levels should be monitored during bisphosphonate therapy. The probability of acute toxicity due to hypocalcaemia is greater with the use of intravenous aminobisphosphonates and supplementation with calcium and vitamin D is recommended [46]. Osteonecrosis of the jaw is a rare but severe complication of aminobisphosphonates [47]. The risk of osteonecrosis seems to be higher with long bisphosphonate treatment duration, poor oral hygiene and tooth operations during the therapy.

Summary

Even though epidemiologic studies show that the risk of breast cancer is greater in women with higher BMD, breast cancer survivors seem to be at increased risk of osteoporosis and fracture as compared with women in general. It is likely that this paradox is explained by oestrogen deficiency that develops in women treated for breast cancer, particularly chemotherapy, which induces early menopause and accelerated bone loss in most premenopausal women, and aromatase inhibitors that inhibit oestrogen synthesis and increase risk of fractures in postmenopausal women. Bisphosphonates are widely used in treatment of osteoporosis. Bisphosphonates also effectively prevent cancer treatment related bone loss and osteoporosis, but no fracture prevention data exist of adjuvant bisphosphonate therapy. Breast cancer patients at risk of osteoporosis seem to be those with osteopenia before adjuvant treatments. In contrast, in women with normal baseline BMD there seems to be no imminent risk of osteoporosis within the next 5–10 years representing the majority of the patients. Therefore initial dual-energy X-ray absorptiometry (DEXA) bone scan is recommended to select breast cancer patients at risk of osteoporosis.

Given that the present adjuvant bisphosphonate trials are inconsistent without any long term disease free or breast cancer specific survival benefit, it remains uncertain whether bisphosphonates are beneficial as adjuvant treatment of breast cancer. Large controlled trials are ongoing. While waiting for the results of these trials the use of adjuvant bisphosphonate treatment outside of the clinical trials is not recommended.

References

1. Coleman RE. Skeletal complications of malignancy. *Cancer*. 1997;80(suppl):1588–94.
2. Pavlakis N, Schmidt R, Stockler M. Bisphosphonates for breast cancer. The Chochrane database of systemic reviews. *The Chocrane library*, Vol 3, 2006.
3. Russell RG, Rogers MJ. Bisphosphonates: From the laboratory to the clinic and back again. Bone 1999;25(1):97–106.
4. Hiraga T, Williams PJ, Ueda A, et al. Zoledronic acid inhibits visceral metastases in the 4T1/luc mouse breast cancer model. *Clin Cancer Res*. 2004;10:4559–67.
5. Boissier S, Ferreras M, Peyruchaud O, et al. Bisphosphonates inhibit breast and prostate carcinoma cell invasion, an early event in the formation of bone metastases. *Cancer Res*. 2000;60:2949–54.
6. Diel I, Solomayer E, Costa SD, et al. Reduction in new metastases in breast cancer with adjuvant clodronate treatment. *N Engl J Med*. 1998;339:357–63.
7. Jaschke A, Baster G, Solomayer E, et al. Adjuvant clodronate treatment improves the overall survival of primary breast cancer patients with micrometastases to bone marrow – a longtime follow-up. *ASCO*. 2004 (abstract 529), 9a.
8. Saarto T, Blomqvist C, Virkkunen P, et al. Adjuvant clodronate treatment does not reduce the frequency of skeletal metastases in node-positive breast cancer patients: 5-year results of a randomized controlled trial. *J Clin Oncol*. 2001;19(1):10–17.
9. Saarto T, Blomqvist C, Virkkunen P, et al. Ten-year follow-up of a randomized controlled trial of adjuvant clodronate treatment in node-positive breast cancer patients. *Acta Oncol*. 2004;43(7)650–6.
10. Powles T, Paterson S, Kanis JA, et al. Randomized, placebo-controlled trial of clodronate in patients with primary operable breast cancer. *J Clin Oncol*. 2002;20(15):3219–24.
11. Powles T, Paterson A, McCloskey E, et al. Reduction in bone relapse and improved survival with oral clodronate for adjuvant treatment of operable breast cancer. *Br Ca Res Treat*. 2006;8:R13.
12. Poole KE, Compston JE. Osteoporosis and its management. *BMJ*. 2006;333:1251–6.
13. Ramaswamy B, Shapiro CL. Osteopenia and osteoporosis in women with breast cancer. *Semin Oncol*. 2003;30:763–75.
14. Chen Z, Maricic M, Bassford TL, et al. Fracture risk among breast cancer survivors: Results from the Women's Health Initiative Observational Study. *Arch Intern Med*. 2005;165:552–8.

15. Bines J, Oleske DM, Cobleigh MA. Ovarian function in premenopausal women treated with adjuvant chemotherapy for breast cancer. *J Clin Oncol.* 1996,14:1718–29.
16. Parulekar WR, Day AG, Ottaway JA, et al. Incidence and Prognostic Impact of Amenorrhea During Adjuvant Therapy in High-Risk Premenopausal Breast Cancer: Analysis of a National Cancer Institute of Canada Clinical Trials Group Study-NCIC CTG MA.5 *J Clin Oncol.* 2005;23(25):6002–8.
17. Martin M, Pienkowski T, Mackey J, et al. Adjuvant docetaxel for node-positive breast cancer. *New Engl J Med.* 2005;352:2302–13.
18. Saarto T, Blomqvist C, Välimäki M, et al. Chemical castration induced by adjuvant CMF therapy causes a rapid bone loss which is reduced by clodronate. A randomized study in premenopausal breast cancer women. *J Clin Oncol.* 1997;15:1341–47.
19. Shapiro CL, Manola J, Leboff M. Ovarian failure after adjuvant chemotherapy is associated with rapid bone loss in women with early-stage breast cancer. *J Clin Oncol.* 2001;19:3306–11.
20. Pouilles JM, Tremollieres F, Ribot C. The effects of menopause on longitudinal bone loss from the spine. *Calcif Tissue Int.* 1993;52:340–3.
21. Vehmanen L, Saarto T, Elomaa I, et al. Long-term impact of chemotherapy-induced ovarian failure on bone mineral density (BMD) in premenopausal breast cancer patients. The effect of adjuvant clodronate treatment. *Eur J Cancer.* 2001;37:2373–8.
22. El-Hajj Fuleihan G, Salamoun M, Mourad YA, et al. Pamidronate in the prevention of chemotherapyinduced bone loss in premenopausal women with breast cancer. *J Clin Endocrinol Metab.* 2005;90:3209–14.
23. Vehmanen L, Saarto T, Blomqvist C, et al. Short-term intermittent intravenous clodronate in the prevention of bone loss related to chemotherapy-induced ovarian failure. *Br Ca Res Treat.* 2004;87:181–8.
24. Genant HK, Cann CE, Ettinger B, et al. Quantitative computed tomography of vertebral spongiosa: A sensitive method for detecting early bone loss after oophorectomy. *Ann Intern Med.* 97:699–705,1982.
25. Fogelman I, Blake GM, Blamey R, et al. Bone mineral density in premenopausal women treated for node-positive early breast cancer with 2 years of goserelin or 6 months of cyclophosphamide, methotrexate and 5-fluorouracil (CMF). *Osteoporos Int.* 2003;14(12):1001–1006.
26. Gnant MF, Mlineritsch B, Luschin-Ebengreuth G, et al. Zoledronic acid prevents cancer treatment-induced bone loss in premenopausal women receiving adjuvant endocrine therapy for hormone-responsive breast cancer: A report from the Austrian Breast and Colorectal Cancer Study Group. *J Clin Oncol.* 2007;25:826–828.
27. Love RR, Mazess RB, Barden HS, et al. Effects of tamoxifen on bone mineral density in postmenopausal women with breast cancer. *N Engl J Med.* 1992;326:852–6.
28. Powles TJ, Hickish T, Kanis JA, et al. Effect of tamoxifen on bone mineral density measured by dual-energy X-ray absorptiometry in healthy premenopausal and postmenopausal women. *J Clin Oncol.* 1996;14:78–84.
29. Vehmanen L, Elomaa I, Blomqvist C, Saarto T. Tamoxifen treatment after adjuvant chemotherapy has opposite effects on bone mineral density in premenopausal patients depending on menstrual status. *J Clin Oncol.* 2006;24(4):675–80.
30. Sverrisdóttir Á, Fornander T, Jacobsson H, et al. Bone mineral density among premenopausal women with early breast cancer in a randomized trial of djuvant endocrine therapy. *J Clin Oncol.* 2004;22:3694–9.
31. Saarto T, Blomqvist C, Välimäki M, et al. Clodronate improves bone mineral density in postmenopausal breast cancer women treated with adjuvant antiestrogens. *Br J Cancer.* 1997;75:602–5.
32. Powles TJ, McCloskey E, Paterson AH, et al. Oral clodronate and reduction in loss of bone mineral density in women with operable primary breast cancer. *J Natl Cancer Inst.* 1998;90:704–8

33. Howell A, Cuzick J, Maum M, et al. Results of the ATAC (Arimidex, Tamoxifen, Alone or in Combination) trial after completion of 5 years' adjuvant treatment for breast cancer. *Lancet*. Jan 1–7, 2005;365(9453):60–2.
34. Breast International Group (BIG) 1-98 Collaborative Group. A comparison of letrozole and tamoxifen in postmenopausal women with early breast cancer. *N Engl J Med*. 2005;353(26):2747–57.
35. Jakesz R, Jonat W, Gnant M, et al. Switching of postmenopausal women with endocrine-responsive early breast cancer to anastrozole after 2 years' adjuvant tamoxifen: Combined results of ABCSG trial 8 and ARNO 95 trial. *Lancet*. 2005;366(9484):455–62.
36. Boccardo F, Rubagotti A, Puntoni M, et al. Switching to anastrozole versus continued tamoxifen treatment of early breast cancer: Preliminary results of the Italian tamoxifen anastrozole trial. *J Clin Oncol*. 2005;23:5138–47.
37. Coombes RC, Hall E, Gibson LJ, et al. A randomized trial of exemestane after two to three years of tamoxifen therapy in postmenopausal women with primary breast cancer. *N Engl J Med*. 2004;350(11):1081–92.
38. Goss PE, Ingle JN, Martino S, et al. Randomized trial of letrozole following tamoxifen as extended adjuvant therapy in receptor-positive breast cancer: Updated findings from NCIC CTG MA.17 *J Natl Cancer Inst*. 2005;97(17):1262–71.
39. Coleman RE, et al. Effect of anastrozole on bone mineral density: 5-year results from the 'Arimidex,' tamoxifen, alone or in combination (ATAC) trial. *Proc Ann Soc Clin Oncol*. 2006;24:511a. Abstract.
40. Perez EA, Josse RG, Pritchard KI, et al. Effect of letrozole versus placebo on bone mineral density in women with primary breast cancer completing 5 or more years of adjuvant tamoxifen: A companion study to NCIC CTG MA.17 *J Clin Oncol*. 2006;24:3629–35
41. Coleman RE, Banks LM, Girgis SI, et al. Intergroup Exemestane Study Group. Skeletal effects of exemestane on bone-mineral density, bone biomarkers, and fracture incidence in postmenopausal women with early breast cancer participating in the Intergroup Exemestane Study (IES): A randomised controlled study. *Lancet Oncol*. 2007;8:89–91.
42. Lonning PE, Geisler JK, Lars E, et al. Effects of exemestane administered for 2 years versus placebo on bone mineral density, bone biomarkers, and plasma lipids in patients with surgically resected early breast cancer. *J Clin Oncol*. 2005;23:5126–37.
43. Brufsky A, Harker WG, Beck JT, et al. Zoledronic acid inhibits adjuvant letrozole–induced bone loss in postmenopausal women with early breast cancer. *J Clin Oncol*. 2007;25:829–36.
44. Lester JE, Gutcher SA, Ellis S, et al. The ARIBON study: Reversal of anastrozole (arimidex) induced bone loss with oral monthly ibandronate (bondronate) treatment during adjuvant therapy for breast cancer. *Ca Treat Reviews*. 2006;32(Suppl 3):121a. Abstract.
45. Saarto T, Vehmanen L, Blomqvist C, et al. 10-year follow-up of the efficacy of clodronate on bone mineral density (BMD) in early stage breast cancer. *Proc Ann Soc Clin Oncol*. 2006;24:676a. Abstract.
46. Conte PF, Guarneri V. Safety of intravenous and oral bisphosphonates and compliance with dosing regimen. *Oncologist*. 2004;4 (Suppl 9):28–37.
47. Woo SB, Hellstein JW, Kalmar JR. Bisphosphonates and osteonecrosis of the jaws. *Ann Intern Med*. 2006;144:753–61.

Part III
New Wind in the Adjuvant Setting

Trastuzumab

Edith A. Perez, Frances M. Palmieri, and Shelly M. Brock

Introduction

Systemic adjuvant therapy is regularly recommended for patients diagnosed with invasive breast cancer based on risk of recurrence and likelihood of benefit from therapy. Progress in molecular biology has resulted in the identification and improved understanding of molecular markers that may have prognostic and predictive value for patients with breast cancer. HER2 (human epidermal growth factor receptor 2) is one of the best characterized of these markers and now plays a critical role in patient management.

HER2 gene amplification or protein overexpression have been reported in 18–30% of all breast cancers [1–4]; however the early reports of 30% may be an overestimation [5]. HER2-positivity is associated with an aggressive disease course, a poor prognosis [2, 6], and relative sensitivity to anthracyclines [7–9]. The anti-HER2 monoclonal antibody trastuzumab specifically targets the HER2 protein, and has proposed cytostatic, cytotoxic, and anti-angiogenic [10] modes of action, reviewed by Baselga et al. [11] and Albanell et al. [12].

Pivotal trials assessing the addition of trastuzumab to standard chemotherapy (doxorubicin plus cyclophosphamide [AC], paclitaxel, or docetaxel) for HER2-positive metastatic breast cancer (MBC) demonstrated that trastuzumab significantly improves clinical outcomes in this patient population compared with chemotherapy alone [13–15]. In addition, trastuzumab has been shown to have activity as a single agent [16–18]. In 1998, the Food and Drug Administration (FDA) in the United States (U.S.) approved trastuzumab for first-line therapy in combination with paclitaxel or as second- or third-line monotherapy for HER2-positive MBC. Other regulatory agencies around the world have also approved trastuzumab for the treatment of HER2-positive MBC. Many studies have now been conducted in the setting of metastatic

E.A. Perez (✉)
Division of Hematology/Oncology, Internal Medicine, Mayo Clinic,
4500 San Pablo Road, Jacksonville, FL 32224.

M. Castiglione, M.J. Piccart (eds.), *Adjuvant Therapy for Breast Cancer*,
Cancer Treatment and Research 151, DOI 10.1007/978-0-387-75115-3_12,

disease, documenting excellent synergistic and additive interactions of this agent with various chemotherapy drugs.

The effectiveness of trastuzumab in the metastatic setting prompted investigators to test trastuzumab in the adjuvant setting to determine whether treating HER2-positive tumors at an earlier stage could improve patient outcomes. These trials have evaluated adding trastuzumab to various chemotherapy and anti-estrogen hormonal approaches.

Four major adjuvant trials collectively enrolled >13,000 women with HER2-positive early breast cancer to investigate different adjuvant treatment approaches with trastuzumab, with enrollment extending from 2000 to 2005. These trials demonstrated that 1 year of trastuzumab significantly improved disease-free survival (DFS) by 33–52% and overall survival (OS) by 34–41%; there were differences in patient population, chemotherapy regimens, and sequencing of treatment across the trials. A small Finnish trial (FinHER) and a pilot U.S. trial (E2198), investigating shorter regimens of trastuzumab, have also shown positive results. Further follow-up of the major adjuvant trials will clarify the long-term survival benefit for women receiving trastuzumab, as well as the optimal treatment duration. In terms of tolerability, cardiac events in the trastuzumab-containing arms of these trials have remained within acceptable levels, with a small increase in the incidence of congestive heart failure (CHF) (0.5–3.0%) that responded to treatment in most cases. Further follow-up will also provide information on long-term cardiac safety. Overall, results from clinical trials are sufficiently compelling to recommend 1 year of adjuvant trastuzumab treatment for women with HER2-positive early breast cancer based on the risk:benefit (therapeutic) ratio and cost-effectiveness demonstrated in these studies.

The Large Phase III Adjuvant Trastuzumab Trials

Trial Designs

Four large phase III randomized trials were conducted to evaluate the efficacy and safety of adding trastuzumab to adjuvant chemotherapy for early breast cancer: National Surgical Adjuvant Breast and Bowel Project (NSABP) B-31 trial (U.S.); North Central Cancer Treatment Group (NCCTG) N9831 Intergroup trial (U.S.); Breast Cancer International Research Group (BCIRG) 006 trial (international); Breast International Group Herceptin Adjuvant (HERA) trial (ex U.S.) (Fig. 1). Each trial included a control chemotherapy-only arm, and either one or two trastuzumab-containing arms, in which trastuzumab was administered concurrently with or following the chemotherapy portion of treatment. Standard chemotherapy regimens were used and these differed between the trials. Cardiac dysfunction has been associated with trastuzumab and anthracycline therapy in the metastatic setting [15, 19] and therefore

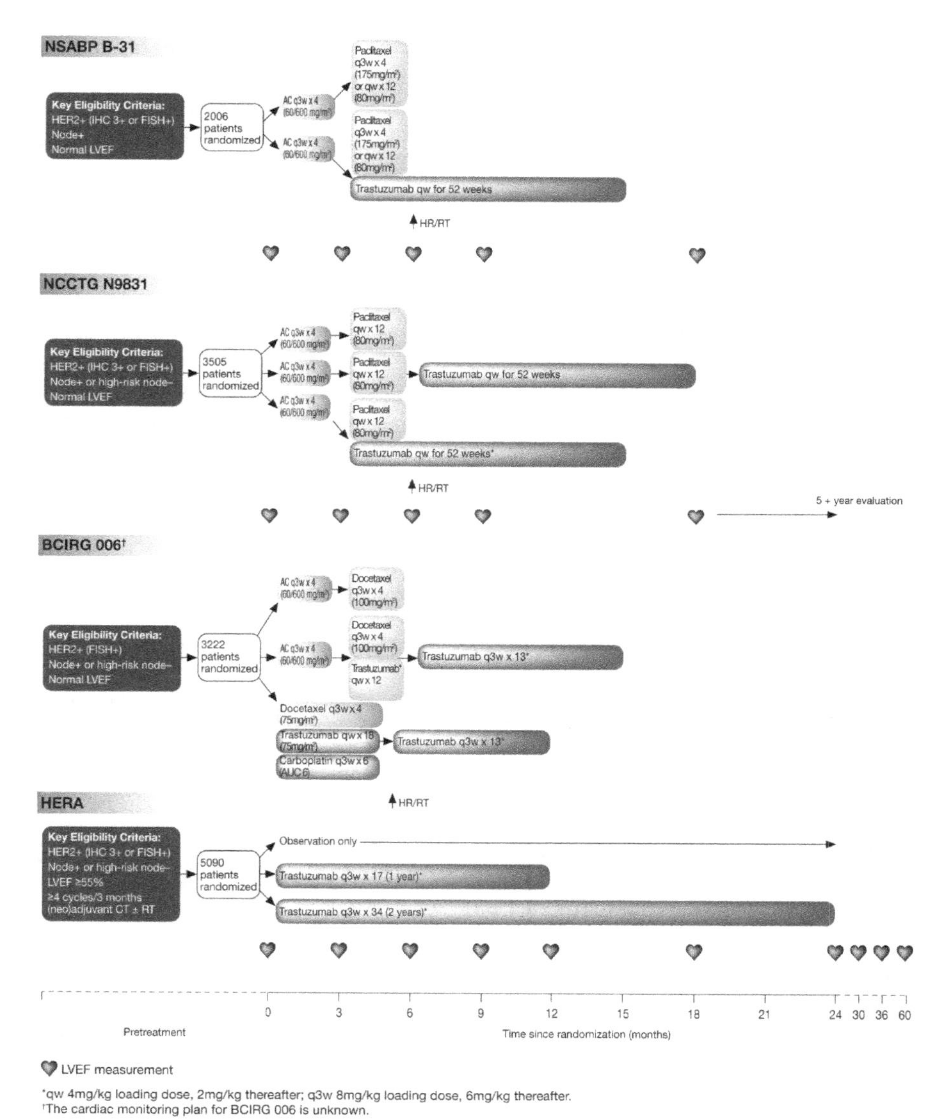

Fig. 1 Designs of the Four Large Phase III Adjuvant Trials
HER2 = human epidermal growth factor receptor 2; IHC = immunohistochemistry; FISH = fluorescence in situ hybridization; node+ = axillary lymph node-positive; node– = axillary lymph node-negative; LVEF = left ventricular ejection fraction; AC = doxorubicin and cyclophosphamide; CT = chemotherapy; HR = hormonal therapy; RT = radiation therapy; q3w = every 3 weeks; qw = weekly

trastuzumab and doxorubicin were not administered concurrently in any of the trials. A non-anthracycline regimen was also assessed in one of the trials. Strict cardiac monitoring plans were implemented in at least three of the four trials

(Fig. 1). Patients received hormonal therapy and/or radiation therapy after chemotherapy, where indicated. The primary endpoint in all the trials was DFS. OS was a secondary endpoint common to all trials. Other secondary efficacy and safety endpoints varied between trials; time to distant recurrence (TTDR) in NSABP B-31, NCCTG N9831, and HERA [20–23], quality of life (QOL) in BCIRG 006 [24, 25], and site of first recurrence in HERA [23].

National Surgical Adjuvant Breast and Bowel Project (NSABP) B-31 Trial

Patients were randomized to receive AC (60 mg/m^2/600 mg/m^2) every 3 weeks for four cycles, followed by paclitaxel (80 mg/m^2 weekly or 175 mg/m^2 every 3 weeks) for a total of 12 weeks, either alone (Arm 1) or concomitantly with weekly trastuzumab for 52 weeks (4 mg/kg loading dose followed by 2 mg/kg thereafter (Arm 2) [20].

North Central Cancer Treatment Group (NCCTG) N9831 Intergroup Trial

Patients were randomized to receive AC (as above), followed by paclitaxel (80 mg/m^{2}weekly for 12 weeks) in one of three subsequent arms; paclitaxel alone (Arm A), paclitaxel followed by weekly trastuzumab (as above for 52 weeks, Arm B), or concurrent paclitaxel and trastuzumab (for 12 weeks), followed by trastuzumab alone (additional 40 weeks, Arm C). The sequential paclitaxel and trastuzumab arm was designed to compare the efficacy and safety of this strategy with the concurrent paclitaxel and trastuzumab regimen [20].

Breast Cancer International Research Group (BCIRG) 006 Trial

BCIRG 006 utilized docetaxel instead of paclitaxel; it is also active and well-tolerated when given in combination with trastuzumab for the treatment of MBC [13]. Patients were randomized onto three arms: AC followed by docetaxel alone (100 mg/m^2 every 3 weeks for 12 weeks, Arm A); AC followed by docetaxel plus weekly trastuzumab (Arm B); or docetaxel (75 mg/m^2), carboplatin (AUC6), and trastuzumab (TCH, Arm C). Trastuzumab was given weekly (4 mg/kg loading dose followed by 2 mg/kg thereafter) with chemotherapy, then every 3 weeks (6 mg/kg) for up to 52 weeks [24, 25]. TCH was included to assess a non-anthracycline chemotherapy regimen. Synergy between docetaxel, carboplatin, and trastuzumab has been demonstrated in the preclinical setting [26] and efficacy observed in the metastatic setting [27]. Earlier studies had shown efficacy with the triple combination of paclitaxel, carboplatin, and trastuzumab [28–31].

Breast International Group Herceptin Adjuvant (HERA) Trial

Patients received predefined neoadjuvant or adjuvant chemotherapy for a minimum of four cycles or 3 months, with or without radiation therapy, as deemed appropriate by the treating oncologist. Patients were then randomized to observation only (Arm A), trastuzumab (every three weeks; 8 mg/kg loading dose followed by 6 mg/kg thereafter) for one (Arm B) or two (Arm C) years [21].

Eligibility Criteria

All eligible patients had HER2-positive early breast cancer. Immunohistochemistry (IHC) and fluorescence in situ hybridization (FISH) assays were used; these are both approved by the U.S. FDA. IHC is a semi-quantitative assay that measures the level of HER2 protein expression on the tumor cell surface. A scoring system of 0 to 3+ is applied; IHC 0/1+ is negative, 2+ is equivocal, and 3+ is strongly positive. Tumors with an IHC 2+ score are retested by FISH to determine HER2 status. FISH is a quantitative assay that measures the number of copies of the HER2 gene within tumor cells. A ratio of HER2 gene copies to the number of chromosome 17 (the chromosome on which HER2 resides) copies is also utilized. A ratio >2 was considered FISH-positive for entry into the trials. In NSABP B-31, NCCTG N9831, and HERA, HER2-positive status was determined using both techniques [20, 21]. In BCIRG 006 all cases had to be FISH-positive [24, 25].

All patients were: ≥18 years (the upper age limit was 70 years in BCIRG 006); with adequate organ function; no prior biologic, chemotherapy, or radiation therapy for breast cancer (except in HERA, and <4 weeks hormonal therapy in NCCTG N9831); no prior taxanes or anthracyclines (except HERA), and no prior platinum agents (BCIRG 006 only) for any malignancy. Only patients with axillary lymph node-positive disease were eligible for NSABP B-31. Patients with node-positive or high-risk (based on tumor size and hormone receptor status) node-negative disease were eligible for NCCTG N9831, BCIRG 006, and HERA. No patients were to have evidence of metastases in any of the trials. Adequate cardiac function, defined as normal left ventricular ejection fraction (LVEF), assessed by echocardiogram (ECHO) or multigated acquisition (MUGA) scan (MUGA only in BCIRG 006), and no history of CHF or current cardiac disease requiring medication was required. All patients provided signed, informed consent.

Cardiac Safety and Monitoring

Stringent cardiac monitoring was applied before, during, and after therapy (Fig. 1). LVEF evaluations by ECHO or MUGA were preformed at registration, and at 3, 6, 9, and 18 months in NSABP B-31 and NCCTG N9831; evaluations were performed at these time points and at 12, 24, 30, 36, and 60 months in HERA. The cardiac monitoring plan for BCIRG 006 is not available.

The definition of a cardiac event differed across the trials and included severe CHF or death from cardiac causes. Severe CHF was classified as either National Cancer Institute Common Toxicity Criteria [NCI-CTC] Grade 3 or 4, or New York Heart Association Class III or IV. Grade 3 or 4 arrhythmia or cardiac ischemia/myocardial infarction were also included as cardiac events in BCIRG 006. Based on the metastatic cardiac event data, an Independent Data Monitoring Committee set a 4% cut-off for the difference in the incidence of cardiac events between the trastuzumab-containing arms and control or observation arms in NSABP B-31, NCCTG N9831, and HERA. A >4% difference would result in suspension of the respective trial.

Trastuzumab was discontinued in patients who developed CHF. If significant decreases in LVEF were observed, treatment was held and cardiac function re-evaluated after 3–4 weeks in NSABP B-31, NCCTG N9831, and HERA. Trastuzumab was discontinued for patients with persistent substantial decreases in LVEF in these trials.

Efficacy and Safety Results

Data are available for all four trials. In the NSABP B-31 and NCCTG N9831 trials, the control arms (Arms 1 and A) and treatment Arms 2 and C were identical, therefore the FDA approved a joint efficacy analysis of the comparable arms [20, 22]. The cardiac safety results of NSABP B-31 and NCCTG N9831 were reported separately [32–34]. The preliminary data of the efficacy results of Arm B in NCCTG N9831 were reported in 2005 [35]; however further follow up is needed before a more definite analysis is reported. The HERA 1-year trastuzumab results are discussed here [23]; the 2-year data are not yet available.

Disease-free Survival

The addition of trastuzumab to adjuvant therapy significantly improved DFS compared with controls in all trials (Table 1). In the second interim joint analysis, DFS was 52% higher in the trastuzumab arm than in the control arm ($p<0.0001$) [22]. A 52% improvement was also observed at the first interim analysis demonstrating consistent benefit [20]. A 36% improvement in DFS was observed in the 1-year trastuzumab group compared with the observation group in HERA ($p<0.0001$) [23]. Both trastuzumab-containing arms in BCIRG 006 showed higher DFS than the control arm, with 39% ($p<0.0001$) and 33% ($p = 0.0003$) improvements in the AC followed by docetaxel plus trastuzumab and TCH arms, respectively [36]. There was no significant difference in DFS between the AC followed by docetaxel plus trastuzumab and TCH arms in BCIRG 006 [36]. A statistically significant improvement in DFS was

Table 1 HER2 Testing criteria and primary efficacy and cardiac safety endpoints

	NCCTG N9831 [22, 32]	NSABP B-31 [32, 33]	BCIRG 006 [36]	HERA [23]
HER2-positive criteria	IHC 3+ (>10%) or FISH-positive (HER2/CEP17 ratio >2)	IHC 3+ (>10%) or FISH-positive (HER2/CEP17 ratio >2)	FISH-positive only	IHC 3+ (>10%) or FISH-positive (HER2/CEP17 ratio >2)
Age limits, years	≥18	≥18	18–70	≥18
Median follow up	2.9 years		3 years	2 years
Primary efficacy endpoint: DFS				
Timepoint for evaluation	4 years		4 years	3 years
Control/observation, % patients disease-free	73.1%		77%	74.3%
Trastuzumab regimen(s), % patients disease-free	AC→T/H: 85.9%		AC→T/H: 83% TCH: 82%	1-year H: 80.6%
Hazard ratio vs control (p value)	0.48 (<0.00001)		AC→T/H: 0.61 (<0.0001) TCH: 0.67 (0.0003)	0.64 (<0.0001)
Protocol-defined cardiac event definition	NCI-CTC Grade 3 or 4 left ventricular dysfunction (CHF) or death from cardiac causes	NYHA Class III or IV CHF or death from cardiac causes	Grade 3 or 4 left ventricular dysfunction (CHF) or death from cardiac causes	Severe (NYHA Class III or IV) CHF or death from cardiac causes
Primary safety endpoint: incidence of protocol-defined cardiac events				
Control/observation	0.3%	0.9%	0.4%	0.06%
Trastuzumab regimen(s)	AC→T/H: 3.3% AC→T→H: 2.8%	AC→T/H : 3.8%	AC→T/H: 1.9% TCH: 0.4%	1-year H: 0.6%

AC = doxorubicin plus cyclophosphamide; CHF = congestive heart failure; DFS = disease-free survival; FISH = fluorescence in situ hybridization; H = trastuzumab; HER2 = human epidermal growth factor 2; IHC = immunohistochemistry; NCI-CTC = National Cancer Institute Common Toxicity Criteria; NYHA = New York Heart Association; T = taxane; TCH = docetaxel, carboplatin, and trastuzumab.

also observed in patients with node-negative disease who received either AC followed by docetaxel plus trastuzumab ($p = 0.0007$) or TCH ($p = 0.0096$) compared with the control.

Improvements in DFS were observed across all subgroups including patients with hormone receptor-positive or negative tumors, all patient age groups ranging from <40 years to >60 years of age, and regardless of tumor size.

Overall Survival

The trastuzumab-containing arms in the joint analysis of NSABP B-31 and NCCTG N9831 showed a significant increase in OS of 35% compared with the control arm (patients alive: 92.6 vs 89.4%; hazard ratio [HR], 0.65; $p = 0.0007$) at the second interim analysis [22]. The improvement in OS was not significant at the first interim analysis [20]. In HERA, 1-year of trastuzumab significantly improved OS by 34% (HR, 0.66; $p = 0.0115$) compared with observation alone (patients alive: 92.4 vs 89.7%) [23]. Significant improvements in OS were also observed in BCIRG 006; 41% in the AC followed by docetaxel plus trastuzumab arm (HR, 0.59; $p = 0.004$) and 34% in the TCH arm (HR, 0.66; $p = 0.017$) compared with the control (patients alive: 92 vs 91% vs 86% [control]) [36].

Other Efficacy Endpoints

The addition of trastuzumab to adjuvant therapy also reduced the incidence of distant recurrences. In the joint analysis of NCCTG N9831 and NSABP B-31, 85.9% of patients in the trastuzumab-containing arm and 73.1% of patients in the control arm were free of distant recurrence at 4 years (HR, 0.48; $p<0.0001$) [20]. First recurrences were more frequent at distant sites than at local or regional sites in both control and trastuzumab-treated groups in both trials. In HERA, TTDR was significantly higher in the trastuzumab arm (HR, 0.60; $p<0.0001$) [23] and approximately 70% of first recurrences were to distant sites in both arms [21].

Cardiac Safety

There was a higher incidence of protocol-defined cardiac events in the trastuzumab-containing arms than in the control or observation arm in all trials but the difference remained <4%, indicating acceptable levels of cardiotoxicity (Table 1). The incidence of cardiac events between the anthracycline-containing and non-anthracycline-containing trastuzumab arms in BCIRG 006 were similar [36]. Results of NSABP B-31 and NCCTG N9831 showed that CHF associated with trastuzumab was generally reversible and manageable with standard medical treatment; the cardiac function improved in the majority of patients who experienced CHF [32–34]. The investigators for both trials found that cardiac events were more frequent among older patients (>50 years), but there was no correlation between radiation therapy and risk of cardiac dysfunction [32, 34, 37]. An association between the LVEF level immediately following AC therapy and risk of cardiac dysfunction was observed in NSABP B-31 [34].

Hematologic and Nonhematologic Safety

The incidences of non-cardiac adverse events were similar between treatment groups in both the NSABP B-31 and NCCTG N9831 trials. An exception was a 0.5% incidence of interstitial pneumonitis that appeared to be related to trastuzumab therapy [20]. Grade 3 or 4 adverse events were significantly higher in the HERA 1-year trastuzumab arm compared with the observation arm (7.9 vs 4.4%, respectively; $p<0.001$) [21]. Infection (1.3 vs 0.4%) and vascular disorder (1.2 vs 0.5%) were the only Grade 3 or 4 events with an incidence >1% in either group in HERA [21].

Additional Adjuvant Trastuzumab Trials

The small FinHER trial and the E2198 pilot trial investigated shorter regimens of trastuzumab in the adjuvant setting [38, 39].

FINHER

Trial Design

Patients ($n=1010$) were randomized to three cycles of docetaxel or vinorelbine, followed by three cycles of fluorouracil, epirubicin, and cyclophosphamide [38]. The primary aim of this trial was to compare treatment with docetaxel vs vinorelbine. The subset of women with HER2-positive tumors ($n=232$) was further randomized to received trastuzumab for 9 weeks concomitantly with docetaxel or vinorelbine or no trastuzumab. The primary end point of FinHer was recurrence-free survival (RFS); secondary end points included adverse events, the effect of treatment on LVEF, time to distant recurrence, and OS.

Eligibility Criteria

All patients had IHC 2+ or 3+ tumors with HER2-positive status confirmed by chromogenic in situ hybridization (CISH). Patients were <66 years of age with either node-positive (≥1 positive node regardless of primary tumor size or hormone receptor status) or node-negative (tumor ≥20 mm diameter and progesterone receptor-negative) disease. Patients with evidence of distant metastases or cardiac disease (within the last 12 months) were excluded.

Efficacy and Safety Results

At 3 years, RFS rates were significantly higher in the trastuzumab arm compared with the non-trastuzumab arm (89.3 vs 77.6%; HR, 0.42; $p = 0.01$); however OS did not differ between the two groups ($p = 0.15$) [38]. There were no cases of CHF among patients who received trastuzumab, and these patients did not experience greater decreases in LVEF than those who did not receive trastuzumab. These data are interesting but only a small number of patients took part in the trial and the follow up is short, so no conclusions regarding duration can be made.

E2198

Trial Design

This was a randomized phase II pilot study evaluating either paclitaxel plus trastuzumab for 10 weeks followed by four cycles of AC (Arm B; $n = 115$) or this regimen followed by an additional 42 weeks of trastuzumab (Arm C; $n = 112$) [39]. The primary endpoint was rate of clinical CHF. DFS and OS were not initial endpoints and this trial was not powered to test trastuzumab duration.

Eligibility Criteria

Patients had HER2-positve tumors defined as IHC 2+ or 3+. Patients also had node-positive disease, no prior history of CHF or recent myocardial infarction, and a resting LVEF >50%.

Efficacy and Safety Results

The DFS (76 vs 75%; $p = 0.55$) and OS (89 vs 83%; $p = 0.29$) at 5 years were similar in both Arms B and C. CHF was observed in 2.6% of patients in Arm B and 3.6% of patients in Arm C [39].

Impact of Trial Results on Clinical Practice

The high efficacy observed with adjuvant trastuzumab compared with that of chemotherapy alone has stimulated the National Comprehensive Cancer Network (NCCN) to update current guidelines to recommend that 1 year of adjuvant trastuzumab be given weekly or every-three-weeks with or following paclitaxel after AC for HER2-positive early breast cancer [40].

It is important that all patients who are likely to benefit from trastuzumab therapy are identified. Patients with HER2-positive disease derive the most benefit from trastuzumab [41], and the American Society of Clinical Oncology (ASCO) and other groups advise that HER2 testing take place at the time of diagnosis in all cases of breast cancer [5, 40]. The ASCO and College of American Pathologists (CAP) Joint Taskforce published new HER2 testing guidelines in 2007, which outline standardization of the testing process to achieve accurate and reproducible assay results [5]. It is important to note that the criteria for entry into the adjuvant trials differ from those outlined in the ASCO/CAP guidelines. An IHC 3+ score was considered to be uniform, intense membrane staining in >10% of tumor cells, however in the ASCO/CAP guidelines it is now >30% of cells [5]. A FISH ratio >2 was considered positive for entry into the four trials; however, FISH-positive is now defined as a ratio >2.2 [5]. In addition, new data suggest that patients whose tumors were deemed to be HER2-negative following central testing derived the same benefit from adjuvant trastuzumab as patients with HER2-positive tumors [22, 42]. HER2 testing is discussed in detail below.

The trials reported here included patients with node-positive and high-risk node-negative disease. General recommendations are that adjuvant trastuzumab be administered to all eligible patients with HER2-positive, node-positive disease, and for those with HER2-positive node-negative tumors >1 cm in diameter, irrespective of hormone receptor status. Data are needed to assess the benefit of trastuzumab for lower-risk (tumor size <1 cm) node-negative patients.

Patients who are eligible for trastuzumab therapy based on the criteria above also need to have adequate baseline cardiac function prior to starting trastuzumab therapy. This includes no history of CHF, no current cardiac disease requiring medication, and an LVEF measurement in the normal range for their treating institution. Risk factors such as age should also be considered, as older patients are more likely to develop cardiac dysfunction. It is important that patients undergo cardiac monitoring (LVEF measurements) before and throughout treatment. NCCN guidelines recommend cardiac monitoring during adjuvant trastuzumab therapy, although methods and procedures for monitoring have not been specified. In the case of the regimen of four cycles of AC followed by paclitaxel plus trastuzumab, as in NSABP B-31 and NCCTG N9831, NCCN recommend cardiac monitoring at baseline, and at 3, 6, and 9 months after treatment initiation [40].

The optimal duration of trastuzumab treatment has yet to be elucidated. Each of the large trials incorporated a 1-year period of trastuzumab treatment. Based on the positive clinical outcomes data from these trials, the NCCN recommends that 1 year of trastuzumab be given in the adjuvant setting [40]. One year of adjuvant trastuzumab is also cost-effective [43–45]. The results of the 2-year trastuzumab arm in HERA are eagerly awaited. Shorter durations of trastuzumab therapy have also been investigated in small trials. Larger trials, with longer follow up, are required before any conclusions regarding optimal duration can be made.

HER2 Testing

The use of laboratory testing for HER2 status as the sole determinant of eligibility for adjuvant trastuzumab, or for patient selection to participate in other anti-HER2 adjuvant studies, poses a significant challenge to pathologists who perform the test and for oncologists who must interpret test results for clinical decision-making. Knowledge of the tumor's HER2 status was a prerequisite of the adjuvant trials evaluating trastuzumab, although the assays used, as well as validation methods for the results initially obtained by local pathologists varied in the different studies.

There is no current single global assay that is considered the 'gold standard' for HER2 testing. Factors that have been identified as potentially leading to inaccuracies in HER2 testing include preparation, fixation, storage of the tissue sections, the antibody or probes used, scoring or result interpretation, and interobserver variability. Given this variability, which has been identified in several of the large adjuvant trials [46, 47], several countries have developed national guidelines for diagnostic centers to follow, including those recently defined by the ASCO and CAP [5]. The guidelines are continuously evolving as we better understand the issues surrounding HER2 testing and as more data on response to anti-HER2 therapies become available.

It is recommended that HER2 status is evaluated on every primary breast cancer at diagnosis. Assays such as IHC and enzyme-linked immunosorbent assay (ELISA) detect HER2 receptor overexpression. FISH, CISH, and polymerase chain reaction measure the level of HER2 gene amplification. The two most commonly used HER2 assays in clinical diagnostic, and recommended by most pathologists and clinicians are IHC and FISH. At present, neither is considered better than the other. CISH is occasionally used in some centers, but is not routinely used for diagnostic or therapeutic decisions in most countries. Any assay used to determine HER2 status should be standardized by adhering to written protocols and be regularly validated, internally and externally, through the implementation of quality control and quality assurance measures [5].

Selection of patients for adjuvant anti-HER2 therapies have been based on HER2 testing of tumor tissue using protein and gene analyses. However, provocative, hypothesis generating data presented at the ASCO 2007 Annual Meeting by investigators from NCCTG [22] and NSABP [42] suggest that central HER2 testing may not be as predictive as previously thought for benefit of adding trastuzumab to chemotherapy. Specifically, the studies raised the question of reliability of HER2 testing and its reliability in the prediction of which patients may benefit from adjuvant trastuzumab. The central testing was conducted at Mayo Clinic (NCCTG N9831) and NSABP by teams of experienced investigators who followed standard guidelines of proficiency testing and have vast experience with both protein and gene analysis for HER2. These groups independently reported a hazard ratio of 0.5 of adding trastuzumab for patients with negative HER2 testing centrally by both IHC and FISH [22, 42]. The reasons for these results are worthy of careful study, as they suggest that central HER2 testing may not be as critically important for predicting benefit of adjuvant trastuzumab. This may be a matter of tumor volume, the ability of trastuzumab to enhance the effectiveness of chemotherapy even at 'normal' levels of HER2 expression, or the fact that the concept of HER2 'positivity' and eligibility for anti-HER2 treatment with adjuvant trastuzumab should be redefined. Follow up of these provocative data will likely lead to the development of further diagnostic analyses and prospective comparative clinical trials.

Future Directions

Further follow up of patients enrolled in the four large trastuzumab adjuvant trials will provide long-term outcomes data. In addition, results comparing the sequential vs concurrent paclitaxel plus trastuzumab arm in NCCTG N9831, and those from the HERA 2-year trastuzumab arm will help define the benefits and safety profiles of these regimens. Future research will investigate various combinations, including trastuzumab with other targeted and non-targeted therapies, and trastuzumab-based regimens with a better cardiac safety profile, for example those that do not include anthracyclines. The other anti-HER2 agent that has already been incorporated in adjuvant trials is lapatinib, as part of the ALTTO (N063D/BIG 2.06) trial. Other ongoing studies are examining the optimal duration of trastuzumab therapy, to determine whether shorter or longer that the standard 1-year therapy may be beneficial. Studies to identify additional factors that may influence trastuzumab-based therapy are ongoing, including other tumor markers that may optimize prediction of benefit (such as topoisomerase II-alpha, c-myc, PTEN, p95, or multigene patterns) or cardiotoxicity (such as troponins, single nucleotide polymorphisms, or metabolomics).

Conclusions

Patients with HER2-positive disease were considered to have a worse prognosis than those with HER2-negative disease. Trastuzumab has now shifted this paradigm to yield a better prognosis in HER2-positive early breast cancer based on the significant improvements in disease-free and overall survival observed with the addition of trastuzumab to standard adjuvant therapy. The survival benefits also outweigh the risk of cardiac dysfunction. Based on these data, it is important to identify all patients who could benefit from trastuzumab therapy.

Acknowledgments Funding partially provided by the Breast Cancer Research Foundation.

References

1. Owens MA, Horten BC, Da Silva MM. HER2 amplification ratios by fluorescence in situ hybridization and correlation with immunohistochemistry in a cohort of 6556 breast cancer tissues. *Clin Breast Cancer*. 2004;5(1):63–9.
2. Slamon DJ, Clark GM, Wong SG, Levin WJ, Ullrich A, McGuire WL. Human breast cancer: Correlation of relapse and survival with amplification of the HER-2/neu oncogene. *Science*. 1987;235(4785):177–82.
3. Slamon DJ, Godolphin W, Jones LA et al. Studies of the HER-2/neu proto-oncogene in human breast and ovarian cancer. *Science*. 1989;244(4905):707–12.
4. Yaziji H, Goldstein LC, Barry TS, et al. HER-2 testing in breast cancer using parallel tissue-based methods. *JAMA*. 2004;291(16):1972–7.
5. Wolff AC, Hammond ME, Schwartz JN, et al. American Society of Clinical Oncology/College of American Pathologists guideline recommendations for human epidermal growth factor receptor 2 testing in breast cancer. *J Clin Oncol*. 2007;25(1):118–45.
6. Paik S, Hazan R, Fisher ER, et al. Pathologic findings from the National Surgical Adjuvant Breast and Bowel Project: Prognostic significance of erbB-2 protein overexpression in primary breast cancer. *J Clin Oncol*. 1990;8(1):103–12.
7. Muss HB, Thor AD, Berry DA, et al. c-erbB-2 expression and response to adjuvant therapy in women with node-positive early breast cancer. *N Engl J Med*. 1994;330(18):1260–6.
8. Paik S, Bryant J, Park C, et al. erbB-2 and response to doxorubicin in patients with axillary lymph node-positive, hormone receptor-negative breast cancer. *J Natl Cancer Inst*. 1998;90(18):1361–70.
9. Thomas E, Berner G. Prognostic and predictive implications of HER2 status for breast cancer patients. *Eur J Oncol Nursing*. 2000;4(Suppl1):10–7.
10. Petit AM, Rak J, Hung MC, et al. Neutralizing antibodies against epidermal growth factor and ErbB-2/neu receptor tyrosine kinases down-regulate vascular endothelial growth factor production by tumor cells in vitro and in vivo: angiogenic implications for signal transduction therapy of solid tumors. *Am J Pathol*. 1997;151(6):1523–30.
11. Baselga J, Albanell J, Molina MA, Arribas J. Mechanism of action of trastuzumab and scientific update. *Semin Oncol*. 2001;28(5 Suppl 16):4–11.
12. Albanell J, Codony J, Rovira A, Mellado B, Gascon P. Mechanism of action of anti-HER2 monoclonal antibodies: Scientific update on trastuzumab and 2C4. *Adv Exp Med Biol*. 2003;532:253–68.
13. Marty M, Cognetti F, Maraninchi D, et al. Randomized Phase II trial of the efficacy and safety of trastuzumab combined with docetaxel in patients with human epidermal growth factor receptor 2-positive metastatic breast cancer administered as first-line treatment: Results of a randomized phase II trial by the M77001 Study Group. *J Clin Oncol*. 2005;23(19):4265–74.
14. Marty M, Cognetti F, Maraninchi D, et al. Superior long-term survival benefits of trastuzumab plus docetaxel compared to docetaxel alone in patients with HER2-positive metastatic breast cancer: Patients surviving more than 4 years in the M77001 study. *Breast Cancer Res Treat*. 2006;100(Suppl 1):S103.
15. Slamon DJ, Leyland-Jones B, Shak S, et al. Use of chemotherapy plus a monoclonal antibody against HER2 for metastatic breast cancer that overexpresses HER2. *N Engl J Med*. 2001;344(11):783–92.
16. Baselga J, Carbonell X, Castaneda-Soto NJ, et al. Phase II study of efficacy, safety, and pharmacokinetics of trastuzumab monotherapy administered on a 3-weekly schedule. *J Clin Oncol*. 2005;23(10):2162–71.
17. Cobleigh MA, Vogel CL, Tripathy D, et al. Multinational study of the efficacy and safety of humanized anti-HER2 monoclonal antibody in women who have HER2-overexpressing metastatic breast cancer that has progressed after chemotherapy for metastatic disease. *J Clin Oncol*. 1999;17(9):2639–48.

18. Vogel CL, Cobleigh MA, Tripathy D, et al. Efficacy and safety of trastuzumab as a single agent in first-line treatment of HER2-overexpressing metastatic breast cancer. *J Clin Oncol.* 2002;20(3):719–26.
19. Seidman A, Hudis C, Pierri MK, et al. Cardiac dysfunction in the trastuzumab clinical trials experience. *J Clin Oncol.* 2002;20(5):1215–21.
20. Romond EH, Perez EA, Bryant J, et al. Trastuzumab plus adjuvant chemotherapy for operable HER2-positive breast cancer. *N Engl J Med.* 2005;353(16):1673–84.
21. Piccart-Gebhart MJ, Procter M, Leyland-Jones B, et al. Trastuzumab after adjuvant chemotherapy in HER2-positive breast cancer. *N Engl J Med.* 2005;353(16):1659–72.
22. Perez EA, Romond EH, Suman VJ, et al. Updated results of the combined analysis of NCCTG N9831 and NSABP B-31 adjuvant chemotherapy with/without trastuzumab in patients with HER2-positive breast cancer. *J Clin Oncol.* 2007;25(18S):6S.
23. Smith I, Procter M, Gelber RD, et al. 2-year follow-up of trastuzumab after adjuvant chemotherapy in HER2-positive breast cancer: A randomised controlled trial. *Lancet.* 2007;369(9555):29–36.
24. Slamon D, Eiermann W, Robert N, et al. Phase III randomized trial comparing doxorubicin and cyclophosphamide followed by docetaxel with doxorubicin and cyclophosphamide followed by docetaxel and trastuzumab with docetaxel, carboplatin and trastuzumab in HER2-positive early breast cancer patients: BCIRG 006 study. *Breast Cancer Res Treat.* 2005;94(Suppl 1):S5.
25. Clinical Trials website. Maintained by the United States National Institutes of Health: National Library of Medicine. National Library of Medicine. 2007. Available at http://www.clinicaltrials.gov. Accessed October 2007.
26. Pegram MD, Konecny GE, O'Callaghan C, Beryt M, Pietras R, Slamon DJ. Rational combinations of trastuzumab with chemotherapeutic drugs used in the treatment of breast cancer. *J Natl Cancer Inst.* 2004;96(10):739–49.
27. Pegram MD, Pienkowski T, Northfelt DW, et al. Results of two open-label, multicenter phase II studies of docetaxel, platinum salts, and trastuzumab in HER2-positive advanced breast cancer. *J Natl Cancer Inst.* 2004;96(10):759–69.
28. Perez EA, Suman VJ, Rowland KM. Two concurrent phase II trials of paclitaxel/carboplatin/trastuzumab (weekly or every-3-week schedule) as first-line therapy in women with HER2-overexpressing metastatic breast cancer: NCCTG study 983252. *Clin Breast Cancer.* 2005;6:425–32.
29. Robert N, Loesch D, Lindquist D. A randomized, phase II trial of weekly paclitaxel vs. weekly paclitaxel + carboplatin for first-line metastatic breast cancer. *Breast Cancer Res Treat.* 2003;77:534.
30. Robert N, Leyland-Jones B, Asmar L, et al. Randomised phase III study of trastuzumab, paclitaxel, and carboplatin versus trastuzumab and paclitaxel in women with HER-2 overexpressing metastatic breast cancer: An update including survival. *Proc Am Soc Clin Oncol.* 2004;23:20.
31. Rowland KM, Suman VJ, Ingle JN, et al. NCCTG 98-32-52: Randomized phase II trial of weekly versus every 3-week administration of paclitaxel, Carboplatin and trastuzumab in women with HER2 positive metastatic breast cancer (MBC). *Proc Am Soc Clin Oncol* 2003;22:8.
32. Perez EA, Suman VJ, Davidson NE, et al. Cardiac safety analysis of doxorubicin and cyclophosphamide followed by paclitaxel with or without wrastuzumab in the North Central Cancer Treatment Group N9831 adjuvant breast cancer trial. *J Clin Oncol.* 2008;26(8):1231–38.
33. Rastogi P, Jeong J, Geyer, et al. CE. Five year update of cardiac dysfunction on NSABP B-31, a randomized trial of sequential doxorubicin/cyclophosphamide (AC)→paclitaxel (T) vs. AC→T with trastuzumab (H). *J Clin Oncol.* 2007;25(18S):513.
34. Tan-Chiu E, Yothers G, Romond E, et al. Assessment of cardiac dysfunction in a randomized trial comparing doxorubicin and cyclophosphamide followed by paclitaxel,

with or without trastuzumab as adjuvant therapy in node-positive, human epidermal growth factor receptor 2-overexpressing breast cancer: NSABP B-31. *J Clin Oncol.* 2005;23(31):7811–9.
35. Perez EA, Suman VJ, Davidson NE, et al. Interim cardiac safety analysis of NCCTG N9831 Intergroup adjuvant trastuzumab trial. *J Clin Oncol, 2005 ASCO Annual Meeting Proceedings* Part I of II. Vol 23, No. 16S (June 1 Suppl), 2005:556.
36. Slamon D, Eiermann W, Robert N. Phase III trial comparing AC-T with AC-TH and with TCH in the adjuvant treatment of HER2-positive early breast cancer patients: Second interim efficacy analysis. *Breast Cancer Res Treat.* 2006;100(Suppl 1):52.
37. Halyard MY, Pisansky TM, Solin LJ, et al. Adjuvant radiotherapy and trastuzumab in stage I–IIA breast cancer: Toxicity data from North Central Cancer Treatment Group Phase III trial N9831. *J Clin Oncol.* 2006;24(18S):8S.
38. Joensuu H, Kellokumpu-Lehtinen PL, Bono P, et al. Adjuvant docetaxel or vinorelbine with or without trastuzumab for breast cancer. *N Engl J Med.* 2006;354(8):809–20.
39. Sledge GW, O'Neill A, Thor AD. Adjuvant trastuzumab: Long-term results of E2198. *Breast Cancer Res Treat.* 2006;100(Suppl 1):S106.
40. NCCN Clinical Practice Guidelines in Oncology: Breast cancer. National Comprehensive Cancer Network 2007. Available at http://www.nccn.org/professionals/physician_gls/PDF/breast.pdf. Accessed May 2007.
41. Chorn N. Accurate identification of HER2-positive patients is essential for superior outcomes with trastuzumab therapy. *Oncol Nurs Forum.* 2006;33(2):265–72.
42. Paik S, Kim C, Jeong J. Benefit from adjuvant trastuzumab may not be confined to patients with IHC 3+ and/or FISH-positive tumors: Central testing results from NSABP B-31. *J Clin Oncol.* 2007;25(18S):511.
43. Garrison L, Lubeck D, Lalla D, Paton V, Dueck A, Perez EA. Cost-effectiveness analysis of trastuzumab in the adjuvant setting for treatment of HER2-positive breast cancer. *Am J Clin Oncol.* 2007;110:489–98.
44. Kurian A, Thompson R, Gaw A, Arai S, Ortiz R, Garber A. A cost-effectiveness analysis of adjuvant trastuzumab regimens in early HER2/neu-positive breast cancer. *J Clin Oncol.* 2007;25(6):634–41.
45. Liberato N, Marchetti M, Barosi G. Cost effectiveness of adjuvant trastuzumab in human epidermal growth factor receptor 2-positive breast cancer. *J Clin Oncol.* 2007;25(6):625–33.
46. Perez EA, Suman VJ, Davidson NE, et al. HER2 testing by local, central, and reference laboratories in the NCCTG N9831 Intergroup Adjuvant Trial. *J Clin Oncol.* 2006;24(19):3032–8.
47. Paik S, Bryant J, Tan-Chiu E, et al. Real-world performance of HER2 testing-National Surgical Adjuvant Breast and Bowel Project experience. *J Natl Cancer Inst.* 2002;94:852–4.

Lapatinib: New Directions in HER2 Directed Therapy for Early Stage Breast Cancer

A. Jo Chien and Hope S. Rugo

Introduction

Research over the last 20 years has resulted in the discovery of a wealth of information with regard to the biology of HER2 and the HER family, as well as convincing evidence supporting the HER2 oncogene hypothesis in the pathogenesis of human breast cancer. HER2 overexpressing tumors are highly addicted to HER2 function and undergo apoptotic cell death if HER2 function is lost. Approximately 25–30% of breast cancers overexpress HER2; clinically these tumors have been shown to have a more aggressive tumor biology and are associated with a worse clinical prognosis [1, 2] (although this has been modified by the use of chemotherapy and targeted therapies). Therefore, HER2 has become one of the most attractive targets in cancer therapeutics.

Efforts to develop HER2-inhibitors have primarily focused on two classes of drugs. The first includes monoclonal antibodies like trastuzumab that bind to the extracellular domain of the HER2 receptor. As discussed in the previous chapter, the administration of trastuzumab has led to significant improvements in disease-free and overall survival when combined with standard chemotherapy in the adjuvant and metastatic settings, and has become a mainstay in the management of HER2-amplified breast cancer. However, in the metastatic setting the majority of tumors that initially respond to trastuzumab will acquire resistance to the drug, and a subset of tumors will not respond to trastuzumab from the outset, demonstrating primary resistance. Furthermore, as the use of trastuzumab expands to the adjuvant setting, identifying and overcoming resistance to this targeted therapy has become an increasing issue. Therefore, HER2-inhibitors that are mechanistically distinct from trastuzumab and effective in trastuzumab-resistant tumors are critically needed. This need has led to the development of tyrosine kinase inhibitors (TKIs), a second class of HER2-inhibitors, which are

A. Jo Chien (✉)
University of California San Francisco, Helen Diller Family Comprehensive Cancer Center
e-mail: kruddy@partners.org

M. Castiglione, M.J. Piccart (eds.), *Adjuvant Therapy for Breast Cancer*, Cancer Treatment and Research 151, DOI 10.1007/978-0-387-75115-3_13,

small molecules that inhibit the catalytic kinase function of HER2. Currently lapatinib is the most specific and potent HER2 tyrosine kinase inhibitor and the furthest along in clinical development. It has shown clinical efficacy in combination with cytotoxic chemotherapy in the metastatic setting, and is currently being actively studied in the adjuvant and neoadjuvant settings.

HER-2 Signaling

HER-2 is a member of the HER family of proteins which consist of four members: EGFR (HER1), HER2, HER3, and HER4. The HER family proteins are type I transmembrane growth factor receptors. Their structure consists of an extracellular ligand-binding domain, a transmembrane domain, and an intracellular catalytic tyrosine kinase domain. Upon ligand binding to the extracellular domains, HER proteins undergo dimerization and transphosphorylation of their c-terminal tails. These phosphorylated tyrosine residues dock numerous intracellular signaling molecules that activate multiple downstream second messenger pathways leading to diverse biological effects [3]. Unlike other HER-family members, HER2 lacks ligand-binding activity, and instead relies on heterodimerization with other members of the HER family in order to activate downstream signaling cascades [4, 5]. Nevertheless, HER2 has the strongest catalytic kinase activity and HER2-containing dimers, in particular HER2-HER3 complexes, have the strongest signaling functions in the family. HER2 activates several downstream signaling cascades including the mitogen-activated protein (MAP) kinase pathway, as well as the phosphatidylinositol-3-OH (PI3K) and AKT pathway which regulates the transcription factors involved in apoptosis and cell cycle arrest and is thought to be the pathway largely responsible for the transforming potential of HER2-overexpressing cancers.

Mechanisms of Trastuzumab Resistance

Although it has been 10 years since the FDA approved trastuzumab for metastatic breast cancer, the mechanisms underlying the anti-tumor activity of trastuzumab are still not completely clear. Several molecular and cellular mechanisms have been described in the literature and include downregulation of surface HER2 expression, inhibition of downstream signaling pathways through the induction of p27 and G1 block, suppressing Akt signaling, increasing plasma phosphatase and tensin (PTEN) localization and activity in cells, and immunological targeting mechanisms [6].

The objective response rate to trastuzumab monotherapy as first-line therapy in patients with HER2-amplified metastatic breast cancer is only ~34% [7]. Furthermore, most patients with metastatic disease who initially respond to trastuzumab will show disease progression within 1 year of therapy [8]. In the adjuvant setting, at least 15% of women who receive trastuzumab either in combination with or following chemotherapy still develop metastatic disease [9, 10], and additional patients present with HER2 positive metastatic disease. Therefore, intrinsic and acquired resistance to trastuzumab severely limits our ability to treat HER2-driven breast cancers and understanding these mechanisms of resistance is critical to improving the survival of patients with HER2-overexpressing tumors.

Blocking Receptor–Antibody Interaction

The mechanisms underlying trastuzumab resistance are likely multifactorial and are equally unclear as are the mechanisms underlying trastuzumab antitumor activity. One proposed mechanism by which cancer cells become resistant to trastuzumab is through the disruption of the interaction between HER2 and trastuzumab. The membrane-associated glycoprotein MUC4 has been shown to bind HER2 and sterically hinder HER2 from binding trastuzumab, and increased MUC4 expression has been associated with increased trastuzumab resistance [11, 12]. Nagy et al. demonstrated an inverse correlation between the level of MUC 4 protein and trastuzumab binding capacity in JIMT-1, a human HER2-overexpressing trastuzumab-resistant cell line [11]. In addition, knockdown of MUC4 increased the sensitivity of JIMT-1 cells to trastuzumab. The possibility that trastuzumab is unable to reach the HER2 receptor because of mutations in the HER2 gene itself or because of decreased HER2 surface expression over time has been proposed but there is currently no evidence to support this.

Truncated HER-2 Protein

Truncated forms of HER2 have been shown to have an effect on trastuzumab response. Matrix metalloproteases cleave the full-length 185-kDa HER2 protein into a 110-kDa extracellular domain (ECD) that circulates in vivo and a 95-kDa membrane-associated C-terminal fragment with increased kinase activity (p95HER-2). The biologic activity of p95HER-2 has not been fully characterized, but breast cancer cell lines stably transfected with p95HER-2 have been shown to be resistant to trastuzumab [13]. Overexpression of p95HER2 causes growth of xenograft tumors in nude mice which do not respond to trastuzumab [14]. In addition to in vivo metalloprotease cleavage, truncated HER2 C-terminal fragments can also result from alternative translation start sites [14]. Moreover, p95HER-2 expression has been found to be an independent prognostic factor in breast cancer and defines a group of patients with HER2-overexpressing tumors that have an even worse clinical outcome [15]. Zabrecky et al reported data suggesting that the presence of HER2 ECD may promote resistance to HER2-targeted antibodies. The authors showed that HER2-targeted monoclonal antibodies bind to circulating HER2 ECD and decrease the level of antibody available for binding to the membrane-bound fragment of HER2, thereby allowing continued signaling through the kinase domain despite HER2 antibody exposure [16]. While studies looking at the predictive value of baseline HER2 ECD in assessing trastuzumab response in metastatic breast cancer have had mixed results, multiple studies have shown that declining ECD levels during trastuzumab therapy correlate with improved disease free survival [17, 18].

Insulin Growth Factor-1 Receptor Signaling

Increased signaling from the insulin-like growth factor-I receptor (IGF-1R) may also contribute to trastuzumab resistance. Overexpression of IGF-IR reduces the growth arrest induced by trastuzumab in HER2-amplified cancer cells while inhibition of IGF-1R activation and signaling restores trastuzumab sensitivity [19]. There are in vitro studies that suggest that trastuzumab-resistance resulting from increased IGF-1R signaling may be mediated by decreased p27 levels [20]. Other studies have shown the IGF-1R to interact directly with and phosphorylate HER2 in trastuzumab-resistant cells but not in trastuzumab-sensitive cells [20].

PTEN and AKT Signaling

Another potential mechanism of trastuzumab resistance includes increased Akt activity, which has been described in BT474 HER2-overexpressing breast cancer cells when compared with parental cells [21]. Nagata et al. showed that down-regulation of PTEN in HER2-overexpressing breast cancer cell lines increases PI3K/Akt signaling and blocks the growth-arrest caused by trastuzumab. Furthermore, the lack of PTEN expression in tumors from patients with HER2-amplified breast cancer is associated with a decreased response to trastuzumab-based therapy compared to those with normal PTEN levels, and therefore the loss of PTEN may be a reasonable predictor of trastuzumab resistance [22]. While these data are compelling, the patients received a combination of trastuzumab and cytotoxic chemotherapy which prevents definitive conclusions about the relationship between PTEN and trastuzumab resistance to be made.

Other Proposed Trastuzumab Resistance Mechanisms

Many other mechanisms of trastuzumab resistance have been implicated including increased signaling by other members of the HER family, increased levels of the ErbB family ligands such as heregulin, EGF, and TGF-α [23–25], and decreased activity of endogenous HER2 inhibitors such as mitogen-inducible gene 6 protein (MIG-6) [26].

Lapatinib

Lapatinib (brand name Tykerb or Tyverb), also known as GW572016, is a 4-anilinoquinazoline class TKI developed at GlaxoSmithKline (GSK) Group Company. It is the TKI furthest along in clinical development for HER2-overexpressing breast cancer. Lapatinib is a reversible small molecule dual-specificity TKI that inhibits both EGFR and HER2 with great specificity and potency (IC50 values of 11 nM and 9 nM, respectively) [27]. Compared to other TKIs in clinical development, lapatinib has a much slower dissociation rate which allows for prolonged inhibition of HER2 catalytic kinase activity.

Theoretical Advantages of Lapatinib over Trastuzumab

TKIs, at least in theory, have certain advantages over antibody therapies for the treatment of HER-2 amplified tumors. While antibody therapies are cell impermeable agents that rely on binding to the ECD of HER2, TKIs are cell-permeable agents that can potentially inhibit the ligand-dependent and -independent kinase activity of HER2 residing within the intracellular domain. This strategy has solid rationale since kinase activity is essential for the oncogenic function of HER2 [28]. TKIs potentially offer the opportunity to fully inactivate HER2 kinase function in patients with HER2-overexpressing cancer, regardless of ligands, protein truncation resulting in lack of ECD, or dimerization status, and to much more directly test the validity of this treatment approach in patients. Furthermore, approximately 30% of breast cancers co-express HER2 and EGFR. Lapatinib offers this subset of patients the theoretical added benefit of inhibiting both receptors, and may be more effective in trastuzumab-resistant cells where compensatory increased EGFR-signaling might contribute to the decreased response to trastuzumab therapy.

It is also possible that a small molecule like lapatinib is more likely to cross the blood-brain barrier than a large antibody like trastuzumab, and therefore may be better at preventing and treating brain metastases in HER2-amplified breast cancer. This would be an important difference between the two agents because patients with HER2-overexpressing disease are known to be at increased risk of developing isolated brain metastases even after treatment with trastuzumab [29]. A phase II trial of lapatinib as first-line therapy in 130 patients with metastatic HER2 positive breast cancer provided unintended data; a single patient was found to have a large occipital metastasis that was missed on screening. At first-follow-up (week 8) [30] on treatment with lapatinib alone, the brain lesion had almost completely resolved. The first hint that lapatinib might prevent CNS metastases came from a randomized phase III study of 321 patients with trastuzumab-refractory metastatic breast cancer who were randomized to receive either single-agent capecitabine or capecitabine with lapatinib [31]. Although the incidence of progressive CNS metastases was not the primary endpoint, the authors reported fewer CNS events as a site of first progression in patients who received lapatinib compared to those who received capecitabine alone (4 (2%) vs 13 (6%), $p = 0.045$) [32]. This hypothesis was further studied in a phase II trial with 39 patients with HER2-positive metastatic breast cancer who had at least 1 progressing CNS metastasis >1 cm in greatest diameter. Women were treated with lapatinib 750 mg twice daily in 4-week cycles. Patients were heavily pre-treated as all patients had developed brain metastases while receiving trastuzumab, and 37 had progressed after prior radiation. One patient (2.6%) achieved a PR in the brain by RECIST criteria, and seven patients (18%) were progression free in both CNS and non-CNS sites at 16 weeks [33]. Although these data did not meet pre-defined criteria for anti-tumor efficacy, there was a suggestion of volumetric reduction in brain tumor burden. These data prompted a large, multi-center, randomized phase II study to further investigate the potential clinical benefit of lapatinib monotherapy on brain metastases using magnetic resonance imaging and volumetric change as a primary endpoint of antitumor efficacy [34]. A total of 241 patients with progressive CNS disease following prior radiation were treated with lapatinib 750 mg twice daily. Partial responses were seen in 15 (6%), and stable disease in an additional 102 (42%). Progression free survival was 15 weeks. Taken together, this data indicates that lapatinib has efficacy in treating and possibly preventing brain metastases in patients with HER2 positive disease, and could be a potential advantage in the adjuvant setting.

Pre-Clinical Studies with Lapatinib

Lapatinib has anti-proliferative and pro-apoptotic activity in EGFR- and HER2-dependent tumor cell lines and xenograft models, and has been shown to inhibit a number of downstream signal transduction pathways deemed to be important in tumor growth, including the MAPK and PI3K/Akt pathways [27]. The PI3K/Akt pathway has anti-apoptotic signaling functions and inhibition of this pathway by lapatinib leads to increased apoptotic signaling and enhanced sensitivity to apoptotic insults [27, 35]. In vitro studies combining lapatinib with trastuzumab and other anti-HER2 antibodies have reported enhanced apoptosis in HER2-overexpressing breast cancer cells compared to cells treated with trastuzumab alone [36]. Moreover, lapatinib has been shown to retain significant in vitro activity against cell lines selected for long-term outgrowth (>9 months) in trastuzumab-containing culture medium [37]. Nahta and colleagues have shown that lapatinib induces apoptosis to the same degree in trastuzumab-resistant cells as it does in trastuzumab-sensitive cells, and propose that this may, at least partially, be due to the concomitant inhibition of IGF-1 signaling [38]. Recent data suggest that lapatinib, unlike trastuzumab, exerts its anti-tumor activity through a PTEN-independent manner. Knockdown of PTEN in HER2-overexpressing breast cancer cell lines with small interfering RNA transfection did not alter lapatinib's ability to induce apoptosis in these cells [39]. As mentioned previously, Scaltriti and colleagues showed that p95HER2-transfected breast cancer cell lines are resistant to trastuzumab. The authors also demonstrated that lapatinib inhibits p95HER2 phosphorylation, reduces downstream phosphorylation of Akt and MAP kinases, and inhibits cell growth in these cells while trastuzumab does not have any effect on these parameters [13]. In sum, these in vitro and in vivo observations provide a clear biological rationale for moving lapatinib forward in the clinical setting and strongly suggest that there is a role for lapatinib in trastuzumab-resistant HER2-dependent breast cancer, and perhaps a role for the prevention of brain metastases as well.

Clinical Trials Testing Lapatinib as Treatment of Advanced and Inflammatory Breast Cancer

Advanced Disease

Currently, the only reported clinical efficacy data for lapatinib is in patients with metastatic or inflammatory breast cancer (IBC), for both treatment refractory and naïve disease. Two phase II trials of lapatinib monotherapy enrolled more than 220 patients with trastuzumab-refractory and heavily pre-treated HER2-overexpressing breast cancer (EGF 20002 and EGF 20008). Modest clinical activity was seen with response rates of 4 and 8%, respectively [30, 40]. Although these results are overall somewhat discouraging, significant variability exists in small reported studies. For example, Iwata et al reported preliminary data at the 2006 San Antonio Breast Cancer Symposium showing an objective response rate of 24% in a cohort of 45 women with metastatic trastuzumab-refractory breast cancer treated with single agent lapatinib [41, 42].

In the first-line setting, EGF20009 evaluated two different schedules of lapatinib as monotherapy in women with HER2-overexpressing metastatic breast cancer [30]. A total of 138 patients were treated with either 1,500 mg once daily or 500 mg twice daily. The overall response rate was 24%, with a 31% clinical benefit rate and progression free survival was 43% at 6 months. The most common adverse events were similar to that seen in single agent studies in heavily pre-treated disease and included diarrhea, rash, pruritis, and nausea; these events were primarily grade 1 or 2. These data suggest that lapatinib may have similar efficacy to trastuzumab in the treatment naïve setting, although with a clearly different toxicity profile.

In addition to the monotherapy of HER2 overexpressing breast cancer, numerous completed or ongoing studies have evaluated the efficacy of lapatinib in combination with various chemotherapeutic agents. Indeed, the first of these trials led to FDA approval of lapatinib in combination with capecitabine for trastuzumab resistant advanced breast cancer. Based on encouraging data from a phase II trial, this large phase III study randomized patients with trastuzumab-refractory, and anthracycline and taxane pre-treated advanced or metastatic breast cancer (EGF 100151) compared capecitabine alone (2,500 mg/m^2 on days 1–14 of a 21-day cycle) to capecitabine combined with lapatinib (capecitabine 2,000 mg/m^2 on days 1–14 of a 21-day cycle and lapatinib 1,250 mg daily). The study planned to enroll

528 patients, however, after the first interim analysis of time-to-progression met specified criteria for early reporting on the basis of superiority in the combination-therapy group enrollment was discontinued. A total of 321 patients were evaluable. Treatment with the combination-therapy arm was associated with a statistically significant 4-month increase in time-to-progression compared to treatment with the monotherapy arm (8.4 vs 4.4 months, respectively) [31]. This improvement in time to progression was achieved without a significant increase in serious toxicities, although treatment with both agents was associated with an increase in grade 1 and 2 diarrhea. Based on this data, lapatinib was approved by the FDA in 2007 in combination with capecitabine for the treatment of patients with HER2 overexpressing, trastuzumab, taxane and anthracycline pre-treated advanced breast cancer.

Based on the known effectiveness of taxanes in the treatment of both HER2 normal and overexpressing breast cancer, a phase III trial treated 579 patients with chemotherapy and trastuzumab naïve advanced breast cancer with every 3 week paclitaxel with or without lapatinib [43]. Diarrhea was more common in the lapatinib treated patients (8 vs <1%), as were all grades of rash, and mucositis. There was an increase in toxic deaths with combination therapy (2.7 vs 0.6%), thought to be due to the initial lack of experience with managing diarrhea, and a pharmacokinetic interaction between lapatinib and paclitaxel that results in ~20% increase in AUC for both drugs. In the entire cohort, lapatinib improved investigator assessed response rate, but not PFS. In contrast, in the 15% (placebo arm) to 19% (lapatinib arm) of patients with HER2+ disease, lapatinib improved TTP (7.9 vs 5.2 months, p=0.007, HR 0.56)) and response rate (60 vs 36%, p=0.027, OR 2.9), with a trend towards improved overall survival. Extensive data has demonstrated there HER2 positive tumors are relatively resistant to hormone therapy. A recently completed phase III trial compared the combination of the aromatase inhibitor letrozole with lapatinib to letrozole alone as first-line therapy for patients with hormone receptor positive advanced breast cancer. Treatment with the combination therapy resulted in a significant improvement in both PFS (3 vs 8.2 months, p = 0.019) and response (15 vs 28%, p = 0.021) in the subset of patients with HER2-positive disease (n=219). Therapy was generally well tolerated, although more patients discontinued therapy in the combination arm due to toxicity. This data compares favorably with hormone therapy combined with trastuzumab, and suggests that HER2 directed therapy can reverse at least a component of hormone resistance in this tumor subset [44].

Lapatinib Combinations

There is reason to believe that a combination of two HER2 directed therapies with different mechanisms of action could result in a synergistic anti-tumor effect, and potentially reverse resistance. An obvious combination with non-overlapping toxicity is lapatinib and trastuzumab. Intriguing data from a phase

I study in women with advanced or metastatic HER2-overexpressing breast cancer has led to a large, randomized trial testing this combination. In the phase I trial, lapatinib was administered in escalating doses (750–1,500 mg/day) in combination with standard weekly dosing of trastuzumab, with expansion at the identified phase II dose for pharmacokinetic studies [45]. A total of 54 patients were treated, 27 in the dose escalation portion, and 27 in the expansion cohort, and the identified phase II dose of lapatinib was 1,000 mg/day with standard weekly trastuzumab. One patient had a complete response, and seven patients had partial responses. Pharmacokinetic studies were not different with the combination compared to monotherapy, and adverse events were mild to moderate in severity with no drug-related grade 4 events. The subsequent phase III trial randomized 296 patients with HER2/neu positive disease refractory to prior chemotherapy (anthracycline and taxane) and trastuzumab to lapatinib (1,500 mg/day) or lapatinib (1,000 mg/day) combined with tratuzumab [46]. Crossover from lapatinib monotherapy to combination therapy was allowed on disease progression. The PFS was significantly longer in patients receiving the combination therapy at 12 vs. 8 weeks ($p = 0.008$), with no significant increase in toxicity. This study provides supportive data for the combination arm of the adjuvant ALTTO trial described below. Multiple phase II trials testing a variety of combinations are ongoing.

Data from human breast cancer lysates has demonstrated a significant positive association between HER-2/neu and VEGF expression, with the majority of HER2/neu overexpressing tumors demonstrating overexpression of VEGF and a poorer prognosis [47]. These studies provided the background for a phase I/II trial testing the combination of trastuzumab with bevacizumab, an antibody to vascular endothelial cell growth factor (VEGF). In the 37 evaluable patients reported to date from the phase II trial, the overall response rate was 54% (3% complete and 51% partial); cardiac toxicity was observed at a low rate [48]. The positive results from this trial have led to two ongoing phase III randomized trials testing the addition of bevacizumab to a combination of chemotherapy and trastuzumab; the BETH trial in the adjuvant setting, and the ECOG 1103 trial in the first-line metastatic setting.

Combinations with oral TKIs have also tested this concept. The combination of lapatinib and bevacizumab is being evaluated in an ongoing phase II clinical trial; preliminary data was presented at ASCO in 2008 in the first 32 patients demonstrating a partial response rate of 13% and a clinical benefit rate of 35% in largely trastuzumab refractory disease [49]. PFS was 63%, and there were no unexpected toxicity signals. Lapatinib alone (1,500 mg/day) was compared to the combination of lapatinib (1,000 mg/day) and the oral VEGFR targeted TKI pazopanib in a randomized phase II trial in 141 patients with trastuzumab and chemotherapy naïve metastatic HER2 positive breast cancer [50]. Two doses of pazopanib improvement in PFS at 12 weeks in the combination arm (63 vs 84%, $p = 0.0091$). Treatment with the lower dose (400 mg/day) also resulted in an improvement in 12 week response rate from 22% with lapatinib alone, to 36% with the combination. There was no further improvement with higher dose pazopanib (800 mg) and lapatinib (1500 mg), and the combination was associated with significant grade 3/4 diarrhea. At the higher dose, about one third of patients were dose reduced or discontinue therapy due to toxicity [51].

Inflammatory Disease

Single agent lapatinib was evaluated in an international multi-center open-label phase II trial (EGF103009) in patients with recurrent or anthracycline-refractory IBC. Patients were divided into two cohorts based on their EGFR and HER2 status. Cohort A included patients with HER2-overexpressing tumors and cohort B included patients with HER2-negative/EGFR-positive tumors. A total of 45 patients (30 in cohort A, 15 in cohort B) received 1,500 mg of lapatinib monotherapy once daily. Fifteen patients (50%) in cohort A, where 75% of patients had previously received trastuzumab, had a clinical response to lapatinib while only one patient responded in cohort B. This finding supports the data that it is the overexpression of HER2 rather than EGFR that determines a tumor's potential susceptibility to lapatinib, and suggests that lapatinib may be more active in the treatment of earlier and less heavily pre-treated disease. Within cohort A, phosphorylated (p) HER-3 and lack of p53 expression predicted for response to lapatinib ($P<0.05$), and neither prior trastuzumab therapy nor loss of PTEN prevented a response [52]. To investigate further the efficacy of lapatinib in IBC, a neoadjuvant phase II trail evaluated the efficacy of lapatinib in combination with paclitaxel [53]. A total of 35 patients with IBC were treated with lapatinib at 1,500 mg once a day for 14 days, with a pre and post-treatment biopsy, followed by lapatinib at the same dose combined with weekly paclitaxel at 80 mg/m^2 for 12 weeks followed by surgery. Thirty patients had HER2 overexpressing disease, and five had non-amplified disease. The overall response rate to the first 2 weeks of lapatinib was 30%, and the overall response rate was 77%. Three out of 18 patients had a pathologic complete response. Toxicity was significant with 60% of patients experiencing at least grade 3 diarrhea, and 20% experiencing at least grade 3 fatigue and/or asthenia. Correlative studies are ongoing to evaluate predictors of response or resistance to lapatinib in this setting, but clearly lapatinib alone as well as in combination with chemotherapy is an active treatment neoadjuvant treatment strategy for HER2 overexpressing IBC.

Toxicities of Lapatinib

Continuous daily dosing of lapatinib is well tolerated and dose escalation studies have determined that lapatinib is tolerable up to 1,800 mg/day given once daily. The most common toxicities of lapatinib are diarrhea, nausea, headache, dyspnea, dehydration, and rash [54, 55].

HER2 function is known to be important in cardiac development and function. Mice lacking the HER2 homologue, *Neu*, die during embryogenesis with multiple abnormalities including cardiac malformation [56]. Mice engineered to lose *Neu* expression during adulthood develop dilated cardiomyopathy [56–58]. Therefore, drugs that inactivate HER2 understandably may lead to cardiac toxicities and warrant close cardiac monitoring. The evaluation of specific cardiac toxicities of HER2-targeted agents in clinical studies is complicated by the widespread use of cardiotoxic chemotherapeutics in these patients, as well as the contribution of these cardiotoxic therapies to resulting toxicities from HER2 directed therapy.

There is now extensive experience with the effect of trastuzumab on cardiac function. The incidence of cardiac dysfunction in studies with either trastuzumab monotherapy or trastuzumab in combination with non-anthracycline chemotherapies is in the range of 3–7% [59], although it may be much higher in patients with pre-existing cardiac damage, exposure to high doses of anthracyclines, and in those with cardiac risk factors. The majority of these events are mild, manageable with standard cardiac medications, and largely reversible upon discontinuation of trastuzumab. Lapatinib appears to have lower rates of cardiac toxicity in clinical studies to date. Perez and colleagues analyzed data from 3,689 patients treated with lapatinib in 43 phases I–III lapatinib clinical trials and showed that 1.6% of patients had a decrease in left ventricular ejection fraction (LVEF) [55]. Only 0.2% of patients had a symptomatic decrease in LVEF. Subgroup analyses showed that the incidence of LVEF depression was similar between patients who had previously received an anthracycline-based therapy but not trastuzumab (2.2%), patients who had previously received trastuzumab and chemotherapy (1.7%), and patients who were trastuzumab- and anthracycline-naïve (1.5%). The cardiac events were generally reversible, of short duration, and non-progressive. Of note, the majority of the patients in this meta-analysis were trastuzumab- and anthracycline-naive and therefore the toxicity rates may be an underestimate. Cardiac safety was monitored in the phase III trial of capecitabine with and without lapatinib and there was no change in mean cardiac ejection fraction or any symptomatic cardiac events from the addition of lapatinib [31]. Continued cardiac evaluation is warranted in current and future lapatinib trials, but thus far it appears that lapatinib-induced cardiac dysfunction is uncommon.

A unique toxicity associated with lapatinib and many other oral TKIs is related to the effect of these agents on metabolism of other drugs, the effect of many drugs and dietary factors on the metabolism of lapatinib. Lapatinib is metabolized through the liver by the cytochrome P450(CYP)3A4 pathways, and to a small degree excreted in feces. Specific dietary recommendations exist to help ensure reproducible absorption, including avoiding agents or foods (grapefruit juice) that increase or lower gastric pH, and lapatinib should be used with caution in patients with hepatic dysfunction. Lapatinib may decrease the metabolism of a variety of agents, and this is thought to be the mechanism of increased toxicity seen when standard doses of paclitaxel and lapatinib are combined. This effect can be reduced by decreasing the dose of lapatinib, a strategy employed in the large international adjuvant trial described below. A similar interaction has been noted when lapatinib is given in combination with irinotecan, with a 50% increase in SN-38, the active metabolite [60].

Ongoing Lapatinib Trials for Early Stage HER2 Overexpressing Breast Cancer

The data reviewed above suggests that lapatinib may be an important addition to adjuvant and neoadjuvant therapy for HER2-overexpressing breast cancer. Preclinical studies have demonstrated activity in trastuzumab resistant cell lines and xenograft models of HER2 overexpressing breast cancer. Lapatinib has shown clinical benefit in combination with chemotherapy in trastuzumab-refractory metastatic disease, as well as low level single agent activity in this setting. As monotherapy in trastuzumab naïve advanced disease, response rates are similar to previous studies with trastuzumab. In combination with paclitaxel, lapatinib improved response rate as well as progression free survival. Preliminary data has demonstrated efficacy in the treatment of inflammatory disease, as well as intriguing responses in trastuzumab refractory disease when combined with trastuzumab. These data provide supporting information for the ongoing adjuvant and neoadjuvant trials outlined below. In addition, the potential of lapatinib to prevent brain metastases is an exciting area of research in the treatment of early stage disease.

Adjuvant Trials

ALLTO Trial

The Adjuvant Lapatinib and/or Trastuzumab Treatment Optimization Study (BIG 2-06/N063D/EGF106708) is an ongoing international cooperative group phase III study for HER2-overexpressing early stage breast cancer. Eligibility includes completion of primary surgery, no prior anti-HER2 therapy, and at least four cycles of an approved anthracycline-based adjuvant chemotherapy regimen. Physicians have the option to enroll patients in one of two designs; design one does not include a taxane, and design 2 allows 12 weeks of concurrent weekly paclitaxel with the start of biologic therapy. A total of 8,000 patients will be randomized to 1 of 4 treatment arms including: (1) trastuzumab alone for a total of 52 weeks (6 mg/kg every 3 weeks in design 1 or 2 mg/kg weekly for 12 weeks followed by 6 mg/kg every 3 weeks for 40 weeks in design 2); (2) lapatinib alone at a dose of 1,500 mg daily for a total of 52 weeks; (3) sequential therapy with trastuzumab 2 mg/kg weekly for 12 weeks followed by a 6-week washout and then lapatinib 1,500 mg daily for 34 weeks; and (4) combination therapy with lapatinib 1,000 mg daily in combination with trastuzumab (6 mg/kg every 3 weeks in design 1 or 2 mg/kg weekly for 12 weeks followed by 6 mg/kg every 3 weeks for 40 weeks in design 2). A recent phase II trial has demonstrated significant toxicity including a 20% rate of grade 3 diarrhea in patients treated with the combination of weekly paclitaxel, trastuzumab and lapatinib at 1,000 mg a day [61]. Based on this data, the dose of lapatinib in the ALTTO trial has been reduced to 750 mg a day during concomitant trastuzumab and paclitaxel, and then is increased again to full dose (1,000 mg/day) at the end of chemotherapy.

The primary endpoint of the study is disease-free survival. The secondary endpoints include overall survival, time to recurrence, and incidence of brain metastases as the first site of recurrence, safety and tolerability. Translational studies including measurements of PTEN, c-Myc, and p95HER2 will be assessed.

TEACH Trial

Many women with HER2-overexpressing breast cancer may not have received adjuvant trastuzumab if their adjuvant chemotherapy was completed prior to May 2005, when the benefits of adjuvant trastuzumab were first established. In addition, a small population of women is unable to receive trastuzumab due to underlying cardiac disease, or hypersensitivity reactions. The TEACH (Tykerb Evaluation After Chemotherapy) trial is a phase III randomized, double-blind, multi-center, placebo-controlled trial assessing the benefit of adjuvant lapatinib therapy in patients with early-stage, trastuzumab-naïve, HER2-overexpressing breast cancer. Eligible women must have trastuzumab or lapatinib naïve stages I–IIIc HER2-positive breast cancer, have completed neoadjuvant or adjuvant chemotherapy prior to enrollment and have no evidence of disease. A total of 3,000 patients have been randomized to 1 year of lapatinib at a dose of 1,500 mg daily or placebo for 1 year. The primary endpoint is disease-free survival. Secondary endpoints include overall survival, rate of CNS recurrence, CNS recurrence-free survival, and safety, and efficacy data is expected over the next several years.

Neoadjuvant Trials

The neoadjuvant approach to chemotherapy has become more commonly used in the treatment of operable breast cancer since large randomized trials have shown no difference in relapse-free and overall survival whether chemotherapy is administered before or after surgery [62–64]. Neoadjuvant therapy increases the opportunity for breast conserving therapy for patients with large or inoperable tumors, allows the anti-tumor efficacy of novel compounds to be tested more efficiently using pathological complete response as a surrogate endpoint for disease free survival [65], and provides an opportunity to obtain serial tissue and imaging for correlative science studies. There are currently a number of ongoing studies evaluating lapatinib in the neoadjuvant setting.

NeoALLTO Trial

The NeoALLTO study is a parallel group, three-arm, randomized, multi-center, open-label phase III neoadjuvant study of women with HER2-overexpressing breast cancer >2.0 cm who have not undergone previous treatment for their invasive cancer. The study will enroll 450 patients and will compare the efficacy and tolerability of: (1) neoadjuvant oral lapatinib (1,500 mg daily) for 6 weeks, followed by lapatinib plus weekly paclitaxel (80 mg/m^2) for an additional 12 weeks; (2) trastuzumab (4 mg/kg load followed by 2 mg/kg weekly) for 6 weeks, followed by trastuzumab plus weekly paclitaxel (80 mg/m^2) for an additional 12 weeks; (3) oral lapatinib (1,000 mg daily) plus trastuzumab (4 mg/kg load followed by 2 mg/kg weekly) for 6 weeks, followed by lapatinib (at 750 mg/day) and trastuzumab plus weekly paclitaxel (80 mg/m^2) for an additional 12 weeks. Definitive surgery will be performed within 4 weeks of the last dose of paclitaxel. Patients will begin adjuvant treatment with three cycles of 5-fluorouracil, epirubicin, and cyclophosphamide (FEC) within 6 weeks of surgery and afterwards will continue on the same anti-HER2 treatment they received in the neoadjuvant setting for an additional 34 weeks. The primary endpoint is pathologic complete response. Secondary endpoints include the safety and tolerability of the three treatment arms, the objective response rates at the end of the of the 6-week biological window and at the time of definitive surgery, the rate of conversion to breast conserving surgery, disease free survival and overall survival. Correlative studies will be performed to identify the molecular characteristics of responding tumors by immunohistochemical, FISH, genomic and proteomic analysis. Circulating tumor cells and the expression of other biomarkers will be assessed before and during therapy to establish correlations with clinical outcome.

NSABP-B41

NSABP-B41 is a randomized phase III study with a design similar to NeoALLTO except for the use of upfront anthracyclines. A total of 522 patients with operable HER2 overexpressing breast cancer >2.0 cm will be treated with doxorubicin 60 mg/m^2 and cyclophosphamide 600 mg/m^2 every 3 weeks for four cycles followed by weekly paclitaxel 80 mg/m^2 on days 1, 8, and 15 of a 28-day cycle for 12 doses (4 cycles) with trastuzumab, lapatinib or the combination. Post-operatively, all patients receive trastuzumab 6 mg/kg every 3 weeks to complete 1 year of anti-HER2 targeted therapy. The primary endpoint is pathologic complete response.

CALGB 40601

CALGB 40601, which will open to enrollment in the later part of 2008, is a randomized phase III trial again similar in design to the NeoALLTO trial with multiple embedded correlative endpoints. A total of 400 patients with newly diagnosed stage II/III HER2-overexpressing breast cancer that is >1 cm will be treated with weekly paclitaxel for 16 weeks and randomized to concurrent weekly trastuzumab, daily lapatinib or the combination. Tissue is obtained at treatment start and at the time of surgery, and the primary endpoint is pathologic complete response. Planned correlative science studies will examine pathways implicated in trastuzumab and lapatinib resistance. Post-operative therapy is left to the discretion of the treating physician but either dose dense or every 3 weeks doxorubicin and cyclophosphamide are recommended as well as 1 year of post-surgical trastuzumab therapy.

Other Ongoing Neoadjuvant Trials

Several investigator initiated trials are ongoing internationally. Two examples are described here. The feasibility and efficacy of using lapatinib in combination with nanoparticle-albumin-bound paclitaxel (nab-paclitaxel) abraxane in the neoadjuvant setting is being investigated at Northwestern University by Gradishar and colleagues. In this study nab-paclitaxel abraxane 260 mg/m^2 is given every 3 weeks of a 4-week cycle in combination with either lapatinib 1,000 mg/day or 1,500 mg/day for a total of four cycles. Stanford University is conducting an open-label phase II trial evaluating pathologic complete response in clinical stage II/III breast cancer following neoadjuvant chemotherapy with sequential doxorubicin 60 mg/m^2 plus cyclophosphamide 600 mg/m^2 every 2 weeks for four cycles followed by docetaxel every 3 weeks with concurrent lapatinib 1,250 mg daily for four cycles. The primary endpoint is pathologic complete response.

Concluding Remarks

While the discovery of trastuzumab has certainly improved the clinical prognosis of a highly aggressive subset of breast cancer, de novo and acquired trastuzumab resistance is a known problem and is clinically an increasing issue with adjuvant use of trastuzumab. Lapatinib has proven to be well-tolerated and active against trastuzumab-resistant tumors both in preclinical and clinical studies, and its efficacy as a single agent in the treatment of inflammatory breast cancer hints that it may be an effective agent in the treatment of early stage breast cancer. Results from numerous ongoing neoadjuvant and adjuvant studies are eagerly awaited.

References

1. Slamon DJ, Clark GM, Wong SG, Levin WJ, Ullrich A, McGuire WL. Human breast cancer: Correlation of relapse and survival with amplification of the HER-2/neu oncogene. *Science*. 1987;235(4785):177–82.
2. Slamon DJ, Godolphin W, Jones LA, et al. Studies of the HER-2/neu proto-oncogene in human breast and ovarian cancer. *Science*. 1989;244(4905):707–12.
3. Barnes CJ, Kumar R. Biology of the epidermal growth factor receptor family. *Cancer Treat Res*. 2004;119:1–13.
4. Cho HS, Mason K, Ramyar KX, et al. Structure of the extracellular region of HER2 alone and in complex with the Herceptin Fab. *Nature*. 2003;421(6924):756–60.
5. Sliwkowski MX. Ready to partner. *Nat Struct Biol*. 2003;10(3):158–9.
6. Valabrega G, Montemurro F, Aglietta M. Trastuzumab: Mechanism of action, resistance and future perspectives in HER2-overexpressing breast cancer. *Ann Oncol*. 2007;18(6):977—84.
7. Vogel CL, Cobleigh MA, Tripathy D, et al. Efficacy and safety of trastuzumab as a single agent in first-line treatment of HER2-overexpressing metastatic breast cancer. *J Clin Oncol*. 2002;20(3):719–26.

8. Slamon DJ, Leyland-Jones B, Shak S, et al. Use of chemotherapy plus a monoclonal antibody against HER2 for metastatic breast cancer that overexpresses HER2. *N Engl J Med.* 2001;344(11):783–92.
9. Piccart-Gebhart MJ, Procter M, Leyland-Jones B, et al. Trastuzumab after adjuvant chemotherapy in HER2-positive breast cancer. *N Engl J Med.* 2005;353(16):1659–72.
10. Romond EH, Perez EA, Bryant J, et al. Trastuzumab plus adjuvant chemotherapy for operable HER2-positive breast cancer. *N Engl J Med.* 2005;353(16):1673–84.
11. Nagy P, Friedlander E, Tanner M, et al. Decreased accessibility and lack of activation of ErbB2 in JIMT-1, a herceptin-resistant, MUC4-expressing breast cancer cell line. *Cancer Res.* 2005;65(2):473–82.
12. Price-Schiavi SA, Jepson S, Li P, et al. Rat Muc4 (sialomucin complex) reduces binding of anti-ErbB2 antibodies to tumor cell surfaces, a potential mechanism for herceptin resistance. *Int J Cancer.* 2002;99(6):783–91.
13. Scaltriti M, Rojo F, Ocana A, et al. Expression of p95HER2, a truncated form of the HER2 receptor, and response to anti-HER2 therapies in breast cancer. *J Natl Cancer Inst.* 2007;99(8):628–38.
14. Anido J, Scaltriti M, Bech Serra JJ, et al. Biosynthesis of tumorigenic HER2 C-terminal fragments by alternative initiation of translation. *Embo J.* 2006;25(13):3234–44.
15. Saez R, Molina MA, Ramsey EE, et al. p95HER-2 predicts worse outcome in patients with HER-2-positive breast cancer. *Clin Cancer Res.* 2006;12(2):424–31.
16. Zabrecky JR, Lam T, McKenzie SJ, Carney W. The extracellular domain of p185/neu is released from the surface of human breast carcinoma cells, SK-BR-3. *J Biol Chem.* 1991;266(3):1716–20.
17. Esteva FJ, Valero V, Booser D, et al. Phase II study of weekly docetaxel and trastuzumab for patients with HER-2-overexpressing metastatic breast cancer. *J Clin Oncol.* 2002;20(7):1800–8.
18. Kostler WJ, Schwab B, Singer CF, et al. Monitoring of serum Her-2/neu predicts response and progression-free survival to trastuzumab-based treatment in patients with metastatic breast cancer. *Clin Cancer Res.* 2004;10(5):1618–24.
19. Lu Y, Zi X, Zhao Y, Mascarenhas D, Pollak M. Insulin-like growth factor-I receptor signaling and resistance to trastuzumab (Herceptin). *J Natl Cancer Inst.* 2001;93(24):1852–7.
20. Nahta R, Yuan LX, Zhang B, Kobayashi R, Esteva FJ. Insulin-like growth factor-I receptor/human epidermal growth factor receptor 2 heterodimerization contributes to trastuzumab resistance of breast cancer cells. *Cancer Res.* 2005;65(23):11118–28.
21. Chan CT, Metz MZ, Kane SE. Differential sensitivities of trastuzumab (Herceptin)-resistant human breast cancer cells to phosphoinositide-3 kinase (PI-3 K) and epidermal growth factor receptor (EGFR) kinase inhibitors. *Breast Cancer Res Treat.* 2005;91(2):187–201.
22. Nagata Y, Lan KH, Zhou X, et al. PTEN activation contributes to tumor inhibition by trastuzumab, and loss of PTEN predicts trastuzumab resistance in patients. *Cancer Cell.* 2004;6(2):117–27.
23. Diermeier S, Horvath G, Knuechel-Clarke R, Hofstaedter F, Szollosi J, Brockhoff G. Epidermal growth factor receptor coexpression modulates susceptibility to Herceptin in HER2/neu overexpressing breast cancer cells via specific erbB-receptor interaction and activation. *Exp Cell Res.* 2005;304(2):604–19.
24. Motoyama AB, Hynes NE, Lane HA. The efficacy of ErbB receptor-targeted anticancer therapeutics is influenced by the availability of epidermal growth factor-related peptides. *Cancer Res.* 2002;62(11):3151–8.
25. Valabrega G, Montemurro F, Sarotto I, et al. TGFalpha expression impairs Trastuzumab-induced HER2 downregulation. *Oncogene.* 2005;24(18):3002–10.
26. Anastasi S, Sala G, Huiping C, et al. Loss of RALT/MIG-6 expression in ERBB2-amplified breast carcinomas enhances ErbB-2 oncogenic potency and favors resistance to Herceptin. *Oncogene.* 2005;24(28):4540–8.

27. Xia W, Mullin RJ, Keith BR, et al. Anti-tumor activity of GW572016: A dual tyrosine kinase inhibitor blocks EGF activation of EGFR/erbB2 and downstream Erk1/2 and AKT pathways. *Oncogene*. 2002;21(41):6255–63.
28. Weiner DB, Kokai Y, Wada T, Cohen JA, Williams WV, Greene MI. Linkage of tyrosine kinase activity with transforming ability of the p185neu oncoprotein. *Oncogene*. 1989;4(10):1175–83.
29. Burstein HJ, Lieberman G, Slamon DJ, Winer EP, Klein P. Isolated central nervous system metastases in patients with HER2-overexpressing advanced breast cancer treated with first-line trastuzumab-based therapy. *Ann Oncol*. 2005;16(11):1772–7.
30. Gomez HL, Doval DC, Chavez MA, et al. Efficacy and safety of lapatinib as first-line therapy for ErbB2-amplified locally advanced or metastatic breast cancer. *J Clin Oncol*. 2008;26(18):2999–3005.
31. Geyer CE, Forster J, Lindquist D, et al. Lapatinib plus capecitabine for HER2-positive advanced breast cancer. *N Engl J Med*. 2006;355(26):2733–43.
32. Geyer CE, Martin A, Newstat B, et al. Lapatinib (L) plus capecitabine (C) in HER2+ advanced breast cancer (ABC): Genomic and updated efficacy data. . *J Clin Oncol*. 2007;25(18S):1035.
33. Lin NU, Carey LA, Liu MC, et al. Phase II trial of lapatinib for brain metastases in patients with human epidermal growth factor receptor 2-positive breast cancer. *J Clin Oncol*. 2008;26(12):1993–9.
34. Lin N, Dieras V, Paul D, et al. EGF105084, a phase II study of lapatinib for brain metastases in patients (pts) with HER2+ breast cancer following trastuzumab (H) based systemic therapy and cranial radiotherapy (RT). *J Clin Oncol*. 2007;25(18S):1012.
35. Zhou H, Kim YS, Peletier A, McCall W, Earp HS, Sartor CI. Effects of the EGFR/HER2 kinase inhibitor GW572016 on EGFR- and HER2-overexpressing breast cancer cell line proliferation, radiosensitization, and resistance. *Int J Radiat Oncol Biol Phys*. 2004;58(2):344–52.
36. Xia W, Gerard CM, Liu L, Baudson NM, Ory TL, Spector NL. Combining lapatinib (GW572016), a small molecule inhibitor of ErbB1 and ErbB2 tyrosine kinases, with therapeutic anti-ErbB2 antibodies enhances apoptosis of ErbB2-overexpressing breast cancer cells. *Oncogene*. 2005;24(41):6213–21.
37. Konecny GE, Pegram MD, Venkatesan N, et al. Activity of the dual kinase inhibitor lapatinib (GW572016) against HER-2-overexpressing and trastuzumab-treated breast cancer cells. *Cancer Res*. 2006;66(3):1630–9.
38. Nahta R, Yuan LX, Du Y, Esteva FJ. Lapatinib induces apoptosis in trastuzumab-resistant breast cancer cells: Effects on insulin-like growth factor I signaling. *Mol Cancer Ther*. 2007;6(2):667–74.
39. Xia W, Husain I, Liu L, et al. Lapatinib antitumor activity is not dependent upon phosphatase and tensin homologue deleted on chromosome 10 in ErbB2-overexpressing breast cancers. *Cancer Res*. 2007;67(3):1170–5.
40. Blackwell KL, Burstein H, Pegram M, et al. Determining relevant biomarkers from tissue and serum that may predict response to single agent lapatinib in trastuzumab refractory metastatic breast cancer. *J Clin Oncol*. 2005;23(S16):3004.
41. Iwata H, Toi M, Fujiwara Y, et al. Phase II clinical study of lapatinib (GW572016) in patients with advanced or metastatic breast cancer. *Breast Cancer Res Treat*. 2006;106:1091.
42. Burstein HJ, Storniolo AM, Franco S, et al. A phase II study of lapatinib monotherapy in chemotherapy-refractory HER2-positive and HER2-negative advanced or metastatic breast cancer. *Ann Oncol*. 2008;19(6):1068–74.
43. DiLeo A, Gomez H, Aziz Z, et al. Lapatinib with paclitaxel versus paclitaxel as first-line treatment for patients with metastatic breast cancer: A phase III randomized, double-blind study in 580 patients. *J Clin Oncol*. 2007;25(18S):1011.

44. Johnston S, Pegram M, Press M, et al. Lapatinib combined with letrozole vs. letrozole alone for front line postmenopausal hormone receptor positive (HR+) metastatic breast cancer (MBC): first results from the EGF30008 trial. *Cancer Res.* 2009; 69(Suppl.)46.
45. Storniolo AM, Pegram MD, Overmoyer B, et al. Phase I dose escalation and pharmacokinetic study of lapatinib in combination with trastuzumab in patients with advanced ErbB2-positive breast cancer. *J Clin Oncol.* 2008;26(20):3317–23.
46. O'Shaughnessy J, Blackwell KL, Burstein H, et al. A randomized study of lapatinib alone or in combination with trastuzumab in heavily pretreated HER2+ metastatic breast cancer progressing on trastuzumab therapy. *J Clin Oncol.* 2008;26:1015.
47. Konecny GE, Meng YG, Untch M, et al. Association between HER-2/neu and vascular endothelial growth factor expression predicts clinical outcome in primary breast cancer patients. *Clin Cancer Res.* 2004;10(5):1706–16.
48. Pegram M, Chan D, Dichmann RA, et al. Phase II combined biological therapy targeting the HER2 proto-oncogene and the vascular endothelial growth factor using trastuzumab (T) and bevacizumab (B) as first line treatment of HER2-amplified breast cancer. *Breast Cancer Res Treat.* 2006;100(S1):301.
49. Rugo HS, Franco S, Munster P, et al. A phase II evaluation of lapatinib (L) and bevacizumab (B) in HER2+ metastatic breast cancer (MBC). *J Clin Oncol.* 2008;26:1042.
50. Slamon D, Gomez HL, Kabbinawar FF, et al. Randomized study of pazopanib + lapatinib vs. lapatinib alone in patients with HER2- positive advanced or metastatic breast cancer. *J Clin Oncol.* 2008;26:1016.
51. Slamon DJ, Stemmer SM, Johnston S, et al. Phase 2 study of dual VEGF/HER2 blockade with pazopanib + lapatinib in patients with first-line HER2 positive advanced or metastatic (adv/met) breast cancer. *Cancer Res.* 2009;69(Suppl.):4114.
52. Johnston S, Trudeau M, Kaufman B, et al. Phase II study of predictive biomarker profiles for response targeting human epidermal growth factor receptor 2 (HER-2) in advanced inflammatory breast cancer with lapatinib monotherapy. *J Clin Oncol.* 2008;26(7):1066–72.
53. Cristofanilli M, Boussen H, Baselga J, et al. A phase II combination study of lapatinib and paclitaxel as a neoadjuvant therapy in patients with newly diagnosed inflammatory breast cancer (IBC). *Breast Cancer Res Treat.* 2006;106:1.
54. Moy B, Goss PE. Lapatinib-associated toxicity and practical management recommendations. *Oncologist.* 2007;12(7):756–65.
55. Perez EA, Koehler M, Byrne J, Preston AJ, Rappold E, Ewer MS. Cardiac safety of lapatinib: Pooled analysis of 3689 patients enrolled in clinical trials. *Mayo Clinic Proceedings* 2008;83(6):679–86.
56. Lee KF, Simon H, Chen H, Bates B, Hung MC, Hauser C. Requirement for neuregulin receptor erbB2 in neural and cardiac development. *Nature.* 1995;378(6555):394–8.
57. Crone SA, Zhao YY, Fan L, et al. ErbB2 is essential in the prevention of dilated cardiomyopathy. *Nat Med.* 2002;8(5):459–65.
58. Ozcelik C, Erdmann B, Pilz B, et al. Conditional mutation of the ErbB2 (HER2) receptor in cardiomyocytes leads to dilated cardiomyopathy. *Proc Natl Acad Sci U S A.* 2002;99(13):8880–5.
59. Smith KL, Dang C, Seidman AD. Cardiac dysfunction associated with trastuzumab. *Expert Opin Drug Saf.* 2006;5(5):619–29.
60. Midgley RS, Kerr DJ, Flaherty KT, et al. A phase I and pharmacokinetic study of lapatinib in combination with infusional 5-fluorouracil, leucovorin and irinotecan. *Ann Oncol.* 2007;18(12):2025–9.
61. Dang CT, Lin NU, Lake D, et al. Preliminary safety results of dose-dense (dd) doxorubicin and cyclophosphamide (AC) followed by weekly paclitaxel (P) with trastuzumab (T) and lapatinib (L) in HER2 overexpressed/amplified breast cancer (BCA). *J Clin Oncol.* 2008;26:518.

62. Bear HD, Anderson S, Smith RE, et al. Sequential preoperative or postoperative docetaxel added to preoperative doxorubicin plus cyclophosphamide for operable breast cancer: National Surgical Adjuvant Breast and Bowel Project Protocol B-27. *J Clin Oncol*. 2006;24(13):2019–27.
63. Fisher B, Bryant J, Wolmark N, et al. Effect of preoperative chemotherapy on the outcome of women with operable breast cancer. *J Clin Oncol*. 1998;16(8):2672–85.
64. van der Hage JA, van de Velde CJ, Julien JP, Tubiana-Hulin M, Vandervelden C, Duchateau L. Preoperative chemotherapy in primary operable breast cancer: Results from the European Organization for Research and Treatment of Cancer trial 10902. *J Clin Oncol*. 2001;19(22):4224–37.
65. Kaufmann M, von Minckwitz G, Smith R, et al. International expert panel on the use of primary (preoperative) systemic treatment of operable breast cancer: review and recommendations. *J Clin Oncol*. 2003;21(13):2600–8.

Part IV
Special Issues

Supportive Care During Adjuvant Treatment

Annabel Pollard

Background: The Context of Supportive Care During Adjuvant Therapy for Breast Cancer

Introduction

The diagnosis and treatment of breast cancer has a substantial impact on health, emotional well-being and quality of life. Adjuvant systemic therapy (the administration of chemotherapy, endocrine or biologic therapy) is a distinct phase of breast cancer treatment following primary treatment [1]. Adjuvant systemic therapy is currently recommended to most women with newly diagnosed breast cancer and is associated with declining mortality for women with breast cancer [2, 3]. Every year in the United States approximately 200,000 women are diagnosed with breast cancer [4].

Most women will be diagnosed with potentially curable early stage disease; however the multimodal nature of adjuvant therapy, including chemotherapy, hormone and radiation treatments, typically extends over several months after primary treatment, and is associated with a variety of acute side effects, delayed toxicities and psychosocial sequelae. Over the past 20 years there has been growing recognition that these side effects and toxicities affect quality of life in both the short and longer term [5]. Thus a substantial, and growing, number of women will be living with the ongoing effects of adjuvant systemic therapy after primary treatment for breast cancer. Factors such as type of adjuvant treatment, psychological morbidity, age at diagnosis, and social situation will all affect how a woman will cope with the challenges associated with a diagnosis of breast cancer and adjuvant treatment.

Supportive care is aimed at ameliorating treatment related side effects and toxicities; unmet needs have been well documented in cancer populations and in women with breast cancer [6, 7]. Supportive care strategies

A. Pollard (✉)
Clinical Psychologist
e-mail: annabel.pollard@petermac.org

M. Castiglione, M.J. Piccart (eds.), *Adjuvant Therapy for Breast Cancer*,
Cancer Treatment and Research 151, DOI 10.1007/978-0-387-75115-3_14,

must be evidence based and should take into account the complex interplay of physical and psychosocial factors that affect women during the course of adjuvant therapy.

The chapter outlines four distinct aspects of supportive care associated with adjuvant therapy. These are: (1) making the decision to have adjuvant therapy post diagnosis and primary treatment; (2) the impact of adjuvant therapy on psychosocial variables; (3) coping with the impact of key treatment related side effects; and (4) follow up and survivorship issues. Implications for supportive care interventions are discussed.

Supportive Care During Adjuvant Breast Cancer Treatment

The Definition Of Supportive Care

Supportive care has been defined as "…the provision of necessary services as defined by those living with or affected by cancer to meet their physical, social, emotional, informational, psychological, spiritual and practical needs during the pre-diagnostic, diagnostic, treatment and follow-up phases of cancer" [8]. Fitch's definition is a broad one; however it encourages a comprehensive approach to service planning and care delivery.

This model suggests that the majority of patients will require less intensive supportive care across the range of known support needs. By predicting the distribution and intensity of supportive care needs this model can be used to identify which resources are required and where resources might need to be positioned, throughout an organisation or cancer service, to enhance provision of supportive care in a sustainable and cost effective manner. For example, in this model *all* women will require information about their treatment and factors such as diet, exercise and emotional adjustment (typically provided by medical and nursing staff) whilst *some* or a *few* might require intensive support from a specialist health professional (dietician, physiotherapist, psychiatrist). Moreover, a breast cancer service will have a different profile of supportive care needs compared to a lung cancer service [9]. Notwithstanding this Fitch, proposes that a significant minority of patients with cancer, about 30–40%, will require specialised or more intensive assistance over the course of cancer diagnosis and treatment [8].

Distress Screening

An important step in the provision of supportive care services in the oncology setting is the identification of the patient and family's specific needs. The systematic identification of need is essential as, for example, studies indicate that health care professionals frequently fail to recognise psychosocial distress [10, 11]. In fact, a number of consensus guidelines now recommend screening as an integral component of cancer care, and ideally patients should be screened across the treatment continuum [12, 13–16]. The presence of an effective screening system and referral process is central to the early identification of unmet needs or morbidity in the cancer patient population, facilitating delivery of effective and timely supportive care interventions to those identified at risk or with sizable needs [6, 16]. Whilst the assessments of quality of life, satisfaction with care and other psychosocial parameters have become more common, few of these assessments clarify which issues are important to the patient [6]. The identification of supportive care needs provides an indication of the incidence of need, allowing targeting of support services to specific needs [17]. A needs screening is a process undertaken to identify patient perceptions of issues for which they may require help to maintain or regain optimal health and quality of life outcomes [18]. Consistent with the Fitch model [8], screening also needs highlights gaps in the overall provision of supportive care services. The Distress Thermometer is an example of a simple tool shown to identify effectively and quickly a range of problems and psychosocial distress and has been well validated in a cancer population [16]. Ideally, screening should be repeated at key points along the treatment continuum.

Referral Pathways

Effective screening identifies patients at increased risk, or those with areas of known unmet need, in a systematic manner (e.g. women at risk of developing lymphedema or at increased risk of distress). However, completion of a screening tool alone does not meet the supportive care needs of oncology patients. For example, a study of 303 breast cancer patients found that 45% had a psychiatric disorder, and 42% had depression, anxiety or both, yet referrals were not made for review of these needs [19]. While a screening tool may capture the patient's need, the screening process must involve a step that translates the need into an action, namely a referral to the appropriate intervention or service. Apart from referrals for treatment of psychosocial distress, few services internationally have described how, once unmet need is identified, patients are referred for supportive care services. Despite many publications now outlining evidence based approaches to supportive care, much more needs to be done to translate research findings into practice [20]. Such an approach might incorporate screening, assessment and referral with a service providing information retrieval and access to reputable internet sites. Another economic perspective might include calculating the downstream effects of expanding medical services such as breast surgery, to ensure sufficient expansion of associated supportive services such as physiotherapy or psychology services.

Issues and Challenges Facing Women During Adjuvant Breast Cancer Treatment

Adjustment to Breast Cancer: The Psychosocial Journey

Cella and Tross [21] likened a person's experience of cancer as a series of multiple stressors. In this model, stressors are conceptualised as traumatic reactions to diagnosis (residual stressors), current day-to-day difficulties of managing a cancer illness (current stressors) and anticipatory stress for an uncertain future health (anticipatory stressors) [21]. Conceptualising the experiences of women recently diagnosed with breast cancer in this way may be useful in guiding supportive care. Initial diagnosis and surgical treatment are usually experienced as a major stressor, both shocking and distressing. Thereafter, most women describe ongoing concerns as a series of stressful experiences, associated with coping with multiple disruptions to everyday life, such as the impositions of attending hospital for regular treatments travel time, financial pressures associated with treatment costs or ceasing employment, making decisions about treatment, coping with acute side effects, as well as other anticipatory stressors including concerns about recurrence, future or mortality. For each woman the cancer experience will vary according to her unique personality, social context and developmental stage. A woman's identity and role(s) as mother, wife, carer or her financial independence remain sources of strength and assist with maintaining a sense of normalcy, and most women find the process of adjusting and coping with the imposition of illness very challenging.

Decision Making, Informational Needs, and Communication

Women with breast cancer are challenged to make a number of complex key decisions about treatment, including seeking confirmation of diagnosis, making decisions about surgery and sentinel node biopsy, and deciding on adjuvant therapy [22]. As treatments have become more complex so has the decision making process for women diagnosed with breast cancer, for example deciding on clinical trial. Adjuvant therapy is known to improve disease-free and overall survival in women with early breast cancer, with greater benefit bestowed on specific groups for example younger women and those in higher risk groups [23]. However, adjuvant treatments are associated with adverse side effects and the anticipated benefits of adjuvant therapy for individual women will depend on a number of complex risk factors such as extent of disease, histology, and receptor status of the cancer [23]. Despite known toxicities, research indicates that few women decline adjuvant therapy, even in low risk groups [24]. Several studies indicate that women judge small benefits to be worthwhile when deciding on adjuvant therapy, making decisions about adjuvant therapy appears to be related to a combination of subjective interpretation, personal circumstances and beliefs and values [25]. There is evidence that some women overestimate survival chances and the risk reduction offered by adjuvant therapies, and many liken their decision to undergo adjuvant therapy as "an insurance policy" [26]. A recent follow up study concluded that making a decision about having adjuvant chemotherapy does not appear to be related to psychosocial factors, such as anxiety or optimism, but rather to parenting concerns, minimising regret, doubts about the information itself, or feeling as if there was no choice [27].

Decision making about adjuvant treatment is generally made in the context of significantly increased distress, and distress can negatively affect information recall in a medical encounter. There is also an association between provision of information and mood; for example, women who feel they have been given inadequate information are more likely to report symptoms of anxiety and depression at 12 months post diagnosis [28].

What are the implications for oncologists and other health care professionals? First, good communication skills are essential to the patient and enhance delivery of information, informed treatment decisions, treatment compliance and adjustment. Evidence shows that oncologists' perceptions of what women want to know do not always match with patient preferences and that physicians frequently do not identify emotional cues very well. Factors such as general interactional skills [29], provision of information, discussing treatment options and providing choice, directing patients to quality information on the internet, and exploring and responding to specific concerns have all been shown to enhance communication between patient and physician [20, 30] and improve adjustment [31]. Patient preferences for information vary significantly and clinicians should establish patient preferences for amount and type of information. Every patient will interpret information differently, and this may impact significantly on their treatment choices; thus tailoring information delivery to patient style can be helpful [32]. In fact, communication skills training has been shown to improve doctor skills [33]. For doctors and health care professionals, routinely seeking patient satisfaction with, and feedback about, consultations could enhance clinician communication skills training and the clinical encounter in the everyday setting [31].

A number of important factors have been shown to influence decision making about cancer treatment. Physician characteristics such as providing support and emphasising hopefulness are judged as helpful when physicians emphasise the content of information rather than just probability [34], and physician's attitudes (confidence, supportive, openness and encouraging) are rated as desirable [35]. Physicians who attend to affective issues are also rated more highly by patients [36]. Use of decision aids in making decisions has been shown to enhance knowledge of disease, and to facilitate informed choices and satisfaction with treatment decisions in women having adjuvant treatment for node negative breast cancer [37, 38]. In summary, the communication style of health care professionals, more especially effective communication, has a significant impact on outcomes for women with breast cancer. Supportive care at this juncture in the treatment of breast cancer is targeted at all women, and encompasses the ability to engage in purposeful and skilled communication including delivering information, discussing treatment choices, and recognising and responding to psychosocial distress. Recommended steps for discussing treatment options are shown in Table 1 [13].

Table 1 Recommended steps for discussing treatment options and encouraging involvement in decision-making

Information About Treatment

- Explain to the person using language that they understand what treatment options are available (including no treatment) and ask how much detail they would like about each option
- Tailor the information to the person's needs and preferences for information content and detail, which may include a discussion of the expected outcomes and major side effects of each treatment option
- Acknowledge the uncertainty of any treatment achieving its aim; explain the pros and cons of each option and then summarise them
- Use a variety of media to provide information about treatment options, eg written information, video tapes, tapes of consultations, etc.
- Ask the person about any questions they may have regarding alternative and complementary therapies
- Ask the person to talk about the concerns they have regarding different options

Making Decisions About Treatment

- Explore at an early stage how the patient would like to be involved in decision-making and adhere to their wishes
- Be aware that the person's preferences may change over time and regularly check the level of involvement they would like
- Ask the patient about their values and life situation in relation to the treatment options
- Use inclusive language (we, our)
- Make it explicit that there is a choice to be made, and that the patient can be involved in the choice
- If the person is unaccompanied ask whether they would like to discuss treatment options with family or friends and tell the person that there is an opportunity for them to be involved in treatment decisions
- Assure the person that there is enough time to consider the treatment options and offer to arrange for them to come back with a decision

Emotional and Supportive Role

- Consider the specific needs related to gender, age and culture
- Give the person the opportunity to discuss and express their feelings, e.g. crying freely, talking about concerns, fears, anger, anxieties, etc. Acknowledge individual differences in emotional impact
- Address disturbing or embarrassing topics directly, and with sensitivity
- Provide information about support services
- Make your own recommendations clear, but offer your willingness to be involved in the ongoing care of the patients (if required) no matter what they decide in response to your recommendation

Adapted with permission, from National Breast Cancer Centre and National Cancer Control Initiative. 2003. Clinical practice guidelines for the psychosocial care of adults with cancer. Table 3.3.2, p 62. National Breast Cancer Centre Camperdown, NSW. Australia

Psychosocial Variables in Breast Cancer

During diagnosis and treatment for breast cancer, the literature suggests that the majority of women will adjust reasonably well; however, a substantial proportion of women will experience some degree of psychological distress and or a psychiatric disorder [28, 39–42]. Distress is associated with a broad range of factors including coping with psychological impact of initial diagnosis, with toxicities and side effects of treatment, with alterations in role and function associated with the former, and with disruptions to social roles and interpersonal relationships. Risk factors for psychosocial adaptation in cancer can be associated with both characteristics of the individual and characteristics of the disease, outlined in Table 2 [13], and may be of predictive value in early identification of those at greater risk. It is helpful to remain aware of these factors in the clinical encounter when assessing risk and needs for additional supportive care interventions.

Table 2 Factors associated with an increased risk of psychosocial problems

Characteristics of the individual:
• Younger
• Single, separated, divorced or widowed
• Living alone
• Children younger than 21 years
• Economic adversity
• Lack of social support, perceived poor social support
• Poor marital or family functioning
• History of psychiatric problems
• Cumulative stressful life events
• History of alcohol or other substance abuse
• Gender
Characteristics/stages of disease and treatment:
• At the time of diagnosis and recurrence
• During advanced stage of the disease
• Poorer prognosis
• More treatment side-effects
• Greater functional impairment and disease burden
• Experiencing lymphoedema
• Experiencing chronic pain
• Fatigue

Adapted with permission, from National Breast Cancer Centre and National Cancer Control Initiative. 2003. Clinical practice guidelines for the psychosocial care of adults with cancer. Table 3.7D, p 98. National Breast Cancer Centre Camperdown, NSW. Australia

Adjustment styles and personality will all play a major role in determining how a woman will respond to and cope with diagnoses and treatment of her breast cancer [43]. In a now classic article, Taylor et al. showed that coping style (an active problem solving approach and decreased avoidance) was associated with improved adjustment and less distress [44]. Conversely, helplessness and hopelessness have been associated with adverse psychological sequelae [45]. Research suggests that in order to be effective, coping efforts are best "matched" to a specific situation [46]. Thus psychological reactions that display flexibility are often more helpful; for example an ability to shift coping approaches from an active style, e.g. information seeking and decision making, at the start of treatment, to a mode of acceptance or 'positive yielding' during times of less control are likely to be adaptive [47]. In practice, individuals who are able to ask for, and accept, assistance and support (from professionals or friends and family) often cope better with diagnosis and treatment; conversely, the rigidly independent person may require coaching to assist them in asking for help.

A diagnosis of cancer is almost always stressful; psychological distress is a common experience during cancer diagnosis and treatment, and distress varies across tumour type [48]. Distress is frequently associated with fear of recurrence, uncertainty, and concerns about ones own mortality. Depression is one of the most prevalent psychological problems for cancer patients [48, 49]. The prevalence of depression in breast cancer has been found to vary from between 1.5% and 46% across studies [50]. Depression of itself causes significant distress and is associated with higher risks of suicide in the breast cancer population [51]. For women with breast cancer, distress rates vary; undergoing adjuvant therapy is frequently a time of increased distress, as women adjust to the impact of diagnosis and surgery and contemplate several further months of treatment. A recent study of newly diagnosed breast cancer patients about to undergo breast surgery indicated that 41% rated their distress as clinically significant on the Distress Thermometer, and a prevalence rate of 11% for depression and 10% for post traumatic stress disorder [52]. Kissane et al. found women with early stage breast cancer (on average 3 months post surgery) had an overall prevalence rate of DSM-IV psychiatric disorder of 45% when diagnosed via structured psychiatric interview [53]. Extensive research now shows that women undergoing treatment for breast cancer experience numerous negative psychological sequelae including depression, anxiety, adjustment reactions and existential distress [54]. Indeed, cancer occurs within the context of ongoing life pressures, and distress and depression during cancer have been shown to be correlated with other concurrent stressful life events [40]. There is evidence that women undergoing adjuvant therapy may experience higher levels of distress and this may be related to the impact of coping with ongoing and often severe treatment related toxicities [55].

Pre-morbid psychiatric disorder including depression or anxiety may indicate previous vulnerability to stress in the individual's genetic or personality orientation or may affect an individuals ability to comply with adjuvant treatment; for example, a past history of trauma, i.e. sexual abuse, may trigger post traumatic reactions, such as re-experiencing traumatic events, which may reduce coping capacity [56, 57]. Concurrent major stressors or history of multiple losses are associated with poorer outcomes [40]. Personality disorders affect a small percentage of the population and may be difficult to diagnose; they are often indicated by the reactions of the treating team to an individual whose behaviours and affect are consistently experienced as challenging – the person is often labelled difficult and referred to the psychiatry. Alcohol or other substance abuse may be indicative of a primary psychiatric disorder, self medication and or ineffective coping under stress [58]. Previous exposure to cancer or family history of experience of breast cancer can colour attitudes and beliefs about cancer, both positively and negatively.

Age related differences are an important consideration in the provision of supportive care in the breast cancer population. Importantly there is a growing body of research that indicates differences in the range of physiological and psychological experiences of older vs younger women, thought in part to be related to developmental or life stage concerns and the differential impacts of treatment. Overall trends of current research now suggest that younger women with breast cancer are more vulnerable to physical and psychological distress [59], and younger women appear to experience greater psychological dysfunction, whereas older women appear to experience greater physical and functional distress [60]. Age is clearly a risk factor that might influence the type and profile of supportive care needs required.

Almost overwhelmingly the presence of adequate social support is linked with improved health outcomes and social support is considered an important factor in mediating the stress of a cancer diagnosis of stressful events such as cancer [61, 62]. Conversely, lack of social support tends to be linked to poor adjustment. Partners and families are frequently cited as the most important sources of support for women with breast cancer.

Partners may be equally distressed by the cancer experience as the patient, and communication is one of the key areas of relationship that is affected; interventions targeting improved communication have been shown to alleviate distress in both partner and patient [63]. Positive couple adaptation is facilitated by intimacy, open communication, emotional closeness, cohesion and flexibility; however, many partners fail to communicate their fears to patients because they worry "they will make things worse" [64]. For example, one study found that 30–40% of couples reported that they did not discuss the cancer prognosis [65]. Even breast cancer patients who report high marital satisfaction report communication difficulties [66, 67]. Barriers to sharing the cancer experience with one's partner may be particularly problematic because of the level of importance the partner has as a source of support [68]. In cancer, couples may experience loss of their sexuality or interruptions to their usual practices of intimacy that can affect the relationship. Breast cancer has sometimes been referred to as the "relationship disease" or the "couple's cancer" indicating its debilitating effect on the sexual component of the couple relationship [69]. Families are affected to the extent that couples cope with the diagnosis of breast cancer together and families who have greater levels of dysfunction do worse [70, 71]. Women with children experience significant distress related to actual or potential alterations in their role as parent, concerns to protect children from cancer related fears, and how to moderate anxiety in the family [72, 73]. However, single women must often cope alone and are likely to experience increased distress [74].

In summary, supportive interventions during adjuvant treatment must take into account key psychosocial variables including psychological distress, information seeking, decision making, coping with psychological distress, age related variables and the impact of roles and relationships.

Social effects and effects on family	Psychological effects
• Role changes	
• Disruption within the family	• Adjustment and coping
• Effects on partner and relationship	• Anxiety
• Effects on children and children's reactions	• Depression
• Impacts on employment	• Distress
• Impact on financial independence	• Fear of recurrence
• Travel to and from treatment centres	• Loss of trust in body
	• Identity
	• Self esteem
	• Sexual dysfunction
	• Fertility

Psychological Impact of Treatment Related Side Effects

Adjuvant systemic therapy is associated with variety of treatment related side effects including ongoing disruptions to quality of life, physical health, psychological well being, social and occupational functioning. Each type of adjuvant therapy has a profile of known toxicities, each of which can adversely impact on overall quality of life and which have implications for supportive care provision, which should be targeted at these core concerns. There are a number of key toxicities that deserve mention in relation to supportive care needs of women undergoing adjuvant treatment. Other chapters will address these issues in more detail. However, it is important to acknowledge that treatment related side effects and physiological/functional losses have a psychological component and are related to psychological distress and the overall experience of cancer. In addition, they require complex support interventions that might require medical psychological and specialist disciplinary input.

Reproductive and Endocrine Effects

The impact of breast cancer adjuvant chemotherapy regimens and endocrine therapy on oestrogen levels is well known. The effects of treatment will vary somewhat, depending on age and type of treatment, but in both pre- and perimenopausal women the endocrine effects of ovarian ablation have been shown to have a significant impact on overall functioning, though the pattern of concerns may vary slightly [75]. For example, risk of menopause varies according to age and type of therapies, and a majority of women over 40 years of age will become permanently menopausal and a substantial minority of women under 40 years will experience permanent menopause [76]. Premature menopause is associated with a variety of unpleasant side effects including psychological distress, loss of menstrual function, vasomotor symptoms (hot flashes, night sweats), fatigue, insomnia, joint pain, vaginal dryness, mood swings and cognitive changes [77]. Younger women tend to report greater impacts on self image identity and life stage interruptions than older women [60, 78]. Taken together these changes often engender significant psychological distress and in a subset of women there may be significant sequelae associated with issues of reproductive losses and other precipitate psychiatric sequelae [53]. Supportive care strategies such as a menopause assessment clinic have been shown to ameliorate symptoms and improve functioning [79, 80]. Biological interventions with selective serotonin reuptake inhibitors have been shown to be useful in suppressing vasomotor symptoms (hot flashes) and exercise may also be an important moderator of symptoms [79].

Lynda: Menopause body image and psychological distress

Lynda is a youthful 60-year-old woman diagnosed with early breast cancer. She underwent surgery, reconstruction with insertion of breast expander and commenced Anastrazole post treatment. She experienced post-operative surgical complications which resulted in several operations and significant scarring of her breast and chest wall region. She was dissatisfied with her cosmetic outcomes and angry with her surgeon whom she blamed. She became increasingly depressed with predominant themes of anger, rumination, despair, and loss of control over the 10 months post treatment. Over this period she also developed Grade 1–2 menopause symptoms (she had been on hormone replacement therapy which was ceased at the time of breast surgery).

Body Image and Self Esteem

The cumulative effects of adjuvant treatment have a significant impact and lasting effect on a woman's body, body image and sense of self. Fobair and colleagues investigated body image and sexual problems in women under 50 years soon after completion of adjuvant treatment [81]. Heightened body image concerns were associated with mastectomy, hair loss from chemotherapy, weight gain, lowered self esteem, and relationship difficulties with partners, and about half the sample experienced some form of sexual problem. Implications for supportive care are that all women could benefit from information about alterations in sexual functioning together with strategies for managing functional changes or losses. Some women and their partners may benefit from additional couples counselling to assist with adjustment to these changes. It is recommended that clinicians ask about current symptomatology and refer women for supportive interventions where appropriate [82].

Weight Gain

Weight gain is another common problem during and after adjuvant treatment for breast cancer and, though its aetiology is not well understood, is thought to be associated with a number of physiological and psychological factors including chemotherapy regime, menopausal status, mood, reduced physical activity during treatment, changes in dietary intake [83]. Clinically women report weight gain as highly distressing, and weight gain impacts negatively on self-esteem and body image at a time of increased psychological vulnerability [81]. Consistent reports of weight gain across a number of studies have shown that between 50% and 96% of women experience some sort of weight gain during adjuvant treatment, average weight gain varies between 2.5 kg and 6.5 kg, and weight gain appears to be more common in premenopausal women [83, 84]. Irrespective of causation, there is increasing evidence that overweight status at diagnosis and increased body mass index (BMI) are associated with increased risk of recurrence [84]. There appears to be enough cumulative evidence to suggest that during adjuvant treatment women require access to information and supportive interventions around diet and regular exercise to minimise weight gain and its associated impact on body image, mood and potential disease risk [85–87].

Neuropsychological Effects

Cognitive impairment in the form of alterations in memory and concentration is frequently described by women undergoing chemotherapy. Often referred to by patients as "chemo-brain", clinically women appear to find this side effect both aversive and unexpected. An association has been found between cytotoxic drugs and cognitive changes; however many studies have been cross sectional and thus conclusions are limited. The phenomenon is not well understood but is reported as a combination of subtle changes in memory and the ability to think clearly [88]. The aetiology is not well described though it has been linked both to mood changes associated with menopause and types and intensity of cytotoxic drug regimens [89]. Brezden et al. found cognitive disturbances in women post standard adjuvant chemotherapy were independent of mood [88]. Stewart et al. in a prospective study showed that women undergoing chemotherapy experienced subtle cognitive deficits greater than those in a hormone therapy control group [90, 91]. The extent of the problem requires further research, is likely to have multifactorial causes and has implications for the type of intervention that might be useful [75]. No treatment has been devised; however, supportive interventions must ensure that all possible causes including mood disturbance and menopause symptoms or insomnia are also treated.

Fatigue

Fatigue is a common yet significant side effect affecting around 70% of cancer patients following adjuvant treatment and can be present up to 5 years post treatment [92]. Fatigue has been extensively researched in women with breast cancer and is thought to be related to a variety of factors associated with treatment, including menopause and depression, although exact mechanisms are not fully understood. It is likely that fatigue has psychogenic as well as physiological causes. The literature suggests that a smaller subset of women will experience more severe fatigue symptoms over a longer period post treatment and that fatigue is correlated with mood disturbance and other symptoms such as pain [92]. Interestingly, fatigue levels in women with breast cancer are comparable to age matched community samples [93]. There is increasing evidence that regular exercise may be a useful treatment for improving cancer related fatigue [94–96].

Side Effects Associated with Psychological Distress	
Acute side effects	**Late effects**
• Menopause • Vasomotor symptoms (hot flashes, night sweats) • Vaginal dryness • Loss of libido • Weight gain • Insomnia • Hair loss • Fatigue • Cognitive changes (concentration and memory)	• Ongoing menopause (loss of libido, vaginal dryness) • Infertility • Osteoporosis • Cardiac toxicities

Survivorship Issues

After completion of several months of adjuvant treatment women are frequently exhausted. The period of early survivorship (first few months after completion of treatment) is often associated with ambivalence as women experience a sense of freedom associated with treatment completion, and yet often report anxiety about the decline in regular medical contact and reassurance. Paradoxically they may experience greater psychological distress at this time as the focus moves away from coping with the practicalities of treatment and side effects. During these periods women finally find the time to process the experience or to contemplate anxieties associated with recurrence or uncertainty about the future. As previously indicated, most women adjust well. However, research indicates that there will be significant variability. Stanton et al. suggest that adaptive tasks post adjuvant treatment can be conceptualised as four domains: emotional, physical, interpersonal relationships, and life perspectives [41]. Fear of recurrence, coping with emotional distress, issues of mortality, dissatisfaction with interpersonal relationships, and reevaluating life priorities are some of the many adaptive concerns post treatment [41, 55]. The IOM report suggests that clinical practice guidelines include plans to support women across a number of survivorship related areas; these include surveillance for recurrence, monitoring for prevention, management of late sequelae, management of psychosocial and physical concerns, management of genetic issues, management of sexuality, fertility issues, and locus of care [97]. There is a substantial period of transition following adjuvant treatment for breast cancer. The literature consistently reports that, whilst all women will experience a degree of impairment across a range of domains, a significant subset will experience a greater complexity and severity of concerns of a more lasting nature. Adjustment to this range of significant health impacts and ongoing concerns is clearly a uniquely personal journey, involving the capacity to assimilate meaningfully and make sense of experience.

Summary

In conclusion, supportive care during the adjuvant phase of breast cancer involves a number of key responses from the health care system and health care professionals. Health care systems can enhance this care by first defining their approach to supportive care and, through conceptualising a comprehensive approach, support provision across an organisation. Key elements of supportive care provision include routine screening for support needs, training of skilled health care professionals in communication and responding to the broader needs of women with breast cancer determined by current research knowledge. Specific initiatives such as systematic provision of information, facilitating the important decision making process are vital when preparing women for adjuvant treatment. Understanding and recognition of psychosocial distress, awareness of those at higher risk and ensuring referral to appropriate resources are key component of effective support. Given the extensive evidence base it is now axiomatic that psychosocial care and supportive care management should be viewed as an integral component of breast cancer treatment and follow up. Finally, the support needs of women with breast cancer and the effects of adjuvant therapy are now well documented – the challenge for all those wishing to demonstrate excellence in cancer care is to incorporate a supportive care framework into everyday clinical practice. For women to survive and thrive, expert medical care is complemented and enhanced by expert supportive care.

Case Study

Libby was diagnosed at the age of 28 years with early breast cancer. Libby recalled finding her diagnosis a "shock" and recalled that at the time she coped well with lumpectomy, chemotherapy and radiation therapy. She underwent four cycles of AC, 6 weeks of radiation treatment, and self funded a course of Herceptin. She was advised by her medical oncologist to take Tamoxifen for 5 years. She viewed her decision to take Tamoxifen as "extra insurance". In the year following treatment completion Libby became increasingly depressed and distressed. The main source of her distress was her inability to start a family. Whilst Tamoxifen treatment was viewed as her insurance policy, it was also the main reason for putting her plans for a family on hold and this caused her some frustration and distress.

When Libby presented for psychological assessment she was experiencing ongoing psychological distress and depression – her mood was affected by repeated pattern of negative intrusive cognitions associated with losses, especially around loss of fertility, this latter being the overt focus of her distress. For Libby, having a family had been her life goal; consequently her distress grew, and over time many of her experiences, social outings, relationships and lifestyle choices were referenced back to this important loss of her life goal.

Libby described ongoing rumination about her losses, fears about not being able to have a family and fears about recurrence. She anticipated grief about the potential loss of family in the future. She felt others could not see or understand her loss. She felt guilty when she found herself feeling envious about other people's good fortune; despite feeling happy for them, her happiness was always tinged with regret about her losses. She felt angry that she must wait to have children and worried that the delay would affect her fertility. She wondered how she would fill her time in. She felt hopeless and without purpose. She felt guilty for feeling this way.

References

1. Osborne C Kent. Adjuvant endocrine therapy. In: Harris JR, Lippman ME, Morrow M, Osborne C Kent, eds. *Diseases of the Breast*. 3rd ed. Philadelphia: Lippincott Williams & Wilkins; 2004:866–91.
2. Stearns V, Davidson NE. Adjuvant Chemotherapy and Chemoendocrine Therapy. In: Harris JR, Lippman ME, Morrow M, Osborne C Kent, eds. *Diseases of the Breast*. 3rd ed. Philadelphia: Lippincott Williams & Wilkins; 2004:893–919.
3. Early Breast Cancer Trialists Collaborative Group. Polychemotherapy for early breast cancer: an overview of the randomised trials – Early Breast Cancer Trialists' Collaborative Group. *Lancet*. 1998;352:930–42.
4. Jemal A, Maurray T, Samuels A, Ghafoor A, Ward E, Thun MJ. Cancer statistics 2003. *Cancer Journal Clinical*. 2003;53:5–26.
5. Shapiro CL, Recht A. Late effects of adjuvant therapy for breast cancer. *Journal of the National Cancer Institute Monographs*. 1994;16:101–12.
6. Sanson-Fisher R, Girgis A, Boyes A, Bonevski B, Burton L, Cook P. The unmet supportive care needs of patients with cancer. Supportive Care Review Group. *Cancer*. 2000;88(1):226–37.
7. Redman S, Turner J, Davis C. Improving supportive care for women with breast cancer in Australia: The challenge of modifying health systems. *Psycho-oncology*. 2003;12(6):521–31.
8. Fitch M. Supportive care for cancer patients. *Hospital Quarterly*. 2000;3(4):39–46.

9. Pigott C, Pollard A, Thomson K, Aranda S. Unmet needs in cancer patients: Development of a supportive needs screening tool (SNST) *Supportive Care in Cancer*. 2009;17(1):33–45.
10. Fallowfield L, Saul J, Gilligan B. Teaching senior nurses how to teach communication skills in oncology. *Cancer Nursing*. 2001;24(3):185–91.
11. Fallowfield L, Ratcliffe D, Jenkins V, Saul J. Psychiatric morbidity and its recognition by doctors in patients with cancer. *British Journal of Cancer*. 2001;84(8):1011–5.
12. National Comprehensive Cancer Network. Distress management clinical guidelines. *J Natl Comp Cancer Network*. 2003;1:344–74.
13. NBCC. *Clinical Practice Guidelines for the Psychosocial Care of Adults with Cancer*. National Breast Cancer Centre and National Cancer Control Initiative, 2003.
14. Jacobsen PB, Ransom S. Implementation of NCCN distress management guidelines by member institutions. *J Natl Comp Cancer Network*. 2007;5(1):99–103.
15. Holland JC, Andersen B, Breitbart WS, Dabrowski M, Dudley MM, Fleishman S, et al. Distress management. *J Natl Comp Cancer Network*. 2007;5(1):66–98.
16. Jacobsen PB, Donovan KA, Trask PC, Fleishman SB, Zabora J, Baker F, et al. Screening for psychologic distress in ambulatory cancer patients. *Cancer*. 2005;103(7):1494–502.
17. Steginga SK, Occhipinti S, Dunn J, Gardiner RA, Heathcote P, Yaxley J. The supportive care needs of men with prostate cancer. *Psycho-Oncology*. 2001;10:66–75.
18. Foot G, Sanson-Fisher R. Measuring the unmet needs of people living with cancer. *Cancer Forum*. 1995;19(2):131–5.
19. Kissane DW, Clarke DM, Ikin J, Bloch S, Smith GC, Vitetta L, et al. Psychological morbidity and quality of life in Australian women with early-stage breast cancer: A cross-sectional survey. *Med J Aust*. 1998;169(4):192–6.
20. Turner J, Zapart S, Pedersen K, Rankin N, Luxford K, Fletcher J. Clinical practice guidelines for the psychosocial care of adults with cancer. *Psycho-Oncology*. Mar 2005;14(3):159–73 (91 ref).
21. Cella DF, Tross S. Psychological adjustment to survival from Hodgkin's disease. *Journal of Consulting and Clinical Psychology*. 1986;54(5):616–22.
22. Rowland JH, Massie MJ. Issues in breast cancer survivorship. In: Harris JR, Lippman ME, Morrow M, Osborne C Kent, eds. Diseases of the Breast. 3rd ed. Philadelphia: Lippincott Williams & Wilkins; 2004:1419–51.
23. Early Breast Cancer Trialists Collaborative Group. Polychemotherapy for early breast cancer: An overview of the randomised trials. *Lancet*. 1998;352:930–42.
24. Duric VM, Fallowfield LJ, Saunders C, Houghton J, Coates AS, Stockler MR. Patients' preferences for adjuvant endocrine therapy in early breast cancer: What makes it worthwhile?. *British Journal of Cancer*. 2005;93(12):1319–23.
25. Duric V, Stockler M. Patients' preferences for adjuvant chemotherapy in early breast cancer: A review of what makes it worthwhile. *Lancet Oncology*. 2001;2(11):691–7.
26. Ravdin PM, Siminoff IA, Harvey JA. Survey of breast cancer patients concerning their knowledge and expectations of adjuvant therapy. *J Clinl Oncol*. 1998;16(2):515–21.
27. Duric VM, Butow PN, Sharpe L, Boyle F, Beith J, Wilcken NR, Heritier S, Coates AS, John Simes R, Stockler MR. Psychosocial factors and patients' preferences for adjuvant chemotherapy in early breast cancer. *Psycho-Oncology*. 2007;16(1):48–59.
28. Fallowfield LJ, Hall A et al. Psychological outcomes of different treatment policies in women with early breast cancer outside a clinical trial. [see comment]. *BMJ*. 1990;301(6752):575–80.
29. Ptacek JT, Ptacek JJ. Patients' perceptions of receiving bad news about cancer. *J Clin Oncol*. 2001;19(21):4160–4.
30. Schofield P, Carey M, Bonevski B, Sanson-Fisher R. Barriers to the provision of evidence-based psychosocial care in oncology. *Psycho-Oncology*. 2006;15(10):863–72.
31. Shilling V, Jenkins V, Fallowfield L. Factors affecting patient and clinician satisfaction with the clinical consultation: Can communication skills training for clinicians improve satisfaction? *Psycho-Oncology*. 2003;12(6):599–611.

32. Lobb EA, Butow P, Tattersall MHN, Girgis A, Mann L, White K, Wilson J, Hobbs K. Talking about prognosis with women who have early breast cancer: What they prefer to know and guidelines to help explain it effectively. Report of *National Breast and Ovarian Cancer Centre and National Library of Australia*. 1998:1–100.
33. Fallowfield L, Jenkins V, Farewell V, Saul J, Duffy A, Eves R. Efficacy of a Cancer Research UK communication skills training model for oncologists: A randomised controlled trial. *Lancet*. 2002;359(9307):650–6.
34. Butow P, Dowsey S, Haggerty R, Tattersall MHN. Communicating prognosis to patients with metastatic disease: What do they really want to know? *Supportive Care Cancer*. 2002;10:161–8.
35. Gray RE, Greenberg M, Fitch M, Sawka C, Hampson A, Labrecque M, Moore B. Information needs of women with metastatic breast cancer. *Cancer prevention & control*. 1998;2:57–62.
36. Dowsett SM, Saul JL, Butow PN, Dunn SM, Boyer MJ, Findlow R, et al. Communication styles in the cancer consultation: preferences for a patient-centred approach. *Psycho-Oncology*. 2000;9(2):147–56.
37. Whelan T, Sawka C, Levine M, Gafni A, Reyno L, Willan A, et al. Helping patients make informed choices: a randomized trial of a decision aid for adjuvant chemotherapy in lymph node-negative breast cancer. *Journal of Nat Cancer Institute*. 2003;95(8):581–7.
38. Siminoff LA, Gordon NH, Silverman P, Budd T, Ravdin PM. A decision aid to assist in adjuvant therapy choices for breast cancer. *Psycho-Oncology*. 2006;15(11):1001–13.
39. **Psychological aspects of breast cancer study group.** (Bloom JR, Cook M, Fotopoulis S, Flamer D, Gates C, Holland JC, Muenz LR, Murawski B, Penman D, Ross RD). Psychological response to mastectomy. A prospective comparison study. *Cancer*. 1987;59(1):189–96.
40. Golden-Kreutz DM, Andersen BL. Depressive symptoms after breast cancer surgery: Relationships with global, cancer-related, and life event stress. *Psycho-Oncology*. 2004;13(3):211–20.
41. Stanton AL, Ganz PA, Rowland JH, Meyerowitz BE, Krupnick JL, Sears SR. Promoting adjustment after treatment for cancer. *Cancer*. 2005;104(11 Suppl):2608–13.
42. Burgess C, Cornelius V, Love S, Graham J, Richards M, Ramirez A. Depression and anxiety in women with early breast cancer: Five year observational cohort study. *BMJ*. 2005;330(7493):702.
43. Watson M, Greer S, Rowden L. et al. Relationships between emotional control, adjustment to cancer and depression and anxiety in breast cancer patients. Psychological Medicine. 1991;21:51–7.
44. Taylor SE, Lichtman RR, Wood JV, Bluming AZ, Dosik GM, Leibowitz RL. Illness-related and treatment-related factors in psychological adjustment to breast cancer. *Cancer*. 1985;55(10):2506–13.
45. Watson M, Greer S, Rowden L, Gorman C, Robertson B, Bliss JM, et al. Relationships between emotional control, adjustment to cancer and depression and anxiety in breast cancer patients. *Psychological Medicine*. 1991;21(1):51–7.
46. Suls J, Fletcher B. The relative efficacy of avoidant and non-avoidant coping strategies: A meta-analysis. *Health Psychology*. 1985;4:249–88.
47. Shapiro SL, Lopez AM. et al. Quality of life and breast cancer: Relationship to psychosocial variables. *Journal of Clinical Psychology*. 2001;57(4):501–19.
48. Zabora J, Brintzenhofeszoc K, Curbow B, Hooker C, Piantadosi S. The prevalence of psychological distress by cancer site. *Psycho-Oncology*. 2001;10(1):19–28.
49. Massie MJ, Holland JC. Depression and the cancer patient. *Journal of Clinical Psychiatry*. 1990;51(Suppl):12–7; discussion 18–19.
50. Massie MJ. Prevalence of depression in patients with cancer. *J Natl Cancer Inst Monogr*. 2004;32:57–71.

51. Schairer C, Brown LM, Chen BE, Howard R, Lynch CF, Hall P, et al. Suicide after breast cancer: An international population-based study of 723,810 women. *Journal of the National Cancer Institute*. 2006;98(19):1416–9.
52. Hegel MT, Moore CP, Collins ED, Kearing S, Gillock KL, Riggs RL, et al. Distress, psychiatric syndromes, and impairment of function in women with newly diagnosed breast cancer. *Cancer*. 2006;107(12):2924–31.
53. David W, Kissane BG, Love A, Clarke DM, Bloch S, Smith GC. Psychiatric disorder in women with early stage and advanced breast cancer: A comparative analysis. *Australian and New Zealand Journal of Psychiatry*. 2004;38(5):320–6.
54. Meyerowitz BE, Watkins IK, Sparks FC. Psychosocial implications of adjuvant chemotherapy. A two-year follow-up. *Cancer*. 1983;52(8):1541–5.
55. Ganz PA, Desmond KA, Leedham B, Rowland JH, Meyerowitz BE, Belin TR. Quality of life in long-term, disease-free survivors of breast cancer: A follow-up study. [erratum appears in *J Natl Cancer Inst*. Mar 2002;20;94(6):463]. *Journal of the National Cancer Institute*. 2002;94(1):39–49.
56. Green BL, Krupnick JL. et al. Trauma history as a predictor of psychologic symptoms in women with breast cancer. *Journal of Clinical Oncology*. 2000;18(5):1084–93.
57. Breitbart W. Identifying patients at risk for, and treatment of major psychiatric complications of cancer. Supportive Care in Cancer. 1995;3(1):45–60.
58. Breitbart W, ed. *Psychiatric Complications of Cancer*. Toronto Philadelphia: Decker, 1988.
59. Northouse L. Breast cancer in younger women: Effects on interpersonal and family relations. *J Natl Cancer Inst Monogr*. 1994;16:183–90.
60. Vinokur AD, Threatt BA, Vinokur-Kaplan D, Satariano WA. The process of recovery from breast cancer for younger and older patients. Changes during the first year. *Cancer*. 1990;65(5):1242–54.
61. Helgeson VS, Cohen S. Social support and adjustment to cancer: Reconciling descriptive, correlational, and intervention research. *Health Psychology*. 1996;15(2):135–48.
62. Ell KO, Mantell JE, Hamovich MB, Nishimoto RH. Social support, sense of control, and coping among patients with breast, lung, or colorectal cancer. *Journal of Psychosocial Oncology*. 1989;7:63–89.
63. Carlson LE, Bultz BD, Speca M, St-Pierre M. Partners of people with cancer: I. Impact, adjustment, and coping across the illness trajectory. *Journal of Psychosocial Oncology*. 2000;18:39–63.
64. O'Mahoney JM, Carroll RA. The impact of breast cancer and its treatment on marital functioning. *Journal of Clinical Psychology in Medical Settings*. 1997;4:397–415.
65. Chekryn J. Cancer recurrence: Personal meaning, communication, and marital adjustment. *Cancer Nursing*. 1984;7:491–498.
66. Lichtman RR, Taylor SE, Wood JV. Social support and marital adjustment after breast cancer. *Journal of Psychosocial Oncology*. 1987;5:47–74.
67. Scott JL, Halford W, Ward BG. United we stand? The effects of a couple-coping intervention on adjustment to early stage breast or gynecological cancer. *Journal of Consulting and Clinical Psychology*. 2004;72:1122–35.
68. Pistrang N, Barker C. The partner relationship in psychological response to breast cancer. *Social Science and Medicine*. 1995;40:789–97.
69. Auchincloss S, McCartney C, eds. *Gynaecologic Cancer*. Oxford: Oxford University Press, 1998.
70. Kissane DW, McKenzie M, Bloch S, Moskowitz C, McKenzie DP, O'Neill I. Family focused grief therapy: a randomized, controlled trial in palliative care and bereavement. *American Journal of Psychiatry*. 2006;163(7):1208–18.
71. Baider L, Koch U, Esacson R, De-Nour AK. Prospective study of cancer patients and their spouses: the weakness of marital strength. *Psycho-Oncology*. 1998;7(1):49–56.

72. Lewis FM, Casey SM, Brandt PA, Shands ME, Zahlis EH. The enhancing connections program: Pilot study of a cognitive-behavioral intervention for mothers and children affected by breast cancer. *Psycho-Oncology*. 2006;15(6):486–97.
73. Lewis FM, Zahlis EH, Shands ME, Sinsheimer JA, Hammond MA. The functioning of single women with breast cancer and their school-aged children.[see comment]. *Cancer Practice*. 1996;4(1):15–24.
74. Watson M, St James-Roberts I, Ashley S, Tilney C, Brougham B, Edwards L, et al. Factors associated with emotional and behavioural problems among school age children of breast cancer patients. *British Journal of Cancer*. 2006;94(1):43–50.
75. Speer JJ, Hillenberg B, Sugrue DP, Blacker C, Kresge CL, Decker VB, et al. Study of sexual functioning determinants in breast cancer survivors. *Breast Journal*. 2005; Nov–Dec; 11(6):440–7 (31 ref).
76. Goodwin PJ, Ennis M, Pritchard KI, Trudeau M, Hood N. Risk of menopause during the first year after breast cancer diagnosis. J Clin Oncol. 1999;17(8):2365–70.
77. Knobf. The influence of endocrine effects of adjuvant chemotherapy on quality of life outcomes in younger breast cancer patients. *Oncologist*. 2006;11:96–110.
78. Bloom JR, Stewart SL, Chang S, Banks PJ. Then and Now: Quality of Life in Young Breast Cancer Survivors. *Psycho-Oncology*. 2004;13(3):147–160.
79. Ganz PA, Greendale GA, Petersen L, Zibecchi L, Kahn B, Belin TR. Managing menopausal symptoms in breast cancer survivors: results of a randomized controlled trial. *Journal of the National Cancer Institute*. 2000;92(13):1054–64.
80. Friedlander M, Thewes B. Counting the costs of treatment: the reproductive and gynaecological consequences of adjuvant therapy in young women with breast cancer. *Internal Medicine Journal*. 2003;33(8):372–9.
81. Fobair P, Stewart SL, Chang S, D'Onofrio C, Banks PJ, Bloom JR. Body image and sexual problems in young women with breast cancer. *Psycho-Oncology*. 2006;15(7):579–94.
82. Ganz PA, Rowland JH, Desmond K, Meyerowitz BE, Wyatt GE. Life after breast cancer: understanding women's health-related quality of life and sexual functioning. *J Clin Oncol*. Feb 1998; 16(2):501–14 (61 ref).
83. Demark-Wahnefried W, Winer EP, Rimer BK. Why women gain weight with adjuvant chemotherapy for breast cancer. *J Clin Oncol*. 1993;11(7):1418–29.
84. Caan BJ, Emond JA, Natarajan L, Castillo A, Gunderson EP, Habel L, et al. Post-diagnosis weight gain and breast cancer recurrence in women with early stage breast cancer. *Breast Cancer Research & Treatment* 2006;99(1):47–57.
85. Markes M, Brockow T, Resch KL. Exercise for women receiving adjuvant therapy for breast cancer. *Cochrane Database of Systematic Reviews*. 2006(4):CD005001.
86. McNeely ML, Campbell KL, Rowe BH, Klassen TP, Mackey JR, Courneya KS. Effects of exercise on breast cancer patients and survivors: A systematic review and meta-analysis. *CMAJ Canadian Medical Association Journal* 2006;175(1):34–41.
87. Galvao DA, Newton RU. Review of exercise intervention studies in cancer patients. *Journal of Clinical Oncology*. 2005;23(4):899–909.
88. Brezden CB, Phillips KA, Abdolell M, Bunston T, Tannock IF. Cognitive function in breast cancer patients receiving adjuvant chemotherapy. *Journal of Clinical Oncology*. 2000;18(14):2695–701.
89. Kayl AE, Wefel JS, Meyers CA. Chemotherapy and cognition: Effects, potential mechanisms, and management. *American Journal of Therapeutics* 2006;13(4):362–9.
90. Angela Stewart BCJMETSVCB. The cognitive effects of adjuvant chemotherapy in early stage breast cancer: A prospective study. *Psycho-Oncology*. 2007;9999(9999):n/a.
91. Stewart A, Collins B, Mackenzie J, Tomiak E, Verma S, Bielajew C. The cognitive effects of adjuvant chemotherapy in early stage breast cancer: A prospective study. *Psycho-Oncology*. 2008;17(2):122–30.

92. de Jong N, Courtens AM, Abu-Saad HH, Schouten HC. Fatigue in patients with breast cancer receiving adjuvant chemotherapy: A review of the literature. *Cancer Nursing*. 2002;25(4):283–97;quiz 298–9.
93. Bower JE, Ganz PA, Desmond KA, Rowland JH, Meyerowitz BE, Belin TR. Fatigue in breast cancer survivors: occurrence, correlates, and impact on quality of life. *Journal of Clinical Oncology*. 2000;18(4):743–53.
94. Mock V, Frangakis C, Davidson NE, Ropka ME, Pickett M, Poniatowski B, et al. Exercise manages fatigue during breast cancer treatment: A randomized controlled trial. *Psycho-Oncology*. 2005;14(6):464–77.
95. Douglas E. Exercise in cancer patients. *Physical Therapy Reviews*. 2005;10(2):71–88.
96. Campbell A, Mutrie N, White F, McGuire F, Kearney N. A pilot study of a supervised group exercise programme as a rehabilitation treatment for women with breast cancer receiving adjuvant treatment. *European Journal of Oncology Nursing*. 2005;9(1):56–63.
97. Institute of Medicine and National Research Council. Meeting psychosocial needs of women with breast cancer. In: Board NCP, ed. Washington DC: National Academies Press, 2004.

Dose in (Adjuvant) Chemotherapy of Breast Cancer

Ulrike. Nitz

Introduction

Dose and dose intensity issues in breast cancer have been extensively discussed during the past few years; however, precise information is rare. Pharmacokinetic data are limited for the majority of the compounds we use. If available at all they show a large interindividual variability. Dose response relationships, even for the most commonly used drugs, have not been well investigated. In general, dosing within given chemotherapy regimens is far more toxicity than efficacy driven. In combinations, tolerable doses of single drugs are generally lower than in sequential regimens. It is therefore difficult to investigate separately the effects of dose intensity, dose density and scheduling. The following text tries to resume the available important clinical data. As remission rates in metastatic disease, especially in high-dose settings, are questionable surrogate parameters for outcome, the text focuses, as far as possible, on survival data from adjuvant randomized trials.

Theoretical Background

The Skipper Schabel Model

The Skipper Schabel [1] model has been one of the most influential models in experimental oncology during the early1970s. It has inspired a lot of clinical trials, not only in leukemia but also in solid tumors. The model as defined by Skipper and Schabel refers to the murine leukemia cell line 1210. This cell line grows in almost perfect exponential fashion from the time of implantation to lethal tumor burden. Over a wide range of growth the sensitivity to neoplastic agents remains stable so that a given number of cycles produce a given number of log kill. The nearly universal use of combinations at fixed intervals for an extended time period is

U. Nitz (✉)
Niderrhein Breast Centre, Mönchengladbach, Germany
e-mail: ulrike.nitz@wsg-online.com

M. Castiglione, M.J. Piccart (eds.), *Adjuvant Therapy for Breast Cancer*,
Cancer Treatment and Research 151, DOI 10.1007/978-0-387-75115-3_15,

traceable to the early L1210 studies. The steep dose response curves for alkylating agents, especially cyclophosphamide, which have been reported by Skipper and Schabel, have determined an entire generation of trials in high dose chemotherapy.

Norton Simon Hypothesis

In contrast to the Skipper Schabel model, the Norton Simon [2] hypothesis refers not to a constant tumor cell growth rate but to a growth rate decreasing with increasing tumor growth. This results in a "Gompertzian" growth curve with steep early tumor growth ending up in a nearly asymptotic curve as the tumor matures. Cure by chemotherapy in this model occurs more probably in the early tumor stage, with the application of multiple ideally rapidly repeated and correctly dosed chemotherapy cycles. Correct dose for a given compound may sometimes be dependent on cross toxicities better realized in a sequential than in a concomitant design. Figure 1 demonstrates the theoretical effects on clinical outcome that the variation of dose (dose intensity) and/or of interval (dose density) may cause. This model has inspired numerous trials in breast cancer.

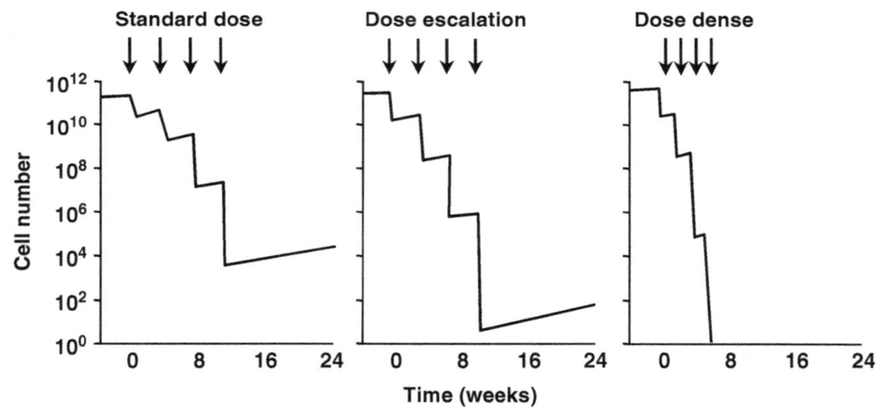

Fig. 1 Dose-Dense Chemotherapy Increase Dose Intensity by Shortening Time Between Cycles

Clinical Data

Retrospective Analyses of the Role of Dose Intensity (Dose per Week) from Levine

Basic research on the role of dose intensity in daily clinical practice has been performed by Levine and Hruniuk [3]. They have investigated dose intensity issues in ovarian cancer, in stage IV breast cancer, and in the adjuvant therapy of breast cancer since the late 1980s. Their early publications refer to retrospective analyses of randomized trials. They choose a given combination like fluorouracil, doxorubicin, and cyclophosphamide (FAC) as standard (standard = 1). All other reported regimens were expressed as a fraction of this standard (X/1) according to the doses reported from different trials. The authors included data about actually given doses, and preferably to intended doses. Later the authors refined their method and they referred to data from metastatic breast cancer trying to evaluate standard doses (= 1) for each compound separately. These data were transferred to the adjuvant setting. Within a given combination the different compounds were weighted according to the results obtained from the metastatic situation. Both methods produced very nice linear curves as demonstrated in Fig. 2.

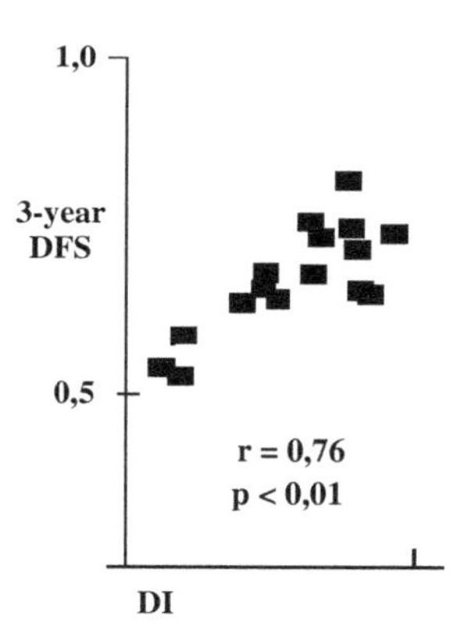

Fig. 2 Dose-intensity and survival

The data strongly suggest that underdosing is a relevant problem in daily routine. In addition the steep and linear dose response effects described by the authors suggested that dose escalations beyond conventional ranges promise proportional increases of survival rates.

Prospective Randomized Clinical Trials

In terms of dose intensity, dose density, influence of total dose, and scheduling, most phase III trials combined different escalation strategies. The following text differentiates trials investigating conventional dose range from those using a dose above the conventional range and tries to identify the corresponding intensification strategies.

Conventional Dose Range

Escalation of Single Dose and Total Dose of One Compound Within a Standard Regimen Cyclophosphamide Within NSABP AC × 4 q3w

Two trials addressed the question of escalation of cyclophosphamide (C) dose within a standard doxorubicin/cyclophosphamide (AC) × 4 regimen given at a standard interval of 3 weeks. The trials were conducted by the NSABP in node positive breast cancer. In all arms doxorubicin was given at a standard dose of 60 mg/m^2 for four cycles at 3-week intervals combined with different doses of cyclophosphamide. NSABP B22 [4] randomized 2,305 patients to three arms with C given either at 600 mg/m^2 × 4 (control), C at 1,200 mg/m^2 × 2 and at 1,200 mg/m^2 × 4. NSABP B25 [5] tested further escalation of C from 1,200 mg/m^2 to 2,400 mg/m^2 in a comparable patient population. A total of 2,548 patients were randomized to either four courses C at 1,200 mg/m^2 × 4 or 2,400 mg/m^2 × 2 or to 2,400 mg/m^2 for four courses.

Severe toxicity correlated with C dose. Neither in NSABP B22 nor in B25 were differences of disease-free or overall survival rates observed. Only one subgroup from B25 (group three receiving 4 × 2,400 mg) had a borderline benefit in terms of disease-free survival but not in terms of overall survival. Overall survival rate within this group at 5 years was 79% and was very similar to that observed in women within the control arm of B22 (78%). Those and other cross-protocol comparisons demonstrated concordant results throughout the six different treatment arms. Thus the findings from these two trials demonstrate that doubling and quadrupling the dose of C does not result in a better outcome.

(Epi) – Doxorubicin Within French Fluorouracil/Epirubicin/ Cyclophosphamide (FEC) × 6 q3w/ NSABP AC × 4 q3w

Fasg 05

The French Adjuvant Study Group 05 [6, 7] compared in 565 node positive epirubicin 50 mg/m^2 (FE50C) vs 100 mg/m^2 (FE100C). The drug was given in a combination with fluorouracil (F) 500 mg/m^2 and C 500 mg/m^2 in both treatment arms for six cycles at 3-week intervals. Patient and treatment characteristics (RT, endocrine therapy) were well balanced in the two treatment arms. After a median follow-up of 110 months the 10-year disease-free (50.7 vs 45.3%) and overall survival rates (54.8 vs 50.0%) were significantly better in the FE100C arm. Careful observation of long term toxicities such as cardiac toxicity and second malignancies confirmed a low risk profile for both regimens. The differences in terms of long term toxicity between the two treatment arms were not significant, so that the authors recommend FE100C in node positive breast cancer patients.

Calgb 9344 [8]

In the late 1990s another trial was designed to evaluate the role of anthracyclines' dose within the AC regimen and the sequential use of taxanes after four courses of AC (two by two design). Doxorubicin was given at three different doses – 60, 75, and 90 mg/m^2 with C at a constant dose of 600 mg/m^2. The trial randomized 3,121 node positive patients; 66% had hormone sensitive disease. Recurrence free survival did not show any differences depending on doxorubicin dose in the range from 60 to 90 mg.

Taxanes

There are no adjuvant phase 3 trials addressing the role of single dose escalation of taxanes. Nevertheless there is an increasing body of evidence that scheduling is a clinically relevant issue (see there).

Paclitaxel/Docetaxel

Winer et al. demonstrated in metastatic breast cancer that doses beyond 175 mg/m^2 of paclitaxel in a 3-week schedule do not improve outcome data.

Escalation of Single Dose and Total Doses of Standard Regimens (CMF, EC, FAC)

CMF (Cyclophosphamide, Methotrexate, Fluorouracil)

In locally advanced breast cancer there is one phase III trial [9] comparing C600M40F600 i.v. given all 3-weeks vs the original regimen used by Bonnadonna with oral cyclophosphamide. The i.v. regimen was inferior to the standard.

In 1995, Bonnadonna [10] et al. published the 20-years follow-up of one of the landmark trials demonstrating a survival benefit associated with adjuvant chemotherapy in breast cancer patients. The data provided clinical evidence that delivering a less-than-standard chemotherapy dose results in suboptimal outcomes. A total of 386 breast cancer patients were randomized to surgery alone (control; n = 179) or surgery followed by 12 monthly cycles of adjuvant chemotherapy (n = 207) consisting of CMF (cyclophosphamide 100 mg/m^2 orally days 1–14 q28d, methotrexate 40 mg/m^2 IV days 1, 8 q28d and 5-fluorouracil 600 mg/m^2 IV days 1, 8 q28d). Patients older than 60 years were given reduced doses (100/30/400); the dose was also reduced in case of myelosuppression. A retrospective analysis showed a dose-response effect, with relapse-free survival at 20 years being 49% in the patients given at least 85% of the planned dose and approximately 30% for all other groups. Compliance with oral medication of cyclophosphamide seems to be a clinically important issue. Inter trial comparisons suggest that 6 courses of CMF are as effective as the originally given 12 cycles.

Epirubicin/Cyclophosphamide (EC) Combinations

Piccart [11] et al. compared in 777-node positive patients 6 courses of classical CMF (oral d1-14) vs 8 courses of E50 C500 vs 8 courses of E100C830(HEC). Patients' and treatment characteristics were well balanced in the three treatment arms. After 4 years of median follow-up the event free and overall survival rates of CMF and HEC did not show any significant differences. The comparison of EC vs HEC demonstrated significant superiority of the HEC arm in terms of event-free survival and overall survival. Though in the combination both drugs were given at different dose levels, the authors attribute the efficacy differences mainly to a steep dose response relationship for E.

Due to sample size considerations, CMF was not compared to EC. The E50C500 arm was considered to be of limited clinical interest. The indirect comparison implies that E50C500 × 8, even if the cumulative dose is clearly higher than for example in the NSABP AC × 4 regime, is less effective than standard CMF.

FAC Combinations

The CALGB 8541 [12] trial randomized 1,572 women with node positive breast cancer to either 6 courses of C400d1, A40 d1 and F400 d1 + 8 repeated every 4 weeks or to 4 courses of C600d1, A60d1 and F600d1 + 8 repeated every 4 weeks or to a third arm receiving half of the total dose used in the other 2 groups and half of the dose intensity of arm 2. After a median follow-up of 3.4 years, both disease free ($p<0.001$) and overall survival ($p = 0.004$) were in favor of the high dose at moderate or high intensity.

Escalation of Single Dose with Constant Total Dose (AC vs A→C)

In trial Int-0137, Linden [13] et al. randomized 3,176 high-risk node negative and low risk node positive patients to either 6 courses of A54/C1200 × 4 q3w or to A40.5 d1 + 2 × 4 q3w followed by C2400 mg × 3 q2w with growth factor support. Total dose and duration were identical in both arms. Dose intensity was substantially higher in the sequential arm (mg/m^2/week was 18 and 27 for A and 400 and 1200 for C). No significant differences in disease-free survival or overall survival were observed. Five-year estimates of overall survival were 88% on AC and 89% on A → C. Grade 4 hematologic toxicity was greater on A → C; other toxicities were similar.

Scheduling (Taxane/Anthracycline Based Regimens)

Recently published trials reveal that, especially for widely used standard third generation taxane/anthracycline based regimens, scheduling and single doses may be clinical relevant variables influencing outcome data.

Total Dose Constant (Dose Density)

There is one specific clinical phase III trial addressing the role of dose density.

Intergroup trial 9741 [14] (CALGB 9741) randomized 2,005 node positive patients to a 2 by 2 design. Patients received either A60 × 4 → paclitaxel (T)175 × 4 → C600 × 4 or A60C600 × 4 → T175 × 4. The chemotherapy courses were given either at 3-weeks interval or at 2-weeks intervals with G-CSF support. As in Int–0137 there was no difference attributable to sequential or concomitant use. At a median follow-up of 36 months, estimated 4-year disease-free survival was 82% for the dose dense regimen and 75% for the other one (RR0.74 ; $p=0.013$). The 3-years overall survival rates were 93% for the dose dense and 90% for the other regimen (RR0.69, $p=0.013$). Disease-free survival and overall survival advantages were not accompanied by increase in toxicity. Further follow-up of this trial confirmed preliminary data.

Total Dose Inconstant

Taxanes – Sequential vs Combination

Tough superiority of taxane based regimens in node positive and recently also in node negative breast cancer is well established, although the optimal mode of application (concurrent vs sequential) remains to be defined. Several trials address this question.

The Breast International Group 02-98 [15] randomized trial tested the effect of incorporating docetaxel into an anthracycline-based adjuvant chemotherapy and compared sequential vs concurrent administration of doxorubicin and docetaxel. A total of 2,887 patients with lymph node–positive breast cancer were randomly assigned to one of four treatments:

1. Sequential control (four cycles of doxorubicin at 75 mg/m^2, followed by three cycles of cyclophosphamide, methotrexate, and 5-fluorouracil (CMF).
2. Concurrent control (four cycles of doxorubicin at 60 mg/m^2 plus cyclophosphamide at 600 mg/m^2, followed by three cycles of CMF).
3. Sequential docetaxel (three cycles of doxorubicin at 75 mg/m^2, followed by three cycles of docetaxel at 100 mg/m^2, followed by three cycles of CMF).
4. Concurrent docetaxel (four cycles of doxorubicin at 50 mg/m^2 plus docetaxel at 75 mg/m^2, followed by three cycles of CMF). Figure 3 outlines the trial design.

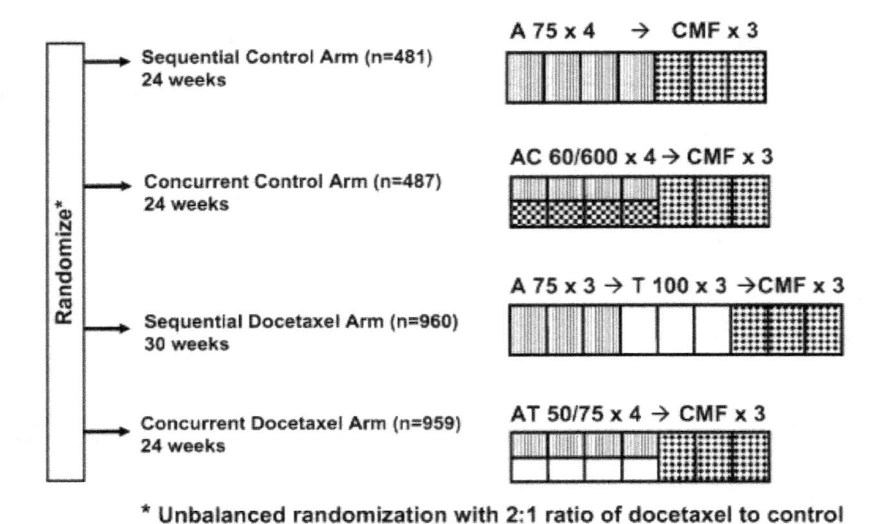

Fig. 3 Resected node positive breast cancer

The primary comparison evaluated the efficacy of including docetaxel regardless of schedule and was planned after 1,215 disease-free survival (DFS) events (i.e., relapse, second primary cancer, or death from any cause). Due to a lower-than-anticipated rate of relapse, this analysis was performed after 5 years with 732 events.

Patients in the control arms had a 5-year DFS of 73% (95% confidence interval [CI] = 70–75%). Docetaxel treatment resulted in an improvement in DFS of borderline statistical significance compared with control treatment (HR = 0.86, 95% CI = 0.74–1.00; p = 0.05). However, DFS in the sequential docetaxel arm was better than that in the concurrent docetaxel arm (HR = 0.83, 95% CI = 60.69–1.00) and in the sequential control arm (HR = 0.79, 95% CI = 0.64–0.98).

In summary, incorporating docetaxel into an anthracycline-based therapy resulted in an improvement in DFS that was of borderline statistical significance. However, important differences may be related to doxorubicin and docetaxel scheduling, with sequential but not concurrent administration, appearing to produce better DFS than anthracycline-based chemotherapy.

Two other trials, not yet published, are evaluating concurrent vs sequential taxanes. The NSABP B30 trial compares AC (60,600 mg/m^2) × 4 followed by docetaxel (100 mg/m^2) × 4 vs AT [60/60 mg/m^2] × 4 vs TAC [60/60/600 mg/m^2] × 4). In this program, a sequence with eight courses is being compared to four courses of docetaxel-doxorubicin based polychemotherapy using the doublet-based docetaxel/doxorubicin at 60/60 mg/m^2 (favoring the increased dose of doxorubicin with 60 mg/m^2 instead of 50 mg/m^2 and decreasing the dose of docetaxel from 75 mg/m^2 to 60 mg/m^2). In parallel to this trial, the BCIRG is conducting a randomized trial (BCIRG 005) comparing the same sequence used in the NSABP B30 trial (AC (60,600 mg/m^2) $\times$ 4 followed by docetaxel (100 mg/m^2) $\times$ 4) to TAC [75/50/500 mg/m^2] given six times in the adjuvant treatment of patients with positive axillary nodes and no amplification of the HER2 gene. Results of these trials will be available in 2008 (SABC).

Taxanes 2 Weekly (q3w) vs Weekly (q1w)

Recently Sparano [16] et al. reported the results of an American Intergroup trial comparing the two different taxanes given either weekly or every 3 weeks in 4,950 women with node positive or high risk node negative disease. Patients received four courses of standard AC followed at 3-week intervals by four courses of paclitaxel (P) 175 mg/m^2 or docetaxel (D) 100 mg/m^2 or by 12 weekly courses of paclitaxel 85 mg/m^2 or docetaxel 35 mg/m^2. The primary endpoint of the trial was disease free survival. The proportion of women who received all doses was 95%(Pq3w), 88% (P q1w), 87% (Dq3w), and 75% (D q1w). The corresponding 5 year-survival rates were 76% (Pq3w), 81.5% (Pq1w), 81.2%(Dq3w), and 77.6% for Dq1w. In terms of schedule these data are clearly in favor of weekly paclitaxel and docetaxel at 3-week intervals. The comparison between the taxanes did not show any significant survival differences. As compared to the standard therapy (4 $\times$ AC $\rightarrow$ 4 $\times$ P q3w) weekly paclitaxel was superior in terms of disease free and overall survival. High grade neurotoxicity was higher with weekly than with 3-weekly paclitaxel.

Beyond Conventional Dose Range....

Steep dose response relationships as investigated by Skipper and Schabel, confirmed by retrospective analyses from Levine and Hruniuk and especially by the early generation of phase I–II high dose chemotherapy trials in metastatic breast cancer influenced a generation of trials testing chemotherapy doses far beyond conventional ranges. These regimens became feasible by evolving supportive therapy strategies integrating G-CSF and/or stem cell support. The trials are homogeneous in terms of patient selection (high-risk groups), but very heterogeneous in terms of dose escalation strategies and control arms, so that few general conclusions can be drawn.

High Dose Chemotherapy with Growth Factor Support

Dose escalation of taxanes and anthracyclines, the most active compounds in breast cancer, is limited mainly by cardiac toxicity and neurotoxicity. Nevertheless, with the use of adequate supportive care including G-CSF and erythropoetin, an important escalation is feasible in an outpatient setting.

The German AGO [17] Group randomized patients with more than four involved lymph nodes to either epirubicin 150 mg/m^2 × 3 q2w → paclitaxel 225 mg/m^2 × 3 q2w → cyclophosphamide 2,500 mg/m^2 × 3 q2w or to a conventional sequential regimen 4 × E90C600 q3w followed by 4 × paclitaxel 175 q3w. The trial design is shown in Fig. 4.

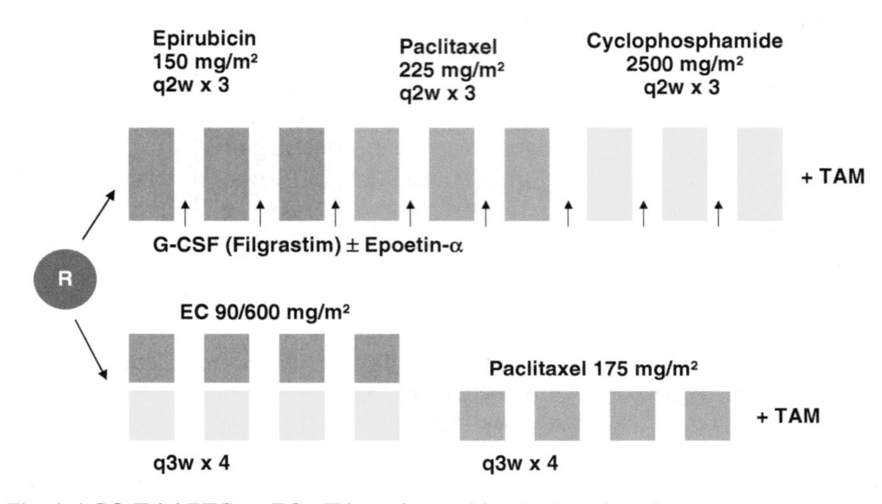

Fig. 4 AGO-Trial ETC vs. EC→T in patients with ≥4 + lymph nodes

Toxicity within the dose-dense dose intense arm was acceptable. Event free and overall survival rates are in favor of the dose-dense dose intense therapy (data submitted in 9/08).

High Dose Chemotherapy with Stem Cell Support

As of dose intensification, high dose chemotherapy trials in early breast cancer historically are in line with the results from Levine and Hruniuk. At least for alkylating agents, laboratory data and in vivo data in metastatic breast cancer demonstrate steep dose response relationships in terms of tumor cell kill and remission rates. Beside this mechanism, it was suggested that by dose escalation far beyond conventional dose ranges, a number of drug resistance mechanisms, especially for alkylating agents, may be overcome. Most regimens have been designed for the whole entity of solid tumors and have not been specifically developed against breast cancer. Within the different combination regimens the most frequently used compounds are alkylating agents. These compounds can be escalated by a factor ranging from × 4 (C) to × 20 (Thiotepa) without being limited by organ toxicity.

Hematoxicity was antagonized by the use of autologous stem cells originating from the marrow in the early trials and from peripheral blood in the recent ones. Peripheral stem cells are collected after adequate stimulation via apheresis and then stored at –80 °C. They are re-transfused after high dose chemotherapy is eliminated from the body. Bone marrow reconstitution in most cases takes 2–3 weeks. During aplasia patients are usually isolated in special units. Therapy related mortality rates of high-dose chemotherapy regimens as used in breast cancer ranged from 7 to 14% in the earlystages. Nowadays therapy related mortality rates are less than 1%. Due to these initial high mortality rates, and due to the considerable toxicity of high dose therapies, there is a selection of high-risk breast cancer patients that have been randomized to the adjuvant trials. The data are unique for this subgroup of patients who generally account only for a small minority of patients within conventional trials, thus making retrospective analyses very difficult.

The existing data refer to three different groups of trials. The first two groups used a late intensification strategy. After a conventional induction regimen consisting of four to six cycles of conventionally dosed chemotherapy there was one myeloablative high dose cycle. They compared either to a classical standard or to some other sort of dose intensified control arm. In the third group two designs foresee an early intensification strategy with a short induction phase followed by repeated high dose cycles (IBCSG, WSG). Table 1 resumes the outlines of the different trials.

A recently presented meta-analysis [30] has included data from 6,210 patients treated in high-dose chemotherapy trials. High dose as identified by the use of stem cell support is compared to the correspondent control arms. In terms of 5-year survival rates, high dose was significantly better than control. The difference did however not translate into a corresponding overall survival benefit. Retrospective subgroup analyses (hormone receptor, HER2 overexpression, nodal involvement, age . . .) do not reveal statistically significant differences in terms of overall survival for any subpopulation.

The pooled analysis does not support the use of stem cell supported high dose chemotherapy in daily routine. Nevertheless the data may help in identifying promising strategies that merit further investigation.

In terms of dose intensification strategy, two trials merit reporting. The first has been conducted by the Scandinavian Breast Cancer Study Group. In 525 patients at high risk of recurrence Bergh, [26] et al. compared six cycles of conventionally dosed FEC followed by one cycle of high-dose chemotherapy (chlorambucil, cyclophosphamide, thiotepa) vs an individually nadir- adapted escalated FEC regimen. Five-year results were in favor of the control arm and overall survival differences were not significant. The second trial was conducted by the West German Study Group [28, 31]. In patients with more than ten involved lymph nodes the Group compared 4 × EC → 3 × CMF at 2-week intervals with growth factor support vs two identical courses of EC followed by

Table 1 Phase III high dose chemotherapy trials

First author	N	Eligibility	Control	High dose (HD)	Result (5 years control vs HD)
"Classical" phase III designs					
Tallman [18]	511	>10 Positive nodes	6 × FAC	6 × FAC → 1HD Cyclo/ Thiotepa	RFS 48 vs 55% (p = 0.12) OS 62 vs 58% (p = 0.32)
Leonard [19]	605	>4 Positive nodes	4 × E → 8 × CMF	4 × E → C → HD Cyclo/ Thiotepa	RFS 54 vs 57% (p = 0.38) OS 64 vs 62% (p = 0.78)
Roche [20]	314	>7 Positive nodes	FEC × 4	3 × FEC → 1HDCyclo/Mel/ Mitoxantron	EFS55 vs77 n% (p = 0.002) OS 84 vs 82% (p = 0.33)
Zander [21]	302	>10 Positive nodes	EC × 4 → CMF ×3 q3w	EC × 4 → HDCyclo/ Thiotepa/Mitoxantron	EFS 42 vs 49% (p = 0.15) OS 62 vs 64% (p = 0.33)
Rodenhuis [24]	885	>4 Positive nodes	FEC × 5	FEC × 4 → HD Cyclo/ Thiotepa/Carbo	DFS 59 vs 64% (p = 0.076) OS 70 vs 73% (p = 0.22)
Dose dense/dose intense vs HD					
Moore [23]	536	>4 Positive nodes	A × 3→ T × 3 → C × 3 di q2w	4 × ACd.i. → STAMP I or V	DFS 80 vs 75% (p = 0.35) OS 88 vs 84% (p = 0.40)
Peters [25]	785	>10 Positive nodes	4 × FAC → di Cyclo/ CDDP/Carmustin	4 × FAC → di Cyclo/CDDP/ Carmustin	EFS 58 vs 61% (p = 0.24) OS 71 vs 71%
Bergh [26]	525	Expected 5 years RFS <30%	9 × tailored FEC	FEC × 6 → 1HD Cyclo/ Carbo/Thiotepa	RFS 72 vs 62% (p = 0.02) OS HR 0.86 (p = 0.287)
Any standard vs multicycle HD					
Gianni [27]	398	>4 Positive nodes	3 × E → 6 × CMF	1 × Cyclo → 1 × MTX → 2 × E → 1 × Thiotepa/Mel	PfS (12 years) 44 vs 52% n.s. OS(12 year) 51 vs 61% n.s.
Nitz [28]	403	>10 positive nodes	EC × 4 → CMF ×3 q2w	2 × EC → 2 × HD E/Cyclo/ Thiotepa	EFS 42 vs 54% (p<0.01) OS 60 vs 72% (p = 0.02)
Basser [29]	344	>9 or >4 and T3 or ER neg	3 × E → 6 × CMF	3 × HD E/cyclo	DFS 43 vs 52% (p = 0.07) OS 61 vs 70% (p = 0.17)

F = 5 fluorouracil; C = Cyclo = cyclophosphamide; A = Adriamycin; E = Epiadriamycin; M = MTX = methotrexate; Mel = melphalan; CDDP = cis; Carbo 0 carboplatinumplatinum, ER = estrogen receptor; RFS = recurrence free survival; EFS = event free survival; pfs = progression free survival; OS = overall survival, n.s. = not significant a rapidly cycled tandem high-dose regimen with thiotepa, cyclophosphamide and epirubicin. The trial is clearly positive for high-dose regime in terms of event free and overall survival. Retrospective subgroup analyses show the maximal benefit in the small group of triple negatives breast cancer patients.

Conclusion

Conventional Dose Range

The most common clinical problem in conventionally dosed chemotherapy is underdosing either by reducing single doses or by prolonging intervals.

In combinations appropriate single doses at 3-week intervals are 60 mg/m^2 for A, 90–100 mg/m^2 for E, and 600 mg/m^2 for cyclophosphamide.

Regimens like CMF 600/40/600 i.v. q3w, F300A30C300 and FE50C are obsolete and should not be used in daily routine because they are inferior to their classical counterparts.

In third generation regimens including anthracyclines and taxanes, scheduling seems to be an important issue. Especially paclitaxel 175 mg/m^2 at 3-week intervals and docetaxel at 35 mg/m^2 weekly bear an important risk of underdosing. After four courses of AC q3w, weekly paclitaxel × 12 is better than 4 × paclitaxel at 3-week intervals. The inverse is true for docetaxel.

In addition, dose-dense application (q2w with G-CSF support) is superior to a 3-week interval in two sequential taxane/anthracycline-based regimens including the original AC × 4 → paclitaxel × 4.

One trial suggests that within a taxane/anthracycline-based regimen sequential use, taxanes may be superior to concomitant use. Data from two other trials addressing this question will be published soon.

High dose range with growth factor/stem cell support

Data refer mainly to patients at high risk of recurrence. The meta-analysis of stem cell supported high dose chemotherapy vs heterogeneous controls does not support the use of high dose chemotherapy in routine settings. Nevertheless, there are single very successful trials supporting the hypothesis that multiple, dose-intensified rapidly cycled chemotherapy courses may improve results in patients with poor outcome after standard regimens.

References

1. Skipper HE, Schabel FM Jr, Mellett LB, et al. Implications of biochemical, cytokinetic, pharmacologic, and toxicologic relationships in the design of optimal therapeutic schedules. *Cancer Chemother Rep*. 1970;54(6):431–50.
2. Norton L, Simon R. The Norton-Simon hypothesis revisited. *Cancer Treat Rep.* 1986;70(1):163–9.
3. Hryniuk W, Frei E III, Wright FA. A single scale for comparing dose-intensity of all chemotherapy regimens in breast cancer: Summation dose-intensity. *J Clin Oncol.* 1998;16(9):3137–47.

4. Fisher B, Anderson S, Wickerham DL, De Cillis A, et al. Increased intensification and total dose of cyclophosphamide in a doxorubicin-cyclophosphamide regimen for the treatment of primary breast cancer: Findings from National Surgical Adjuvant Breast an Bowel Project B22. *J Clin Oncol.* 1997;15:1858–69.
5. Fisher B, Anderson S, Wickerham DL, De Cillis A, et al. Further evaluation of intensified and increased total dose of cyclophosphamide for the treatment of primary breast cancer: Findings from National Surgical Adjuvant Breast an Bowel Project B25, *J Clin Oncol.* 1999;17:3374–88.
6. Bonneterre J, Rochè H, Kerbrat P, et al. Epirubicin increases long-term survival in adjuvant chemotherapy of patients with poor-prognosis, node-positive, early breast cancer: 10-Year Follow-Up Results of the French Adjuvant Study Group 05 Randomized Trial. *J Clin Oncol.* 2005;23(12):2686–93.
7. French Adjuvant Study Group, Benefit fo a High-Dose Epirubicin regimen in adjuvant chemotherapy for node-positive breast cancer patients with poor prognostic factors: 5-Year Follow-Up Results of French Adjuvant Study Group 05 Randomized Trial. *J Clin Oncol.* 2001;19(3):602–11.
8. Henderson IC, Berry DA, Demetri GD, et al. Improved outcomes from adding sequential paclitaxel but not from escalating doxorubicin dose in an adjuvant chemotherapy regimen for patients with node positive primary breast cancer. *J Clin Oncol.* 2003;21:976–83.
9. Engelsman E, Klijn JCM, Rubens RD, et al. "Classical" CMF versus a 3-weekly intravenous CMF schedule in postmenopausal patients with advanced breast cancer. *Eur J Cancer.* 1991;27(8):966–70.
10. Bonnadonna G, Valagussa P, et al. Dose-response effect of adjuvant chemotherapy in breast cancer. *New Engl J Med.* 1981;304:10–5.
11. Piccart, MJ, Di Leo A, Beauduin M, et al. Phase III trial comparing two dose levels of epirubicin combined with cyclophosphamide with cyclophosphamide, methotrexate, and fluorouracil in node-positive breast cancer. *J Clin Oncol.* 2001;19(12):3103–10.
12. Wood WC, Budman DR, Korzun AH, et al. Dose and dose intensity of adjuvant chemotherapy for Stage II, node-positive breast carcinoma. *N Engl J Med.* 1994;330(18):1253–9.
13. Linden HM, Haskell CM, Green SJ, et al. Sequenced compared with simultaneous anthracycline and cyclophosphamide in high-risk Stage I and II breast cancer: Final Analysis from INT-0137 (S9313). *J Clin Oncol.* 2007;25(6):656–61.
14. Citron ML, Berry DA, Cirrincione C, et al. Randomized trial of dose-dense conventionally scheduled and sequential versus concurrent combination chemotherapy as postoperative adjuvant treatment of node-positive primary breast cancer: First report of intergroup Trial C 9741/ Cancer and Leukemia Group B Trial 9741. *J Clin Oncol.* 2003;21(8):1431–9.
15. Francis P, Crown J, Di Leo A, et al. Adjuvant chemotherapy with sequential or concurrent anthracycline and docetaxel: Breast International Group 02 98 Randomized Trial. *J Natl Cancer Inst.* 2008;100(2):121–33.
16. Sparano JA, Wang M, Martino S, et al. Weekly paclitaxel in the adjuvant treatment of breast cancer. *N Engl J Med.* 2008;358(16):1663–71.
17. Moebus V, Lueck HJ, Thomssen C, et al. Dose-dense sequential chemotherapy with epirubicin (E), paclitaxel (T) and cyclophosphamide (C) (ETC) in comparison to conventional dosed chemotherapy in high breast cancer patients (4 + LN). Mature results of an AGO trial. San Antonio Breast cancer symposium (2006).
18. Tallman MS, Gray R, Robert NJ, et al. Conventional adjuvant chemotherapy with or without high-dose chemotherapy and autologous stem-cell transplantation in high-risk breast cancer. *N Engl J Med.* 2003;349(1):17–26.
19. Leonard R, Lind M, Twelves C, et al. Conventional adjuvant chemotherapy versus single-cycle, autograft-supported, high-dose, late-intensification chemotherapy in high-risk breast cancer patients: A randomized trial. *J Natl Cancer Inst.* 2004;96(14):1076–83.

20. Roché H, Viens P, Biron P, et al. High-dose chemotherapy for breast cancer: the French PEGASE experience. *Cancer Control*. 2003;10(1):42–7.
21. Zander AR, Kroeger N, Schmoor C, et al. High-dose chemotherapy with autologous hematopoietic stem-cell support compared with standard-dose chemotherapy in breast cancer patients with 10 or more positive lymph nodes: First results of a randomized trial. *J Clin Oncol*. 2004;22(12):2273–83.
22. Zander AR, Schmoor C, Kröger N, et al. Randomized trial of high-dose adjuvant chemotherapy with autologous hematopoietic stem-cell support versus standard-dose chemotherapy in breast cancer patients with 10 or more positive lymph nodes: overall survival after 6 years of follow-up. *Ann Oncol*. 2008;19(6):1082–9.
23. Moore HCF, Green SJ, Gralow JR, et al. Intensive dose-dense compared with high-dose adjuvant chemotherapy for high-risk operable breast cancer: Southwest Oncology Group/Intergroup Study 9623. *J Clin Oncol* 2007;25(13):1677–82.
24. Rodenhuis S, Bontenbal M, Beex LV, et al. High-dose chemotherapy with hematopoetic stem-cell rescue for high risk breast cancer. *N Engl J Med*. 2003;349(1):7–16.
25. Peters W, Rosner GL, Vredenburgh JJ, et al. Prospective, randomized comparison of high-dose chemotherapy with stem-cell support versus intermediate-dose chemotherapy after surgery and adjuvant chemotherapy in women with high-risk primary breast cancer: A report of CALGB 9082, SWOG 9114, and NCIC MA-13. *J Clin Oncol*. 2005;23(10):2191–200.
26. Bergh J, Wiklund T, Erikstein B, et al. Tailored fluorouracil, epirubicin and cyclophosphamide compared with marrow-supported high-dose chemotherapy as adjuvant treatment for high-risk breast cancer: A randomised trial. *Lancet*. 2000;356(9239):1384–91.
27. Gianni A, Sienna S, Bregni M, et al. Efficacy, toxicity, and applicability of high-dose sequential chemotherapy as adjuvant treatment in operable breast cancer with 10 or more involved axillary nodes: Five-year results. *J Clin Oncol*. 1997;15(6):2312–21.
28. Nitz U, Mohrmann S, Fischer J, et al. Comparison of rapidly cycled tandem high-dose chemotherapy plus peripheral-blood stem-cell support versus dose-dense conventional chemotherapy for adjuvant treatment of high-risk breast cancer: Results of a multicentre phase III trial. *Lancet*. 2005;366(9501):1935–44.
29. Basser R, O'Neill A, Martinelli G, et al. Multicycle dose-intensive chemotherapy for women with high-risk primary breast cancer: Results of International Breast Cancer Study Group Trial 15-95. *J Clin Oncol*. 2006;24(3):370–8.
30. Berry D, Ueno N, Johnson MM, et al. High-dose chemotherapy with autologous stem-cell support versus standard-dose chemotherapy: Meta-analysis of individual patient data from 15 randomized adjuvant breast cancer trials. *Breast Cancer Res Treat*. 2007;106(Suppl 1):Abstr 11.
31. Gluz O, Nitz UA, Harbeck N, et al. Triple-negative high-risk breast cancer derives particular benefit from dose intensification of adjuvant chemotherapy: Results of WSG AM-01 trial. *Ann Oncol*. 2008;19(5):861–70.

Timing of Adjuvant Therapy

O. Pagani

Timing of Risk and Benefit

Breast cancer (BC) mortality rates in the United States, as assessed by the National Cancer Institute's Surveillance Epidemiology and End Results (SEER) program, declined to 25 per 100,000 woman-years in 2003. Mathematical models and clinical trial results suggest that mammography screening and adjuvant systemic therapy are largely responsible for the overall decline in mortality. Recently, population-based mortality rates in subgroups of BC patients have also been systematically described. Annual hazard rates (HR) for BC mortality during the years 1990–2003 have been different and non-proportional according to oestrogen receptor (ER) expression. Hazard rates in ER negative patients rise to a sharp peak of 7–8% per year approximately 2 years after initial BC diagnosis, and then decline. In contrast, ER-positive HR lack a sharp peak but have a stable long-term rate of 1–2% per year (Fig. 1) [1]. This means that patients with endocrine unresponsive tumours are at much greater risk of recurrence and death during the early years after diagnosis, whereas patients with ER-positive tumours have a fairly consistent long-term risk of BC death. In addition, the magnitude of the peak in the risk of death is far greater for women with ER-negative than with ER-positive tumours: interestingly, hazard curves cross for ER-negative and ER-positive tumours approximately 6–8 years after diagnosis.

Gene expression studies have also recently identified three major subtypes of BC (basal-like, HER2+/ER–, and luminal) associated with different prognoses [2]. A particularly poor outcome is seen among the two hormone receptor–negative subtypes (i.e., basal-like and HER2+/ER–). HER2 overexpression in particular is associated with earlier and greater likelihood of

O. Pagani (✉)
Institute of Oncology of Southern Switzerland, Ospedale Italiano, Viganello, Lugano, Switzerland, International Breast Cancer Study Group (IBCSG) and Swiss Group for Clinical Cancer Research (SAKK), Bern, Switzerland
e-mail: olivia.pagani@ibcsg.org

M. Castiglione, M.J. Piccart (eds.), *Adjuvant Therapy for Breast Cancer*,
Cancer Treatment and Research 151, DOI 10.1007/978-0-387-75115-3_16,

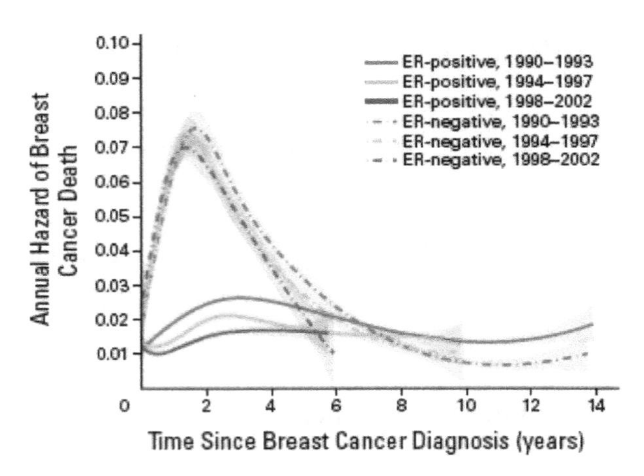

Fig. 1 Annual hazard rates of breast cancer death according to estrogen receptor (ER) status Jatoi I et al. *J Clin Oncol.* 25:1683–90, 2007

tumour recurrence [3, 4] with a distinctive pattern of short term, and largely distant, relapse and with a higher rate of disease recurrence in the central nervous system, occurring approximately in one-third of patients [5].

Taken together this information strongly favours a differential impact of adjuvant treatments, not only in terms of quantitative effects but also of time of benefit, in different biological subtypes of BC. In particular, the high risk of an event in the first 2–3 years after diagnosis for ER-negative patients coincides with the period of time when the benefits of the more effective chemotherapy regimens become evident [6]. On the other hand, the benefit of adjuvant chemotherapy in women with ER-positive tumours is far less dramatic: in this period, the risk of recurrence is so small in ER-positive patients who receive adequate endocrine treatment that any additional risk reduction due to chemotherapy would be very difficult to detect statistically [7].

Timing of Surgery

The results of several studies, assessing the effect on prognosis of the hormonal milieu at the time of surgery, have been conflicting [8–10]. Comparisons among studies of menstrual timing of surgery have been complicated by differences in cycle divisions, extent of primary surgery, frequency of adjuvant therapy, duration of follow-up and analytic procedures [11]. Some but not all reports have shown improved survival and decreased risk of vascular invasion among patients with positive axillary lymph nodes surgically treated in the luteal phase of the menstrual cycle, when progesterone levels are elevated (i.e. >4 ng/mL) [12]. Some evidence also exists of molecular, genetic and cellular changes in BC according to the phases of the menstrual cycle when biopsy was performed [13].

Multidisciplinary and well designed prospective studies should be developed to characterize adequately the influence of the menstrual cycle and of other aspects of women's reproductive physiology on BC management and outcome.

Timing of Sentinel Node Biopsy

Information on the feasibility and accuracy of sentinel node (SLN) biopsy following preoperative systemic therapy (PST) is still quite limited. The American Society of Clinical Oncology (ASCO) panel recently concluded that current data are insufficient to recommend SLN biopsy after PST, although the technique has proven to be technically feasible after chemotherapy [14]. The available data report an identification rate of 77–98%, an accuracy of 77–100%, and a false-negative rate of up to 33% but this information is prejudiced by the small numbers of patients, treated in single institutions. The National Surgical Adjuvant Breast and Bowel Project (NSABP) has evaluated the method in one of its neoadjuvant trials and found the data comparable to those obtained from multicenter studies evaluating SLN biopsy before systemic therapy [15]. A recent systematic review of 24 trials (1799 subjects), published between 2000 and 2007, demonstrates both successful identification (90%) and false-negative rates (8%) [16]. With adequate technical experience and standardization of the procedure, SLN biopsy after PST could therefore be discussed and might be a reasonable approach in selected patients who have shown a treatment response, except for patients with inflammatory disease [17]. The need for an SLN biopsy before preoperative treatment is debatable despite small series have reported an identification rate of almost 100% with different techniques [18].

Timing of Pathology

The accurate pathological assessment of any residual disease after PST is crucial, being complete pathological response (pCR) positively correlated with long term survival [19]. In presence of extensive regression of the primary tumour it may be difficult to estimate the real tumour size, especially if there are residual cells scattered over the original tumour area. The histo-pathological findings should be assessed using established regression criteria [20]: a pCR is achieved when no histological evidence of residual tumour cells, including non-invasive foci, is found, either in the breast or the axillary lymph nodes, after extensive microscopic examination. Immunohistochemical markers, such as the hormone receptor and Her2/*neu*status, should be determined both before and after PST if residual tumour is present. Standard pathologic terms and the same criteria used in the assessment of primary tumours without PST should be adopted. Recent data suggest that gene expression profiling might have the potential to identify and select patients most likely to achieve a pCR [21].

Timing of Radiotherapy

Radiotherapy Initiation and Duration

The optimal timing of adjuvant radiotherapy (RT) after BC surgery and its sequencing with systemic treatments (chemotherapy and/or endocrine treatment) is controversial. Overall, the available evidence from patients treated within controlled randomised trials suggests that, in node positive patients who receive up to 6 months of adjuvant chemotherapy, postponing RT is not associated either with a higher local recurrence rate [22] or with a significant difference in the medium-term (48 months of median follow-up) incidence of distant metastases, or overall survival [23, 24]. Somewhat contradictory results are on the contrary available in node-negative patients who do not receive any adjuvant systemic treatment [25, 26].

Accelerated partial-breast irradiation (APBI) is a group of RT techniques that deliver higher daily doses of radiation to the surgical cavity over a shorter time than whole-breast irradiation (WBI), reducing total treatment time from 6–6.5 weeks to 1–2 weeks. Phase III randomized clinical trials are currently underway to assess local control, acute and chronic toxicities, and quality of life associated compared to WBI [27].

Hypofractionated WBI also applies higher doses per fraction reducing overall treatment duration: the approach is feasible but appropriate patient selection is mandatory as well as long-term toxicity assessment [28]. These modern techniques potentially increase the use of breast-conservation, the longer 6- to 7-week standard regimen inducing many women, especially elderly patients, to choose mastectomy.

Radiotherapy in Combination with Systemic Treatments

The concurrent administration of cyclophosphamide, methotrexate, and 5-fluorouracil (CMF) with RT is associated with a low risk of serious toxicity [29, 30]. As regards anthracycline-containing regimens, the risk of increasing the well known cardiac toxicity has prevented the concomitant administration with RT: early experience in limited sets of patients seems to suggest that this approach could be revisited [31].

Preliminary data from small series show that combining RT and taxanes is apparently not associated with increased toxicity, in particular radiation pneumonitis or brachial plexopathy [32, 33]. This observation, if confirmed by additional data, would allow anticipation of RT in high risk patients receiving long-lasting chemotherapy regimens, thus avoiding the possible negative impact on outcome of late RT administration.

The data available from the randomised adjuvant trials in >13,000 HER-2 positive women show no apparent mid-term detrimental effect of the combination of trastuzumab and RT [34]. Early evidence also suggests that the inclusion of concurrent trastuzumab in radio-chemotherapy protocols does not seem to increase radiation or systemic toxicity but this approach still needs further evaluation and longer follow up [35].

The optimal sequencing of Tamoxifen (TAM) and RT remains controversial. The concurrent use of TAM with RT may theoretically reduce sensitivity to RT by arresting BC cells in the relatively radio-resistant G0/G1 phases of the cell cycle [36], and some evidence has been reported of increased pulmonary and breast fibrosis from the combination [37, 38]. The interpretation of this data is limited by the small numbers of patients and the lack of a randomised comparison to sequential treatment. A retrospective analysis of 1,649 patients treated in a single institution suggested that, with a median follow-up of 10 years, concurrent TAM with RT does not compromise local control (HR, 0.932; 95% CI, 0.42–2.05; $p = 0.86$) or overall survival (HR, 1.234; 95% CI, 0.42–2.05; $p = 0.45$) [39]: this data were confirmed in a smaller series of 279 patients treated at the University of Pennsylvania between 1980 and 1995 [40] and by a retrospective analysis of 309 high-risk node-negative patients treated within the Intergroup trial 0102 [41].

On the other hand, timing of RT did not adversely affect the 10-year local relapse-free survival in 1446 stage I–II node negative patients, not receiving adjuvant systemic therapy, treated prospectively in a single institution, but had a significant impact on the 10-year distant metastasis-free survival with a 40–70% relative survival benefit when RT was delivered from 36 to 112 days after breast conserving surgery as compared to early treatment (within 36 days) [25].

In the absence of any randomized trial, no firm conclusions regarding the relative effectiveness of sequential or concurrent TAM and RT can be drawn. The general question of sequencing of hormonal therapy and radiation is likely to remain relevant and open also with the increasing use of the third-generation aromatase inhibitors (AIs) and APBI. Aromatase inhibitors cause G1 cell cycle arrest like TAM but recent preclinical data suggest that BC cells pretreated with modern AIs may have increased radiation sensitivity [42].

Timing of Adjuvant Systemic Therapy

The latency between BC diagnosis and disease relapse after initial treatment, often lasting several years or even decades, has led to the hypothesis that a state of cancer dormancy could at least in part explain this phenomenon. Research on tumour dormancy, a complex and still poorly understood biological process, has been limited due to the scarcity of appropriate models and clinical correlates. Preclinical models designed to compare the biological behaviour of metastatic vs non-metastatic variants of tumour cells provide some evidence that tumour dormancy may depend upon a reciprocal dialogue between the tumour cell and the tissue microenvironment and have in particular stressed the role of cell adhesion in the balance between proliferation and dormancy [43]. Cancer cells degrade the extracellular matrix by controlled proteolysis to spread into lymphatic and blood vessels and form metastases at distant sites. One proteolytic system involved in these processes is the urokinase-type plasminogen activator (uPA) system which has been recently claimed to exert a biological role in tumour dormancy in solid cancer [44]. The ras-mitogen-activated protein kinase (MAPK) signal transduction pathway has multiple roles in biological processes such as cell cycling. The interaction between p38 MAPK phosphorylation and the uPA system is under investigation as a possible mechanism for the maintenance of the BC invasive phenotype during dormancy and its modulation might become a therapeutic target [45]. The transition between dormant and proliferating cells is also influenced by growth stimulating factors [46] and withdrawal of angiogenesis inhibitors [47]. Circulating tumour cells (CTCs) have been identified in a significant proportion of BC patients with no evidence of clinical disease as long as 22 years after mastectomy [48]. Their replication appears to be balanced by cell death/apoptosis: the mechanisms underlying this control could be represented either by immune responses, or angiogenic suppression. The impact of CTCs in early BC [49] is currently less well established than the presence of micrometastases in bone marrow which has been clearly associated with poor prognosis [50]. Surgical trauma and removal of the primary tumour has also been postulated to act as "angiogenic switch" [51]. The different temporal patterns of recurrence after primary BC removal could at least in part be explained by distinct tumour dormancy models which show selective sensitivity to adjuvant chemotherapy [52]. In premenopausal node-positive patients dormant micrometastases triggered by surgery have been supposed to synchronize into a temporal highly chemosensitive state which, if confirmed by additional data, could explain both the benefit of adjuvant chemotherapy and the tumour aggressiveness in younger patients [53]. Comparative genomic studies also showed that dormant CTCs displayed significantly fewer chromosomal aberrations than those from patients with manifest metastases, suggesting that dissemination occurs very early in the process of accumulation of genetic changes [54]. The recognition of all these steps might reveal novel homeostatic mechanisms that could lead to development of new drugs and therapeutic approaches to be tested in clinical trials [55].

Preoperative (Neoadjuvant) Systemic Therapy

Preoperative systemic therapy (PST) is used either to improve the surgical options (i.e. to reduce the frequency of mastectomies), to obtain information on disease response as a predictor of long-term outcome and of efficacy of subsequent adjuvant therapies or to achieve long-term disease-free survival by complete eradication of distant micrometastatic disease [56]. Overall, disease-free survival (DFS) and overall survival (OS) are equivalent in patients treated with the same adjuvant or neoadjuvant regimen [57].

Primary Endocrine Therapy

Primary endocrine therapy has been tested only in postmenopausal patients with endocrine responsive disease, showing moderate activity [58] but information is lacking on the comparative efficacy of hormonal agents administered pre- and postoperatively. Endocrine sensitive tumours have also generally shown a poor response to primary chemotherapy (CT) [59].

Primary Chemotherapy

Patients with endocrine-unresponsive disease benefit most from preoperative CT, the response being significantly higher in this subset of women [60] who can nowadays also be identified by gene expression profiles [19, 21, 61, 62].

Overall, the preliminary results of targeted PST with trastuzumab in combination with CT show promising activity in patients with confirmed HER-2-positive breast cancer, achieving high clinical and pCR rates, with a favourable safety profile [63–66]. Response rates to single-agent trastuzumab range from 12 to 34% in metastatic breast cancer and preliminary data also report encouraging antitumour activity as neoadjuvant treatment [67]. The relative benefits of administering trastuzumab alone, concurrently with or sequentially after CT in the preoperative setting, still need to be investigated.

Duration of Preoperative Systemic Treatment

The optimal duration of PST has not been established, the length of therapy having varied from 8 weeks to 36 weeks and being different in almost all trials, with some trials splitting the systemic therapy into a preoperative and post-operative part. In addition, recent data suggest that longer treatment compares favourably with shorter treatment [68, 69]. Nonetheless, at least four cycles of CT and at least 3–4 months of endocrine therapy are recommended in the absence of disease progression.

Postoperative (Adjuvant) Systemic Therapy

Chemoendocrine Treatment

Preclinical data suggest that in ER positive BC cells TAM and other selective ER modulators (SERMs) could exert an antagonistic effect when combined with some cytotoxic drugs: endocrine treatment slows tumour growth by causing a G-transition delay which may make tumour cells less susceptible to cell cycle-specific cytotoxic agents. Furthermore, TAM may alter membrane lipids, thereby changing diffusion rates of some drugs and it also seems to inhibit CA^{++}-dependent cellular processes potentially modifying drug uptake. This antagonism seems to be drug-specific and even alkylating-agent specific, since it was demonstrated with melphalan and fluorouracil but not with 4-hydroxy-cyclophosphamide, the active metabolite of cyclophosphamide, or doxorubicin [70, 71]. Definitive interpretation of these somewhat contradictory observations is confounded by the fact that most experiments were conducted with very high (supra-pharmacologic) concentrations of TAM for only a short duration exposure, which is probably insufficient to achieve an antiestrogen-induced effect on tumour cell kinetics before exposure to the cytotoxic agent. Furthermore, this strategy may not accurately mimic in vivo chemo-endocrine therapy in which tumour cells are exposed to a prolonged clinically relevant TAM concentration with the cytotoxic chemotherapy given in intermittent "bursts" over the course of treatment. Little or no information is available with other endocrine agents such as medroxyprogesterone acetate or AIs.

A possible detrimental effect of the concurrent administration of adjuvant melphalan and fluorouracil with TAM was observed in node positive patients treated in the NSABP Trial B-09 [72] and in node positive postmenopausal patients treated with TAM in combination with oral CMF in the International (former Ludwig) Breast Cancer Study Group (IBCSG) trial VII [73], in particular in women with low ER expression. Recent studies on the administration of anthracycline-containing adjuvant chemotherapy either concurrent or sequential with TAM favoured sequential administration [74–76] but these trials were not designed to evaluate the effect of chemoendocrine therapy separately according to the degree of endocrine-responsiveness of the tumour. On the other hand, no major difference in 5 years OS was reported between concomitant and sequential administration of TAM and anthracycline-based adjuvant chemotherapy in the retrospective analysis of two consecutive trials in node positive BC patients [77]. A potential advantage with concomitant treatment observed in young patients (<40 years) and in patients with high ER level tumours needs to be further addressed in prospective trials.

A significant higher incidence of thromboembolic events has also been reported by the National Cancer Institute of Canada Clinical Trials Group in node positive postmenopausal women randomised to concurrent TAM and CMF as compared to women receiving TAM alone [78].

In the absence of any conclusive data a safe attitude could be to sequence the two treatment modalities by completing adjuvant chemotherapy before starting prolonged TAM treatment.

Only limited information is also available on the effectiveness of delayed chemotherapy to patients already receiving TAM. In the previously mentioned IBCSG trial VII, 1212 node-positive postmenopausal patients were randomized to receive either TAM for 5 years or TAM plus three concurrent courses of 'classical' CMF, either early, delayed (on months 9, 12 and 15) or both [79]. The late reintroduction approach was based on the mathematical model developed by Speer in which breast tumours grow by alternating periods of fast proliferation to phases of slower or no progression [80]. Since cancer cells are more likely to be sensitive to chemotherapy during phases of fast growth, and to be resistant during periods of quiescence, the timing of cytotoxic agent administration could influence treatment efficacy. The selection of the same regimen as reintroduction was based on the empirical observation in advanced disease that patients could achieve a clinical response when given the same chemotherapy they received as adjuvant therapy. Patients with endocrine responsive tumours (ER-moderate or -high) gained a substantial benefit from the combination of chemotherapy and TAM regardless of when the concurrent chemotherapy was administered, as opposed to patients with ER-absent or ER-low expression tumours in whom delayed chemotherapy seemed to be detrimental. The retrospective nature of these results should be viewed as hypothesis-generating, prompting the evaluation of delayed chemotherapy for patients with endocrine-responsive disease and high risk of relapse within tailored treatment trials using novel endocrine agents.

Chemotherapy (CT)

CT Initiation

The demonstration of a survival benefit from adjuvant CT in early-stage BC is based on the results of randomised trials in which a selected time interval, usually $\leq$12 weeks, from surgery to the start of CT was allowed: whether equivalent benefit can be obtained when CT is started beyond this time window is still not known. Only one randomised trial has specifically investigated the timing of CT delivery: RT followed by CT (median time to CT start 17 weeks) was not associated with inferior OS compared with CT followed by RT (median time to CT 7.4 weeks) [81].

Overall, several retrospective analyses have also shown equivalent outcomes when CT was started up to 13 weeks from surgery [82–85] but none of them had enough statistical power to detect possible differences among different prognostic groups (i.e. age, tumour size, vascular invasion, histological grade, number of involved nodes, hormonal receptor status and co-administration of hormone therapy).

Data are on the contrary accumulating on the possible benefit on disease outcome by an early initiation of CT after definitive surgery. Two small clinical studies [86, 87] have suggested that patients who received CT within 28 to 35 days from surgery had improved DFS compared with those who received CT later. Perioperative CT, i.e. within 3 days after surgery, can be used as a useful model for identifying subgroups of patients according to biological features that could benefit the most from early initiation of adjuvant treatment. Overall, the results of a meta-analysis of trials on perioperative CT showed a reduced risk of relapse by 11%, but no impact on OS, compared with the usual delayed administration [88]. In addition, the European Organization for Research and Treatment of Cancer (EORTC) demonstrated a long-term benefit (11 years median follow-up) in terms of progression-free survival (PFS) and locoregional control by one course of perioperative anthracycline-containing polychemotherapy in 2,795 patients with early BC [89]. Data on treatment effect according to different predictive features, such as c-*erb*B-2, steroid hormone receptor expression, or grading, were not analysed.

The IBCSG conducted a randomized clinical trial (Trial V) to evaluate the role of the addition of perioperative CT (within 36 h after mastectomy) [90] in node-positive premenopausal patients with early BC. A total of 475 patients were randomised to receive either perioperative CMF followed by conventionally timed CT given for 6 months or the conventional CT alone. At a median follow-up of 11 years, among the small subset of women (101) with ER-absent tumours, the 10-year DFS rate was 48% for those who received perioperative CMF compared with 38% for those who received conventionally timed CT alone (HR, 0.80; 95% CI, 0.48 to 1.34; $p=0.40$). Despite the small number of patients, the 20% reduction in the risk of recurrence provided motivation to investigate whether early initiation of CT might be beneficial at least for the endocrine unresponsive subgroup of premenopausal patients. The subsequent analysis of all IBCSG trials of classical CMF CT in premenopausal patients (Trials I, II, and VI) confirmed that, in the small subset of node-positive patients with ER-absent tumours, early initiation (within 21 days) of systemic CT after primary surgery was associated with a significant and clinically striking improvement in 10-year DFS (60 vs 34%; $p=0.0003$) [91].

In addition, within IBCSG Trial V, a total of 1,275 patients with node-negative disease were also stratified by menopausal status and randomised to receive perioperative CMF (PeCT) or no adjuvant treatment. In premenopausal patients the 10-year DFS percentage did not significantly differ between the PeCT and no-adjuvant-treatment groups (61 and 59%, respectively, $p=0.70$) and no predictive factors were identified. In postmenopausal patients the 10-year DFS percentages were 63 and 58%, respectively ($p=0.03$) with the absence of expression of ER, PgR, or both being the most important factor predicting improved outcome with PeCT. The 10-year DFS percentages were 85 and 53% for the steroid hormone receptor–absent cohort of treated and untreated patients, respectively ($p=0.0009$) [92]. These findings provide strong support for the hypothesis that endocrine factors related to both menopausal and steroid hormone receptor status, considered together, play a key role in influencing response to CT.

In summary, early start of CT is unlikely to be clinically significant in patients with tumours expressing some ER: in this subset of patients CT exerts some of its effect via an endocrine mechanism and as a consequence the impact of early initiation of CT may not be as relevant as opposed to patients with ER-absent tumours who benefit exclusively from the cytotoxic mechanisms of CT.

CT Duration

Adjuvant CT is generally administered for 6–12 months after definitive surgical treatment. Several trials in the past have directly compared the duration of adjuvant CT but most of them were not sufficiently sized to detect modest differences in the outcome. An overview of six such trials showed that shorter treatment duration (6 months) was as effective as longer duration therapy (12–24 months) [93].

The previously mentioned IBCSG trial V demonstrated that overall a single course of perioperative CMF was associated with a significantly shorter DFS and OS compared with a total of six or seven courses of the same treatment in patients with node-positive disease [90].

The IBCSG also conducted a randomized trial in 1,475 node-positive pre- and peri-menopausal women (Trial VI) comparing three and six cycles of classical adjuvant CMF. Patients who received the shorter duration of CT had a 5-year DFS rate of 53% compared with 58% in women in the longer duration treatment arm ($p = 0.04$). The increased risk of relapse was more marked for women aged less than 40 years and for patients with ER-negative tumours [94].

This observation was in contrast to that of the German Breast Cancer Group (GBSG) trial in which 3 and 6 cycles of modified CMF were compared in 483 node-positive patients and yielded a similar event-free survival (EFS) after a median follow-up of 10 years [95]. In the German trial only 42% of randomised patients were premenopausal and no analysis according to age was undertaken. A subsequent joint analysis of the two studies [96] showed that three cycles of CMF were adequate, and even slightly more effective in both studies for patients at least 40-years-old with ER-positive tumours ($n = 594$; HR, 0.86; 95% CI, 0.68–1.08; $p = 0.19$). In contrast, three cycles were possibly inferior to six cycles for women less than 40-years-old ($n = 190$; HR, 1.25; 95% CI, 0.87–1.80; $p = 0.22$) and for women with ER -negative tumours ($n = 302$; HR, 1.15; 95% CI, 0.85–1.57; $p = 0.37$).

IBCSG Trial VI also addressed the question of late re-introduction of CT by adding three single courses of CMF given on months 6, 9, and 12 [97]. The possibility that a single cycle of CMF could by itself have some influence on disease recurrence was demonstrated in the previously illustrated IBCSG Trial V for node-negative patients with a presumed low burden of disease. The reintroduction showed a trend to therapeutic effect, but this was not statistically significant. Patients who were randomized to receive reintroduction had a reduced risk of relapse (14% estimated reduction) whether the initial CT consisted of three or six cycles. Several contrasting and confounding factors could have interfered with the overall results, such as to one side the longer treatment duration in the reintroduction group and on the other side the decreased ability to deliver all prescribed cycles of CT with a possible dilution of the therapeutic effect. In addition, the choice of single cycles of reintroduction CT administered 3 months apart might not represent the most effective approach. As a consequence, two subsequent IBCSG trials in node positive patients (13–93 and 14–93) compared classical adjuvant CT with four cycles of AC/EC (cyclophosphamide plus either doxorubicin or epirubicin) followed by immediate CMF given for three cycles vs a 16-week gap between the two regimens. Overall, the gap and no-gap groups had similar DFS and OS but exploratory subgroup analysis noted a trend towards decreased DFS for gap compared with no-gap for women with ER-negative tumours, especially evident during the first 2 years (HR 1.36; 95% CI = 0.92, 2.02, $p = 0.12$) [98].

Insufficient scientific evidence is available in women age 70 and older who are under represented in most BC treatment trials [99, 100] but emerging data suggest lymph node-positive, ER-negative patients as the subgroup possibly benefiting from CT [101, 102]. Considerable uncertainty remains regarding the risk/benefit ratio in elderly women, based mainly on co-morbidities, functional status, future life expectancy and the expected physical and psychological tolerability of CT [103, 104]. A shorter duration (12–16 weeks) of a less intensive CT could therefore be reasonable for elderly patients: the IBCSG attempted to investigate such an approach in the CASA trial, designed for older patients (≥66 years) with endocrine non responsive BC and not suitable for standard combination regimens. The study aimed to test two complementary options (4 months of low dose pegylated liposomol doxorubicin given every 2 weeks vs observation and pegylated liposomal doxorubicin vs 16 weeks of low dose, oral metronomic cyclophosphamide and methotrexate) in a quality-of-life targeted approach, but was prematurely closed due to insufficient accrual.

Endocrine Treatment

The role of adjuvant endocrine therapy in women with endocrine responsive BC has been re-emphasized during the last St. Gallen Consensus Conference [105]. The new paper will be published soon, maybe in time to be incorporated.

Ovarian Function Ablation/Suppression (OFS)

The role of OFS and TAM has been clearly established in premenopausal women with hormone receptors positive early BC [99]. A recent meta-analysis substantially updated and refined the results of the last Early Breast Cancer Trialists' Collaborative Group (EBCTCG) overview (based on data up to the year 2000) by dealing only with trials of OFS by LHRH agonists (thus excluding radiation or surgical menopause), and focusing specifically on hormone-receptor-positive patients [106]. Sixteen trials were available for the current overview, for a total of 9,022 patients and a median follow-up of·6.8 years: duration of LHRH treatment was 2 years in most trials, but 18 months, 3 years, or 5 years were also used. Overall, LHRH agonists, when used as the only systemic adjuvant treatment, significantly reduced the risk of recurrence (28%, $p = 0{\cdot}08$) or death after recurrence (17·8%, $p = 0.49$), but the number of patients included in this comparison was very small, as reflected by the borderline p value. The addition of LHRH agonists to TAM, CT, or both, further reduced recurrence by 13% ($p = 0{\cdot}02$); and death after recurrence by 15% ($p = 0{\cdot}03$). In addition LHRH agonists showed similar efficacy to CT but no trials had assessed an LHRH agonist vs CT with TAM in both arms. Not surprisingly, the effects of LHRH analogues were greater in younger women than in those older than 40 years (Fig. 2).

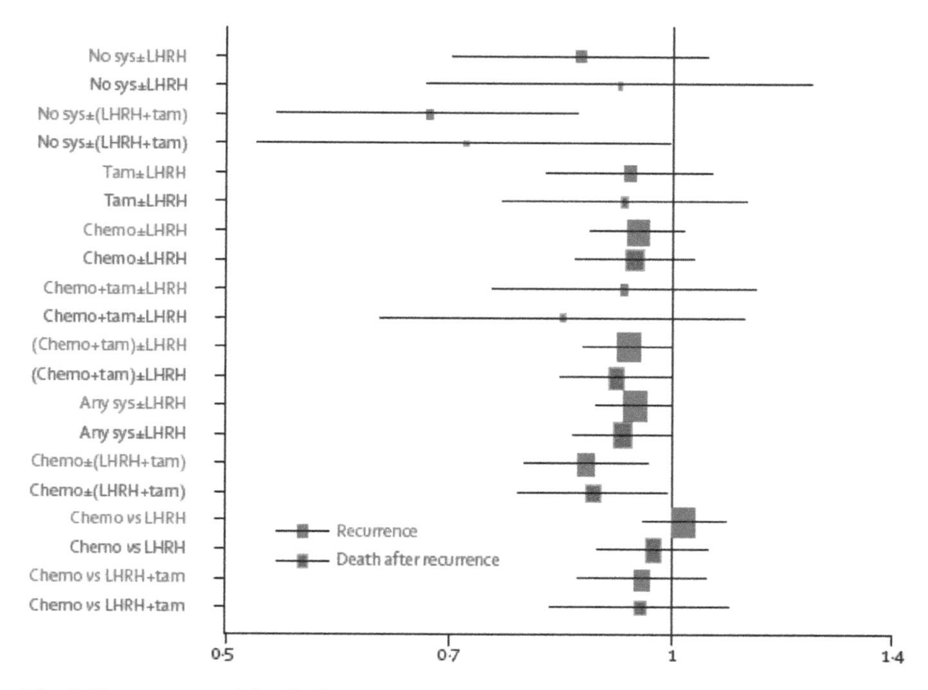

Fig. 2 Recurrence and death after recurrence
Cuzick J et al: *Lancet*. May 19, 2007;369:1711–23

The optimal duration of LHRH administration, which induces reversible ovarian failure, remains unknown as no clinical trial directly compared different treatment durations. In absence of any data on a possible carryover effect of OFS this information would be of extreme importance especially when discussing adjuvant strategies with very young women who possibly have still to make their personal child bearing decisions.

Selective ER Modulators (SERMS): Tamoxifen

The 2005 report from the EBCTCG overview [99] shows, after 15 years of follow-up, that 5 years of TAM induce a 12% absolute reduction in BC recurrence and a 9% reduction in BC mortality in women with ER-positive tumours, irrespective of age and nodal status. Overall, longer treatment appears to be more effective at controlling BC than shorter treatment, the reduction in both recurrence and mortality being significantly higher in women who had 5 years of adjuvant TAM therapy compared with those who received only 1–2 years (recurrence rate ratio 0·82, 2p<0·00001, breast cancer death rate ratio 0·91, 2p = 0·01). The value of extending adjuvant TAM therapy beyond 5 years has been investigated so far in small trials which have not demonstrated any benefit, although longer treatment appears to involve slightly lower recurrence and BC mortality rates in the most recent studies. With longer treatment, a slight and non-significant excess mortality rate from other causes (i.e., thromboembolism, stroke, other vascular causes but not uterine cancer) was reported. Two ongoing large (>18,000 women enrolled) randomized clinical trials, Adjuvant Tamoxifen Treatment-Offer More (aTTom) [107] and Adjuvant Tamoxifen-Longer against Shorter (ATLAS) [108], randomized patients who had completed ~5 years of adjuvant TAM between continuing for another 5 years and stopping. The combined preliminary results indicate that continuation of TAM beyond the first 5 years reduces recurrence over the next few years, but further follow-up is needed to assess reliably the longer-term effects on recurrence and the net effects, if any, on mortality. No significant differences in mortality from any other non-breast cancer cause have been reported so far.

The benefits associated with TAM treatment are not only substantial but also persistent. In women receiving 5 years of TAM an additional one third annual reduction in the recurrence rate was shown within 10 years, which indicates a protective carryover effect over the next few years after treatment interruption. In addition, despite no further reduction in the recurrence rates was observed after 10 years, no net loss of the earlier gains emerged, confirming a persisting long-lasting effect. For BC mortality the persistence of the effects of about 5 years of treatment is even more remarkable with a steady divergence between treatment and control throughout the first 15 years in both BC related and overall mortality (Fig. 3).

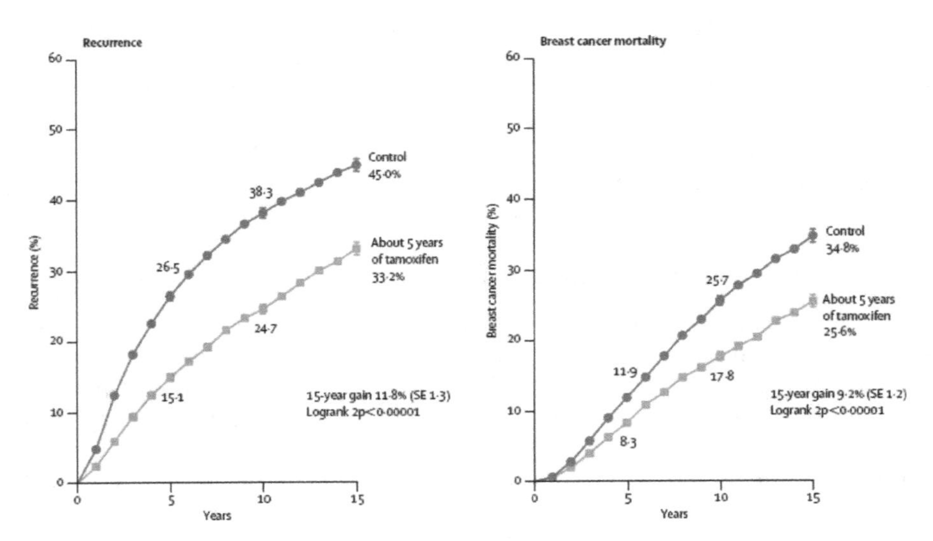

Fig. 3 About 5 years of tamoxifen vs not in ER-positive (or ER-unknown) disease: 15-year probabilities of recurrence and of breast cancer mortality
EBCTCG Overview: *Lancet*. 365:1687–717, 2005

On the other hand, a sustained significant benefit, in terms of prolonged DFS, is evident, after a median follow-up of 25 years, in older ($\geq$65 years) node-positive patients treated for 1 year with TAM alone as compared to control (IBCSG Trial III and IV), with no additional impact on recurrence by the addition of chemotherapy (CMF) (Pagani). These long-term results suggest short-term endocrine treatment could be a safe and effective treatment option for frail elderly women.

Aromatase Inhibitors (AIs)

Overall, several large clinical trials involving several thousands of postmenopausal patients have shown that third generation AIs are superior to TAM in preventing contralateral BC and improving DFS. Mature results are currently available with several schedules: upfront treatment; sequencing treatment either after 2–3 years of TAM or followed by TAM for 3 years; and extended treatment after 5 years of TAM [109–114]. Larger reductions in the hazard ratio for recurrence have been reported in the sequencing and extended treatment regimens, but a proper evaluation of the overall impact on recurrence needs to account for the higher recurrence rates that occurred in the period before switching to an AI. Multivariate and subgroup analyses within the BIG1-98 trial seem to indicate that patients with high risk for early relapse (four or more positive nodes, tumours >2 cm, presence of vascular invasion, HER-2 overexpression/amplification and high values of Ki-67) may benefit most from upfront letrozole, while sequential therapy might be reserved for patients with intermediate risk, in whom TAM did not differ significantly from letrozole [115–117].

Optimal duration of treatment with an AI is one key outstanding question for which there are currently no data: at this time, there is no evidence to suggest that a longer than 5-year treatment with an AI is of benefit and extended treatment with AIs beyond the initial 5 years should only be administered as part of a clinical trial. A second randomization is now planned in patients who received 2 years of exemestane after 5 years of TAM (NSABP B-33 trial) and in patients who were treated with extended letrozole (MA-17 trial) to continue the same AI vs placebo for 5 more years (years 11–15).

An additional question is how long the effect will be maintained after treatment is stopped: the only data on a possible carryover effect by AIs come from the ATAC trial where the same magnitude of reduction was seen in year 6 as in previous years [110].

Information on the use of TAM after an AI and on the comparison of an AI upfront versus sequencing after TAM is now available with the recently presented results of the BIG 1-98 trial which compared letrozole and TAM given in either sequence with letrozole alone. Overall, the sequential treatments did not improve DFS compared with letrozole alone but the data suggest initial use of letrozole could be beneficial in patients at higher risk of relapse (e.g., node positive) and patients commenced on letrozole can be safely switched to TAM [114].

No trial did compare starting an AI at 2.5 years versus starting following 5 years of TAM and thus, the optimal moment of transition from TAM to an AI will probably not be known.

Recent evidence suggests that estradiol is capable of inducing apoptosis in aromatase resistant BC cells [118]. High dose estradiol showed an antitumour activity in patients with advanced BC progressing under oestrogen deprivation [119]. Low-dose oestrogen levels (achievable through interruptions of treatment with AIs) could therefore induce apoptosis in BC cells become resistant under long-term therapy with AIs, making residual disease susceptible to subsequent reintroduction. The IBCSG is comparing extended continuous treatment with letrozole for 5 years with intermittent therapy in women with endocrine-responsive node-positive disease after completion of prior adjuvant SERM/AI endocrine therapy (SOLE trial).

A large population of postmenopausal women with hormone sensitive early BC, treated with 5 years of adjuvant TAM remain disease-free 6–15 years after diagnosis [99] (Fig. 3). Overall, these women have a significant persisting risk of later BC related events with an annual risk of about 1–3% per year: women with endocrine responsive disease in particular have an annual risk or relapse >10–20% in the first 10 years and of 1–4% annually from year 15 to year 20 after diagnosis with 60% of recurrences occurring >6 years post surgery (Fig. 4) [120]. The Australia and New Zealand Breast Cancer Trials Group (ANZ BCTG) is running within BIG a late intervention trial with an AI (LATER) with the aim of preventing new BC events and reducing mortality.

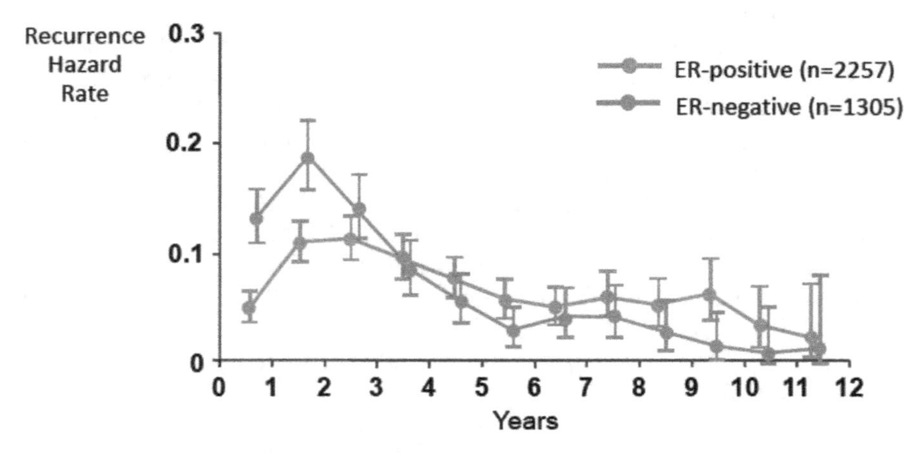

Fig. 4 Annual Recurrence Hazard Rates for by endocrine responsiveness
Saphner T et al. *J Clin Oncol.* 14:2738–46, 1996

AIs are contraindicated in women with functioning ovaries because the reduced feedback of oestrogen to the hypothalamus and pituitary leads to an increase in secretion of gonadotrophins. Many premenopausal women who developed permanent amenorrhoea after CT have recently been offered adjuvant AIs: the preliminary experience in this subset of patients, the majority of whom is older than age 40, has pointed out that a significant proportion of these women (as high as 27%) may regain ovarian function while receiving AIs and even become pregnant [121]. Estradiol, LH, and FSH levels, using validated and accurate assays, should be monitored serially when giving adjuvant AIs in these patients and treatment should be administered only if levels are consistent with postmenopausal status (elevated gonadotropin levels and estradiol <10 pmol/L) and under serial monitoring.

Targeted Therapies

Up to one quarter of women with early BC have HER-2 positive tumours, characteristic which is associated with a high risk of early relapse and death [3–5].

Four major adjuvant trials—HERA, NSABP B-31, NCCTG N9831, and BCIRG 006—including >13,000 HER-2 positive women overall, have investigated different adjuvant treatment approaches with trastuzumab and have shown that the addition of trastuzumab significantly reduces the risk of recurrence and death. A small Finnish trial, FinHer, investigating a shorter trastuzumab regimen, also confirmed similar positive results [34].

Whereas further follow-up will provide information on long-term cardiac safety and clarify the survival benefit, a number of questions remain unanswered. The first is whether trastuzumab started concurrently with taxane CT (as in the USA and FinHer trials) is better than trastuzumab starting sequentially after completion of CT (as in the HERA approach). The NCCTG N9831 trial addressed this issue by including a third arm with sequential trastuzumab: preliminary data suggest that sequential treatment might be less effective than concurrent treatment [122], but this was an unplanned comparison with low statistical power, and longer follow-up is needed for assessing the relative benefits of administering trastuzumab concurrently with or sequentially after paclitaxel. It could also be noted that the median time from diagnosis to starting trastuzumab in the HERA trial was 8·5 months, which could have affected efficacy in patients with high risk of early relapse. The second issue concerns the duration of trastuzumab treatment. In this context, a third arm in the HERA trial, in which patients are treated with trastuzumab for 2 years, addresses the impact of longer trastuzumab administration: data comparing the 1- and 2-year arms will provide information on whether extending treatment beyond 1 year offers additional benefit. On the other hand, in the Finnish trial, involving only 232 women, a DFS benefit within the same range as those recorded in trials of trastuzumab treatment for 1 year has been reported with 9 weeks only of trastuzumab (HR 0·42, 95% CI 0·21–0·83; $p = 0·01$), but the small sample size, together with the wide CI, require confirmatory data. The Finnish group is now conducting a subsequent trial in 3000 patients comparing a shorter (9 weeks) and longer (1 year) duration of adjuvant trastuzumab (SOLD trial).

Clinical data about sequencing or combining trastuzumab with RT and/ or hormone therapy in the adjuvant treatment setting are still immature. Patients in the adjuvant trials received adjuvant RT upon completion of CT, during maintenance trastuzumab with no apparent detrimental effect [34]. At a median follow-up time of 3.7 years, concurrent adjuvant RT and trastuzumab in the NCCTG trial was not associated with increased acute adverse events, including cardiac events, but further follow-up is required to assess potential late toxicity (Halyard). Endocrine therapy for patients with hormone receptor-positive disease was begun at the completion of either CT or RT.

Conclusion

Timing is one of the important variables which should be taken into account when tailoring adjuvant treatments for the individual patient. The process is not trivial given the different patterns of treatment responsiveness and recurrence with respect to the biological subtypes of BC, the complexity of modern therapies and the number of open questions, i.e., the biological mechanisms underlying tumour dormancy, the potential for overlapping and unexpected toxicities when combining different therapies, the long-term follow up required to properly assess efficacy and safety. Innovative research programs should therefore address not only the integration of different therapeutic strategies in terms of biological targets and synergisms but also in view of their potential temporal interactions.

References

1. Jatoi I, Chen BE, Anderson WF, Rosenberg PS. Breast Cancer Mortality Trends in the United States According to Estrogen Receptor Status and Age at Diagnosis. *J Clin Oncol.* 2007;25:1683–90.
2. Sorlie T. Molecular classification of breast tumors: Toward improved diagnostics and treatments. *Methods Mol Biol.* 2007;360:91–114.
3. Ross JS, Fletcher JA, Linette GP, et al. The Her-2/neu gene and protein in breast cancer 2003: Biomarker and target of therapy. *Oncologist.* 2003;8:307–25.
4. Slamon DJ, Godolphin W, Jones LA, et al. Human breast cancer: correlation of relapse and survival with amplification of the HER2-2/neu proto-oncogene in human breast and ovarian cancer. *Science.* 1989;244:707–12.
5. Burstein HJ, Lieberman G, Slamon DJ, et al. Isolated central nervous system metastases in patients with HER2-overexpressing advanced breast cancer treated with first-line trastuzumab-based therapy. *Ann Oncol.* 2005;16:1772–7.
6. Early Breast Cancer Trialists' Collaborative Group (EBCTCG). Adjuvant polychemotherapy in oestrogen-receptor-poor breast cancer: meta-analysis of individual patient data from the randomised trials. Submitted to The Lancet 10 April 2007.

7. Berry DA, Cirrincione C, Henderson IC, et al. Estrogen-receptor status and outcomes of modern chemotherapy for patients with node-positive breast cancer. *JAMA*. 2006;295:1658–67.
8. Pujol P, Daures JP, Brouillet JP, et al. A prospective prognostic study of the hormonal milieu at the time of surgery in premenopausal breast carcinoma. *Cancer*. 2001;91(10):1854–61.
9. Milella M, Nistico C, Ferraresi V, et al. Breast cancer and timing of surgery during menstrual cycle: A 5-year analysis of 248 premenopausal women. *Breast Cancer Res Treat*. 1999;55(3):259–66.
10. Thorpe H, Brown SR, Sainsbury JR et al. Timing of breast cancer surgery in relation to menstrual cycle phase: No effect on 3-year prognosis: The ITS Study. BJC. 2008;98:39–44.
11. Chaudhry A, Puntis ML, Gikas P, Mokbel K. Does the timing of breast cancer surgery in pre-menopausal women affect clinical outcome? An update. *International Seminars in Surgical Oncology*. 2006;3:37.
12. Goldhirsch A, Gelber RD, Castiglione M, et al. Menstrual cycle and timing of breast surgery in premenopausal node-positive breast cancer: results of the International Breast Cancer Study Group (IBCSG) Trial VI. *Ann Oncol*. 1997;8:751–6.
13. Macleod J, Fraser R, Horeczko N. Menses and breast cancer: Does timing of mammographically directed core biopsy affect outcome? *J Surg Oncol*. 2000;74(3):232–6.
14. Lyman GH, Giuliano AE, Somerfield MR, et al. American Society of Clinical Oncology guideline recommendations for sentinel lymph node biopsy in early-stage breast cancer. *J Clin Oncol*. 2005;23:2540–5.
15. Mamounas EP, Brown A, Anderson S, et al. Sentinel node biopsy after neoadjuvant chemotherapy in breast cancer: Results from national surgical adjuvant breast and bowel project protocol B-27. *J Clin Oncol*. 2005;23:2694–702.
16. Kelly AM, Dwamena B, Cronin P, Carlos RC. Breast cancer sentinel node identification and classification after neoadjuvant chemotherapy-systematic review and meta analysis. *Acad Radiol*. 2009;16(5):551–63.
17. Stearns V, Ewing CA, Slack R, et al. Sentinel lymphadenectomy after neoadjuvant chemotherapy for breast cancer may reliable represent the axilla except for inflammatory patients. *Ann Surg Oncol*. 2002;9:235–42.
18. Jones JL, Zabicki K, Christian RL, et al. A comparison of sentinel node biopsy before and after neoadjuvant chemotherapy: Timing is important. *Am J Surg*. 2005;190(4):517–20.
19. Sataloff DM, Mason BA, Prestipino AJ, et al. Pathologic response to induction chemotherapy in locally advanced carcinoma of the breast: A determinant of outcome. *J Am Coll Surg*. 1995;180:297–306.
20. Ogston KN, Miller ID, Payne S, et al. A new histological grading system to assess response of breast cancers to primary chemotherapy: Prognostic significance and survival. *Breast*. 2003;12:320–7.
21. Ayers M, Symmans WF, Stec J, et al. Gene expression profiles predict complete pathological response to neoadjuvant paclitaxel and fluorouracil, doxorubicin, and cyclophosphamide chemotherapy in breast cancer. *J Clin Oncol*. 2004;22:2284–93.
22. Benchalal M, Le Prise E, de Lafontan B, et al. Influence of the time between surgery and radiotherapy on local recurrence in patients with lymph node-positive, early-stage, invasive breast carcinoma undergoing breast-conserving surgery: Results of the French Adjuvant Study Group. *Cancer*. 2005;104(2):240–50.
23. Wallgren A, Bernier J, Gelber RD, et al. Timing of radiotherapy and chemotherapy following breast-conserving surgery for patients with node-positive breast cancer. International Breast Cancer Study Group. *Int J Radiat Oncol Biol Phys*. 1996;35(4):649–59.
24. Arcangeli G, Pinnaro P, Rambone R, et al. A phase III randomized study on the sequencing of radiotherapy and chemotherapy in the conservative management of early-stage breast cancer. *Int J Radiat Oncol Biol Phys*. 2006;64(1):161–7.

25. Jobsen JJ, van der Palen J, Ong F, Meerwaldt JH. Timing of radiotherapy and survival benefit in breast cancer. *Breast Cancer Res Treat*. 2006;99(3):289–94.
26. Vujovic O, Yu E, Cherian A, et al. Eleven-year follow-up results in the delay of breast irradiation after conservative breast surgery in node-negative breast cancer patients. *Int J Radiat Oncol Biol Phys*. 2006;64(3):760–4.
27. Fearmonti RM, Vicini FA, Pawlik TM, Kuerer HM. Integrating partial breast irradiation into surgical practice and clinical trials. *Surg Clin North Am*. 2007;87(2):485–98.
28. Arthur DW, Morris MM, Vicini FA. Breast cancer: new radiation treatment options. *Oncology*. 2004;18(13):1621–9.
29. Isaac N, Panzarella T, Lau A, et al. Concurrent cyclophosphamide, methotrexate, and 5-fluorouracil chemotherapy and radiotherapy for breast carcinoma: a well tolerated adjuvant regimen. *Cancer*. 2002;95(4):696–703.
30. Montemurro F, Gatti M, Redana S, et al. Concurrent radiotherapy does not affect adjuvant CMF delivery but is associated with increased toxicity in women with early breast cancer. *J Chemother*. 2006;18(1):90–7.
31. Luini A, Gatti G, Zurrida S, et al. The evolution of the conservative approach to breast cancer. *Breast*. 2007;16(2):120–9.
32. Taghian AG, Assaad SI, Niemierko A, et al. Risk of pneumonitis in breast cancer patients treated with radiation therapy and combination chemotherapy with paclitaxel. *J Natl Cancer Inst*. 2001;93(23):1806–11.
33. Ellerbroek N, Martino S, Mautner B, et al. Breast-conserving therapy with adjuvant paclitaxel and radiation therapy: Feasibility of concurrent treatment. *Breast J*. 2003;9(2):74–8.
34. Baselga J, Perez EA, Pienkowski T, Bell R. Adjuvant Trastuzumab: A Milestone in the Treatment of HER-2-Positive Early Breast Cancer. *The Oncologist*. 2006;11(suppl 1):4–12.
35. Koukourakis MI, Manavis J, Simopoulos C, et al. Hypofractionated accelerated radiotherapy with cytoprotection combined with trastuzumab, liposomal doxorubicine, and docetaxel in c-erbB-2-positive breast cancer. *Am J Clin Oncol*. 2005;28(5):495–500.
36. Schmidberger H, Hermann RM, Hess CF, Emons G. Interactions between radiation and endocrine therapy in breast cancer. *Endocr Relat Cancer*. 2003;10(3):375–88.
37. Koc M, Polat P, Suma S. Effects of tamoxifen on pulmonary fibrosis after cobalt-60 radiotherapy in breast cancer patients. *Radiother Oncol*. 2002;64:171–5.
38. Wazer D, DiPetrillo T, Schmidt-Ullrich R, et al. Factors influencing cosmetic outcome and complication risk after conservative surgery and radiotherapy for early-stage breast carcinoma. *J Clin Oncol*. 1992;10:356–63.
39. Ahn PH, Vu HT, Lannin D, et al. Sequence of radiotherapy with tamoxifen in conservatively managed breast cancer does not affect local relapse rates. *J Clin Oncol*. 2005;23(1):17–23.
40. Harris EER, Christensen VJ, Hwang WT, et al. Impact of concurrent versus sequential tamoxifen with radiation therapy in early-stage breast cancer patients undergoing breast conservation treatment. *J Clin Oncol*. 2005;23:11–16.
41. Pierce LJ, Hutchins LF, Green SR, et al. Sequencing of tamoxifen and radiotherapy after breast-conserving surgery in early-stage breast cancer. *J Clin Oncol*. 2005;23:24–9.
42. Azria D, Larbouret C, Cunat S, et al. Letrozole sensitizes breast cancer cells to ionizing radiation. *Breast Cancer Res*. 2005;7(1):R156–63.
43. White DE, Rayment JH, Muller WJ. Addressing the role of cell adhesion in tumour cell dormancy. *Cell Cycle*. 2006;5(16):1756–9.
44. Laufs S, Schumacher J, Allgayer H. Urokinase-receptor (u-PAR): An essential player in multiple games of cancer: a review on its role in tumour progression, invasion, metastasis, proliferation/dormancy, clinical outcome and minimal residual disease. *Cell Cycle*. 2006;5(16):1760–71.
45. Ranganathan AC, Adam AP, Aguirre-Ghiso JA. Opposing roles of mitogenic and stress signaling pathways in the induction of cancer dormancy. *Cell Cycle*. 2006;5(16):1799–807.
46. Fisher B, Saffer EA, Rudok C, et al. Presence of a growth-stimulating factor in serum following primary tumour removal in mice. *Cancer Res*. 1989;49:1996–2001.

47. Naumov GN, Akslen LA, Folkman J. Role of angiogenesis in human tumour dormancy: Animal models of the angiogenic switch. *Cell Cycle*. 2006;5(16):1779–87.
48. Marches R, Scheuermann R, Uhr J. Cancer dormancy: From mice to man. *Cell Cycle*. 2006;5(16):1772–8.
49. Muller V, Hayes DF, Pantel K. Recent translational research: circulating tumour cells in breast cancer patients. *Breast Cancer Res*. 2006;8(5):110.
50. Braun S, Vogl FD, Naume B, et al. A pooled analysis of bone marrow micrometastasis in breast cancer. *N Engl J Med*. 2005;353(8):793–802.
51. McCulloch P, Choy A, Martin L. Association between tumour angiogenesis and tumour cell shedding into effluent venous blood during breast cancer surgery. *Lancet*. 1995;346:1334–1335.
52. Demicheli R, Miceli R, Moliterni A, et al. Breast cancer recurrence dynamics following adjuvant CMF is consistent with tumour dormancy and mastectomy-driven acceleration of the metastatic process. *Ann Oncol*. 2005;16:1449–57.
53. Retsky M, Bonadonna G, Demicheli R, et al. Hypothesis: induced angiogenesis after surgery in premenopausal node-positive breast cancer patients is a major underlying reason why adjuvant chemotherapy works particularly well for those patients. *Breast Cancer Res*. 2004;6(4):R372–R374.
54. Klein CA. The systemic progression of human cancer: A focus on the individual disseminated cancer cell–the unit of selection. *Adv Cancer Res*. 2003;89:35–67.
55. Uhr JW, Scheuermann RH, Street NE, Vitetta ES. Cancer dormancy: Opportunities for new therapeutic approaches. *Nat Med*. 1997;3:505–9.
56. Kaufmann M, Hortobagyi GN, Goldhirsch A, et al. Recommendations from an International Expert Panel on the Use of Neoadjuvant (Primary) Systemic Treatment of Operable Breast Cancer: An Update. *J Clin Oncol*. 2006;24:1940–9.
57. Mauri D, Pavlidis N, Ioannidis JP. Neoadjuvant versus adjuvant systemic treatment in breast cancer: A meta-analysis. *J Natl Cancer Inst*. 2005;97:188–94.
58. Macaskill EJ, Dixon JM. Neoadjuvant use of endocrine therapy in breast cancer. *Breast J*. 2007;13(3):243–50.
59. Semiglazov VF, Semiglazov VV, Dashyan GA, et al. Phase 2 randomized trial of primary endocrine therapy versus chemotherapy in postmenopausal patients with estrogen receptor-positive breast cancer. *Cancer*. 2007 May 30.
60. Colleoni M, Viale G, Zahrieh D, et al. Expression of ER, PgR, HER1, HER2, and response: A study of preoperative chemotherapy. *Ann Oncol*. 2008;19:465–72.
61. Carey LA, Dees EC, Sawyer L, et al. The Triple Negative Paradox: Primary Tumor Chemosensitivity of Breast Cancer Subtypes. *Clin Cancer Res*. 2007;13(8):2329–34.
62. Rouzier R, Perou CM, Symmans WF, et al. Breast cancer molecular subtypes respond differently to preoperative chemotherapy. *Clin Cancer Res*. 2005;11:5678–85.
63. Montemurro F, Aglietta M. Incorporating trastuzumab into the neoadjuvant treatment of HER2-overexpressing breast cancer. *Clin Breast Cancer*. 2005;6:77–80.
64. Coudert BP, Largillier R, Arnould L, et al. Multicenter phase II trail of neoadjuvant therapy with trastuzumab, docetaxel, and carboplatin for human epidermal growth factor receptor-2-overexpressing stage II or III breast cancer: results of the GETN(A)-1 trial. *J Clin Oncol*. 200;25(19):2678–84.
65. Limentani SA, Brufsky AM, Erban JK, et al. Phase II study of neoadjuvant docetaxel, vinorelbine, and trastuzumab followed by surgery and adjuvant doxorubicin plus cyclophosphamide in women with human epidermal growth factor receptor 2– overexpressing locally advanced breast cancer. *J Clin Oncol*. 2007;25:1232–8.
66. Hurley J, Doliny P, Reis I, et al. Docetaxel, Cisplatin, and Trastuzumab as primary systemic therapy for human epidermal growth factor receptor 2–positive locally advanced breast cancer. *J Clin Oncol*. 2006;24:1831–8.
67. Gennari R, Menard S, Fagnoni F, et al. Pilot study of the mechanism of action of preoperative trastuzumab in patients with primary operable breast tumours overexpressing HER2. *Clin Cancer Res*. 2004;10(17):5650–5.

68. von Minckwitz G, Blohmer JU, Raab G, et al. In vivo chemosensitivity-adapted preoperative chemotherapy in patients with early-stage breast cancer: The GEPARTRIO pilot study. *Ann Oncol.* 2005;16:56–63.
69. Therasse P, Mauriac L, Welnicka-Jaskiewicz M, et al. Final results of a randomized phase III trial comparing cyclophosphamide, epirubicin, and fluorouracil with a dose-intensified epirubicin and cyclophosphamide ± filgrastim as neoadjuvant treatment in locally advanced breast cancer: An EORTC-NCIC-SAKK multicenter study. *J Clin Oncol.* 2003;21:843–50.
70. Osborne CK, Kitten L, Arteaga CL. Antagonism of chemotherapy-induced cytotoxicity for human breast cancer cells by antiestrogens. *J Clin Oncol.* 1989;7(6):710–17.
71. Berman E, Adams M, Duigou-Osterndorf R, et al. Effect of tamoxifen on cell lines displaying the multidrug-resistant phenotype. *Blood.* 1991;77:818–25.
72. Fisher B, Redmond C, Brown A, et al. Adjuvant chemotherapy with and without tamoxifen: Five-year results from the National Surgical Adjuvant Breast and Bowel Project trial. *J Clin Oncol.* 1986;4:459–71.
73. The International Breast Cancer Study Group. Effectiveness of adjuvant chemotherapy in combination with tamoxifen for node-positive postmenopausal breast cancer patients. *J Clin Oncol.* 1997;15:1385–93.
74. Pico C, Martin M, Jara C. Epirubicin-cyclophosphamide adjuvant chemotherapy plus tamoxifen administered concurrently versus sequentially: Randomized phase III trial in postmenopausal node-positive breast cancer patients. A GEICAM 9401 study. *Ann Oncol.* 2004;15:79–87.
75. Sertoli MR, Pronzato P, Venturini M, et al. A randomized study of concurrent versus sequential adjuvant chemotherapy and tamoxifen in stage II breast cancer. *Proc Am Soc Clin Oncol.* 2002;21:182.
76. Albain K, Barlow W, O'Malley F, et al. Concurrent (CAFT) versus sequential (CAF-T) chemohormonal therapy (cyclophosphamide, doxorubicin, 5-fluorouracil, tamoxifen) versus T alone for postmenopausal, node-positive, estrogen (ER) and/or progesterone (PgR) receptor-positive breast cancer: mature outcomes and new biologic correlates on phase III intergroup trial 0100 (SWOG-8814). Breast Cancer Res Treat. 2004;88:(abstr 37).
77. Del Mastro L, Dozin B, Aitini E, et al. Timing of adjuvant chemotherapy and tamoxifen in women with breast cancer: findings from two consecutive trials of Gruppo Oncologico Nord-Ovest–Mammella Intergruppo (GONO-MIG) Group. Ann Oncol. 2008; 19:299–307.
78. Pritchard KI, Paterson AH, Paul NA, et al. Increased thromboembolic complications with concurrent tamoxifen and chemotherapy in a randomized trial of adjuvant therapy for women with breast cancer. National Cancer Institute of Canada Clinical Trials Group Breast Cancer Site Group. *J Clin Oncol.* 1996;14:2731–7.
79. M. Colleoni M, Li S, Gelber RD, et al. Timing of CMF chemotherapy in combination with tamoxifen in postmenopausal women with breast cancer: Role of endocrine responsiveness of the tumor. *Ann Oncol.* 2005;16(5):716–25.
80. Speer JF, Petrosky VE, Retsky MW, et al. A stochastic numerical model of breast cancer growth that simulates clinical data. *Cancer Res.* 1984;44:4124–30.
81. Bellon JR, Come SE, Gelman RS. Sequencing of Chemotherapy and Radiation Therapy in Early-Stage Breast Cancer: Updated Results of a Prospective Randomized Trial. *J Clin Oncol.* 2005;23:1934–40.
82. Cold S, During M, Ewertz M, et al. Does timing of adjuvant chemotherapy influence the prognosis after early breast cancer? Results of the Danish Breast Cancer Cooperative Group (DBCG). *Br J Cancer.* 2005;93:627–32.
83. Jara Sanchez C, Ruiz A, Martin M, et al. Influence of Timing of Initiation of Adjuvant Chemotherapy Over Survival in Breast Cancer: A Negative Outcome Study by the Spanish Breast Cancer Research Group (GEICAM). *Breast Cancer Res Treat.* 2007;101(2):215–23.

84. Lohrisch C, Paltiel C, Gelmon K, et al. Impact on survival of time from definitive surgery to initiation of adjuvant chemotherapy for early-stage breast cancer. *J Clin Oncol*. 2006;24:4888–94.
85. Shannon C, Ashley S, Smith IE. Does timing of adjuvant chemotherapy for early breast cancer influence survival? *J Clin Oncol*. 2003;21:3792–97.
86. Brooks RJ, Jones SE, Salmon SE, et al. Adjuvant chemotherapy of axillary node-negative carcinoma of the breast using doxorubicin and cyclophosphamide. *NCI Monogr*. 1986;(1):135–7.
87. Pronzato P, Campora E, Amoroso D, et al. Impact of administration related factors on outcome of adjuvant chemotherapy for primary breast cancer. *Am J Clin Oncol*. 1989;12:481–5.
88. Clahsen PC, van de Velde CJH, Goldhirsch A, et al. Overview of randomized perioperative polychemotherapy trials in women with early stage breast cancer. *J Clin Oncol*. 1997;15:2525–35.
89. van der Hage JA, van de Velde CJ, Julien JP, et al. Improved survival after one course of perioperative chemotherapy in early breast cancer patients. long-term results from the European Organization for Research and Treatment of Cancer (EORTC) Trial 10854. *Eur J Cancer*. 2001;37(17):2184–93.
90. The Ludwig Breast Cancer Study Group. Combination adjuvant chemotherapy for node-positive breast cancer: Inadequacy of a single perioperative cycle. *N Engl J Med*. 1988;319:677–83.
91. Colleoni M, Bonetti M, Coates AS, et al. Early start of adjuvant chemotherapy may improve treatment outcome for premenopausal breast cancer patients with tumors not expressing estrogen receptors: The International Breast Cancer Study Group. *J Clin Oncol*. 2000;18:584–90.
92. Colleoni M, Gelber S, Coates AS, et al. Influence of endocrine-related factors on response to perioperative chemotherapy for patients with node–negative breast cancer. *J Clin Oncol*. 2001;19:4141–9.
93. Henderson IC, Gelman RS, Harris JR, et al. Duration of therapy in adjuvant chemotherapy trials. NCI Monogr. 1986;1:95–8.
94. International Breast Cancer Study Group: Duration and reintroduction of adjuvant chemotherapy for node-positive premenopausal breast cancer patients. *J Clin Oncol*. 1996;14:1885–94.
95. Sauerbrei W, Bastert G, Bojar H, et al. for the German Breast Cancer Study Group. Randomized 2 3 2 trial evaluating hormonal treatment and the duration of chemotherapy in node-positive breast cancer patients: An Update Based on 10 Years' Follow-Up. *J Clin Oncol*. 2000;18:94–101.
96. Colleoni M, Litman HJ, Castiglione-Gertsch M, et al. Duration of adjuvant chemotherapy for breast cancer: A joint analysis of two randomised trials investigating three versus six courses of CMF. International Breast Cancer Study Group; German Breast Cancer Study Group. *Br J Cancer*. 2002;86(11):1705–14.
97. Ludwig Breast Cancer Study Group: Prolonged disease-free survival after one course of perioperative adjuvant chemotherapy for node-negative breast cancer. *N Engl J Med*. 1989;320:491–6.
98. International Breast Cancer Study Group. Effects of a treatment gap during adjuvant chemotherapy in node-positive breast cancer: results of International Breast Cancer Study Group (IBCSG) Trials 13–93 and 14–93. *Ann Oncol*. Apr 11, 2007.
99. Early Breast Cancer Trialists' Collaborative Group. Effects of chemotherapy and hormonal therapy for early breast cancer on recurrence and 15-year survival: An overview of the randomized trials. *Lancet*. 2005;365:1687–717.
100. Silliman RA, Ganz PA. Adjuvant chemotherapy use and outcomes in older women with breast cancer: What have we learned? *J Clin Oncol*. 2006;24(18):2697–9.
101. Muss HB, Woolf S, Berry D, et al. Adjuvant chemotherapy in older and younger women with lymph node-positive breast cancer. *JAMA*. 2005;293:1073–81.

102. Elkin EB, Hurria A, Mitra N, et al. Adjuvant chemotherapy and survival in older women with hormone receptor-negative breast cancer: Assessing outcome in a population-based, observational cohort. *J Clin Oncol.* 2006;24:2757–64.
103. Extermann M, Balducci L, Lyman GH. What threshold for adjuvant therapy in older breast cancer patients? *J Clin Oncol.* 2000;18:1709–17.
104. Giordano SH, Duan Z, Kuo Y-F, et al. Use and outcomes of adjuvant chemotherapy in older women with breast cancer. *J Clin Oncol.* 2006;24:2750–6.
105. Goldhirsch A, Wood WC, Gelber RD, et al. and Panel Members. Progress and Promise: International Expert Consensus on the Primary Therapy of Early Breast Cancer 2007. *Ann Oncol* (submitted).
106. Cuzick J, Ambroisine L, Davidson N, et al. Use of luteinising-hormone-releasing hormone agonists as adjuvant treatment in premenopausal patients with hormone-receptor-positive breast cancer: A meta-analysis of individual patient data from randomised adjuvant trials LHRH-agonists in Early Breast Cancer Overview group. *Lancet.* 2007;369:1711–23.
107. Gray RG, Rea DW, Handley K, et al. aTTom (adjuvant Tamoxifen–To offer more?): Randomized trial of 10 versus 5 years of adjuvant tamoxifen among 6,934 women with estrogen receptor-positive (ER+) or ER untested breast cancer–Preliminary results. J Clin Oncol. 2008;26 (May 20 suppl; abstr 513)
108. Peto R, Davies C on Behalf of the ATLAS Collaboration. ATLAS (Adjuvant Tamoxifen, Longer Against Shorter): international randomized trial of 10 versus 5 years of adjuvant tamoxifen among 11 500 women – preliminary results. SABCS 2007 (abstr 48).
109. Coates AS, Keshaviah A, Thürlimann B, et al. Five Years of Letrozole Compared With Tamoxifen As Initial Adjuvant Therapy for Postmenopausal Women With Endocrine-Responsive Early Breast Cancer: Update of Study BIG 1-98. *J Clin Oncol.* 2007;25:486–92.
110. Arimidex, Tamoxifen, Alone or in Combination (ATAC) Trialists' Group: Effect of anastrozole and tamoxifen as adjuvant treatment for early-stage breast cancer: 100-month analysis of the ATAC trial. Lancet Oncol. 2008;(1):45–53.
111. Coombes RC, Kilburn LS, Snowdon CF, et al. Survival and safety of exemestane versus tamoxifen after 2–3 years' tamoxifen treatment (Intergroup Exemestane Study): A randomised controlled trial. *Lancet.* 2007;369:559–70.
112. Jonat W, Gnant M, Boccardo F, et al. Effectiveness of switching from adjuvant tamoxifen to anastrozole in postmenopausal women with hormone sensitive early-stage breast cancer: a meta-analysis. *Lancet Oncol.* 2006;7:991–6.
113. Goss PE, Ingle JN, Martino S, et al. Efficacy of letrozole extended adjuvant therapy according to estrogen receptor and progesterone receptor status of the primary tumor: National Cancer Institute of Canada Clinical Trials Group MA.17. *J Clin Oncol.* 2007;25:2006–11.
114. Mouridsen HT, Giobbie-Hurder A, Mauriac L, et al. BIG 1-98: A randomized double-blind phase III study evaluating letrozole and tamoxifen given in sequence as adjuvant endocrine therapy for postmenopausal women with receptor-positive breast cancer. SABCS 2008, (abstr 13).
115. Mauriac L, Keshaviah A, Debled M, et al. Predictors of early relapse in postmenopausal women with hormone receptor-positive breast cancer in the BIG 1-98 trial. *Ann Oncol.* 2007;18:859–67.
116. Viale G, Giobbie-Hurde Ar, Regan MM, et al. Prognostic and predictive value of centrally reviewed Ki-67 labeling index in postmenopausal women with endocrine-responsive breast cancer: Results from breast international group trial 1-98 comparing adjuvant tamoxifen with letrozole. J Clin Oncol 2008;26:5569–75.
117. Rasmussen BB, Regan MM, Lykkesfeldt AE, et al. Adjuvant letrozole versus tamoxifen according to centrally-assessed ERBB2 status for postmenopausal women with endocrine-responsive early breast cancer: supplementary results from the BIG 1-98 randomised trial. Lancet Oncol. 2008;9:23–8.

118. Lewis JS, Osipo C, Meeke K, et al. Estrogen-induced apoptosis in breast cancer model resistant to long-term estrogen withdrawal. *J Steroid Biochem Mol Biol.* 2005;94:131–41.
119. Lonning PE, Taylor PD, Anker G, et al. High-dose estrogen treatment in postmenopausal breast cancer patients heavily exposed to endocrine therapy. *Breast Cancer Res Treat.* 2001;67:111–6.
120. Saphner T, Tormey DC, Gray R. Annual recurrence hazard rates for breast cancer after adjuvant therapy annual hazard rates of recurrence for breast cancer after primary therapy. *J Clin Oncol.* 1996;14:2738–46.
121. Smith IE, Dowsett M, Yap YS, et al. Adjuvant aromatase inhibitors for early breast cancer after chemotherapy-induced amenorrhoea: Caution and Suggested Guidelines. *J Clin Oncol.* 2006;24:2444–7.
122. Perez EA, Suman VJ, Davidson N, et al. Advances in monoclonal therapy for breast cancer: Further analysis of NCCTG N9831. 41st Annual Meeting of the American Society of Clinical Oncology; Orlando: FL; May 16, 2005.
123. Halyard MY, Pisansky TM, Dueck AC, et al. Radiotherapy and adjuvant trastuzumab in operable breast cancer: Tolerability and adverse event data from the NCCTG phase III trial N9831. J Clin Oncol. 2009;27. Published Ahead of Print on April 6th.

Sequencing of Systemic Treatment and Radiotherapy

Pia Ursula Huguenin[†]

Introduction

The mortality of breast cancer is mainly due to metastatic disease, and the majority of clinical trials are aimed at the optimization of systemic treatments in order to reduce the risk for the development of a systemic disease. In early years, following the observation of outcome in large numbers of patients with specific disease profiles supposed to be risk factors, surgery was supplemented by orthovoltage radiotherapy and ovarian ablation as the first form of systemic treatment. The efficacy of radiotherapy was analyzed in very early randomized trials. The question of sequencing was addressed only later, with the availability of many active drugs and the establishment of breast-conserving therapy including radiotherapy to the remaining breast.

Efficacy of Radiotherapy in the Concept of Treatment of Early Breast Cancer

Radiotherapy plays an important role in the curative treatment of operable breast cancer. Adjuvant postoperative radiotherapy reduces the annual odds of local recurrence by a factor of three [1]. Despite some extra mortality as consequence of poor radiotherapy techniques in the earliest trials, a decrease in cancer-related deaths with radiation therapy was observed in a meta-analysis [2]. The improvement of loco-regional control translated into a significant reduction of deaths due to cancer: for every 100 patients receiving radiotherapy, 20 loco-regional failures were prevented and five deaths due to cancer were avoided [1].

P.U. Huguenin[†] (✉)
Radiation Therapy Department, Kantonsspital Graubünden, Chur, Switzerland

M. Castiglione, M.J. Piccart (eds.), *Adjuvant Therapy for Breast Cancer*,
Cancer Treatment and Research 151, DOI 10.1007/978-0-387-75115-3_17,

Current Practice of Combined Modality Treatment Including Radiotherapy Outside of Clinical Trials

Following breast conserving surgery, all patients should undergo radiotherapy irrespective of systemic treatment; so far, no patients' subgroup was identified that would not profit in terms of reduction of the local failure rate [3]. Patients requiring adjuvant polychemotherapy usually get this soon following surgery and before radiotherapy, as microscopic tumor burden would be treated more efficiently by systemic treatment than by radiotherapy [4].

The International Breast Cancer Study Group (IBCSG) investigated the timing of radiotherapy in two trials, one for pre/perimenopausal patients with involved nodes, one for node-positive postmenopausal patients [5]. Systemic treatment consisted of 6 cycles of cyclophosphamide, methotrexate and 5-fluoro-uracil (CMF) or, in receptor-positive postmenopausal patients, in tamoxifen only (146/718 patients). There was no difference in ipsilateral breast recurrence or disease-free survival at 4 years for both groups receiving radiotherapy early or later at the end of chemotherapy. Free resection margins were required for the inclusion into these trials; whether close or involved margins would favor early radiotherapy remains unanswered.

Recommendations for radiotherapy with or without inclusion of nodal areas following mastectomy are based on less sound data [3]. Postmastectomy radiotherapy is a generally accepted standard for tumor stages pT3 or pT4 and /or for ≥pN2a [3]. An intergroup study is currently running for patients with one to three involved axillary nodes and/or tumor stage pT2 with histologically poor differentiation and/or lymphovascular invasion ("SUPREMO", selective use of postoperative radiotherapy after mastectomy).

Are There Reasons to Re-investigate Current Practice of Radiotherapy?

Yes, there are at least two reasons: delay of radiotherapy may decrease the chance of cure and concurrent radiotherapy with systemic therapy has been shown to be superior to sequential application of radiation and drugs in many other solid tumors.

In addition, with the sequential application of postoperative systemic treatment followed by radiation and later by hormonal treatment, overall treatment time is considerably prolonged as compared to concomitant therapy, and the radiosensitizing effect in tumor cells is not used.

Potential Impact of Delay of Radiotherapy on Outcome

Delay of radiotherapy following breast surgery may have different reasons; the discussion is restricted to postoperative adjuvant radiotherapy.

Delay by any reason may negatively affect treatment outcome in several malignant tumors, as systematically summarized based on retrospective data by a Canadian research group [6]. Most studies on breast cancer dealt with a cutoff point of 8 weeks following surgery and restricted the analysis to local control. The pooled data showed a superior local relapse-free rate using early radiotherapy, compared to postoperative full chemotherapy followed by radiotherapy (eleven studies; odds ratio 2.28, 95% confidence interval 1.45–3.57, corresponding to a local relapse rate of 6% with postoperative radiotherapy, compared to a relapse rate of 16% using chemotherapy before radiation).

Comparable results with a significant loss in disease-specific survival associated with a delay of 3 months or more until beginning of postoperative radiotherapy have been shown in a recent report by the Surveillance, Epidemiology, and End Results (SEER)-Medicare database 1991–1999 in patients over 65 years who did not receive chemotherapy [7].

Concomitant Chemo- and Radiotherapy

For some solid tumors, concomitant chemo-radiation has been demonstrated as the most efficient way of treatment (uterine cervix [8]; carcinomas of the head and neck [9, 10]) with respect to loco-regional tumor control rates, compared to radiotherapy alone. Simultaneous radio-immunotherapy was effective in the same order [11]. However, a potential increase in acute and late toxicity may be prohibitive for a simultaneous application of radiation with some of the frequently used drugs such as anthracyclines and taxanes. Cyclophosphamide, methotrexate and fluorouracil (CMF) combined with postmastectomy radiation of the chest wall and lymph nodes have been reported to be superior to radiotherapy alone in two randomized trials [12, 13]. However, the "CMF" regimen used in these trials was different from the "CMF" originally reported to improve disease-free and overall survival, and modifications may reduce the optimal efficacy even in presence of an additive effect of RT and chemotherapy [14].

The concomitant chemo-radiotherapy using the original CMF and a carefully fractionated radiotherapy at a rather low total dose has been shown to be feasible without impact on dose intensity or toxicity in a pilot trial [15].

Concomitant, most often preoperative chemo-radiation is established and, outside clinical trials, reserved for locally advanced and inoperable or inflammatory breast cancer. Details on this combined modality treatment for primarily inoperable extensive breast cancers are beyond the scope of this chapter. However, long-term locoregional control may be achieved in two thirds of patients using an appropriate systemic treatment and radiotherapy [16]. A breast conserving treatment was possible in 70% of the cases in a French Series with a documented rate of pathological response of 27%; a grade 4 hematological toxicity rate was observed in 22% [17].

Randomized Trials on Sequencing of Postoperative Concomitant Adjuvant Radiotherapy and Systemic Polychemotherapy Treatment

In a small trial at the Joint Center in Boston run between 1984 and 1992, 244 patients with considerable risk to develop distant metastases were randomized to chemotherapy over 12 weeks first (methotrexate, folinic acid, fluorouracil, prednisone, cyclophosphamide and doxorubicin) followed by tamoxifen, or radiotherapy first (45 Gy in 25 fractions to the whole breast) followed by a boost dose of 16–18 Gy [18]. Local recurrences were marginally reduced in the arm starting with radiation therapy (55 vs 14%, $p = 0.007$) but a re-analysis of this series after a follow-up of 135 months showed no significant difference in the rates of freedom from any event, including ipsi- or contralateral breast cancer, secondary malignancy, death, freedom from metastasis or overall survival [19].

Concomitant vs sequential application of CMF chemotherapy and radiotherapy in a small Italian trial in 206 patients found no significant difference in outcome at 5 years including late toxicity [20]. In contrast in the French ARCOSEIN Trial, where 716 patients were randomized to radiation therapy plus chemotherapy (mitoxantrone, fluorouracil and cyclophosphamide) or to the sequential application starting with six courses of systemic treatment following breast conserving surgery, the 5-year locoregional recurrence-free survival was in favor of the concomitant treatment in the node-positive subgroup (97 vs 91%, $p = 0.02$) [21]. Unfortunately, the incidence of grade 2 or more late effects was increased following concomitant chemo-radiotherapy [21].

Based on biological considerations and on retrospective analysis of early clinical data, the combined use of tamoxifen and radiotherapy seemed to increase the risk of lung fibrosis following local/locoregional surgery [22]. However, in the randomized NSABP-B21 Trial, late toxicity following simultaneous application of radiotherapy and tamoxifen was not described in detail [23] and two other trials, one retrospective analysis [24] and a randomized SWOG trial [25] did not demonstrate any increase in late toxicities. All these trials reported an improved local control rate for patients receiving concurrently radiotherapy and tamoxifen.

Many additional drugs are now applied in the adjuvant setting, especially the taxanes, new hormonal agents and antibodies against the ErbB-2 receptor. Based on experimental and clinical data, some of these drugs are potential radiosensitizers, and the therapeutic gain depends on the sensitizing effect in tumor compared to normal tissues [26–28].

One of the recently introduced new drugs, trastuzumab, an antibody against ErbB2 (member of the epidermal growth factor receptor (EGFR) family), may act as radiosensitizer similarly to other antibodies or molecules that interfere with signal transduction. An abstract publication of toxicity data on a recent phase III North Central Cancer Treatment Group trial did not show increased acute toxicity for radiotherapy with simultaneous application of trastuzumab [29].

Open Questions

Several items for which we have no or insufficient clinical data remain open.

There is no doubt about the importance of clear surgical margins in primary treatment of breast cancer. However, it is not known whether a higher local dose of radiotherapy can compensate for poor surgery; probably not.

Hypofractionated radiotherapy with less fractions may be given without increase in late toxicity and with the same probability of local tumor control, in order to shorten overall treatment time [30]; a short or even only one radiation fraction applied intraoperatively focally to the breast bed [31] may allow to postpone the systemic adjuvant treatment for a short time without loss in systemic efficacy (distant disease-free survival).

Conclusion

Radiation therapy after breast surgery has been shown to dramatically decrease local relapses. Delays in radiation therapy start after surgery may well lead to a reduced disease-free survival. The concurrent application of multiple drugs and radiotherapy may enhance the toxicity of both modalities and, moreover is more intensive and time consuming for the patients who need some time after surgery in order to recover physically and mentally. Outside of clinical trials, the sequential application of drugs and radiotherapy is still recommended.

References

1. Kurtz J. The curative role of radiotherapy in the treatment of operable breast cancer. *Eur J Cancer*. 2002;38:1961–74.
2. Group EBCTsC: Favourable and unfavourable effects on long-term survival of radiotherapy for early breast cancer: An overview of the randomised trials. Early breast cancer trialists' collaborative group. *Lancet*. 2000;355:1757–70.
3. Poortmans P. Evidence based radiation oncology: Breast cancer. *Radiother Oncol*. 2007;84:84–101.
4. Beil DR, Wein LM: Sequencing surgery, radiotherapy and chemotherapy: Insights from a mathematical analysis. *Breast Cancer Res Treat*. 2002;74:279–86.
5. Wallgren A, Bernier J, Gelber RD, Goldhirsch A, Roncadin M, Joseph D, Castiglione-Gertsch M: Timing of radiotherapy and chemotherapy following breast-conserving surgery for patients with node-positive breast cancer. International breast cancer study group. *Int J Radiat Oncol Biol Phys*. 1996;35:649–59.
6. Huang J, Barbera L, Brouwers M, Browman G, Mackillop WJ. Does delay in starting treatment affect the outcomes of radiotherapy? A systematic review. *J Clin Oncol*. 2003;21:555–63.
7. Hershman DL, Wang X, McBride R, Jacobson JS, Grann VR, Neugut AI. Delay in initiating adjuvant radiotherapy following breast conservation surgery and its impact on survival. *Int J Radiat Oncol Biol Phys*. 2006;65:1353–60.
8. Thomas GM. Improved treatment for cervical cancer – concurrent chemotherapy and radiotherapy. *N Engl J Med*. 1999;340:1198–200.

9. Auperin A, Le Pechoux C, Pignon JP, Koning C, Jeremic B, Clamon G, Einhorn L, Ball D, Trovo MG, Groen HJ, Bonner JA, Le Chevalier T, Arriagada R. Concomitant radiochemotherapy based on platin compounds in patients with locally advanced non-small cell lung cancer (nsclc): A meta-analysis of individual data from 1764 patients. *Ann Oncol.* 2006;17:473–83.
10. Pignon JP, Bourhis J, Domenge C, Designe L. Chemotherapy added to locoregional treatment for head and neck squamous-cell carcinoma: Three meta-analyses of updated individual data. Mach-nc collaborative group. Meta-analysis of chemotherapy on head and neck cancer. *Lancet.* 2000;355:949–55.
11. Bonner JA, Harari PM, Giralt J, Azarnia N, Shin DM, Cohen RB, Jones CU, Sur R, Raben D, Jassem J, Ove R, Kies MS, Baselga J, Youssoufian H, Amellal N, Rowinsky EK, Ang KK. Radiotherapy plus cetuximab for squamous-cell carcinoma of the head and neck. *N Engl J Med.* 2006;354:567–78.
12. Overgaard M, Hansen PS, Overgaard J, Rose C, Andersson M, Bach F, Kjaer M, Gadeberg CC, Mouridsen HT, Jensen MB, Zedeler K. Postoperative radiotherapy in high-risk premenopausal women with breast cancer who receive adjuvant chemotherapy. Danish breast cancer cooperative group 82b trial. *N Engl J Med.* 1997;337:949–55.
13. Ragaz J, Jackson SM, Le N, Plenderleith IH, Spinelli JJ, Basco VE, Wilson KS, Knowling MA, Coppin CM, Paradis M, Coldman AJ, Olivotto IA. Adjuvant radiotherapy and chemotherapy in node-positive premenopausal women with breast cancer. *N Engl J Med.* 1997;337:956–62.
14. Goldhirsch A, Colleoni M, Coates AS, Castiglione-Gertsch M, Gelber RD. Adding adjuvant cmf chemotherapy to either radiotherapy or tamoxifen: Are all cmfs alike? The international breast cancer study group (ibcsg). *Ann Oncol.* 1998;9:489–93.
15. Dubey A, Recht A, Come SE, Gelman RS, Silver B, Harris JR, Shulman LN. Concurrent cmf and radiation therapy for early stage breast cancer: Results of a pilot study. *Int J Radiat Oncol Biol Phys.* 1999;45:877–84.
16. Liao Z, Strom EA, Buzdar AU, Singletary SE, Hunt K, Allen PK, McNeese MD. Locoregional irradiation for inflammatory breast cancer: Effectiveness of dose escalation in decreasing recurrence. *Int J Radiat Oncol Biol.* Phys 2000;47:1191–2000.
17. Bollet MA, Sigal-Zafrani B, Gambotti L, Extra JM, Meunier M, Nos C, Dendale R, Campana F, Kirova YM, Dieras V, Fourquet A. Pathological response to preoperative concurrent chemo-radiotherapy for breast cancer: Results of a phase ii study. *Eur J Cancer.* 2006;42:2286–95.
18. Recht A, Come SE, Henderson IC, Gelman RS, Silver B, Hayes DF, Shulman LN, Harris JR. The sequencing of chemotherapy and radiation therapy after conservative surgery for early-stage breast cancer. *N Engl J Med.* 1996;334:1356–61.
19. Bellon JR, Come SE, Gelman RS, Henderson IC, Shulman LN, Silver BJ, Harris JR, Recht A. Sequencing of chemotherapy and radiation therapy in early-stage breast cancer: Updated results of a prospective randomized trial. *J Clin Oncol.* 2005;23:1934–40.
20. Arcangeli G, Pinnaro P, Rambone R, Giannarelli D, Benassi M. A phase iii randomized study on the sequencing of radiotherapy and chemotherapy in the conservative management of early-stage breast cancer. *Int J Radiat Oncol Biol. Phys.* 2006;64:161–7.
21. Toledano A, Garaud P, Serin D, Fourquet A, Bosset JF, Breteau N, Body G, Azria D, Le Floch O, Calais G. Concurrent administration of adjuvant chemotherapy and radiotherapy after breast-conserving surgery enhances late toxicities: Long-term results of the arcosein multicenter randomized study. *Int J Radiat Oncol Biol Phys.* 2006;65:324–32.
22. Bentzen SM, Skoczylas JZ, Overgaard M, Overgaard J. Radiotherapy-related lung fibrosis enhanced by tamoxifen. *J Natl Cancer Inst.* 1996;88:918–22.
23. Fisher B, Bryant J, Dignam JJ, Wickerham DL, Mamounas EP, Fisher ER, Margolese RG, Nesbitt L, Paik S, Pisansky TM, Wolmark N. Tamoxifen, radiation therapy, or both for prevention of ipsilateral breast tumor recurrence after lumpectomy in women with invasive breast cancers of one centimeter or less. *J Clin Oncol.* 2002;20:4141–9.

24. Harris EE, Christensen VJ, Hwang WT, Fox K, Solin LJ. Impact of concurrent versus sequential tamoxifen with radiation therapy in early-stage breast cancer patients undergoing breast conservation treatment. *J Clin Oncol.* 2005;23:11–16.
25. Pierce LJ, Hutchins LF, Green SR, Lew DL, Gralow JR, Livingston RB, Osborne CK, Albain KS. Sequencing of tamoxifen and radiotherapy after breast-conserving surgery in early-stage breast cancer. *J Clin Oncol.* 2005;23:24–29.
26. Horsman MR, Bohm L, Margison GP, Milas L, Rosier JF, Safrany G, Selzer E, Verheij M, Hendry JH. Tumor radiosensitizers – current status of development of various approaches: Report of an international atomic energy agency meeting. *Int J Radiat Oncol Biol Phys.* 2006;64:551–61.
27. Tannock IF. Treatment of cancer with radiation and drugs. *J Clin Oncol.* 1996;14:3156–74.
28. Wardman P. Chemical radiosensitizers for use in radiotherapy. *Clin Oncol. (R Coll Radiol).* 2007;19:397–417.
29. Halyard MY, Pisansky TM, Solin LJ, Marks LB, Pierce LJ, Dueck A, Perez EA. Adjuvant radiotherapy (rt) and trastuzumab in stage i–iia breast cancer: Toxicity data from north central cancer treatment group phase iii trial n9831. *J Clin Oncol* (Meeting Abstracts). 2006;24:523.
30. Dewar JA, Haviland JS, Agrawal RK, Bliss JM, Hopwood P, Magee B, Owen JR, Sydenham MA, Venables K, Yarnold JR, on behalf of the STc. Hypofractionation for early breast cancer: First results of the UK standardization of breast radiotherapy (start) trials. *J Clin Oncol* (Meeting Abstracts). 2007;25:LBA518.
31. Holmes DR, Baum M, Joseph D. The targit trial: Targeted intraoperative radiation therapy versus conventional postoperative whole-breast radiotherapy after breast-conserving surgery for the management of early-stage invasive breast cancer (a trial update). *Am J Surg.* 2007;194:507–10.

Part V
Special Populations

Young Patients with Breast Cancer

P.A. Francis

Incidence and Prognosis

Among women diagnosed with early breast cancer, one in four will be premenopausal. In relation to breast cancer, the term "young" typically refers to patients aged less than 40 years. While breast cancer in young women is not common, breast cancer remains the leading cause of cancer deaths among young women. Only about 1 in 40 women diagnosed with breast cancer will be very young (defined here as <35 years).

Women aged younger than 35 years diagnosed with early breast cancer have been shown in a number of series to have a poorer prognosis and higher risk of relapse. In a Swedish data set, the relative survival among patients <50 years decreased with younger age. Patients younger than 35 years had a much lower relative survival than those aged 44–49 years, with a 13% absolute difference at 5 years [1]. In a large single institution French study of premenopausal women, the relationship between hazard of recurrence and age indicated a 4% decrease in recurrence for every additional year of age [2]. Younger patients tend to present more frequently with unfavorable histologic features, with more positive lymph nodes, larger tumors, negative hormone receptors and high S-phase fractions or elevated Ki67 in their tumors [3, 4]. The St. Gallen International Expert Consensus on the Primary Therapy of Early Breast Cancer excludes women <35 years of age with resected breast cancer from the "low risk" category [5].

Endocrine Considerations

While the Early Breast Cancer Trialists' Collaborative Group (EBCTCG) overview analyses have provided important information regarding treatment effects, small sub-groups such as very young women may not be well

P.A. Francis (✉)
Breast Medical Oncology, Peter MacCallum Cancer Center, Melbourne, Australia

M. Castiglione, M.J. Piccart (eds.), *Adjuvant Therapy for Breast Cancer*,
Cancer Treatment and Research 151, DOI 10.1007/978-0-387-75115-3_18,

represented in overall data. Emerging data suggest that breast cancer outcomes in this age group may have some unique aspects. EBCTCG overview data suggest that women <40 years and women aged 40–49 years derive a similar proportional reduction in risk from polychemotherapy [6]. However, when the International Breast Cancer Study Group (IBCSG) analyzed outcomes for very young women (<35 years) in a series of trials testing adjuvant CMF chemotherapy in premenopausal women, they found that women <35 years had a higher risk of relapse and death than the older premenopausal women (≥35 years) when treated with CMF alone [7]. The 10-year disease-free survival (DFS) of 35% in women <35 years was significantly worse than the DFS of 47% in the older premenopausal women ($p<0.001$). The relapse and death rate in the women <35 years was particularly high in those with estrogen receptor positive (ER + ve) tumors, who paradoxically had a worse outcome than women <35 years with estrogen receptor negative tumors. The 10-year DFS was 25% for ER positive compared with 47% for ER negative among the very young ($p = 0.014$). When major North American Cooperative Groups (NSABP, ECOG, and SWOG) were invited to study the outcomes of very young women compared with older premenopausal women treated in their chemotherapy only trials, a similar phenomenon was seen, with the worst outcome in women <35 years with ER + ve breast cancer [8]. Interestingly, among women with ER negative tumors, the outcome in women <35 years was similar to that for older premenopausal women >35 years. Thus, very young women with hormone receptor positive breast cancer are a subgroup who appear to deserve special attention because of their poorer outcome when treated with chemotherapy alone.

For premenopausal women with hormone receptor positive breast cancer who receive chemotherapy and no other systemic treatment, the outcome is significantly better when the chemotherapy results in amenorrhea, even if the amenorrhea is temporary [9]. The risk of amenorrhea following chemotherapy is age dependent, with more than 80% of women ≥40 years developing amenorrhea with six cycles of classic CMF. For women <40 years, less than half develop amenorrhea, while for women <35 years of age, less than one in three develop amenorrhea with CMF [10, 11]. Among premenopausal women, four cycles of doxorubicin and cyclophosphamide (AC) results in less amenorrhea than CMF [12]. Patients aged 35–39 years have a greater chance of developing amenorrhea after CMF or CEF chemotherapy than those aged <35 years [13]. The poor outcome for very young women with resected estrogen receptor positive tumors, when treated with chemotherapy alone, may be explained at least in part by the failure to achieve amenorrhea in this age group, resulting in a potential ongoing estrogenic stimulus to occult tumor cells. The older premenopausal women who achieve amenorrhea after chemotherapy derive an indirect endocrine benefit from the chemotherapy in addition to its direct cytotoxic effects.

EBCTCG data show that ovarian ablation or suppression is an effective adjuvant treatment for women under 50 years and significantly reduces recurrence and breast cancer mortality [6]. However, in women who also receive chemotherapy, ovarian ablation or suppression provides a smaller benefit of questionable significance, even for women <40 years. Some women <40 years who receive adjuvant chemotherapy become menopausal and these women are unlikely to derive additional benefit from ovarian ablation or suppression. The EBCTCG data on efficacy of ovarian ablation/suppression also include many women unselected for hormone receptor status. Therefore the overview data on the efficacy of ovarian ablation or suppression in the presence of chemotherapy may underestimate the potential benefit for the subgroup of very young women with hormone receptor positive breast cancer.

The question of whether ovarian suppression adds to the benefits of adjuvant chemotherapy was tested in an ECOG led Intergroup Trial 0101 for premenopausal women with node positive hormone receptor positive breast cancer. Women were randomized to receive chemotherapy with CAF alone, CAF followed by goserelin (CAF-Z), or CAF followed by goserelin plus tamoxifen (CAF-ZT). While the addition of tamoxifen to CAF-Z improved DFS, there was no significant effect on disease free survival (DFS) with addition of goserelin to CAF (9 years DFS: CAF = 57%, CAF-Z = 60%, CAF-ZT = 68%) [14]. However in an unplanned retrospective analysis in the subgroup of women <40 years there was a trend to benefit from goserelin when added to CAF (HR for DFS = 0.78; 95% CI, 0.56–1.08), while no effect was seen in the subgroup ≥40 years (HR for DFS = 1.0). These data again suggest overall results from chemo-endocrine trials in premenopausal women may not be applicable to the very young subgroup.

IBCSG randomized premenopausal women with node negative breast cancer to treatment with CMF chemotherapy, treatment with goserelin (Zoladex) for 2 years, or a sequential combination of CMF then goserelin for 18 months [15]. Overall the addition of goserelin after CMF resulted in a small improvement in 5-year DFS that did not reach significance (HR for DFS = 0.80, 95% CI, 0.57–1.11). However, in an unplanned subgroup analysis according to age, it appeared that the subgroup who were estrogen receptor positive and <40 years of age, derived benefit from the addition of goserelin after CMF (HR for DFS = 0.34, 95% CI, 0.14–0.87) while the group who were estrogen receptor positive and aged ≥40 years had no benefit from the addition of goserelin after CMF (HR for DFS = 1.00). Presumably the high frequency of permanent amenorrhea that occurred after CMF in the older age group, negated the potential additional benefit of goserelin. Treatment for 2 years with goserelin alone in the subgroup who were <40 years and ER +ve did not result in a good outcome in this node-negative study (5 year DFS of 62%), suggesting that ovarian suppression treatment alone may not be an optimal treatment for the young hormone receptor positive subgroup.

The EBCTCG overview data suggests that the reduction in the risk of breast cancer recurrence with adjuvant tamoxifen is similar for all age groups, including those younger than 40 years [6]. However, outcomes for premenopausal women treated with tamoxifen alone in NSABP trials showed a significantly higher relative risk of relapse for those under 35 years compared with those aged 35–49 years (RR 1.91; 95% C.I. 1.21–3.01) [8]. Cooperative group data (NSABP, ECOG and SWOG) were analyzed to assess the outcomes of the very young ER +ve women compared with their older premenopausal counterparts, from randomized trials in which they received chemotherapy followed by tamoxifen. The results again suggest a significantly increased relative risk of relapse for those less than 35 years of age [8].

In a randomized trial performed in Asia, premenopausal women were randomized to receive no adjuvant therapy vs a combination of oophorectomy plus tamoxifen. The combined endocrine treatment was clearly superior to no adjuvant therapy. In a subsequent analysis according to age, it was shown that among the women randomized to the combination endocrine treatment, there was a significantly worse outcome for those <40 years of age vs those ≥ 40 years of age [16].

In combination the above data suggest that, for very young women with hormone receptor positive breast cancer who typically remain premenopausal after chemotherapy, consideration to combining maximal endocrine treatment with chemotherapy may prove to be the optimal strategy. This strategy is being tested in a randomized trial known as "SOFT" (*S*uppression of *O*varian *F*unction *T*rial) conducted by the IBCSG. The SOFT trial is relevant for clinicians who choose chemotherapy followed by tamoxifen as the standard of care for premenopausal hormone receptor positive breast cancer. The SOFT trial tests the role of adding ovarian function suppression to tamoxifen and the role of substituting an aromatase inhibitor (exemestane) combined with ovarian function suppression. Only women who remain premenopausal (after chemotherapy if chemotherapy is given) are eligible.

The SOFT trial is one of a tailored-treatment suite of trials developed by the IBCSG for premenopausal women with hormone receptor positive breast cancer. The trials are being conducted with the support of Breast International Group (BIG) and the North American Breast Intergroup co-operative groups. Clinicians and patients can select from the trials according to their treatment preferences in this situation. For those who routinely choose ovarian suppression as an initial part of the systemic treatment for this patient group, an alternate trial called "TEXT" (*T*amoxifen and *EX*emestane *T*rial) has been developed. The TEXT trial tests the substitution of an aromatase inhibitor (exemestane) for tamoxifen, with each hormone given in combination with ovarian suppression. Chemotherapy is optional per clinician/patient preference. It is hoped that results of these important trials will provide answers regarding chemo-endocrine questions in the treatment of very young women with early breast cancer.

While aromatase inhibitors (AI) are playing an increasingly important role in the adjuvant hormonal treatment of postmenopausal women, there is concern that younger women who appear to be "post-menopausal" after adjuvant chemotherapy, are being prescribed AIs outside of a trial setting. This may not be an effective therapy because chemotherapy induced menopause is frequently reversible in younger women, and premenopausal estradiol levels may occur in the absence of menses. Trials testing the use of aromatase inhibitors as adjuvant hormonal therapy in postmenopausal women typically excluded women under age 45 with chemotherapy induced menopause for this reason.

Loco-regional Therapy

Randomized clinical trials have shown equivalent survival outcomes for mastectomy vs breast conserving surgery plus radiation for women with operable breast cancer. While age is not a contraindication to breast conserving surgery, young women have been shown to have a higher risk of local recurrence following breast conserving surgery compared with older women. In a very young woman with a conserved breast, there maybe 50 or more years during which additional ipsilateral events could occur. In young patients, very careful attention to obtaining clear surgical margins with regard to both invasive cancer and DCIS is crucial to minimize this risk and consideration to re-excision should be given where doubt exists. When mastectomy is deemed appropriate, young women should be offered the opportunity for reconstruction. A randomized trial conducted by the EORTC in women undergoing breast conserving surgery and receiving a radiation dose of 50 Gy has demonstrated the value of a 16-Gy boost radiation dose, which was particularly beneficial in young patients. For women aged ≤40 years, the local recurrence rate was reduced from 24% to 14% at 10 years, with the addition of the boost [17]. For women over 60 years, the comparable rates of local recurrence at 10 years were 7% without and 4% with the boost. Thus even with a boost dose of radiation, young women have a higher risk of local recurrence than their older counterparts. Whether an even higher dose boost would provide additional risk reduction will be the subject of further investigation. The clinical importance of avoiding local recurrence has been underscored by the recent EBCTCG overview which postulated that differences in local treatment that substantially affect local recurrence rates could theoretically avoid one breast cancer death over the subsequent 15 years, for every four local recurrences avoided [18].

Pregnancy, Fertility and Menopause

The management of (1) breast cancer diagnosed during pregnancy, (2) menopausal problems due to adjuvant therapy and (3) the preservation of fertility in relation to adjuvant therapy and pregnancy after a breast cancer diagnosis are discussed in separate chapters. These issues may be of great importance for young women who value informed discussion and advice from their treating team when deciding upon adjuvant therapy for early breast cancer. American Society of Clinical Oncology (ASCO) has developed Clinical Oncology

Recommendations on fertility preservation in cancer patients [19]. It should be noted that fertility and ovarian reserve maybe reduced in women who receive adjuvant chemotherapy, even if menstrual cycles continue and young patients may not be aware of this. While pregnancy after a diagnosis of early breast cancer is not thought to have an adverse effect on breast cancer outcome, there is data which suggests that women diagnosed with breast cancer either during or within a few years after pregnancy, have a worse prognosis independent of tumor characteristics [20, 21].

Specific intergroup collaborations/clinical trials in these areas have been developed to help better inform future care for young patients. A study led by the German Breast Group (BIG 2-03) is prospectively assessing the treatment and outcomes of breast cancer during pregnancy. An NCCTG led trial (NCCTG 9431/ IBCSG 21) is studying any association between disease free survival and the timing of breast cancer surgery in relation to menstrual cycle phase. A study led by the EORTC (BIG 3-98) is assessing attitudes to loss of fertility in women less than 35 years. A randomized trial led by Southwest Oncology Group (SWOG 0230/ IBCSG 34) is testing whether administration of goserelin during adjuvant chemotherapy can reduce the risk of premature ovarian failure in women with hormone receptor negative breast cancer. For women with hormone receptor positive breast cancer, however, it is possible that strategies which reduce the risk of premature ovarian failure may ultimately have a detrimental effect on breast cancer outcome through ongoing estrogen production.

Genetic Considerations

A diagnosis of breast cancer at a young age increases the likelihood of a specific genetic mutation (e.g. BRCA1 or BRCA2) being found compared with breast cancer at an older age; however, most women diagnosed with breast cancer under 40 years will not have a specific mutation identified if tested. In a population-based Australian study of women diagnosed with breast cancer before age 40 years, a germline mutation in BRCA1 or BRCA2 was found in 42 (5.3%) of 788 cases [22]. Additional factors that may increase the likelihood of a genetic predisposition should be sought in the history and include personal or family history (particularly at younger age) of breast or ovarian cancer, male breast cancer, bilateral breast cancer, and Ashkenazi Jewish heritage. Family history of malignancies (breast, brain, sarcoma, adrenocortical cancer, etc.) at younger age may be associated with inherited p53 mutation. Apart from identification of mutations for future risk reducing strategies and optimal screening, preferences for breast cancer therapy may differ in the case of known mutations. For example, in the case of a premenopausal woman with BRCA2 mutation and early breast cancer which is endocrine responsive and not considered high risk, salpingo-oophorectomy could reduce the risk of ovarian cancer and new breast cancers in the future, but might also be an appropriate alternative adjuvant therapy to chemotherapy, when combined with oral adjuvant hormonal therapy.

Psycho-social Considerations

Women diagnosed with breast cancer at a very young age are at greater risk for psycho-social distress [23]. Women at this stage of life typically have demands upon them from family and/or work. Fertility concerns, altered perception of body image or femininity, sexuality and fears of recurrence maybe factors relevant to difficult adjustment after diagnosis at a young age. Age appropriate supports maybe helpful.

Conclusions

Young patients diagnosed with breast cancer deserve special attention from all members of the multidisciplinary team because there are differences in the incidence, prognostic factors, systemic and loco-regional treatments, and outcomes for this age group. In addition, young women may require special assessment for issues such as preservation of fertility, desire for future pregnancy, or management of premature menopause. Consideration of the possible role of genetic factors should be considered when diagnosis occurs at a young age. Due to potential for increased distress in younger patients, attention to appropriate psycho-social support is needed. Specific trials designed to test the optimal adjuvant treatment strategies appropriate for young patients are important.

References

1. Adami HO, Malker B, Holmberg L, et al. The relation between survival and age at diagnosis in breast cancer. *NEJM*. 1986;315:559–63.
2. De la Rochefordiere A, Asselain B, Campana F, et al. Age as a prognostic factor in premenopausal breast cancer. *Lancet*. 1993;341;1039–43.
3. Albain K, Allred C, Clark G. Breast cancer outcome and predictors of outcome: Are there age differentials? *JNCI monographs*. 1994;16:35–42.
4. Colleoni M, Rotmensz N, Peruzzotti G, et al. Role of endocrine responsiveness and adjuvant therapy in very young (below 35 years) with operable breast cancer and node negative disease. *Ann Oncol*. 2006;17:1497–503.
5. Goldhirsch A, Glick JH, Gelber RD, et al. Meeting Highlights: International expert consensus on the primary therapy of early breast cancer 2005. *Ann Oncol*. 2005;16:1569–83.
6. Early Breast Cancer Trialists' Collaborative Group (EBCTCG). Effects of chemotherapy and hormonal therapy for early breast cancer on recurrence and 15-year survival: an overview of the randomized trials. *Lancet*. 2005;365:1687–717.

7. Aebi S, Gelber S, Castiglione-Gertsch M, et al. Is chemotherapy alone adequate for young women with oestrogen-receptor positive breast cancer? *Lancet*. 2000;355:1869–74.
8. Goldhirsch A, Gelber RD, Yothers G, et al. Adjuvant therapy for very young women with breast cancer: Need for tailored treatments. *JNCI Monographs*. 2001;30:44–51.
9. Pagani O, O'Neill A, Castiglione M, et al. Prognostic impact of amenorrhoea after adjuvant chemotherapy in premenopausal breast cancer patients with axillary node involvement: Results of the International Breast cancer Study Group (IBCSG) Trial VI. *Eur J Cancer*. 1998;34:632–40.
10. Goldhirsch A, Gelber RD, Castiglione M. The magnitude of endocrine effect of adjuvant chemotherapy for premenopausal breast cancer patients. *Ann Oncol*. 1990;1:183–8.
11. Tancini G, Valagussa P, Bajetta E, et al. Preliminary 3-year results of 12 versus 6 cycles of surgical adjuvant CMF in premenopausal breast cancer. *Cancer Clin Trials*. 1979;2:285–92.
12. Cobleigh M et al. *Proc Am Soc Clin Oncol*. 1995;14:A158.
13. Goodwin PJ, Ennis M, Pritchard KI, et al. Risk of menopause during the first year after breast cancer diagnosis. *J Clin Oncol*. 1999;17:2365–70.
14. Davidson N, O'Neill AM, Vukov AM, et al. Chemoendocrine therapy for premenopausal women with axillary lymph node-positive, steroid hormone receptor-positive breast cancer: Results form INT 0101 (E5188). *J Clin Oncol*. 2005;23:5973–82.
15. International Breast Cancer Study Group. Adjuvant Chemotherapy followed by goserelin versus either modality alone for premenopausal lymph node-negative breast cancer: A randomized trial. *JNCI*. 2003;95:1833–46.
16. Love RR, Nguyen BD, Nguyen VD, et al. Young age as an adverse prognostic factor in premenopausal women with operable breast cancer. *Clin Breast Cancer*. 2002;2:294–8.
17. Bartelink H, Horiot JC, Poortmans P, et al. Impact of radiation dose on local control, fibrosis and survival after breast conserving treatment:10 year results of the EORTC Trial 22881-10882. *Breast Cancer Res and Treat*. 2006;100(suppl 1, S8).
18. Early Breast Cancer Trialists' Collaborative Group. Effects of radiation and of differences in the extent of surgery for early breast cancer on local recurrence and 15-year survival: An overview of randomised trials. *Lancet*. 2005;366:2087–106.
19. Lee SJ, Schover LR, Partridge AH, et al. American Society of Clinical Oncology Recommendations on Fertility Preservation in Cancer Patients. *J Clin Oncol*. 2006;24:2917–31.
20. Guinee VF, Olsson H, Moller T, et al. Effect of pregnancy on prognosis for young women with breast cancer. *Lancet*. 1994;343:1587–1589.
21. Phillips KA, Milne RL, Friedlander ML, et al. Prognosis of premenopausal breast cancer and childbirth prior to diagnosis. *J Clin Oncol*. 2004;22:699–705.
22. Dite GS, Jenkins MA, Hocking JS, et al. Familial risks, early onset breast cancer, and BRCA1 and BRCA2 germline mutations. *JNCI*. 2003;95:448–57.
23. Ganz PA, Greendale GA, Petersen L, et al. Breast cancer in younger women: Reproductive and late health effects of treatment. *J Clin Oncol*. 2003;21:4184–93.

Special Populations: Elderly Patients

Diana Crivellari and Lucia Fratino

Introduction

The ageing of the population and the increase of life expectancy have put new social and health questions into the public health agenda of Western countries. In Europe, the median life expectancy at birth in the 1990s has reached 72.7 years among men (ranging from 75.1 in Sweden to 64.4 in Estonia) and 79.5 years among women (ranging from 82 in France to 75 in Estonia). Globally, the segment aged 65 years and over constitutes about 14.0% of the European populations, though wide geographic variations are recorded (from 17.8% in Sweden to 10.1% in Poland). [1] Moreover, time patterns show that the population group over 75 years of age is rapidly increasing in size and that life expectancy in men at age 65 increases by nearly 3 years. In elderly women, such a gain seems to be more pronounced, i.e. 6 years (from 11.9 to 17.9 years). The longest life expectancy at 65 years was registered in Japan (15.7 in men and 19.3 in women) and in Nordic European countries (14.6 in men and 18.7 in women). The larger improvement registered among women, as compared to men, is mainly due to the marked reduction in maternal mortality and to the lower impact of smoking-related deaths recorded since the 1950s. For the future, it has been estimated that in developed countries life expectancy at birth may reach 90 years for women [2].

The ageing of the population heavily affects the hardship of chronic diseases, including cancer which is primarily a disease of older people and a leading cause of death. As seen for the vast majority of carcinomas, the incidence rates for breast cancer also steadily increase with age [3]. After 70 years of age, between 280 (United Kingdom) and 427 new cases of breast cancer/100,000 women are registered each year in Western countries reaching a peak of 443/100,000 women aged 75–79 years in the SEER registry of the United States (IARC).

D. Crivellari (✉)
Division of Medical Oncology C, Centro di Riferimento Oncologico National Cancer Institute, Aviano (PN), Italy

M. Castiglione, M.J. Piccart (eds.), *Adjuvant Therapy for Breast Cancer*, Cancer Treatment and Research 151, DOI 10.1007/978-0-387-75115-3_19,

With regard to mortality, after earlier rises in most areas, breast cancer mortality in women aged 65–84 declined by 8% in the US and by 3% in the EU to reach 106/100,000 in both areas whereas it rose from 80 to 90/100,000 in Eastern Europe and from 19 to 24/100,000 in Japan [4]. Although population-based screening are not recommended over 70 years of age, at least part of these favourable trends in mortality reflect advancement in early diagnosis, in addition to improved treatment. Elderly women have experienced a less significant decline in mortality rates than the one recorded in younger women by approximately 15–20%. This difference highlights a well known debate on the opportunity of expanding the screening to older groups and on the need of improving the offer of optimal treatments to elderly women.

Assessment of Older Patients

The ageing process is characterized, for both acute and chronic diseases, by a progressive decline in physical and cognitive functions whose underlying causes are only partially understood. As a consequence, one of the most characteristic aspects of ageing is the great variability from person to person: some persons maintain their physical and cognitive abilities throughout their lifetimes (successful ageing), while others lose these abilities rather early in adult life. In a very small subgroup of individuals, the functional status even appears to improve over time [5]. The basis for this heterogeneity is largely unknown, and probably influenced by the interaction of genetic, environmental, functional, social and psychological factors that make up the individual aging process.

Modern geriatrics is the study of the complexity of many aspects of old age and the application of knowledge related to the biological, biomedical, behavioural and social aspects of ageing to perception, diagnosis, treatment and care of older persons. The geriatric approach is specifically targeted towards patients with multiple, interacting problems brought on by disease or ageing and resulting in a progressive reduction in reserve of multiple organ systems, disability (i.e., functional impairment and dependency), co-morbidity, frailty and geriatric syndromes. Such patients are not simply elderly, but are "geriatric" patients because of interacting psychosocial and physical problems. In addiction, diseases in the elderly may appear with atypical signs and symptoms, a silent presentation may occur and aged persons are extremely susceptible to iatrogenic disease. Co-morbid diseases are common and their contribution makes the picture more complex [6].

As a consequence, the health status of elderly persons cannot be evaluated by merely describing the single disease, and/or by measuring their response or survival after treatment. Conversely, it is necessary to conduct a more comprehensive investigation of the 'functional status' of the aged person. The assessment of the functional status is defined as the measurement of a patient's ability to complete functional tasks; these range from simple self care in activities of daily living (ADL) [7] to more complex instrumental activities of daily living and fulfilling social roles (IADL) [8]. ADL includes feeding, grooming, transferring and toileting. IADL includes shopping, managing finances, housekeeping, laundry, meal preparation, ability to use transportation and communicating by telephone, as well as the ability to take medications. Independence, or the degree of dependence in the ADL and IADL scales, determines whether an older person can eventually live alone without a caregiver. As for social roles, these include the ability to use transportation, the ability of requiring help in cases of urgent need and the ability of living in an interpersonal context. Each impairment in the physical, social or psychological dimension which gives rise to functional limitations is defined as disability.

As age from a clinical perspective is highly heterogeneous and poorly reflected by chronological age, the clinical evaluation of the older person is influenced by several factors and is a key step in the clinical decision process. A geriatric consultation provides a significant amount of relevant information and enables the health-care team to manage the complexity of health-care in the elderly [9]: this process is referred to as the Comprehensive Geriatric Assessment (CGA). CGA is defined as a multidimensional, often interdisciplinary, diagnostic process aimed at determining the medical, psychological and functional capabilities of elderly persons in order to develop an overall plan for treatment and long-term follow-up. It differs from the standard medical evaluation in the following ways: (1) it focuses on frail elderly people with their complex problems; (2) it emphasizes their functional status and their quality of life; and (3) it benefits from the use of an interdisciplinary team. In the geriatric setting, several studies have supported the effectiveness of CGA in improving functional status, reducing hospitalization, decreasing medical costs and prolonging survival. The meta-analysis by Stuck and colleagues showed a positive effect of the CGA, and the authors recommended its use within interdisciplinary units [10].

Due to the increasing advanced age composition of the population affected by cancer, the oncologist needed an evaluation tool to assess the older patient's overall health other than Karnofsky or ECOG performance status, as well as a scheme that provided information regarding the "biological age" in comparison to the "chronological age" of the older patient. In the early 1990s, Monfardini and colleagues designed and validated a comprehensive geriatric assessment instrument tailored on the oncological setting [11]. Such an instrument included the evaluation of functional status (ECOG performance status, ADL, IADL), co-morbidity condition (Satariano Index), cognitive function (Mini-mental state evaluation) [12], depressive symptoms, poly-pharmacy, and nutrition. The second step was the application of these assessment tools in observational studies to evaluate the usefulness of CGA in evaluating the association between PS, co-morbidity and the other dimensions of CGA [13]. The main findings were that such a "geriatric" approach may help in the management of older individuals with cancer in at least three areas: detection of frailty, treatment of unsuspected conditions, and removal of social barriers to treatment [13].

In the case of the older cancer patient, the CGA demonstrates the following advantages:

- Gross estimate of life-expectancy
- Gross estimate of functional reserve and tolerance of chemotherapy
- Recognition of reversible comorbid conditions that may interfere with cancer treatment
- Recognition of special social economic needs that may interfere with cancer treatment
- Management of nutrition and medications

In addition, it indicates the adoption of a common language in the management of older cancer patients; this is essential both for the retrospective evaluation of quality of care and for the prospective assessment of outcome in clinical trials.

In 2000, Balducci and Yates included CGA in the guidelines for the management of elderly cancer patients [14]: the main recommendation was that these scales should be applied to all elderly cancer patients regardless of age to estimate functional status in order to determine a treatment course, assess eligibility for clinical trials and predict treatment toxicity.

A further evolution on the application of said approach was to use the Geriatric Multidimensional Assessment as a milestone in the screening process and in decision-making. Oncologists should be able to intervene and target interventions by choosing between aggressive or palliative treatments, and prevent toxicity. Elderly cancer patients could be stratified upon entering optimal treatment strategies and/or clinical trials by means of their global health assessment and age related issue recognition. Usually according to CGA standards, the evaluation of elderly cancer patients for a course of treatment results in classification into three risk groups: fit, unfit, and frail patients.

Since the CGA is a time-consuming approach, Overcash and colleagues proposed an abbreviated CGA (aCGA) for use in the onco-geriatric setting consisting in applying only selected items from the main domains scored by CGA with the aim of pre-screening older cancer patients who would benefit from a more complex assessment [15]. Another approach consisted in a partially self- administered CGA tool that was designed by Hurria and colleagues [16].

A key step in the patient evaluation in the onco-geriatric setting is the definition and identification of frailty (this represents a major issue in clinical geriatrics). Although the term frailty has been increasingly used since the 1980s in medical literature, its actual meaning is still not well defined.

Different authors emphasize different aspects of frailty, [17] and frailty includes the following notions:

- Being dependent on others
- Being at a substantial risk of dependency and other adverse health outcomes
- Experiencing the loss of 'physiological reserves'

- Having many chronic illnesses
- Having complex medical and psycho–social problems
- Having 'atypical' disease presentations

In the oncological setting, Balducci firstly defined frailty as the condition of being over 80 years old, or having some ADL disability or being affected by more than three co-morbidities or a geriatric syndrome [18]. Frailty is a reversible condition characterized by a high degree of susceptibility to external changes that require adaptation and compensation. On these bases, when cancer is the "external change" the main objective of frailty detection is to adopt compensatory strategies acting at different levels. For instance, the cellular biology level (e.g., growth factors, erythropoietin), the physiological level (e.g., supportive therapies), and the metabolic pathways (nutritional support) interplay between functional status and social behaviours. With regard to social behaviours, a particular role is played by care-givers whose presence assures adherence to therapeutic plans. Oncologists with poor experience in the assessment of older individuals are even led to consider as frail those persons with moderate disability who may benefit from aggressive cancer treatments.

Certain older cancer patients are frail and effectively need palliation; this may include treatment with low doses of chemotherapy. Due to demographic and epidemiological considerations, frail patients have become the new target of onco-geriatrics, especially in a sub-set of breast cancer patients [19]. Thus, as the frail population increases, clinical trials including this subgroup are needed. The usefulness of these trials requires a consensus on the definition of frailty.

To date, most data concerning older women with breast cancer are derived from retrospective studies, which are often affected by a selection bias [20]. These studies do not provide adequate information on the global health status of older women. Therefore, such results cannot be applied to the older population as a whole.

Biological Aspects

Breast cancer is a heterogeneous disease and approximately 70–80% of all breast tumors in elderly patients express ER protein, thus representing an endocrine-responsive disease. These tumors tend to grow slowly, are usually better differentiated, respond to hormonal drugs, and are associated with longer disease-free interval and a slightly better overall prognosis [21]. The findings that the age-specific breast cancer rates are composed of at least two different patterns one for ER+ and another for ER– have been recently confirmed in a large SEER data-base [22]. These data indicated that the ER+ cancer rates increase with age, but at a slower pace after age 50–54, while the ER– cancer rates do not increase after age 50–54, suggesting that breast cancer is composed of two or more different subgroups and should be examined separately in future clinical studies. Furthermore, from the molecular point of view the ER+ cancers are characterized by relatively high expression of many genes expressed by breast luminal cells, with little to no Erb-B2 expression, while the ER– cancers are characterized by two subgroups, one involving basal epithelial cells and another involving high Erb-B2 expression.

The results of the largest biological study, confirming the clinical impression of a more indolent disease and a favourable outcome in the elderly, were reported some years ago by Diab [23]. These data were recently also confirmed in two large Italian data-bases [24, 25].

There is, however, a 20–30% rate of patients who remain at high risk of relapse because of extensive nodal involvement or estrogen receptor negative disease. Genetic profile will provide us with new insight on the aggressiveness of the tumor, while the ongoing studies on host-influence, such as those on immune-senescence and cytokines of aging, should provide us with new ideas on the mechanisms of tumor growth that are still poorly understood. These may help us to understand why in some patients, even if the biology of the tumor seems favourable, the disease has in the individual patient an aggressive behaviour.

Treatment

Surgery

The surgical approach can easily be used in the majority of patients [26] considering that co-morbidities and not age are the main factors influencing morbidity or mortality [27]. However, in the case of a very old woman, the first question to ask is, for sure, whether it is possible to spare this stress to our patient? The studies that are currently in the literature document attempt to use tamoxifen instead of surgery, but even though there were no differences in terms of overall survival, all studies reported a significant increase in local relapses [28–31]. Disease-free survival and quality of life become the principal end-points, and we know that quality of life is very different when a woman lives with or without a growing cancer. A Cochrane review finally concluded that primary endocrine therapy alone was inferior to surgery (with or without endocrine therapy) for the local control of breast cancer(http://www.cochrane.org/reviews/en/ab004272.html). Data are summarized in Table 1.

Table 1 Cochrane Review of seven trials comparing surgery vs primary endocrine therapy for operable elderly women

Treatment	PFS Hazard ratio	95% Confidence interval	p Value	OS Hazard ratio	95% Confidence interval	p Value
Surgery alone vs TAM	0.55	0.39–0.77	0.0006	0.98	0.74–1.30	0.9
Surgery + TAM vs TAM	0.65	0.53–0.81	0.0001	0.86	0.73–1.00	0.06

Surgery therefore remains a valid landmark in the treatment of early breast cancer and should be offered to medically fit older patients, while alternative therapies should be reserved for those patients unfit or not eligible for surgery, or who refuse this treatment option. A recent paper, however, showed a strongly impaired survival for women who refuse surgery for their breast cancer: they had a 2.1-fold increased risk of dying of breast cancer compared with operated women [32].

With the advent of a new generation of aromatase inhibitors, which proved to be more effective than tamoxifen in advanced disease [33–36], especially in older women and in those who have an overexpression of HER2/*neu* [37], this scenario will be reassessed.

Axillary surgery has had an established role in the staging and cure of breast cancer, but recently, mainly due to the widespread use of sentinel node biopsy, its role was questioned by many surgeons. The magnitude of the therapeutic benefit of removing axillary lymph nodes is now debated [38]. The results of the International Breast Cancer Study Group Trial 10-93 performed in women older than 60 years with clinically node negative operable breast cancer and comparing axillary clearance vs no axillary dissection followed by 5 years of tamoxifen in endocrine responsive patients are reassuring. There is a reported very low local relapse rate (2% at 5 years median follow-up), at least in endocrine responsive patients also treated with 5 years of tamoxifen adjuvant therapy (median age in both arms was 74 years) [39].

Radiotherapy

Even if there is a consensus that postoperative radiotherapy decreases local recurrences following breast-conserving surgery [40], the lower ability for independent living or the need for assistance of frail patients questioned the avoidance of postoperative radiotherapy at least in selected older patients.

A Canadian trial showed a local recurrence rate of 0.6% in the tamoxifen plus radiotherapy group at 5 years vs 7.7% in the tamoxifen only group ($p<0.001$), indicating a greater benefit from radiation therapy in the former. This study included patients older than 50 years with tumors up to 5 cm (T1-2) [41]. A second study was limited to breast tumors up to 2 cm (T1 N0 and ER+) in women older than 70 years [42]. In this case, the advantage of giving radiotherapy was smaller (only a 3% difference in relapse rate), showing that there may be a group of women at sufficiently low risk for local recurrence that do not require breast irradiation. An update at 7.9 years median follow-up showed that radiation produces a 5.3% absolute difference in breast recurrence but without any impact on breast conservation, distant metastases or death due to other causes. Therefore, this would confirm at a longer follow-up that avoiding radiotherapy is reasonable for T1 N0 ER positive older women [43].

Breast irradiation following breast-conserving surgery remains part of standard therapy, but in older women a careful balance between life-expectancy and possible serious adverse effects (usually less than 1%) which include radiation' pneumonitis, pericarditis and rib fracture, has to be taken into account when recommending postoperative radiotherapy. Ongoing trials such as PRIME (Postoperative Radiotherapy In Minimum-risk Elderly) are addressing issues of local control, morbidity, and quality of life in low-risk patients [44]. A new option is now used: it consists of a single-fraction treatment targeted to the tumor bed (IORT), done intra-operatively immediately after the lesion removal, and preliminary data showed comparable results with conventional external radiotherapy [45]. This new approach may be particularly interesting for elderly patients for whom the risk of local recurrence is very low and two randomized trials are ongoing in a large patient population not selected for age [46, 47] in order to confirm the equivalence of these methods with conventional techniques.

Hormonal Treatment

Adjuvant hormonal therapy should be recommended to women whose breast tumors contain hormone receptor proteins, regardless of age, menopausal status, involvement of axillary lymph nodes, or tumor size according to current recommendations by the National Institute of Health (NIH) [48]. As up to 80% of elderly breast cancer patients have endocrine responsive tumors, hormonal treatment is extremely important in this setting. Tamoxifen is still the most commonly used hormonal therapy in endocrine responsive patients, with data supporting a 5-year course rather than shorter periods [49]. However, only 1 year of treatment has a significant effect on disease-free and overall survival up to 21 years in an elderly population, as demonstrated by the recently re-evaluated IBCSG Trial IV data [50]. With the advent of the innovative aromatase inhibitors (anastrozole, letrozole, exemestane) a new era has opened.

The 2005 St Gallen consensus meeting [51] extended the therapeutic window of hormonal drugs active in the adjuvant setting to aromatase inhibitors. This was due to the data gathered on 9,366 patients accrued in the ATAC trial (Arimidex, Tamoxifen, alone or in combination as adjuvant therapy in post-menopausal women) [52] data recently revisited [53]. This is a demonstration of a disease free survival advantage of anastrozole over tamoxifen, with a hazard ratio of 0.83 ($p = 0.005$) and a longer time to recurrence (HR 0.74; $p = 0.0002$) in hormone-receptor-positive patients. Furthermore, this 26% risk reduction over tamoxifen for time-to-recurrence occurs in addition to the 47% risk reduction previously reported with 5 years of tamoxifen vs placebo. In comparison with tamoxifen, a reduced toxicity was noted for thrombo-embolic events, ischaemic cerebrovascular events, as well as endometrial cancer, vaginal bleeding, hot flashes and vaginal discharge; on the other hand, an increase in bone events was recently reported with anastrozole [54].

Data on 5 years of letrozole as part of the BIG 1-98 Trial were updated [55] regarding 4,922 out of 8,028 patients treated with continuous adjuvant therapy with either letrozole or tamoxifen (the remainder received the agents in sequence) at a median follow-up of 51 months. A significant benefit in favor of letrozole was noted (with an 18% reduction in the risk of an event (hazard ratio of 0.82; 95% CI, 0.71–0.95; $p = 0.007$). This protective effect was seen for local failure, but it is worth noting that it was reported also for distant recurrence. The analysis of adverse events showed the same kind of events as in the ATAC trial with fewer thrombo-embolic events but more frequent bone fractures and cardiovascular events; factors that need to be better evaluated in all trials with aromatase inhibitors.

Hence, a 5-year course of adjuvant tamoxifen as standard therapy is challenged by the introduction of aromatase inhibitors, even if uncertainty persists about the optimal time to introduce these drugs. The American Society of Clinical Oncology Technology Assessment published new recommendations for adjuvant treatments [56] that included aromatase inhibitors in the treatment of postmenopausal women with ER-positive breast cancer. Trials of switching to an aromatase inhibitor after 2–3 years of tamoxifen [57–61] showed larger reductions in hazard ratios, partly due to the fact that early relapses are not calculated since the drug is introduced after 2–3 years (Table 2). This matter raises the question of whether a sequential approach should be a better hormonal approach not only for reducing events but also the side effects of both tamoxifen and aromatase inhibitors. The response to this issue will probably be answered in the next few years by receiving results from two trials: the BIG 1-98 protocol which has a sequence of tamoxifen and letrozole or the inverse and the TEAM trial (Tamoxifen Exemestane Multinational).

Table 2 Aromatase inhibitors trials as adjuvant therapy

				Hazard Ratio for recurrence		
Trial	Median ageyears	Sample size	Median FU (ms)	All ER+	ER+/ PgR+	ER+/ PgR–
ATAC	64	5216	68	0.74	0.84	0.43
BIG 1-98	61	8028	51	0.82	0.83	0.92
IES	64	4742	56	0.76	0.77	0.73
ITA	63	448	64	0.57	Nr	Nr
ABCSG/8 ARNO	63	3224	28	0.60	0.66	0.42
MA.17	62	5157	30	0.59	Nr	Nr
ABCSG 6a	63	856	60	0.64	Nr	Nr

Nr = not reported

Hence, the problems in the choice of upfront adjuvant treatment of ER positive elderly women must currently take into account a better selection of patients according to hormone-responsiveness (ER + PgR + vs ER + PgR–) and overexpression of HER2 as well as a careful attention to the presence of co-morbidities and risk factors for toxicity in individual patients. The most common co-morbidities reported in postmenopausal women are cardiovascular diseases and alterations in lipid metabolism, pre-existent osteoporosis and joint pain and menopausal symptoms. Although the long-term effects of both steroidal and non-steroidal aromatase inhibitors are yet to be determined, the safety profile of the drugs is in favour of their use also in the elderly population.

Chemotherapy

Numerous randomized controlled trials have demonstrated that chemotherapy improves both recurrence-free and overall survival for women with early breast cancer, but a lesser absolute benefit from chemotherapy has been observed with increasing age [21, 62]. In fact, the proportional reduction in the risk of recurrence and mortality seems to decrease with the increase of age, even if only about 600 patients (3%) were 70 years or older. Data on the results of the last two overviews are summarized in Table 3. Combined chemotherapy followed by treatment with tamoxifen was confirmed in the last overview to be superior to tamoxifen alone in node-positive postmenopausal patients with tumor expressing estrogen and/or progesterone receptors [21]. However, the optimal chemotherapy regimens, doses, and schedules for the adjuvant treatment of elderly patients have not yet been defined, while concern is increasing regarding the toxicity associated with cytotoxic regimens in this patient population [63]. Furthermore, in this retrospective review of data on four randomized trials of CALGB for node-positive breast cancer patients during the period 1975–1999, disease-free survival, overall survival and treatment-related mortality were analyzed among three different age groups (50 years or younger, 51–64 years, and 65 years or older). Among 6,487 women, only 542 (8%) were 65 years or older and only 159 (2%) were 70 years or older; the significance of their conclusions that older and younger women derived similar reductions in breast cancer mortality and recurrence from chemotherapy regimens must be taken with caution. We emphasize prudence as these data are not only derived from a small minority of elderly patients, but, more importantly, they are derived from patients that were highly selected and therefore probably not representative of the entire elderly population.

Table 3 Chemotherapy data on metanalysis[a]

Age	10 years (1998) DFS%	10 years (1998) OS%	15 years (2005) DFS%	15 years OS%
<50	34	27	36	30
50–59	22	14	23	15
60–69	18	8	13	9
>70	–	–	12	13

[a]EBCTCG *Lancet*. 1998 and 2005 (21,62) references

More recently, Elkin et al. [64] published the results of their study conducted on a population-based, observational cohort of older women to evaluate the relationship between adjuvant chemotherapy use and survival in breast cancer patients with hormone receptor-negative tumors. They identified 5,051 elderly patients and 1,711 of them (34%) received adjuvant chemotherapy within 6 months of cancer diagnosis. As expected, chemotherapy use decreased with increasing age and co-morbidity, while it increased in the successive years of diagnosis, tumor size number of positive nodes and higher tumor grade. Approximately 15% of mortality reduction was observed with the greatest benefit reported in node-positive patients or node-negative ones with high risk disease characteristics. In parallel, the study of Giordano et al. was published [65]. It evaluated the patterns and outcomes of adjuvant chemotherapy use in a population-based cohort of older women with primary breast cancer (both ER+ and ER–). In this larger study a total of 41,390 women were detected and 4,500 of them (10.9%) received chemotherapy. The use of adjuvant chemotherapy increased during the years spanning from 7.4% in 1991 to 16.3% in 1999 ($p<0.0001$) and also with a significant shift toward anthracyclines use. Chemotherapy was not associated with improved survival among women with node-negative disease or node-positive and ER positive disease (HR 1.05; 95% CI 0.85–1.31), while there was a significant reduction in breast cancer mortality in node-positive and ER negative patients (HR 0.72; 95% CI 0.54–0.96) also evident in the subset of women over 70 years (HR 0.74; 95% CI 0.56–0.97).

Non-anthracycline-containing regimens were thought to be preferable given the fear of cardiac toxicity in older patients, but regimens such as CMF showed no significant advantage over tamoxifen in different trials involving older women [66, 67]. Anthracyclines seems to be more effective as was reported in the NSABP B-16 trial [68], with a short course (four cycles) of doxorubicin and cyclophosphamide combined with tamoxifen that was superior to tamoxifen alone. The International Collaborative Cancer Group reported a benefit in terms of disease free survival with Epirubicin in 604 patients [69], confirmed by a recent French study on 338 elderly women with node-positive disease, which showed a significant disease free survival benefit with weekly Epirubicin and tamoxifen over tamoxifen alone at a 6-year median follow-up [70]. Unfortunately, this trial is underpowered to draw definite conclusions on the advantage of anthracyclines, even if it represents a further suggestion in this direction. There is the possibility that healthy elderly women might benefit from a combined modality treatment regimen and therefore an anthracycline-based regimen should be favoured.

On the other hand, we know that age is the main important risk factor for doxorubicin-related congestive heart failure [71] with older patients (>65 years) showing a greater incidence of CHF after a cumulative dose of 400 mg/m^2. This dose is superior to what is expected with four standard doses of adjuvant treatment, but Li et al. [72] have recently shown that the initial concentrations of doxorubicin following intravenous administration are higher in older people because of a decrease in the distribution clearance, related to altered regional blood flow, and these changes could contribute to age-related doxorubicin-induced cardiotoxicity.

New drugs such as liposomal doxorubicin, capecitabine, gemcitabine, taxanes, and oral vinorelbine are now available, possibly becoming useful tools for the treatment of older patients. New targeted therapies with monoclonal antibodies like trastuzumab proved extremely effective in the adjuvant setting [73] but only few and highly selected patients were treated so far.

The need for chemotherapy trials is becoming more and more important for people older than 65 years, as they represent the fastest growing segment of the population in Western countries. Two main questions should be answered as soon as possible: first, whether adjuvant chemotherapy works in the older group of patients with endocrine unresponsive disease, and second, which is the best treatment regimen, also in terms of quality of life.

Conclusions and Future Perspectives

Molecular biology is going to challenge surgical staging with axillary clearance; the treatment plan for early breast cancer will probably change in the next few years. The stage of disease remains an important variable, but increasingly, hormone receptor status (ER and PgR) and HER-2 status are defining distinct biological subtypes of breast cancer. Even if it is clear that enormous work has to be done on the molecular sub-classification of ER-positive breast cancer [74].

The use of micro-array technology, able to identify a limited number of genes that can predict disease-free survival in a much more accurate way than nodal status, is of particular interest and importance for elderly patients. One such assay generated a recurrence score of low, intermediate, and high risk patients based on a 21-gene panel [75]. This assay proved useful to determine the value of adjuvant chemotherapy in an NSABP B-20 study where only patients with a high risk score seemed to benefit from addition of chemotherapy. This observation may be particularly useful for elderly patients who are at higher risk of having co-morbidities or developing impaired organ functions, and for whom sparing morbidity and mortality due to different therapies is the major issue.

A better evaluation of the heterogeneity of older patients requires the incorporation of geriatric screening measurements possibly able to predict not only treatment toxicities, but also the risk of dying from other causes. These tests have to be validated in different cancer patients and need to be easily performed not only in dedicated cancer centers, but, possibly, in every single institution if we want elderly patients to be evaluated and treated in the best way. Considering the burden of having to travel far from their homes and all the associated problems that this may create for them, the availability of these tests nearby could resolve a number of the issues regarding the patients' quality of life and logistic problems for their families.

The challenge for the future is, therefore, to identify better treatments and decrease cancer-specific mortality, also in this group of patients.

References

1. Socio-economic factors and health care system characteristics related to cancer survival in the elderly A population-based analysis in 16 European countries (ELDCARE project) Quaglia A, Vercelli M, Lillini R, Mugnoc E, Coebergh JW, Quinn M, Martinez-Garcia C, Capocaccia R, Micheli A on behalf of the ELDCARE Working Group *Crit Rev Oncol Hematol.* 2005;54:117–28.
2. Yancik RM, Ries L. Cancer and age: Magnitude of the problem. In Balducci L, Lyman GH, Ershler WB, eds. *ComprehensiveGeriatric Oncology*, 2nd ed. London: Harwood Academic; 1998:95–103.
3. Franceschi S, La Vecchia C. Cancer epidemiology in the elderly. *Crit Rev Oncol Hematol.* 2001;39:219–26.
4. Levi F, Lucchini F, Negri E, Boyle P, La Vecchia C. Changed trends of cancer mortality in the elderly. *Ann Oncol.* 2001;12:1467–77.
5. Stuck AE, Aronow HU, Steiner A, et al. A trial of annual inhome comprehensive geriatric assessment for elderly people living in the community. *N Engl J Med.* 1995;333:1184–9.
6. Satariano WA, Ragland DR. The effect of Comorbidity on 3 year survival of women with primary breast cancer. *ANN Int Med.* 1994;120(2):104–10.
7. Katz S, Downs TD, Cash HR, Grotz RC. Progress in development of the index of ADL. *Gerontologist.* 1970;10:20–30,73.
8. Lawton MP, Brody E. Assessment of older people: Self-maintaining and instrumental activities of daily living. *Gerontologist.* 1969;9:179–86.
9. Fratino L, Ferrario L, Redmond K, Audisio RA. Global Health care: The role of geriatrician, general practitioner and oncology nurse. *Crit Rev Oncol Hematol.* 1998;27:101–9.
10. Stuck AK, Siu AL, Wieland DG, Adams J, Rubenstein LZ. Comprehensive geriatric assessment. A meta-analysis of controlled trials. *Lancet.* 1993;342:1032–6.
11. Monfardini S, Ferrucci L, Fratino L, Del Lungo I, Serraino D, Zagonel V. Validation of a multidimensional evaluation scale for use in elderly cancer patients. *Cancer.* 1996;77:395–401.
12. Folstein ME, Folstein SE, McHugh PR. A mini mental state: a practical method for grading the cognitive status of patients for the clinician. *J Psychiatr Res.* 1975;12:189–98.
13. Repetto L, Fratino L, Audisio RA, Venturino A, Gianni W, Vercelli M, Parodi S, Dal Lago D, Gioia F, Monfardini F, Aapro MS, Serraino D, Zagonel V. Comprehensive Geriatric Assessment Adds Information to Eastern Cooperative Oncology Group Performance Status in Elderly Cancer Patients An Italian Group for Geriatric Oncology Study. *J Clinl Oncol.* 2002;20(Issue 2):494–502.
14. Balducci L, Beghè C. The application of the principlesof geriatrics to the management of the older person with cancer. *Crit Rev Oncol Hematol.* 2000;35:147–54.
15. Balducci L, Yates J. General guidelines for the management of older patients with cancer. *Oncology.* 2000;14(11A):221–7.
16. Overcash JA, Beckstead J, Extermann M, Cobb S. The abbreviated comprehensive geriatric assessment (aCGA): A retrospective analysis. *Crit Rev Oncol Hematol.* 2005;54:129–36.
17. Hurria A, Lachs MS, Cohenc HJ, Mussd HB, Kornblith AB. Geriatric assessment for oncologist: rationale and future directions. *Crit Rev Oncol Hematol.* 2006;59:211–7.
18. Fried LP, Tangen C, Walston J, et al. Frailty on older adults: Evidence for a phenotype. *J Gerontol Med Sci.* 2001;56:M146–M156.

19. Balducci L, Stanta G. Cancer in the frail patient: a coming epidemic. *Hematol Oncol Clin North Am*. 2000;14:235–50.
20. Sweeney C, Schmitz KH, Lazovich D, Virgin BA, Wallace RB, Folsom AR. Functional limitation in elderly female cancer survivors. *J Natl Cancer Inst*. 2006;98:521–9.
21. Early Breast Cancer Trialists' Collaborative Group (EBCTCG). Effects of chemotherapy and hormonal therapy for early breast cancer on recurrence and 15-year survival: An overview of the randomised trials. *Lancet*. 2005;365:1687–717.
22. Chu KC, Anderson WF. Rates for breast cancer characteristics by estrogen and progesterone receptor status in the major racial/ethnic groups. *Breast Canc Res Treat*. 2002;74:199–211.
23. Diab SG, Elledge RM, Clark GM. Tumor characteristics and clinical outcome of elderly women with breast cancer. *J Natl Cancer Inst*. 2000;92:550–6.
24. Daidone MG, Coradini D, Martelli G, et al. Primary breast cancer in elderly women: Biological profile and relation with clinical outcome. *Crit Rev Oncol Hematol*. 2003;45:313–25.
25. Molino A, Giovannini M, Auriemma A, et al. Pathological, biological and clinical characteristics, and surgical management of elderly women with breast cancer. *Crit Rev Oncol Hematol*. 2006;59:226–33.
26. Audisio RA, Bozzetti F, Gennari R, et al. The surgical management of elderly cancer patients: recommendations of the SIOG surgical task force. *Eur J Cancer*. 2004;40:926–38.
27. Ramesh HS, Jain S, Audisio RA. Implications of age in surgical oncology. *Cancer*. 2005;11(6):488–94.
28. Gazet JC, Ford H, Coombes RC. Prospective randomised trial of tamoxifen versus surgery in elderly patients with breast cancer. *Eur J Surg Oncol*. 1994;20:207–14.
29. Robertson JFR, Todd JH, Ellis IO, et al. Comparison of mastectomy with tamoxifen for treating elderly patients with operable breast cancer. *BMJd*. 1998;297:917–8.
30. Mustacchi G, Ceccherini R, Dilani S, et al. Tamoxifen alone versus adjuvant tamoxifen for operable breast cancer of the elderly: Long term results of the phase III randomized controlled multicenter GRETA trial. *Ann Oncol*. 2003;14:414–20.
31. Bates T, Riley DL, Houghton J, et al. Breast cancer in elderly women: A Cancer Research Campaign trial comparing treatment with tamoxifen and optimal surgery with tamoxifen alone. The Elderly Breast Cancer Working Party. *Br J Surg*. 1991;78:591–4..
32. Verkooijen HM, Fioretta GM, Rapiti E, et al. Patient's refusal of surgery strongly impairs breast cancer survival. *Ann Surg*. 2005;242:276–80.
33. Mouridsen H, Gershanovich M, Sun Y, et al. Phase III study of letrozole versus tamoxifen as first-line therapy of advanced breast cancer in postmenopausal women: Analysis of survival and update of efficacy from the International Letrozole Breast Cancer Group. *J Clin Oncol*. 2003;21:2101–9.
34. Paridaens R, Therasse P, Dirix L, et al. First line hormonal treatment (HT) for metastatic breast cancer (MBC) with exemestane or tamoxifen in postmenopausal patients – A randomized phase III trial of the EORTC Breast Group. *Proc Am Soc Clin Onco*l. 2004;23:6(abs 515).
35. Nabholtz JM, Buzdar A, Pollak M, et al. Anastrozole is superior to tamoxifen as first-line therapy for advanced breast cancer in postmenopausal women: Results of a North American multicenter randomized trial. Arimidex Study Group. *J Clin Oncol*. 2000;18:3758–67.
36. Eiermann W, Paepke S, Appfelstaedt J, et al. Preoperative treatment of postmenopausal breast cancer patients with letrozole: A randomized double-blind multicenter study. *Ann Oncol*. 2001;12:1527–32.
37. Mouridsen H, Chaudri-Ross HA. Efficacy of first-line letrozole versus tamoxifen as a function of age in postmenopausal women with advanced breast cancer. *Oncologist*. 2004;9:497–506.

38. Veronesi U, Boyle P, Goldhirsch A, et al. Breast Cancer. *Lancet*. 2005;365:1727–41.
39. International Breast Cancer Study Group. Randomized trial comparing axillary clearance versus no axillary clearance in older patients with breast cancer: First results of International Breast Cancer Study Group Trial 10–93. *J Clin Oncol*. 2006;24:337–44.
40. Vinh-Hung V, Verschraegen C. Breast conserving surgery with or without radiotherapy: Pooled-analysis for risks of ipsilateral breast tumor recurrence and mortality. *J Natl Cancer Inst*. 2004;96:115–21.
41. Fyles A, McCready D, Manchul L, et al. Tamoxifen with or without breast irradiation in women 50 years of age or older with early breast cancer. *N Engl J Med*. 2004;351:1021–3.
42. Hughes KS, Schnaper LA, Berry D, et al. Lumpectomy plus tamoxifen with or without irradiation in women 70 years of age or older with early breast cancer. *N Engl J Med*. 2004;351:971–7.
43. Hughes KS, Schnaper LA, Berry D, et al. Lumpectomy plus tamoxifen with or without irradiation in women 70 years of age or older with early breast cancer: A report of further follow-up. SABCS (abs December 2006).
44. Prescott RJ, Hunkler IH, Williams LJ, et al. PRIME I: Assessing the impact of adjuvant breast radiotherapy on quality of life in low risk older patients following breast conservation. *Breast*. 2007;(16):S35.
45. Veronesi U, Orecchia R, Luini A. A preliminary report of intraoperative radiotherapy (IORT) in limited-stage breast cancers that are conservatively treated. *Eur J Cancer*. 2001;37:2178–83.
46. Vaidya JS, Baum M, Tobias JS, et al. Targeted Intraoperative Radiotherapy (TARGIT)-trial protocol. *Lancet* online (1999). Available at: http://www.thelancet.com/journals/lancet/misc/protocol/99PRT-47.
47. Orecchia R, Ciocca M, Lazzari R. Intraoperative radiation therapy with electrons (ELIOT) in early stage breast cancer. *Breast*. 2003;12:483–90.
48. Eifel P, Axelson JA, Costa J, et al. National Institute of Health Consensus Development Conference Statement: Adjuvant therapy for breast cancer, November 1–3 (2000). *J Natl Cancer Inst*. 2001;93:979–89.
49. Early Breast Cancer Trialists' Collaborative Group (EBCTCG). Effects of chemotherapy and hormonal therapy for early breast cancer on recurrence and 15-year survival: An overview of the randomised trials. *Lancet*. 2005;365:1687–717.
50. Crivellari D, Price K, Gelber RD, et al. Adjuvant endocrine therapy compared with no systemic therapy for elderly women with early breast cancer. 21-year results of International Breast Cancer Study Group Trial IV. *J Clin Oncol*. 2003;21:4517–23.
51. Goldhirsch A, Glick JH, Gelber RD, et al. Meeting highlights: Updated international expert consensus on the primary therapy of early breast cancer 2005. *Ann Oncol*. 2005;16:1569–83.
52. ATAC Trialists Group. Anastrozole alone or in combination with tamoxifen versus tamoxifen alone for adjuvant treatment of postmenopausal women with early breast cancer: First results of the ATAC randomised trial. *Lancet*. 2002;359:2131–9.
53. ATAC Trialists Group. Results of the ATAC (Arimidex, Tamoxifen, Alone or in Combination) trial after completion of 5 years' adjuvant treatment for breast cancer. *Lancet*. 2005;365:60–2.
54. Coleman RE on behalf of the ATAC Trialists' Group. Effect of anastrozole on bone mineral density: 5-year results from the "Arimidex, tamoxifen, Alone or in combination (ATAC) trial. *Proc Am Soc Clin Oncol*. 2006 (abs 511).
55. Coates A, Keshaviah A, Thurlimann B, et al. Five years of letrozole compared with tamoxifen as initial adjuvant therapy for postmenopausal women with endocrine-responsive early breast cancer: Update of study BIG 1–98. *J Clin Oncol*. 2007;25:486–92.
56. Winer EP, Hudis C, Burstein HJ, et al. American Society of Clinical Oncology Technology Assessment on the use of Aromatase Inhibitors as adjuvant therapy for

postmenopausal women with hormone-receptor-positive breast cancer: Status Report 2004. *J Clin Oncol*. 2005;3:1–11.
57. Coombes RC, Hall E, Gibson LJ, et al. A randomised trial of exemestane after two to three years of tamoxifen therapy in postmenopausal women with primary breast cancer. *N Engl J Med*. 2004;350:1081–92.
58. Boccardo F, Rubagotti A, Puntoni M, et al. Switching to anastrozole versus continued tamoxifen treatment of early breast cancer: preliminary results of the Italian Tamoxifen Anastrozole (ITA) trial. *J Clin Oncol*. 2005;23:5138–47.
59. Jakesz R, Jonat W, Gnant M, et al. Switching of postmenopausal women with endocrine-responsive early breast cancer to anastrozole after 2 years adjuvant tamoxifen: Combined results of ABCSG trial 8 and ARNO 95 trial. *Lancet*. 2005;366:455–62.
60. Goss P, Ingle J, Martino S, et al. A randomized trial of letrozole in postmenopausal women after 5 years of tamoxifen therapy for early breast cancer. *N Engl J Med*. 2003;349:1793–802.
61. Jakesz R, Samonigg H, Greil R, et al. Extended adjuvant treatment with anastrozole: Results from the Austrian Breast and Colorectal Cancer Study Group Trial 6a (ABCSG 6a). *Proc Am Soc Clin Oncol*. 2005;23(abs 105).
62. Early Breast Cancer Trialists' Collaborative Group: Polychemotherapy for early breast cancer: An overview of the randomised trials. *Lancet*. 1998;352:930–42.
63. Muss HB, Woolf S, Berry D, et al. Adjuvant chemotherapy in older and younger women with lymph node-positive breast cancer. *JAMA*. 2005;293:1073–81.
64. Elkin EB, Hurria A, Mitra N, et al. Adjuvant chemotherapy and survival in older women with hormone receptor-negative breast cancer: Assessing outcome in a population-based, observational cohort. *J Clin Oncol*. 2006;24:2757–64.
65. Giordano SH, Duan Z, Kuo F-Y, et al. Use and outcomes of adjuvant chemotherapy in older women with breast cancer. *J Clin Oncol*. 2006;24:2750–6.
66. Pritchard KI, Paterson AH, Fine S, et al. Randomized trial of cyclophosphamide, methotrexate, and fluorouracil chemotherapy added to tamoxifen as adjuvant therapy in postmenopausal women with node-positive estrogen and/or progesterone receptor-positive breast cancer: A report of the National Cancer Institute of Canada Clinical Trials Group. Breast Cancer Site Group. *J Clin Oncol*. 1997;15:2302–11.
67. Crivellari D, Bonetti M, Castiglione-Gertsch M, et al. Burdens and benefits of adjuvant cyclophosphamide, methotrexate, fluorouracil and tamoxifen for elderly patients with breast cancer: The International Breast Cancer Study Group Trial VII. *J Clin Oncol*. 2000;18:1412–22.
68. Fisher B, Redmond C, Legault-Poisson S, et al. Postoperative chemotherapy and tamoxifen compared with tamoxifen alone in the treatment of positive-node breast cancer patients aged 50 years and older with tumors responsive to tamoxifen: Results from the National Surgical Adjuvant Breast and Bowel Project B-16. *J Clin Oncol*. 1990;8:1005–18.
69. Wils JA, Bliss JM, Marty M, et al. Epirubicin plus tamoxifen vs tamoxifen alone in node-positive postmenopausal patients with breast cancer: A randomized trial of the International Collaborative Cancer Group. *J Clin Oncol*. 1999;17:1988–98.
70. Fargeot P, Bonneterre J, Rochè H, et al. Disease-free survival advantage of weekly Epirubicin plus tamoxifen versus tamoxifen alone as adjuvant treatment of operable, node-positive, elderly breast cancer patients: 6-year follow-up results of the French Adjuvant Study Group 08 trial. *J Clin Oncol*. 2004;23:4622–30.
71. Swain SM, Whaley FS, Ewer MS. Congestive heart failure in patients treated with doxorubicin: A retrospective analysis of three trials. *Cancer*. 2003;97:2869–79.
72. Li J, Gwilt PR. The effect of age on the early disposition of doxorubicin. *Cancer Chemother Pharmacol*. 2003;51:395–402.
73. Romond EH, Perez EA, Bryant J, et al. Trastuzumab plus adjuvant chemotherapy for operable HER2-positive breast cancer. *N Engl J Med*. 2005;353:1673–84.

74. Winer EP, Carey LA, Dowsett M, et al. Beyond anatomic staging: Are we ready to take the leap to molecular classification? *ASCO Proc*. 2005;46–59.
75. Paik S, Shak S, Tang G, et al. A multigene assay to predict recurrence of tamoxifen treated, node negative breast cancer. *N Engl J Med*. 2004;351:2817–26.

Adjuvant Therapy in Patients with Breast Cancer During Pregnancy

Sibylle Loibl

Introduction

Breast cancer is one of the most commonly diagnosed cancers during pregnancy accounting for 1/3,000 pregnancies. It is believed that the incidence of breast cancer during pregnancy (BCP) will increase as more women delay child-bearing and because the incidence of breast cancer increases with increasing age.

The predominant histology is invasive ductal [1–3]. Invasive lobular carcinoma has been diagnosed infrequently in pregnant women and in young non-pregnant women [4]. The majority of breast tumours in pregnant women are high grade and lymphovascular invasion is common [5–7]. Moreover, most tumours are hormone independent as demonstrated in the series by Middleton et al. [7]. In this series of women with BCP, 28% of the tumours were ER-positive and 24% were PR-positive by immunohistochemistry compared to 45% and 36% respectively of non-pregnant young women with breast cancer studied by Maru et al. [8]. Hormone positive disease is age-related and is seen more often in postmenopausal women.

While Elledge et al. [9] found 7 out of 12 pregnant patients (58%) to be positive for Her2/neu, Middleton et al. [12] did not find any difference in Her2/neu expression rate (28%) in the M.D. Anderson series of pregnant women with breast cancer compared to that reported in young non-pregnant women [7, 10].

It appears that the histopathological and immunohistochemical findings of the tumours of pregnant women with breast cancer are similar to those of non-pregnant young women with breast cancer. Thus it is more likely that age at diagnosis rather than the pregnancy determines the biological features of the tumour.

There is almost always a perceived conflict between the optimal therapy of the mother with breast cancer and the wellbeing of the foetus. The pregnant

S. Loibl (✉)
Ambulantes Krebszentrum Frankfurt, Germany, J.W. Goethe-University, Frankfurt am Main, Germany, German Breast Group, Neu-Isenburg,
e-mail: sibylle.loibl@germanbreastgroup.de

M. Castiglione, M.J. Piccart (eds.), *Adjuvant Therapy for Breast Cancer*, Cancer Treatment and Research 151, DOI 10.1007/978-0-387-75115-3_20,

breast cancer patient, her family, and her medical team may be in conflict because treatment of the cancer may compromise the foetus. However, insufficient treatment of the breast cancer, presumed to protect the foetus, may compromise the health of the mother.

Systemic Therapy

The largest series of prospective cases has been reported by the MD Anderson Cancer Centre first in 1999 and an update has been published recently. The authors have evaluated a prospective protocol with 5-fluorouracil, doxorubicin, cyclophosphamide (F: 500 mg/m^2 day 1 + 4; A: 50 mg/m^2 continuous 72 h day 1, C: 500 mg/m^2 day 1 of a 3-week cycle) and did not observe any negative outcome of the infants [11,12]. No major foetal complications have been described. Nevertheless only limited data on the use of chemotherapy in pregnancy is available.

The risk for morbidities of the newborn due to preterm delivery is approaching the expected after the 34th week of gestation. Therefore the last cycle of chemotherapy should be given around the 34th week of gestation to allow delivery from the 37th week onward.

Chemotherapy

The teratogenic and mutagenic effects of cytotoxic drugs have been well described in animals, but extrapolation of data from animals to human organogenesis is difficult. Clear evidence of toxicity to human embryos exists for only a few drugs. Officially all cytotoxic agents belong to class C of the drugs (Table 1). Nonetheless, the risk appears to be significantly lower than is commonly expected, and the overall incidence of major congenital malformations after using cytotoxic drugs has been quoted as approximately 3% [13].

The risk of teratogenicity of drugs used in breast cancer chemotherapy depends on multiple factors like the time of application, the amount, the frequency, and the agent itself. There is no increased risk during the preimplantation period. Previous epidemiological data from case series and various registries indicate that the risk of malformation increases in the first trimester to 10–20%, whereas in the second and third trimester the risk declines to 1.3% [14–16]. However, foetal exposure of antineoplastic agents may lead to growth retardation and haematologic cytotoxicity [17].

The antimetabolite methotrexate has been shown to cause foetal death in mammals. A syndrome caused by methotrexate has been reported which consists of cranial dysostosis (delay in ossification of the bones of calvarium), hypertelorism, a wide nasal bridge, ear anomalies, micrognathia, abnormalities of the external ears, limb deformities and cerebral anomalies [18]. However,

Table 1 Safety of drugs according to the FDA [62]

A	"Controlled studies in women fail to demonstrate a risk to the foetus..."	There are practically no category A drugs
B	"Either animal reproduction studies have not demonstrated a foetal risk or there are no controlled studies in pregnant women"	Category B drugs are, e.g., vitamins, acetaminophen...if there is a clinical need for category B drug, it is considered to be safe
C	"Studies in animals have revealed adverse effects on the foetus and there are no controlled studies in women and animals are not available"	Category C drugs have not been shown to be harmful to the foetus. Drugs should be given only if the potential benefit justifies the potential risk to the foetus
D	"There is positive evidence of human foetal risk"	Category D drugs have some significant risks. They should be used during pregnancy only when the alternatives are worse
X	"Studies in animal or human beings have demonstrated foetal abnormalities...and the risk of the use of the drug in pregnant women clearly outweighs any possible benefit"	The drug is contraindicated in women who are or may become pregnant

there are also reports on healthy offspring after the use of methotrexate. Those reports suggest that methotrexate is not always teratogenic when given in the first trimester and that there might be a critical dose (10 mg per week with a maximum of 6–8 weeks treatment) above which foetal malformations occur [19]. Other antimetabolites have rarely been associated with foetal malformations. Exposure to 5-fluorouracil in the second trimester or later singly or in combination with other agents has not resulted in adverse effects [20]. Alkylating agents seem less toxic than antimetabolites [21]. Doxorubicin has been shown to produce congenital defects in animals but has not been associated with birth defects in human embryos when used either alone or in combination. There are several reports that describe safe application even in the first trimester [22, 23]. Thus far data on the use of newer therapeutic agents such as docetaxel and paclitaxel in pregnant breast cancer patients is limited to case reports, but their application seems safe [24–27]. Pregnancy is associated with several physiologic changes that may at least theoretically affect the pharmacokinetic behaviour of a drug [28]. The renal blood flow increases by 50%, leading to an increased glomerular filtration rate, and consequently an increased elimination of agents excreted by the kidney. The increase of the total body water and plasma volume results in changes in the distribution volume for water-soluble drugs and leads to a decrease in serum levels of several agents. In contrast, albumin and other plasma protein level decline by approximately 30%, which leads to an increase in the free fraction of drugs with low lipid solubility that are tightly bound to plasma proteins [29]. Generally, lipophylic drugs with a low molecular weight, which are non-ionised and loosely bound to plasma proteins, cross the placental barrier more easily. However, the syncytiotrophoblast contains a variety of drug- extruding transporters like P-glycoprotein (PGP) [30] and others (e.g. BCRP-1), for which several antineoplastic agents (vinca-alcaloids, anthracycline derivatives, taxanes and topotecan) are proven substrates. From experimental studies with a perfused placenta model or trophoblast tissue, it has been shown that these drug transporters are able to reduce the drug concentrations at the foetal side to perhaps non-toxic levels. On the other side, drugs which inhibit the P-GP transport system or which compete with cytotoxic drugs for the transport (like tamoxifen or verapamil) might counteract this protection [31–33].

However, pharmacokinetic data on antineoplastic agents are in general rare, especially in (non-pregnant) women. At the moment, it is recommended to use the same agents and dosages for the treatment of pregnant breast cancer patients as in non-pregnant patients and to monitor strictly and report adverse events.

PK samples for a population analysis would be helpful for future dosing recommendations, if appropriate.

There are no data on dose-dense or high dose chemotherapy in pregnant breast cancer patients. Generally, the dose-dense has so far not been a standard treatment for breast cancer patients despite showing promising effects. Therefore it is recommend to use the standard therapy dose.

Children with In Utero Exposure to Chemotherapy

Early toxicities of the cytotoxic treatment on the foetus are principally anaemia, neutropenia and alopecia depending on the timing of the therapy in relation to delivery [58]. Usually newborns will recover from these side effects. However, the neonatologist should be aware of these possible complications and should monitor the newborn carefully.

Little is known about the possible delayed effects of exposure to antineoplastic agents in utero. Major concerns include physical and mental development, heart function, secondary malignancies, and infertility. A large study, with a median follow-up of 18.7 years on 84 children who were born to mothers who received chemotherapy during pregnancy for haematological malignancies, did not show any congenital neurological and psychological abnormalities including normal learning and educational behaviour [34].

Some data can be extrapolated from children who have received chemotherapy for leukaemia. However, the amount and type of drugs given in children is comparatively high and in the pregnant breast cancer patient only a percentage of the delivered drug will reach the foetus.

In a study by Kremer et al. [35] which investigated the anthracycline-induced clinical heart failure in a cohort of 607 children, a rate of 5% has been detected 15 years after therapy. The incidence increased with the cumulative dose given and the follow up period. In two reviews by the same authors the incidence of subclinical cardiotoxicity and heart failure after anthracycline containing chemotherapy ranged from 0% to 57% and 0% to 16%, respectively [36, 37]. However, most of the trials had limitations and therefore new studies with well defined patient groups were recommended by the authors. A case report of foetal echocardiography sequences during a maternal anthracycline containing chemotherapy revealed no changes of the shortening fractions as well as the biometry [38].

Hormonal Therapy

Hormone treatment, if indicated, is to be started after delivery and after completion of chemotherapy. Neonatal defects by tamoxifen have been described in the genital tract in female mice [39]. Although tamoxifen has been safely given in patients with metastatic breast cancer without damage to the child [40, 41], there are other reports of birth defects such as Goldenhar-Syndrome [42], ambiguous genitalia [43] in human embryos [57].

Treatment with Trastuzumab

A limited number of case reports have been published where trastuzumab has been given in pregnant patients with breast cancer. In one of those cases a reversible anhydramnios has been reported [44] In two cases there was no detrimental effect for the pregnancy [45,46]. So far it is strongly advised not to use trastuzumab in pregnant breast cancer patients. Trastuzumab has been labelled as a pregnancy category B drug by the United States Food and Drug Administration. Studies in monkeys showed a placental transfer but no harm to the foetuses was observed.

New Drugs

New drugs will enter the breast cancer scene. None of them will be tested in breast cancer patients who are pregnant. It is believed that antiangiogenic drugs like bevacizumab or new tyrosine kinase inhibitors should not be used during pregnancy at any stage. Thalidomide is an antiangiogenic drug which can cause severe teratogenic effects.

Bisphosphonates

So far bisphosphonates have not been approved for the use in the adjuvant treatment for breast cancer. However, some comments should be made at this point. There is limited number of cases reported in human beings. One has to be aware of the effects of bisphosphonates: they can induce hypocalcaemia, possibly affecting the contractility of the uterus which was associated with neonatal deaths and which can be overcome by i.v. calcium supplementation [47]; as an additional process, the osteoclast activity is inhibited and this might theoretically lead to skeletal abnormalities which have so far not been reported. However, given the small numbers of patients who have been treated during pregnancy, it does not necessarily mean this effect does not exist [48]. Therefore, the use of bisphosphonates cannot be recommended during pregnancy.

Supportive Therapy

Supportive treatment can be given according to the general recommendations consisting of a 5HT3-serotonin antagonist and steroids. Pyridoxine has been described as alternative treatment for radiation and pregnancy-induced nausea and vomiting [49–51].

One case control study found a statistically significant association between first-trimester exposure to corticosteroids and cleft palate in newborns, even when controlled for potential confounding factors [52, 53]. Thereafter, their application seems safe.

No developmental toxicity was seen in rats and rabbits exposed to the 5HT3-antagonist ondansetron, at doses 70 times higher than that used in humans [54]. The application of ondansetron during first trimester did not cause malformations in humans [55, 56]. Tropisetron is the only 5HT3-antagonist which is listed as a category C drug due to its teratogenicity in rodent models. In the case of the use of granisetron the oral formulation should be preferred because the i.v. formulation contains benzyl alcohol.

Granulocyte colony stimulating factor (G-CSF) and erythropoietin stimulating factors (ESF) have been used safely in pregnant patients [57, 58]. Maternally administered G-CSF has been shown to cross the placenta during the third trimester and induce granulopoiesis in neonatal rats [59]. No teratogenicity was observed in animal models. G-CSF and ESF belong to the C category of drugs. Erythropoietin as a glycoprotein with a molecular weight of 30 kD and is therefore not expected to cross the placenta. No large controlled studies exist and no teratogenic effects have been reported so far [60, 61].

Summary

The initial assessment and management of women who have suspected breast cancer during pregnancy requires a multidisciplinary approach, with special attention to the use of appropriate investigations during diagnosis and staging. The treatment of the cancer needs to be carefully planned with consideration given to the potential risks to the developing foetus. Pregnant women with

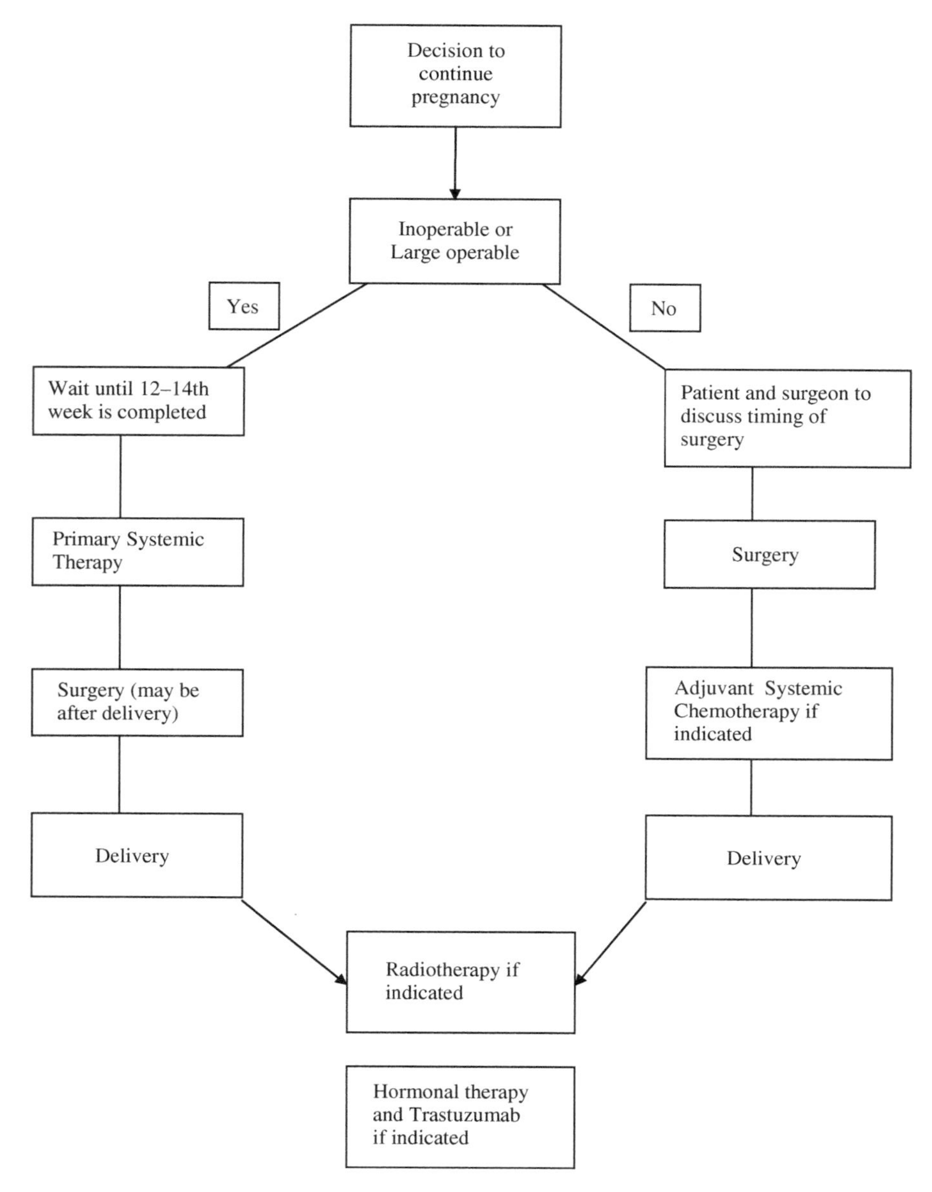

Fig. 1 Algorithm for decision making in pregnant breast cancer patients. Adapted from Loibl et al. **a** <12th to 14th week of gestation at histological diagnosis. **b** 12–34 weeks at histological confirmed diagnosis. **c** > 34 week of gestation at histological diagnosis. Immediate delivery in case of inflammatory or highly aggressive disease. Otherwise, plan delivery when foetal maturation is appropriate

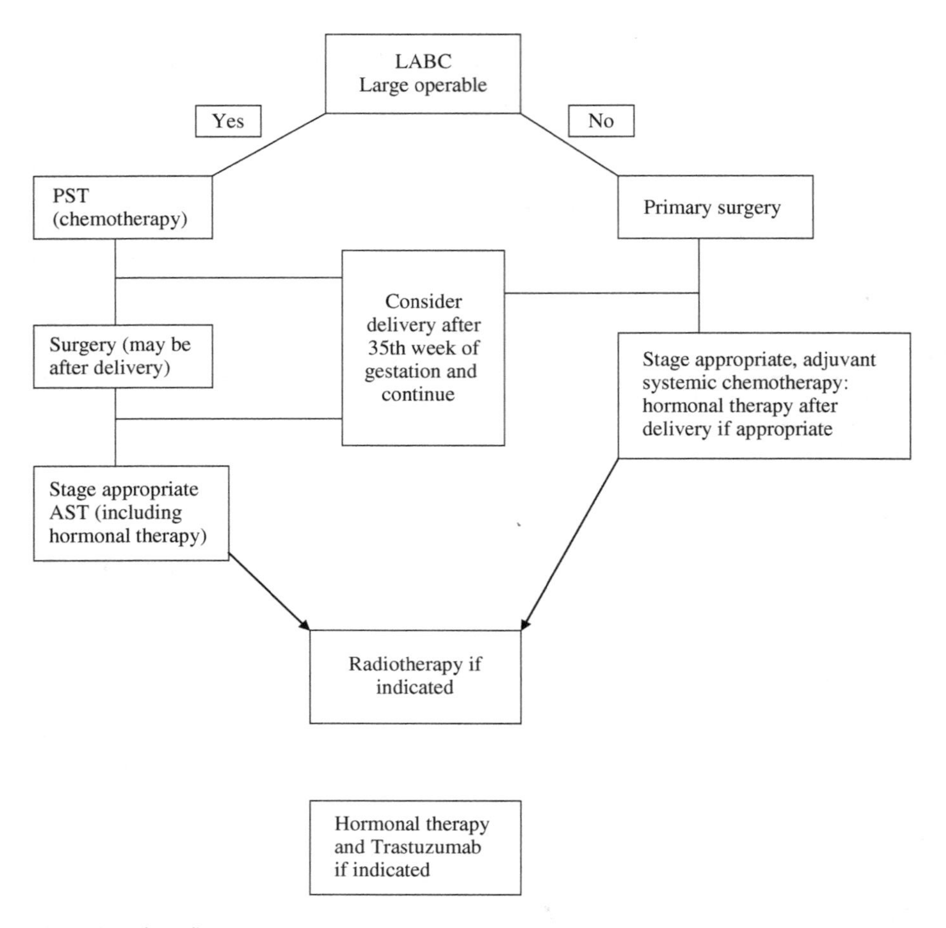

Fig. 1 (continued)

breast cancer can be treated with anthracycline-based chemotherapy such as FA(E)C in the second and third trimesters of pregnancy with minimal risk to the foetus. While breast surgery, mastectomy or breast conservation can be performed with relative safety during pregnancy, patients who are clinically node-negative need to be counselled regarding the use of sentinel lymph node biopsy. Radiation therapy should be delayed until after delivery. The routine use of other systemic treatment such as the taxanes, trastuzumab and tamoxifen is not recommended during pregnancy given the limited data available.

The treatment should nevertheless be as close to the standard as possible to ensure the best treatment for the mother. Sometimes the worse outcome of patients with breast cancer during pregnancy might be due to insufficient therapy given. However, there should always be a careful balancing between the necessity of treating the patient with potentially harmful drugs during pregnancy and postponing treatment after delivery. Nevertheless, the basis for adjuvant treatment with cytotoxic drugs during pregnancy is quite solid, but should be performed in referral centres. It is always an individual decision which should be made involving the partner/family and an interdisciplinary team.

In the treatment of the pregnant breast cancer patient, the evidence upon which we base our decisions has been largely limited to case reports, case-control studies and retrospective cohorts. Thus, it is critical that prospective data such as those collected by the German Breast Group (www.germanbreastgroup.de/pregnancy)/Breast International Group be continued and developed.

References

1. Parente JT, Amsel M, Lerner R, Chinea F. Breast cancer associated with pregnancy. *Obstet Gynecol.* 1988;71:861–4.
2. Tobon H, Horowitz LF. Breast cancer during pregnancy. *Breast Dis.* 1993;6:127–34.
3. King RM, Welch JS, Martin JK Jr, Coulam CB. Carcinoma of the breast associated with pregnancy. *Surg Gynecol Obstet.* 1985;160:228–32.
4. Fisher CJ, Egan MK, Smith P, Wicks K, Millis RR, Fentiman IS. Histopathology of breast cancer in relation to age. *Br J Cancer.* 1997;75:593–6.
5. Shousha S. Breast carcinoma presenting during or shortly after pregnancy and lactation. *Arch Pathol Lab Med.* 2000;124:1053–60.
6. Ishida T, Yokoe T, Kasmu F, et al. Clinicopathologic characteristics and prognosis of breast cancer patients associated with pregnancy and lactation: Analysis of case-control study in Japan. *Jpn J Cancer Res.* 1992;83:1143–9.
7. Middleton LP, Amin M, Gwyn K, Theriault R, Sahin A. Breast carcinoma in pregnant women: Assessment of clinicopathologic and immunohistochemical features. *Cancer.* 2003;98;1055–60.
8. Maru D, Middleton LP, Wang S, Valero V, Sahin A. HER-2/neu and p53 overexpression as biomarkers of breast carcinoma in women age 30 years and younger. *Cancer.* 2005;103:900–5.
9. Elledge RM, Ciocca DR, Langone G, McGuire WL. Estrogen receptor, progesterone receptor, and HER-2/neu protein in breast cancers from pregnant patients. *Cancer.* 1993;71:2499–506.
10. Lebeau A, Deimling D, Kaltz C, Sendelhofert A, Iff A, Luthardt B, et al. Her-2/neu analysis in archival tissue samples of human breast cancer: Comparison of immunohistochemistry and fluorescence in situ hybridization. *J Clin Oncol.* 2001;19: 354–63.
11. Berry DL, Theriault RL, Holmes FA, Parisi VM, Booser DJ, Singletary SE, Buzdar AU, Hortobagyi GN. Management of breast cancer during pregnancy using a standardized protocol. *J Clin Oncol.* 1999;17:855–61.
12. Hahn K, Johnson PE, Gordon N, Kuerer H, Middleton L, Ramirez M, Yang W, Perkins G, Hortobagyyi GN, Theriault RL. Treatment of pregnant breast cancer patients and outcomes of children exposed to vhemotherapy in utero. *Cancer* 2006;upub ahead of print
13. Kalter H, Warkany J. Congenital malformations. *N Engl J Med.* 1983;308:424–31,491–7.
14. Doll DC, Ringenberg QS. Yarbro JW. Antineoplastic Agents in Pregnancy. *Sem Oncol.* 1989;16:337–46.
15. Ebert U, Löffler H, Kirch W. Cytotoxic therapy and pregnancy. *Pharmacol Ther.* 1997;74:207–20.
16. Woo JC, Yu T, Hurd TC. Breast Cancer in pregnancy: A literature review. *Arch Surg.* 2003;138:91–8.

17. Giacalone PL, Laffargue F, Benos P. Chemotherapy for breast carcinoma during pregnancy: A French national survey. *Cancer*. 1999;86:2266–72.
18. Warkany J. Aminopterin and methotrexate: Folic acid deficiency. *Teratology*. 1978;17:353–7.
19. Feldkamp M, Carey JC. Clinical teratology counseling and consultation case report: Low dose methotrexate exposure in the early weeks of pregnancy. *Teratology*. 1993;47:533–9.
20. Maghfoor I, Doll DC. Chemotherapy in pregnancy. In: Perry MC, ed. *The chemotherapy source book*. 3rd ed. 537–46.
21. Glantz JC. Reproductive toxicology of alkylating agents. *Obstet Gynecol Surv*. 1994;49:709–15.
22. Garcia V, Miguel JS, Borrasca AL. Doxorubicin in the first trimester of pregnancy. *Ann Intern Med*. 1981;94:547.
23. Germann N, Goffinet F, Goldwasser F. Anthracyclines during pregnancy: Embryo-fetal outcome in 160 patients. *Ann Oncol*. 2004;15:146–50.
24. De Santis M, Lucchese A, De Carolis S, Ferrazani S, Caruso A. Metastatic breast cancer in pregnancy: first case of chemotherapy with docetaxel. *Eur J Cancer Care*. 2000;9:235–7.
25. Gadducci A, Cosio S, Fanucchi A, et al. Chemotherapy with epirubicin and paclitaxel for breast cancer during pregnancy: Case report and review of the literature. *Anticancer Res*. 2003;23:5225–9.
26. Gonzalez-Angulo AM, Walters RS, Carpenter RJ, et al. Paclitaxel chemotherapy in a pregnant patient with bilateral breast cancer. *Clin Breast Cancer*. 2004;5:317–9.
27. Nieto Y, Santiseban M, Aramendia JM, Fernandez-Hidalgo O, Garcia-Manerom, Lopez G. Docetaxel administered during pregnancy for inflammatory breast carcinoma. *Clin Breast Cancer*. 2006;6:533–4.
28. Little BB. Pharmacokinetics during pregnancy: Evidence-based maternal dose formulation. *Obstet Gynecol*. 1999;93:658–68.
29. Mucklow JC. The fate of drugs in pregnancy. *Clin Obstet Gynecol*. 1986;13:161–75.
30. Arceci RJ, Croop JM, Horwitz SB, Housman D. The gene encoding multidrug resistance is induced and expressed at high levels during pregnancy in the secretory epithelium of the uterus. *Proc Natl Acad Sci U S A*. 1988;85:4350–4.
31. Smit JW, Huisman MT, van Tellingen O, Wiltshire HR, Schinkel AH. Absence or pharmacological blocking of placental P-glycoprotein profoundly increases fetal drug exposure. *J Clin Invest*. 1999;104:1441–7.
32. Gedeon C, Koren G. Designing pregnancy centered medications: drugs which do not cross the human placenta. *Placenta*. 2006;27:861–8.
33. Evseenko DA, Paxton JW, Keelan JA. ABC drug transporter expression and functional activity in trophoblast-like cell lines and differentiating primary trophoblast. *Am J Physiol Regul Intergr Comp Physiol*. 2006;290:R1357–65.
34. Aviles A, Neri N. Hematological Malignancies and Pregnancy: A Final Report of 84 children who received chemotherapy in utero. *Clin Lymphoma*. 2001;2:173–7.
35. Kremer LC, van Dalen EC, Offringa M, Ottenkamp J, Voute PA. Anthracycline-induced clinical heart failure in a cohort of 607 children: Long-term follow-up study. *J Clin Oncol*. 2001;19:191–6.
36. Kremer LC, van der Pal HJ, Offringa M, van Dalen EC, Voute PA. Frequency and risk factors of subclinical cardiotoxicity after anthracycline therapy in children: A systematic review. *Ann Oncol*. 2002;13:819–29.
37. Kremer LC, van Dalen EC, Offringa M, Voute PA. Frequency and risk factors of anthracycline-induced clinical heart failure in children: A systematic review. *Ann Oncol*. 2002;13:503–12
38. Meyer-Wittkopf M, Barth H, Emons G, Schmidt S. Fetal cardiac effects of doxorubicin therapy for carcinoma of the breast during pregnancy: Case report and review of the literature. *Ultrasound Obstet and Gynecol*. 2001;18:62–6.

39. Cunha GR, Taguchi O, Namikawa R, Nishizuka Y, Robboy SJ. Teratogenic effects of clomiphene, tamoxifen, and diethylstilbestrol on the developing human female genital tract. *Hum Pathol.* 1987;18:1132–43.
40. Oksuzoglu B, Guler N. An infertile patient with breast cancer who delivered a healthy child under adjuvant tamoxifen therapy. *Eur J Obstet Gynecol Reprod Biol.* 2002;104:79.
41. Isaacs RJ, Hunter W, Clark K. Tamoxifen as systemic treatment of advanced breast cancer during pregnancy-case report and literature review. *Gynecologic Oncology.* 2001;80:405–8.
42. Cullins SL, Pridjian G, Sutherland CM. Goldenhar's syndrome associated with tamoxifen given to the mother during gestation. *JAMA.* 1994;271:1905–6.
43. Tewari K, Bonebrake RG, Asrat T, Shanberg AM. Ambiguous genitalia in infant exposed to tamoxifen in utero. *Lancet.* 1997;350:183.
44. Watson WJ. Herceptin (trastuzumab) therapy during pregnancy: Association with reversible anhydramnios. *Obstet Gynecol.* 2005;105:642–3.
45. Fanale MA, Uyei AR, Theriault RL, Adam K, Thompson RA. Treatment of metastatic breast cancer with trastuzumab and vinorelbine during pregnancy. *Clin Breast cancer.* 2005;6:354–6.
46. Waterston AM, Graham J. Effect of adjuvant trastuzumab on pregnancy. *J Clin Oncol.* 2006;24:321–2.
47. Culbert EC, Schfirin BS. Malignant hypercalcemia in pregnancy: Effect of pamidroinate on uterine contractions. *Obstet Gynecol.* 2006;108:789–91.
48. Illidge TM, Hussey M, Godden CW. Malignant hypercalcemia in pregnancy and antenatal administration of intravenous pamidronate. *Clin Oncol.* 1996;8:257–8.
49. Bsat FA, Hoffman DE, Seubert DE. Comparison of three outpatient regimens in the management of nausea and vomiting in pregnancy. *J Perinatol.* 2003;23:531–5.
50. Mahajan MK, Singh V. Assessment of efficacy of pyridoxine in control of radiation induced sickness. *J Indian Med Assoc.* 1998;96:82–3.
51. Sahakian V, Rouse D, Sipes S, Rose N, Niebyl J. Vitamin B6 is effective therapy for nausea and vomiting of pregnancy: A randomized, double-blind placebo-controlled study. *Obstet Gynecol.* 1991;78:33–36.
52. Rodriguez-Pinilla E, Martinez-Frias ML. Corticosteroids during pregnancy and oral clefts: A case-control study. *Teratology.* 1998;58:2–5.
53. Magee LA, Mazzotta P, Koren G. Evidence based view of safety and effectiveness of phamarcologic therapy for nausea and vomiting of pregnancy. *Am J Obstet Gynecol.* 2002;186:256–61.
54. Tincello DG, Johnstone MJ. Treatment of hyperemesis gravidarum with the 5-HT3 antagonist ondansetron (Zofran). *Postgrad Med J.* 1996;72:688–9.
55. Sullivan CA, Johnson CA, Roach H, Martin RW, Stewart DK, Morrison JC. A pilot study of intravenous ondansetron for hyperemesis gravidarum. *Am J Obstet Gynecol.* 1996;174:1565–8.
56. Briggs GC, Freeman RK, Yaffee SM. A reference guide to fetal and neonatal risk: Drugs in pregnancy and lactation. Philadelphia (PA): Lippincott Williams & Wilkins; 1998.
57. Ozer H, Armitage JO, Bennett CL, Crawford J, Demetri GD, Pizzo PA, et al. American Society of Clinical Oncology. 2000 update of recommendations for the use of hematopoietic colony-stimulating factors: evidence-based, clinical practice guidelines. American Society of Clinical Oncology Growth Factors Expert Panel. *J Clin Oncol.* 2000;18:3558–85.
58. Medlock ES, Kaplan DL, Cecchini M, Ulich TR, Del Castilo J, Anderson J. Granulocyte colony-stimulating factor crosses the placenta and stimulates fetal rat granulopoiesis. *Blood.* 1993;81:916–22.
59. Scott LL, Ramin SM, Richey M, Hanson J, Gilstrap LC. Erythropoietin use in pregnancy: Two cases and a review of the literature. *Am J Perinatol.* 1995;12:22–24.

60. Sifakis S, Angelakis E, Vardaki E, Koumantaki Y, Matalliotakis I, Koumantakis E. Erythropoietin in the treatment of iron deficiency anemia during pregnancy. *Gynecol Obstet Invest*. 2001;51:150–6.
61. FDA. *Federal Register*. 1980;44:37434–67.
62. Loibl S, von Minckwitz G, Gwyn K, Ellis P, Blohmer JU, Schlegelberger B, Keller M, Harder S, Theriault RL, Crivellari D, Klingebiel T, Louwen F, Kaufmann M. Breast Cancer During Pregnancy. *Cancer*. 2006;106:237–46.

Part VI
After Breast Cancer and Treatment, Sequelae of Adjuvant Treatment Social Issues

Investigations After Adjuvant Therapy

Silvia Dellapasqua

"As the morning progresses the hospital waiting area fills up with anxious, mostly gray haired women. They have been treated for breast cancer in the past and are attending for "routine" follow up. For those who are apparently free of disease, what is the purpose of follow up, how often should it be done, and by whom, and what investigations, if any, should be performed routinely?"

[Dewar J. Follow up in breast cancer: A suitable case for reappraisal. BMJ. *1995;310:685.]*

More than 2 million women in the US alone are living with a history of breast cancer. Most women in whom breast cancer is diagnosed do not die of the disease: of the 180,000 women who receive a diagnosis of invasive breast cancer in the US every year, more than 80% can expect to survive for at least 5 years [1].

Routine follow up after adjuvant treatment for breast cancer is standard practice in most countries, and it usually involves visits to hospital outpatient clinics [2]. The usual basic components of the routine follow-up are regular history and physical examinations, annual mammography, and blood tests, radiologic and scintigraphic examinations at varying intervals. Blood tests usually include complete blood counts, liver function tests, serum calcium and bone enzyme measurements, as well as determination of tumor marker levels. Radiologic and scintigraphic examinations performed routinely at some centers include chest X-ray, bone scan, liver ultrasound, or CT scan. This choice of examinations reflects the well established pattern of first recurrence following primary therapy for breast cancer: locoregional in 15–40% (expressed as

S. Dellapasqua (✉)
Assistant, Medical Senology Research Unit, Division of Medical Oncology, European Institute of Oncology, Milan, Italy
e-mail: silvia.dellapasque@ieo.it

M. Castiglione, M.J. Piccart (eds.), *Adjuvant Therapy for Breast Cancer*, Cancer Treatment and Research 151, DOI 10.1007/978-0-387-75115-3_21,

percentage of all recurrences), bone in 30–60%, bone in combination with another site in 10–15%, isolated lung in 5–1 5%, and isolated liver in 3–10%. The choice of interval between assessments has been arbitrary but based on our knowledge of timing of first relapses: the rates are highest within the first 5 years following primary treatment, but the patient remains at risk for the rest of her life [3].

Women with breast cancer present with several unique health issues. Not only do they require regular follow-up to detect recurrences of their breast cancer and/or second primary cancers, but they may suffer from local complications after breast surgery and radiation therapy, as well as long-lasting side effects of treatment, including premature menopause [1]. Close follow-up might also serve a psychosocial function [4]. The most frequently recorded problems during follow-up are anxiety and unrelated medical problems. Anxiety and depression tend to present relatively soon and are often enduring, since patients are especially worried of recurrence, whereas concomitant medical problems tend to present later [5].

There are clearly limitations associated with close follow-up of breast cancer patients. An obvious limitation is the cost in terms of patient and physician time and other monetary costs. Follow-up visits can provide marked anxiety for many patients. None of the follow-up testing procedures has neither optimal sensitivity nor specificity with regard to determination of whether a patient has recurrent breast cancer. In addition, there are marked limitations with regard to instituting treatment for recurrent breast cancer. For virtually all patients who have had a mastectomy, recurrent breast cancer is not a curable disease. In addition, there is no convincing evidence that particularly early institution of "salvage" therapy is more efficacious than using the "salvage" therapy at a future time point in the disease course. There might be a few exceptions with regard to isolated locoregional disease recurrences, but this only applies to a minority of patients. Patients who have undergone lumpectomy plus primary radiation therapy are an exception to the above, because an isolated breast recurrence seems to be potentially curable with salvage mastectomy [4].

Historically, breast cancer follow-up has used a conservative approach based on clinical examination and mammography, but variations in practice patterns exist and have significant cost implications. Mille et al. studied the impact of clinical practice guidelines (CPG) on follow-up of patients with localized breast cancer. A before-and-after analysis of the records of patients who received post-therapeutic follow-up for localized breast cancer as of either 1993 or 1995 was performed. Two hundred records were chosen at random, 100 from 1993 and 100 from 1995. Follow-up was continued for as long as possible and CPG compliance was studied for each year of the follow-up periods. Follow-up that was not guideline compliant cost 2.2–3.6 times more than guideline-compliant follow-up as a result of non-mammographic examinations performed in the absence of any warning signs or symptoms of recurrence. After the introduction of surveillance guidelines in 1994, there was a one-third decrease in expenditures per patient, with no change in health outcomes expected [6].

Detection of Breast Cancer Recurrences

For the rest of their lives, women with a history of breast cancer are at risk for recurrence. Most recurrences are detected within 5 years, but later recurrences are not uncommon. Symptoms suggestive of recurrence are not specific and, even in survivors of cancer, are frequently due to benign conditions. Because more than 75% of recurrences are heralded by symptoms or by findings on physical examination, symptoms should be carefully evaluated and physical examination should aim to detect local or regional recurrences in the breast, chest wall, or lymph nodes [1].

There has been much controversy about the routine use of laboratory tests, chest roentgenography, and bone scanning, which rarely identify metastatic disease in asymptomatic patients: more than half of breast cancer recurrences are symptomatic and detected by patients themselves, who frequently present at unscheduled visits in the interval between follow up appointments [2].

A meta-analysis by de Bock et al. on 12 studies involving 5,045 patients found that approximately 40% of isolated locoregional recurrences were diagnosed during routine visits and routine tests in asymptomatic patients treated for early-stage invasive breast cancer, whereas the remainder (approximately 60%) developed symptomatic recurrences before their scheduled clinical visits [7].

Even with intensive surveillance, asymptomatic recurrences constitute only the 15–25% of all cases of metastatic disease [1]. Two randomized trials conducted in Italy failed to show any impact of intensive diagnostic follow-up on 5-year mortality for patients with early breast cancer: more intensive follow-up resulted in a slightly earlier detection of tumor recurrence, but there was no difference in overall survival [8]. In the first of such trials, 1,243 consecutive patients surgically treated for unilateral invasive breast carcinoma with no evidence of metastases were randomized in a 2-year period by 12 participating centers in Italy either to the intensive follow-up group (n = 622) – in which patients were invited to have a periodic physical examination (every 3 months in the first 2 years and every 6 months thereafter) and annual mammography as well as a biannual chest X-ray and bone scan – or to the clinical follow-up group (n = 621) – in which patients were offered physical examination and mammography with the same schedule but no other routine diagnostic tests. The two study groups were well balanced in terms of clinical and prognostic characteristics. Overall, 393 recurrences (104 local and 289 distant) were observed. Increased detection of isolated intrathoracic and bone metastases was evident in the intensive follow-up group compared with the clinical follow-up group (112 vs 71 cases), while no difference was observed for other sites and for local and/or regional recurrences. The 5-year relapse-free survival rate was significantly higher for the clinical follow-up group, with patients in the intensive follow-up group showing earlier detection of recurrences. No difference in 5-year overall mortality (18.6 vs 19.5%) was observed between the two follow-up groups [9]. After a longer follow up, 343 deaths were identified (222 in the intensive follow-up group and 212 in the clinical follow-up group). Estimated 10-year mortality cumulative rates were not different for the clinical (31.5%) and intensive (34.8%) follow-up groups. No survival advantage was revealed for the intensive protocol (hazard ratio, 1.05; 95% confidence interval, 0.87–1.26) [8, 10]. In the second trial, conducted by 26 general hospitals in Italy, 1,320 consecutive patients younger than 70 years with stage I–III unilateral primary breast cancer were randomly assigned to an intensive surveillance, which included physician's visits and performance of bone scan, liver echography, chest roentgenography, and laboratory tests at predefined intervals (655 patients), or to a control regimen (665 patients), in which patients were seen by their physicians at the same frequency but only clinically indicated tests were performed. Both groups received a yearly mammogram aimed at detecting contralateral breast cancer. Compliance to the two follow-up policies was more than 80%. After a median follow-up of 71 months, no difference was apparent in overall survival with 132 deaths (20%) in the intensive group and 122 deaths (18%) in the control group. No significant differences were apparent for the time to detection of recurrence between the two groups. Measurements of health-related quality of life (i.e., overall health and quality-of-life perception, emotional well-being, body image, social functioning, symptoms, and satisfaction with care) at different time-points did not show differences by type of care received [11, 12]. The two trials suggest that periodic intensive follow-up should not be recommended as a routine policy because, despite periodic examinations allow earlier detection of distant metastases, anticipated diagnosis is the only effect of intensive follow-up, and no impact on prognosis can be seen after 5 years [9].

Reducing the frequency of routine follow up has also proved popular among patients with a history of breast cancer. Gulliford et al. conducted a trial in Great Britain and randomized 196 patients with a history of breast cancer to conventionally scheduled follow-up visits vs less frequent visits only after mammography. Both cohorts received identical mammography and were invited to telephone for immediate appointments if they detected symptoms. Twice as many patients in both groups expressed a preference for reducing rather than increasing follow up. No increased use of local practitioner services or telephone triage was apparent in the cohort randomized to less frequent follow up by specialists [13, 8].

The American Society of Clinical Oncology (ASCO) updated its recommended breast cancer surveillance guidelines in 1998 to establish an evidence-based, postoperative surveillance strategy for the detection and treatment of recurrent breast cancer [14]. Since the last update in 1998, there has been an increase in the availability of diagnostic testing for breast cancer patients, and therefore ASCO guidelines were updated in 2006, considering that the clinical outcomes that justify the use of a technology or drugs in the guideline development process should include improvements in overall or disease-free survival, improvement in quality of life, reduced toxicity, and improved cost effectiveness [15].

The 2006 ASCO recommended investigations in breast cancer surveillance include the following:

- *History, physical examination, and patient education regarding symptoms of recurrence*. All women should have a careful history and physical examination every 3–6 months for the first 3 years after primary therapy, then every 6–12 months for the next 2 years, and then annually. Physicians should counsel patients about the symptoms of recurrence including new lumps, bone pain, chest pain, dyspnea, abdominal pain, or persistent headaches [16].

  Several studies have reported that 75–85% of breast cancer recurrences are detected only with history and physical examination (even when frequent additional tests are performed) [4].
- *Genetic counseling*. Women at high risk for familial breast cancer syndromes should be referred for genetic counseling in accordance with clinical guidelines recommended by the US Preventive Services Task Force. Criteria to recommend referral include the following: Ashkenazi Jewish heritage; history of ovarian cancer at any age in the patient or any first or second-degree relatives; any first-degree relative with a history of breast cancer diagnosed before the age of 50 years; two or more first- or second-degree relatives diagnosed with breast cancer at any age; patient or relative with diagnosis of bilateral breast cancer; and history of breast cancer in a male relative [16]. Patients with node-negative breast cancer who are carriers of a *BRCA1* or *BRCA2* mutation may have gains in life expectancy from prophylactic contralateral mastectomy [17]. In addition, the family members of affected patients may want to consider intensive surveillance or prophylactic surgery [18].
- *Breast self-examination*. All women should be counseled to perform monthly breast self-examination (BSE). However, women should be made aware that monthly BSE does not replace mammography as a breast cancer screening tool [16].
- *Mammography*. Women treated with breast-conserving therapy should have their first post-treatment mammogram no earlier than 6 months after definitive radiation therapy. Subsequent mammograms should be obtained every 6–12 months for surveillance of abnormalities. Mammography should be performed yearly if stability of mammographic findings is achieved after completion of locoregional therapy [16]. In patients who have undergone breast conservation surgery and primary radiation therapy, mammography is important for detecting clinically asymptomatic recurrent disease in the treated breast. In women who have undergone a unilateral mastectomy, mammograms are primarily helpful for detecting evidence of a clinically asymptomatic new primary breast cancer in the contralateral breast [4]. The risk of a second primary cancer in the contralateral breast is estimated

to be 0.5–1% per year [19] and is greater in women diagnosed at a younger age, with heritable or familial breast cancer, and with radiation therapy for primary breast cancer, particularly if less than 45 years old at the time of treatment [20, 21]. The lack of high-level evidence supporting current practice of mammography surveillance has been reported by Grunfeld [22]. Despite the lack of randomized controlled trial data, observational studies suggest that the method of detection (physical examination or mammography), when reported, did not seem to influence survival. Acknowledging the barriers to designing a prospective randomized trial to answer such a question, routine mammography continues to be recommended for breast cancer surveillance [16].

Data are still insufficient to recommend the routine use of the following investigations in the follow up of early breast cancer patients [16]:

- *CBC testing and automated chemistry studies*. A chemistry group can be the first evidence of recurrent breast cancer approximately 1–12% of the times, when obtained on a frequent basis, whereas a hematology group very rarely is the first indicator of recurrent breast cancer [4].
- *Chest radiographs*. A chest x-ray can be the first evidence of recurrent breast cancer in 0–5% of patients when obtained on a frequent basis [4].
- *Bone scan*. Bone is the most common site to which breast cancer metastasizes. No consensus exists as to the best modality for diagnosing bone lesions among skeletal scintigraphy, plain radiography, computed tomography, or magnetic resonance imaging. Despite the many descriptive studies indicating its limited accuracy, the first choice for screening in common practice is usually bone scan. However, bone scan often needs to be followed by other modalities (X-ray, CT, or MRI) for an accurate diagnosis because it reflects only bone metabolism [23]. Bone scans can detect recurrent breast cancer 0–8% of the time when they are obtained as routine follow-up tests. However, it has been estimated that less than 1% of bone scans will be positive in patients who have no evidence of recurrent breast cancer by history, physical examination, chemistry evaluation, or chest X-ray [4].
- *Ultrasound of the liver*.
- *Computed tomography*. Drotman et al. retrospectively reviewed 6,628 CT scans of the pelvis in 2,426 patients with breast cancer over a 9-year period. Pelvic metastases were the only site of metastases in 13 patients (0.5%) and 4 other patients (0.2%) had new or enlarging pelvic metastases despite the presence of stable extrapelvic metastases. This led to over 200 additional radiographic examinations, including 186 pelvic sonographic examinations, and 50 surgical procedures; 84% of the additional procedures (radiographic and surgical) yielded normal, benign or indeterminate results [24]. Another retrospective study evaluated 250 patients with early-stage breast cancer over a 2-year period. All patients had chest radiographs (74%) or CT scans (26%) for screening purposes or to evaluate symptoms. Of the 10 patients (4%) who developed metastatic disease, only 2 (0.8%) had metastatic disease

diagnosed by chest radiograph. No patients were found to have metastatic disease by routine chest CT scanning [25].

- *[18F]Fluorodeoxyglucose–positron emission tomography (FDG-PET) scanning.* Available data on FDGPET scanning in breast cancer surveillance come from retrospective cohort studies; there are no prospective randomized trial data. Although FDG-PET scanning may have more sensitivity than conventional imaging in diagnosing recurrent disease, there is no evidence that there is an impact on survival, quality of life, or cost effectiveness [16]. In a cohort study of 61 patients comparing FDG-PET scanning to conventional imaging for detecting residual or recurrent breast cancer, sensitivity of FDG-PET vs conventional imaging was slightly improved (93 vs 79%, respectively; $p<.05$), but there was no difference in positive predictive value or specificity. The negative predictive value of FDG-PET compared with conventional imaging was also improved (84 vs 59%, respectively; $p<.05$), but the impact of these results on survival, quality of life, and cost was not evaluated [26]. Another study evaluated the efficacy of whole-body FDG-PET scanning in 60 women with clinical or radiographic suspicion of recurrent breast cancer. Forty women had histologically proven relapsed disease. PET scanning was sensitive and specific for locoregional and distant relapse and seemed to be more sensitive than tumor marker CA 15-3 for detecting recurrence [27]. A meta-analysis of 16 studies comprising 808 patients demonstrated a median sensitivity and specificity of 92.7 and 81.6%, respectively, for FDG-PET scanning. The pooled sensitivity was 90% (95% CI, 86.8–93.2%), and the pooled false-positive rate was 11% (95% CI, 86.0–90.6%) [28]. Thus, although FDG-PET scanning seems to be a useful tool to diagnose suspected breast cancer recurrence, there are no data to support its role in routine breast cancer surveillance in asymptomatic patients [16].
- *Breast magnetic resonance imaging.* A cohort study of 529 women at high risk for breast cancer based on family history found that MRI offered higher sensitivity than mammography (91 vs 33%, respectively) at detecting breast cancer, whereas specificity was similar (97.2 vs 96.8%, respectively) [29]. Another cohort study of 649 women at high familial risk for breast cancer demonstrated similar results in sensitivity (MRI: 77%; 95% CI, 60–90%; mammography: 40%; 95% CI, 24–58%) and specificity (MRI: 81%; 95% CI, 80–83%; mammography: 93%; 95% CI, 92–95%) for detecting breast cancer [30]. Although screening breast MRI seems to be more sensitive than conventional imaging at detecting breast cancer in high-risk women, there is no evidence that breast MRI improves outcomes when used as a breast cancer surveillance tool during routine follow-up in asymptomatic patients. The decision to use breast MRI in high-risk patients should be made on an individual basis [16].
- *Breast cancer tumor markers (CEA, CA 15-3 and CA 27.29).* The use of breast cancer tumor markers such as CEA, CA 15-3 or CA 27.29 is not recommended for routine surveillance of breast cancer patients after primary

therapy [16]. There are no randomized data to address the value of specific serum tumor markers in this context, but the available uncontrolled data do not suggest that tumor markers would lead to survival benefit in patients with curatively treated primary breast cancer [14]. In a recent review of the literature relevant to serum tumor markers in breast cancer, none of the available markers was found to be of value for the detection of early breast cancer due to the lack of sensitivity for early disease and lack of specificity. Although serial determinations of tumor markers after primary treatment for breast cancer can preclinically detect recurrent/metastatic disease with lead times of about 2–9 months, the clinical value of this lead time remains to be determined [31].

One of the reasons for continuing routine follow-up examinations, in the absence of data supporting their value, is the common thought that such tests are reassuring to patients with a history of breast cancer.

One prospective study carried out in Helsinki concluded that follow-up was associated with a feeling of security despite transient anxiety caused by the visits. Most patients criticized the lack of psychological support provided by physicians, while more than 80% of patients were satisfied with the frequency of radiologic examinations [32].

In a survey conducted in the US, women also tended to overestimate the importance of radiographs, scans, and blood tests in detecting recurrence. Over 90% believed that early detection improved long-term outlook, a chance for cure, or the chance to respond to therapy. Few patients were aware of the limitations of routine follow-up investigations [33].

Without formal, country-specific evaluations of patients' perceptions of the value of follow-up programs, it is difficult to judge the ability of such programs to provide emotional support for patients. Some women may be reassured by extensive negative investigations, others may view these tests as anxiety-provoking, still others who have a false positive test result, may be subject to costly, time-consuming, uncomfortable and anxiety-provoking investigations without any positive benefit [3].

Although survivors of breast cancer may find laboratory and radiologic tests reassuring [33], most patients respond well to less intense surveillance once physicians explain the rationale [1].

Moreover, surveillance tests might negatively influence quality of life. In fact, although it is often claimed that follow-up surveillance tests can be reassuring for patients, this may be true if all of the tests are completely normal every time. In the opposite case, which is not an uncommon one, patients are not at all reassured during the waiting time from a test to another. Patients should be informed that presently available data fail to suggest that surveillance tests improve survival or quality of life. Instead, patients should be informed that, since breast cancer recurrences in an irradiated breast, or new contralateral primary breast cancers, are curable – especially if they are caught early-yearly mammograms are important, as well as evaluation of new symptoms and evaluating psychosocial and other health concerns. The best use of resources would be to ensure that all breast cancer survivors be taught signs or symptoms of recurrence, do breast self-examination, and get mammograms. Finally, it is important to stress to patients that not performing blood tests is not therapeutic nihilism. There simply are not blood tests shown to improve quality or quantity of life. It is important to make sure those things that work – mammograms, good preventive care, and healthy lifestyle, including diet and exercise – are performed regularly [34].

Local Complications After Breast Surgery and Radiation Therapy for Breast Cancer

Breast surgery and radiation therapy can be associated with long-lasting side effects. The vast majority of complications are mild, but they may interfere with normal functioning or quality of life [35]. Local complications are worse with more extensive surgery, more extensive radiation, or both and may be aggravated by adjuvant chemotherapy [1].

There are no data suggesting that immediate or delayed *breast reconstruction* alters the long-term outcome of breast cancer or that it impedes or delays the detection of local or regional recurrence [36, 37]. The reconstructed breast should be examined for nodular, erythematous, or rashlike changes in the skin or subcutaneous tissues that might indicate recurrence [1].

Lymphedema affects 10–25% of breast cancer patients, its risk being directly related to the extent of axillary surgery and radiation treatment [38–40]. Sentinel node biopsy is likely to be associated with a lower risk of lymphedema than axillary dissection [1]. Obesity, weight gain, and infection in the arm are additional risk factors for lymphedema. Patients should be taught that usually lymphedema responds to conservative management, such as arm elevation and the use of compression gloves or sleeves [41]. Appropriate physical therapy may relieve those cases that do not respond to conservative treatment. Patients should also be told that, to minimize the chance of lymphedema, they should protect the ipsilateral arm from infection, compression, venipuncture, exposure to intense heat, and abrasion [42].

Long-lasting Side Effects of Systemic Adjuvant Treatment for Breast Cancer

Chemotherapy for breast cancer can have many adverse effects, most of which resolve after treatment has been completed. The most serious, even life-threatening, late sequelae are secondary leukemias and cardiac impairment, both of which are rare [1].

Clinically significant *congestive heart failure* develops in 0.5–1.0% of women treated with standard anthracycline-based chemotherapy regimens [43, 44]. Risk factors for cardiac toxicity include older age, pre-existing cardiac disease, higher cumulative dose of anthracycline, and irradiation of the heart [45, 46]. Symptoms usually develop within several months after chemotherapy, although they may develop later. Non-specific electrocardiographic or echocardiographic abnormalities may arise during long-term follow-up in patients without symptoms of cardiac disease. At present, routine screening of cardiac function is not recommended, although patients with symptoms suggestive of cardiac disease should be evaluated with electrocardiography and echocardiography [1].

Myelodysplastic syndromes or *acute myeloid leukemias* can occur after chemotherapy. The risk is 0.2–1.0% after standard chemotherapy with cyclophosphamide, methotrexate, and fluorouracil or anthracycline-based adjuvant chemotherapy [47, 48]. Two secondary leukemia syndromes have been described; they are associated with exposure to different classes of chemotherapy and are characterized by different latency periods and cytogenetic findings. Leukemias that are associated with exposure to alkylating agents may arise 5–7 years after treatment with agents such as cyclophosphamide and are frequently preceded by a myelodysplastic syndrome. Topoisomerase inhibitors, such as anthracyclines, can give rise to secondary leukemias 6 months to 5 years after therapy. Risk factors for secondary leukemias include high-dose chemotherapy, irradiation, and treatment with older regimens based on alkylating agents. Currently, there are no methods of screening for these disorders in survivors of breast cancer, although they should be considered in the evaluation of patients in whom cytopenia develops after the treatment of breast cancer [1].

Adjuvant chemotherapy may cause temporary or permanent *amenorrhea* in premenopausal women. The risk of chemotherapy-related amenorrhea is directly related to age at time of treatment and varies with type, dose, and duration of chemotherapy. Less than 50% of women younger than 40 years of age will achieve menopause after adjuvant chemotherapy, whereas the majority of women aged 40 years or older will become permanently menopausal. Rates of permanent amenorrhea range from about 40% after four cycles of doxorubicin and cyclophosphamide (AC) with or without four cycles of paclitaxel to nearly 70% for six cycles of oral CMF, with a lower likelihood of becoming amenorrheic with six cycles of intravenous CMF compared with six cycles of oral CMF [49–53]. Chemotherapy-induced ovarian failure is characterized by diminished circulating levels of estrogen and progesterone and elevated levels of follicle-stimulating hormone and luteinizing hormone; these changes are similar to the changes seen in natural menopause and have the same effects. Because of the rapid change in menopausal status, symptoms can be more severe than those associated with the more gradual lowering of estrogen levels that occurs with normal aging [1].

Tamoxifen is a mixed estrogen agonist and antagonist that has a variety of effects on *gynecologic function* [54]. It may cause hot flashes, night sweats, and vaginal discharge, itching, or dryness, and may contribute to dyspareunia and loss of libido [55–57]. Patients should be advised that vasomotor symptoms become less pronounced after several months of tamoxifen therapy. Women who have menstrual dysfunction while taking tamoxifen may resume normal menses after drug therapy stops [58, 59]. Patients taking tamoxifen should be advised to adopt adequate contraception and, in those who wish to become pregnant, to discontinue tamoxifen therapy several months before conceiving because the drug causes urogenital abnormalities when given to neonatal laboratory rodents, and its effects on human fetal development are not known [1, 60].

Tamoxifen increases the risk of *endometrial cancer*, owing to its estrogenic effects on the endometrium [54]. The risk is more pronounced among postmenopausal women, obese women, and women who have had hormone-replacement therapy [61]. Endometrial cancer develops in 0.5–1.0% of women who take tamoxifen for 5 years, as compared with one third as many women taking placebo, but most of these are early-stage and low-grade tumors [62, 63]. Regular gynecologic follow-up is recommended for all women. Patients who receive tamoxifen therapy should be advised to report any vaginal bleeding to their physicians and they should undergo prompt and thorough evaluation, including endometrial biopsy. Tamoxifen causes changes in the uterus that reduce the specificity of screening measures such as ultrasonography and endometrial biopsy. Fortunately, the vast majority of cases of uterine bleeding in patients taking tamoxifen are due to benign processes [1, 16].

Breast cancer patients achieving menopause as a result of adjuvant treatment for early breast cancer may be at higher risk of developing *osteoporosis*, with a loss of bone mineral density of 2–7%, similar to that which occurs during natural menopause [64, 65]. As with normal menopause, trabecular bone (such as the lumbar spine) is affected more than cortical bone (such as the femoral neck). Tamoxifen preserves bone density in postmenopausal women by its estrogenic effects and may reduce the incidence of osteoporotic fractures of the hip, spine, and radius [54, 63]. In premenopausal women, however, tamoxifen therapy has been associated with varying degrees of loss of bone mineral density. Bisphosphonates may prevent the loss of bone mineral density associated with chemotherapy-induced menopause, as they do in the general population of postmenopausal women [64, 65]. To minimize the risk of osteoporosis, breast cancer patients should be encouraged to stop smoking, treat any metabolic or endocrine disorders, perform regular weight-bearing exercise, and receive adequate intakes of calcium (1,000–1,500 mg per day) and vitamin D (400 to 800 IU per day) [66]. Evaluation of bone mineral density within 6–12 months may be warranted in patients in whom adjuvant therapy induces menopause and in premenopausal women taking tamoxifen because these women are at higher risk for osteoporosis. Therapy to prevent further bone loss should be considered for women found to have bone mineral density 1–2 SD below the mean bone mineral density of young women. Women with less pronounced bone loss may also benefit from treatment, particularly if other risk factors for osteoporosis are present [1].

There is concern that prolonged estrogen deprivation may put survivors of breast cancer at greater risk for *heart disease*. Patients should be encouraged to manage possible risk factors for cardiovascular disease, such as hypertension, diabetes, and elevated lipid levels, and to quit smoking. With modern techniques of radiation therapy, the risk of cardiac disease due to irradiation of the left side of the chest appears to be minimal [67, 68]. Women treated according to older radiation protocols and with older equipment may have a slightly increased long-term risk of cardiac complications from irradiation of the breast or chest wall [69]. Tamoxifen lowers the levels of total and low-density lipoprotein cholesterol in postmenopausal women without affecting high-density lipoprotein cholesterol, but it has minimal effects on the lipid profiles of premenopausal women [54]. Some, but not all, randomized trials of adjuvant tamoxifen have suggested a slight reduction in the incidence of coronary events with the use of tamoxifen [70]. The Scottish Trial has reported a decrease of death from myocardial infarction for patients treated with tamoxifen [71]. More recently, a report at the 2004 ESMO Congress from the Swedish tamoxifen trial of 5 years vs 2 has confirmed that the mortality from coronary heart disease was significantly reduced in the 5-year group [72]. On the other hand, the National Surgical Adjuvant Breast and Bowel Project prevention trial did not find a reduction in the risk of coronary events associated with use of tamoxifen [63].

Tamoxifen therapy is associated with an increased risk of *thromboembolic events*, including deep venous thrombosis, pulmonary embolism, and stroke. The absolute risk is small (these events occur in 0.5% of patients) but is higher among women receiving concurrent chemotherapy. Women who have even minimal symptoms suggesting thromboembolic disease should be carefully evaluated [1].

Psychosocial Issues

The diagnosis and treatment of breast cancer are life-altering events, with significant psychological impact on patients, families, and friends. Specific treatments for cancer and the experience of having a serious illness contribute to psychosocial difficulties. During follow-up visits clinicians should inquire about mood disorders, fatigue, anxiety, impaired cognitive performance, and sexual dysfunction, since these problems are prevalent among survivors of breast cancer. Psychosocial distress and problems are most intense during the first year after diagnosis and therapy, and they tend to improve over time. Risk factors for more pronounced psychological and social distress include preexisting psychosocial, family, or marital stress; a more intense initial response to diagnosis and treatment; younger age; negative body image; and treatment-related side effects, such as menopause or lymphedema. The use of dietary or nutritional supplements and complementary or alternative therapies among survivors of breast cancer is quite common and may be a marker of an impaired quality of life.

Although the impact of breast cancer on psychological well-being and social functioning can be profound, patients and clinicians can take heart from several observations. First, most of these impairments resolve with time. Studies find that the long-term quality of life among survivors of breast cancer is quite high, with the large majority of patients functioning at levels similar to those for age-matched controls. Second, survivors of breast cancer identify many positive aspects of life after the diagnosis of cancer, including an optimistic outlook on life and a renewed sense of confidence, purpose, and vitality [1].

Coordination of Care

With the increasing number of patients being followed-up after adjuvant treatment for early breast cancer, there has been much debate about whether follow-up visits should be performed by the hospital-based specialist or if patients – in countries with a strong primary care base – should be referred to the general practitioner for routine follow up, with the option to reinitiate specialist hospital care if problems develop [2].

In 1996, Grunfeld et al. published the results of a randomized trial, conducted in Great Britain, on 296 women with breast cancer in remission (stage I–III) comparing follow-up in hospital clinics according to the usual practice (control group, n = 148), vs follow-up from their own general practitioners (GPs, n = 148), with referral back to hospital clinics if any breast cancer related problems developed (experimental group). Patients who were eligible but declined to participate in the trial were significantly older than participants (mean age 64.3 vs 60.7 years). The two groups were similar in clinical characteristics and quality of life [73]. The recommended frequency of routine visits in general practice was the same as for women remaining in hospital follow up and depended on the time since breast cancer had been diagnosed. In the trial, most recurrences (18/26, 69%) were detected by women themselves in the interval between follow up appointments, and almost half (7/16, 44%) of the recurrences in the hospital group presented first to general practice, irrespective of continuing hospital follow up. The median time to hospital confirmation of recurrence was 21 days in the hospital group (range 1–376 days) and 22 days in the general practice group (range 4–64 days). No significant differences in time to detection of recurrence and quality of life (defined with scores for social functioning, mental health and general health perception) emerged. The trial suggests that there is no reason to believe that the place of follow up will affect recurrence rates or survival. However, delay in confirming a diagnosis of recurrence and reinitiating specialist care may result in an increase in morbidity: in all three cases of purely local recurrence in the general practice group, re-entry to the hospital system from general practice took 4 weeks or more. In every case the delay was primarily administrative. Such administrative delays can be avoided by good organization and quality control, particularly if the pressure on outpatient clinics can be relieved by reducing the burden of routine follow up. The vast majority of general practitioners wish to provide follow up for their patients with breast cancer if their concerns about increased workload can be met, if clear guidelines for follow up can be given, and if assurances are given that patients will be seen urgently by the specialist on an open access basis [2, 8]. In the same trial, patient satisfaction was measured by a self-administered questionnaire supplied three times during the 18-month study period. Patients were more satisfied with follow-up in general practice than in hospital outpatient departments. Furthermore, in the general practice group there was a significant increase in satisfaction over baseline; a similar significant increase in satisfaction over baseline was not found in the hospital group [74]. Moreover, follow-up by general practitioners led to lower health service and patient costs [75].

The above-mentioned report suggests an approach to follow up that can be considered in the future. For women who are willing to consider follow up in a general practice setting (one third were not) and for GPs who are willing to accept this responsibility (in an Ontario survey 10% were reportedly unwilling) [76], general practice is a possible option. However, whether sufficient unused general practice resources exist to meet this demand has not been addressed. Patients who have strong preferences for follow up in specialist settings and for whom follow up in such settings would be most appropriate (e.g., those with treatment related complications) will continue to exist. Furthermore, patient preferences and satisfaction with care may differ considerably in health care systems other than those of the British National Health Service; therefore satisfaction measured by other groups and in the health care systems of other countries should also be evaluated [77].

Possible limits of this trial were short follow up (18 months) and small number of patients involved; moreover, women randomized to follow up by their general practitioner knew that they were under special surveillance, which is different from being "discharged" from hospital; finally, the detection of recurrence is often difficult, particularly after breast surgery and radiation therapy [78]. In addition, a report by Dixon and Norman suggests that regular clinical follow up allows to detect local recurrence after breast conservation. Among 55 patients treated by wide local excision and radiotherapy, 10 breast recurrences were detected by patients themselves, 23 by regular clinical examination in follow up clinic, and 22 by annual mammography. Recurrences detected by patients were larger than those in the two other groups. Of the 23 detected by regular clinical examination, 8 were not visible on mammography. All but one patient with an asymptomatic recurrence were free of metastatic disease and were suitable for a further excision or a mastectomy, compared with 6 of the 10 with symptoms. Since over 80% of recurrences that develop after breast conservation are detected by regular hospital visits, before regular hospital follow up is abandoned for patients with breast cancer a further study looking specifically at the problem of local recurrence is clearly required [79].

In 2006, Grunfeld and colleagues published the results of a multicenter, randomized, controlled trial conducted in Canada involving 968 patients with early-stage breast cancer who had completed adjuvant treatment, were disease free, and were between 9 and 15 months after diagnosis. Patients were randomly allocated to follow-up in the cancer center according to usual practice (CC group) or follow-up from their own family physician (FP group). In the FP group, there were 54 recurrences (11.2%) and 29 deaths (6.0%). In the CC group, there were 64 recurrences (13.2%) and 30 deaths (6.2%). In the FP group, 17 patients (3.5%) compared with 18 patients (3.7%) in the CC group experienced a recurrence-related serious clinical event (0.19% difference; 95% CI, –2.26% to 2.65%). No statistically significant differences ($p<.05$) were detected between groups on any of the health-related quality of life questionnaires. The authors concluded that breast cancer patients can be offered follow-up by their family physician without concern that important recurrence-related serious clinical events will occur more frequently or that health-related quality of life will be negatively affected [80].

Similarly rigorous evaluations of this same surveillance question for breast cancer patients in the Unites States are not currently available. There is no a priori reason to expect that patients in the United States would want different follow-up schedules, and the demand for medically inappropriate testing may be reduced by patient education about the specificity, sensitivity, and usefulness of the available tests [34].

Data suggest that current follow-up procedures could be improved. However, there are substantial issues that have not yet been addressed. First of all, there are no data that show how frequently oncologists or primary care physicians inquire about some of the "softer" but important issues of body image, sexuality, sexual functioning, adaptation back to normal life, cognitive dysfunction, neuropathic pain, bone health, depression, menopause, or all the other symptoms left after treatment: a prospective study of a one-page follow-up check list would give the answers. Second, there are no data assessing if patient outcomes for specific symptoms due to treatment, such as chronic breast pain, sexual function, menopause symptoms, depression, and so on vary between the two groups, because the Hospital Anxiety and Depression Scale (HADS) and 36-item short form (SF-36) are good instruments for global function, but are not designed for breast cancer survivor symptoms. Oncologists are not very good at assessing emotional health. In a study of 204 patients and 5 oncologists, patients reported many more symptoms than their oncologists perceived, and the oncologists had better sensitivity and specificity for physical symptoms than psychosocial. The oncologists had sensitivity rates up to 80% for fatigue, nausea, vomiting, and hair loss, but recognized only 17% of the patients with anxiety and only 6% of those with clinical depression [81]. Finally, there are concerns about the way to educate all who follow breast cancer patients in the many issues that are present during survivorship in a rapidly changing oncology practice. There are some practical steps that can be taken to improve follow-up of women with breast cancer: working with patient advocacy groups to educate their members; give the family physician a sort of one-page follow-up guideline to help improve communication about important health issues; in the absence of a single electronic medical record, providing patients with a USB flash drive with a form for the health care professional to complete each time, that could list the most common concerns and practical tips for fixing them, along with allergies, problem list, radiographs, and so on; following the guidelines we already have in place. The evidence from multiple randomized clinical trials suggests that ASCO should begin partnering with our primary care colleagues and our shared patients to better improve the follow-up process [82].

The 2006 ASCO Guidelines underline that continuity of care for breast cancer patients is recommended and should be performed by a physician experienced in the surveillance of cancer patients and in breast examination, including the examination of irradiated breasts. Follow-up by a primary care physician (PCP) seems to lead to the same health outcomes as specialist follow-up with good patient satisfaction. If a patient with early-stage breast cancer (tumor <5 cm and less than four positive nodes) desires follow-up exclusively by a PCP, care may be transferred to the PCP approximately 1 year after diagnosis. If care is transferred to a PCP, both the PCP and the patient should be informed of the appropriate follow-up and management strategy. This approach will necessitate referral for oncology assessment if a patient is receiving adjuvant endocrine therapy [16]. In fact, follow-up of a patient by multiple specialists after initial therapy is costly, has not been shown to improve outcomes, and may represent duplication of effort. A recently published overview [83] by the Early Breast Cancer Trialists' Collaborative Group reported 15-year breast cancer recurrence and survival rates. Although hazard ratios for recurrence are highest during the first few years after diagnosis, there seems to be a steady relapse rate through 15 years and beyond. In women with estrogen receptor–positive breast cancer treated with tamoxifen for 5 years, the 15-year probability of death from breast cancer is more than three times as great as the 5-year probability. This suggests that the majority of breast cancer recurrences occur more than 5 years after diagnosis when patients are observed for more than 15 years. These findings have implications for long-term breast cancer surveillance and for choice of adjuvant endocrine therapy, which will be required in most patients with hormone receptor-positive cancer. This latter issue is of particular interest in the current era of changing endocrine therapy strategies, and a number of clinical trials continue to address this matter. A variety of care models have been proposed to coordinate follow-up care between oncologists and PCPs. The Institute of Medicine's recent report "From Cancer Patient to Cancer Survivor: Lost in Transition" [84] contains recommendations for improving survivorship care including a shared-care model that could be integrated across different specialties. If agreed by the patient and treating oncologist, a shared-care model would provide treatment summary information and a plan for follow-up care for the patient and PCP;

the level of shared follow-up provided by the oncologist and PCP would depend on patient and provider preferences. This is an evolving field of evidence-based practice; the mechanism of care transfer, level of shared care among providers, and likelihood of success of this strategy will depend on the characteristics of the local clinical setting [16].

Conclusions

Some women certainly seem reassured after a follow up visit (even if they find the days before the visit stressful). This reassurance may be less solidly based than they imagine, given that routine follow up has not been shown to improve survival. Conversely, some women may find that the visits serve only to remind them of their disease and remain a continuing source of anxiety. There is a paucity of data on the effect of follow up on the quality of patients' lives, plus there are certainly financial costs for the patients – such as time off work and the costs of travel – and also for any accompanying relatives or friends.

For the medical and nursing staff, the sheer numbers of patients attending follow up clinics can reduce the time available for patients with problems. Conversely, the presence of fit women in the clinic may serve as a useful counterbalance to the negative effect of their continuously seeing patients whose disease has relapsed. In addition, data on the morbidity of treatment can be acquired only if all patients are seen [85].

With the lack of any convincing data to suggest significant survival benefits from early detection of distant metastases and with increasing awareness of financial constraints, more and more oncologists are abandoning the traditional follow-up practices established in the last few decades. Routine follow-up visits including yearly mammography are of value to patients completing local and adjuvant therapies for early breast cancer. They allow detection of isolated locoregional recurrences, new primaries in the conservatively treated breast, and new contralateral breast primaries. They may be of significant psychological value. They provide the oncologist with an excellent opportunity for lifestyle, family risk and pregnancy counseling and for monitoring of long-term complications of combined modality therapy (including accelerated bone loss and, rarely, long-term cardiovascular sequelae or secondary malignancies). All these are worthy goals and should not be neglected [3].

References

1. Burstein HJ, Winer EP. Primary care for survivors of breast cancer. *NEJM*. 2000;343(15):1086–94
2. Grunfeld E, Mant D, Yudkin P, Adewuyi-Dalton R, Cole D, Stewart J, Fitzpatrick R, Vessey M. Routine follow up of breast cancer in primary care: Randomised trial. *BMJ*. Sep 1996;14;313(7058):665–9

3. Tomiak E, Piccart M. Routine follow-up of patients after primary therapy for early breast cancer: Changing concepts and challenges for the future. *Ann Oncol.* 1993;4:199–204
4. Loprinzi CL. It is now the age to define the appropriate follow-up of primary breast cancer patients. *J Clin Oncol.* 1994;12(5):881–3.
5. Jiwa M, Thompson J, Coleman R, Reed M. Breast cancer follow-up: Could primary care be the right venue? *Curr Med Res Opin.* 2006;22(4):625–30.
6. Mille D, Roy T, Carrère M, Ray I, Ferdjaoui N, Späth H, Chauvin F, Philip T. Economic impact of harmonizing medical practices: Compliance with clinical practice guidelines in the follow-up of breast cancer in a French Comprehensive Cancer Center. *J Clin Oncol*, April 2000;18(8):1718–24.
7. de Bock GH, Bonnema J, van der Hage J, et al. Effectiveness of routine visits and routine tests in detecting isolated locoregional recurrences after treatment for early-stage invasive breast cancer: A meta-analysis and systematic review. *J Clin Oncol.* 2004;22:4010–8.
8. Rojas MP, Telaro E, Russo A, et al. Follow-up strategies for women treated for early breast cancer. Oxford, United Kingdom, Cochrane Library, CD001768, 1, 2005.
9. Rosselli Del Turco M, Palli D, Cariddi A, Ciatto S, Pacini P, Distante V. Intensive diagnositic follow up after treatment of primary breast cancer. *JAMA.* 1994;271:1593–7.
10. Palli D, Russo A, Saieva C, Ciatto S, Rosselli Del Turco M, Distante V, Pacini P, for the National Research Council Project on Breast Cancer Follow-up. Intensive vs clinical follow-up after treatment of primary breast cancer: 10-year update of a randomized trial. *JAMA.* 1999;281(17):1586.
11. GIVIO Investigators. Impact of follow up testing on survival and health-related quality of life in breast cancer patients. *JAMA.* 1994;271:1587–92.
12. Liberati A. The GIVIO trial on the impact of follow-up care on survival and quality of life in breast cancer patients. Interdisciplinary Group for Cancer Care Evaluation. *Ann Oncol.* 1995;6(Suppl 2):41–6.
13. Gulliford T, Opomu M, Wilson E, et al. Popularity of less frequent follow up for breast cancer in randomised study: Initial findings from the hotline study. *BMJ.* 1997;314:174–7.
14. American Society of Clinical Oncology: 1997 update of recommendations for the use of tumor markers in breast and colorectal cancer: Adopted on November 7, 1997, by the American Society of Clinical Oncology. *J Clin Oncol.* 1998;16:793–5.
15. American Society of Clinical Oncology: Outcomes of cancer treatment for technology assessment and cancer treatment guidelines. *J Clin Oncol.* 1996;14:671–9.
16. Khatcheressian JL, Wolff AC, Smith TJ, et al. American Society of Clinical Oncology 2006 Update of the Breast Cancer Follow-Up and Management Guidelines in the Adjuvant Setting. *J Clin Oncol.* 24(31):1–7.
17. Schrag D, Kuntz KM, Garber JE, Weeks JC. Life expectancy gains from cancer prevention strategies for women with breast cancer and BRCA1 and BRCA2 mutations. *JAMA.* 2000;283:617–24.
18. Hartmann LC, Schaid DJ, Woods JE, et al. Efficacy of bilateral prophylactic mastectomy in women with a family history of breast cancer. *N Engl J Med.* 1999;340:77–84.
19. Dawson LA, Chow E, Goss PE. Evolving perspectives in contralateral breast cancer. *Eur J Cancer.* 1998;34:2000–9.
20. Bernstein JL, Thompson WD, Risch N, Holford TR. The genetic epidemiology of second primary breast cancer. *Am J Epidemiol.* 1992;136:937–48.
21. Boice JD Jr, Harvey EB, Blettner M, Stovall M, Flannery JT. Cancer in the contralateral breast after radiotherapy for breast cancer. *N Engl J Med.* 1992;326:781–5.
22. Grunfeld E, Noorani H, McGahan L, et al. Surveillance mammography after treatment of primary breast cancer: A systematic review. *Breast.* 2002;11:228–35.
23. Hamaoka T, Madewell JE, Podoloff DA, Hortobagyi GN, Ueno NT. Bone Imaging in Metastatic Breast Cancer. *J Clin Oncol.* 2004;22:2942–53.

24. Drotman MB, Machnicki SC, Schwartz LH, et al. Breast cancer: Assessing the use of routine pelvic CT in patient evaluation. *Am J Roentgenol.* 2001;176:1433–6.
25. Hurria A, Leung D, Trainor K, et al. Screening chest imaging studies are not effective in the follow-up of breast cancer patients. *J Oncol Manag.* 2003;12:13–5.
26. Vranjesevic D, Filmont JE, Meta J, et al. Whole-body (18)F-FDG PET and conventional imaging for predicting outcome in previously treated breast cancer patients. *J Nucl Med.* 2002;43:325–9.
27. Kamel EM, Wyss MT, Fehr MK, et al. [18F]-Fluorodeoxyglucose positron emission tomography in patients with suspected recurrence of breast cancer. *J Cancer Res Clin Oncol.* 2003;129:147–53.
28. Isasi CR, Moadel RM, Blaufox MD. A metaanalysis of FDG-PET for the evaluation of breast cancer recurrence and metastases. *Breast Cancer Res Treat.* 2005;90:105–12.
29. Kuhl CK, Schrading S, Leutner CC, et al. Mammography, breast ultrasound, and magnetic resonance imaging for surveillance of women at high familial risk for breast cancer. *J Clin Oncol.* 2005;23:8469–76.
30. Leach MO, Boggis CR, Dixon AK, et al. Screening with magnetic resonance imaging and mammography of a UK population at high familial risk of breast cancer: A prospective multicenter cohort study (MARIBS). *Lancet.* 2005;365:1769–78.
31. Duffy MJ. Serum tumor markers in breast cancer: Are they of clinical value? *Clin Chem.* 2006;52(3):345–51.
32. Hietanen P. Response to follow-up of breast cancer. *Strahlentherapie.* 1985;161:678–80.
33. Muss HB, Tell GS, Case LD, Robertson P, Atwell BM. Perceptions of follow-up care in women with breast cancer. *Am J Clin Oncol.* 1991;14:55–9.
34. Loprinzi CL, Hayes D, Smith T. Doc, shouldn't we be getting some tests? Classic Papers, suppl to *J Clin Oncol.* 2003, 21(9):108–11.
35. Warmuth MA, Bowen G, Prosnitz L, et al. Complications of axillary lymph node dissection for carcinoma of the breast: A report based on a patient survey. *Cancer.* 1998;83:1362–8.
36. Johnson CH, van Heerden JA, Donohue JH, Martin JK Jr, Jackson IT, Ilstrup DM. Oncological aspects of immediate breast reconstruction following mastectomy for malignancy. *Arch Surg* 1989;124:819–23.
37. Slavin SA, Love SM, Goldwyn RM. Recurrent breast cancer following immediate reconstruction with myocutaneous flaps. *Plast Reconstr Surg.* 1994;93:1191–204.
38. Petrek JA, Lerner R. Lymphedema. Harris JR, Lippman ME, Morrow M, Osborne K, eds. *Diseases of the Breast.* 2nd ed. Philadelphia: Lippincott Williams & Wilkins; 2000:1033–40.
39. Larson D, Weinstein M, Goldberg I, et al. Edema of the arm as a function of the extent of axillary surgery in patients with stage I–II carcinoma of the breast treated with primary radiotherapy. *Int J Radiat Oncol Biol Phys.* 1986;12:1575–82.
40. Pezner RD, Patterson MP, Hill LR, et al. Arm lymphedema in patients treated conservatively for breast cancer: Relationship to patient age and axillary node dissection technique. *Int J Radiat Oncol Biol Phys.* 1986;12:2079–83.
41. Bertelli G, Venturini M, Forno G, Macchiavello F, Dini D. Conservative treatment of postmastectomy lymphedema: a controlled, randomized trial. *Ann Oncol.* 1991;2:575–8.
42. Rockson SG. Precipitating factors in lymphedema: Myths and realities. *Cancer.* 1998;83:2814–6.
43. Valagussa P, Zambetti M, Biasi S, Moliterni A, Zucali R, Bonadonna G. Cardiac effects following adjuvant chemotherapy and breast irradiation in operable breast cancer. *Ann Oncol.* 1994;5:209–16.
44. Hortobagyi GN, Buzdar AU, Marcus CE, Smith TL. Immediate and long-term toxicity of adjuvant chemotherapy regimens containing doxorubicin in trials at M. D. Anderson Hospital and Tumor Institute. Lippman ME, ed. National Institutes of Health Consensus Development Conference on Adjuvant Chemotherapy and Endocrine Therapy for Breast

Cancer. NCI monographs. No. 1. Washington, D.C.: Government Printing Office, 1986:105-9. (NIH publication no. 86–2860.)
45. Shapiro CL, Hardenbergh PH, Gelman R, et al. Cardiac effects of adjuvant doxorubicin and radiation therapy in breast cancer patients. *J Clin Oncol.* 1998;16:3493–501.
46. Shan K, Lincoff AM, Young JB. Anthracycline-induced cardiotoxicity. *Ann Intern Med.* 1996;125:47–58.
47. Valagussa P, Moliterni A, Terenziani M, Zambetti M, Bonadonna G. Second malignancies following CMF-based adjuvant chemotherapy in respectable breast cancer. *Ann Oncol.* 1994;5:803–8.
48. Diamandidou E, Buzdar AU, Smith TL, Frye D, Witjaksono M, Hortobagyi GN. Treatment-related leukemia in breast cancer patients treated with fluorouracil-doxorubicin-cyclophosphamide combination adjuvant chemotherapy: the University of Texas M.D. Anderson Cancer Center experience. *J Clin Oncol.* 1996;14:2722–30.
49. Davidson NE. Ovarian ablation as adjuvant therapy for breast cancer. *J Natl Cancer Inst Monogr.* 2001;30:67–71.
50. Bines J, Oleske DM, Cobleigh MA. Ovarian function in premenopausal women treated with adjuvant chemotherapy for breast cancer. *J Clin Oncol.* 1996;14:1718–29.
51. Davidson NE. Ovarian ablation as treatment for young women with breast cancer. *J Natl Cancer Inst Monogr.* 1994;16:95–99.
52. Stone ER, Slack RS, Novielli A, et al. Rate of chemotherapy related amenorrhea (CRA) associated with adjuvant adriamycin and cytoxan (AC) and adriamycin and cytoxan followed by taxol (ACT) in early stage breast cancer. *Breast Cancer Res Treat.* 2000;64:61(abstr 224).
53. Minton SE, Munster PN. Chemotherapy induced amenorrhea and fertility in women undergoing adjuvant treatment for breast cancer. *Cancer Control.* 2002;9:466–72.
54. Osborne CK. Tamoxifen in the treatment of breast cancer. *N Engl J Med.* 1998;339:1609–18.
55. Love RR, Cameron L, Connell BL, Leventhal H. Symptoms associated with tamoxifen treatment in postmenopausal women. *Arch Intern Med.* 1991;151:1842–7.
56. Day R, Ganz PA, Costantino JP, Cronin WM, Wickerham DL, Fisher B. Health-related quality of life and tamoxifen in breast cancer prevention: A report from the National Surgical Adjuvant Breast and Bowel Project P-1 Study. *J Clin Oncol.* 1999;17:2659–69.
57. Mortimer JE, Boucher L, Baty J, Knapp DL, Ryan E, Rowland JH. Effect of tamoxifen on sexual functioning in patients with breast cancer. *J Clin Oncol.* 1999;17:1488–92.
58. Goodwin PJ, Ennis M, Pritchard KI, Trudeau M, Hood N. Risk of menopause during the first year after breast cancer diagnosis. *J Clin Oncol.* 1999;17:2365–70.
59. Chang J, Powles TJ, Ashley SE, Iveson T, Gregory RK, Dowsett M. Variation in endometrial thickening in women with amenorrhea on tamoxifen. *Breast Cancer Res Treat.* 1998;48:81–5.
60. Wolf DM, Jordan VC. Gynecologic complications associated with long-term adjuvant tamoxifen therapy for breast cancer. *Gynecol Oncol.* 1992;45:118–28.
61. Bernstein L, Deapen D, Cerhan JR, et al. Tamoxifen therapy for breast cancer and endometrial cancer risk. *J Natl Cancer Inst.* 1999;91:1654–62.
62. Fisher B, Costantino JP, Redmond CK, Fisher ER, Wickerham DL, Cronin WM. Endometrial cancer in tamoxifen-treated breast cancer patients: Findings from the National Surgical Adjuvant Breast and Bowel Project (NSABP) B-14. *J Natl Cancer Inst.* 1994;86:527–37.
63. Fisher B, Costantino JP, Wickerham DL, et al. Tamoxifen for prevention of breast cancer: report of the National Surgical Adjuvant Breast and Bowel Project P-1 Study. *J Natl Cancer Inst.* 1998;90:1371–88.

64. Saarto T, Blomqvist C, Valimaki M, Makela P, Sarna S, Elomaa I. Chemical castration induced by adjuvant cyclophosphamide, methotrexate, and fluorouracil chemotherapy causes rapid bone loss that is reduced by clodronate: a randomized study in premenopausal breast cancer patients. *J Clin Oncol.* 1997;15:1341–7.
65. Powles TJ, McCloskey E, Paterson AHG, et al. Oral clodronate and reduction in loss of bone mineral density in women with operable primary breast cancer. *J Natl Cancer Inst.* 1998;90:704–8.
66. Eastell R. Treatment of postmenopausal osteoporosis. *N Engl J Med.* 1998;338:736–46.
67. Nixon AJ, Manola J, Gelman R, et al. No long-term increase in cardiac-related mortality after breast-conserving surgery and radiation therapy using modern techniques. *J Clin Oncol.* 1998;16:1374–9.
68. Hojris, I, Overgaard M, Christensen JJ, Overgaard J. Morbidity and mortality of ischaemic heart disease in high-risk breast-cancer patients after adjuvant postmastectomy systemic treatment with or without radiotherapy: analysis of DBCG 82b and 82c randomised trials. *Lancet.* 1999;354:1425–30.
69. Paszat LF, Mackillop WJ, Groome PA, Boyd C, Schulze K, Holowaty E. Mortality from myocardial infarction after adjuvant radiotherapy for breast cancer in the Surveillance, Epidemiology, and End-Results cancer registries. *J Clin Oncol.* 1998;16:2625–31 (Erratum, *J Clin Oncol.* 1999;17:740.
70. Ragaz J, Coldman A. Survival impact of adjuvant tamoxifen on competing causes of mortality in breast cancer survivors, with analysis of mortality from contralateral breast cancer, cardiovascular events, endometrial cancer, and thromboembolic episodes. *J Clin Oncol.* 1998;16:2018–24.
71. Stewart HJ. The Scottish trial of adjuvant tamoxifen in node negative breast cancer. *J Natl Cancer Inst Monogr.* 1992, 11, 117–20.
72. Nordenskjöld B, Rosell J, Rutqvist LE, et al. The Swedish Breast Cancer Group trail of two versus five years of adjuvant tamoxifen: reduced coronary heart disease death rate in the five years group. *Ann Oncol.* 2004, 15(Suppl. 3), iii54–iii55 (Abstract 2060).
73. Grunfeld E, Mant D, Vessey MP, Yudkin P. Evaluating primary care follow-up of breast cancer: Methods and preliminary results of three studies. *Ann Oncol.* 1995;6(Suppl 2):47–52.
74. Grunfeld E, Fitzpatrick R, Mant D, et al. Comparison of breast cancer patient satisfaction with follow-up in primary care versus specialist care: Results from a randomized controlled trial. *Br J Gen Pract.* 1999 Sep;49(446):705–10.
75. Grunfeld E, Gray A, Mant D, et al. Follow-up of breast cancer in primary care vs specialist care: Results of an economic evaluation. *Br J Cancer.* 1999;79:1227–33.
76. Worster A, Bass MJ, Wood ML. Willingness to follow breast cancer. Survey of family physicians. *Can Fam Physician.* 1996;42:263–8.
77. Goodwin PJ. Women with breast cancer were more satisfied with general practitioner care than with outpatient clinic care. *Evid Based Med.* May 1,2000; 5(3):89.
78. Rainsbury D. Routine follow up of breast cancer in primary care. *BMJ.* 1996 313:1547.
79. Dixon JM, Norman B. Most recurrences after breast conservation are detected by regular hospital visits. *BMJ.* 1996;313:1548.
80. Grunfeld E, Levine MN, Julian JA, et al. Randomized Trial of Long-Term Follow-Up for Early-Stage Breast Cancer: A Comparison of Family Physician versus Specialist Care. *J Clin Oncol.* 2006;24(6):848–55.
81. Newell S, Sanson-Fisher RW, Girgis A, et al. How well do medical oncologists' perceptions reflect their patients' reported physical and psychosocial problems? Data from a survey of five oncologists. *Cancer.* 1998; 83:1640–51
82. Khatcheressian JL, Smith TJ. Randomized trial of long-term follow-up for early-stage breast cancer: A comparison of family physician versus specialist care. *J Clin Oncol.* 20 February 2006;24(6):835–7.

83. Early Breast Cancer Trialists' Collaborative Group: Effects of Chemotherapy and Hormonal therapy for early breast cancer on recurrence and 15-year survival: An overview of the randomised trials. *Lancet*. 2005;365:1687–717.
84. Institute of Medicine and National Research Council, Committee on Cancer Survivorship: Improving care and quality of life, National Cancer Policy Board. From Cancer Patient to Cancer Survivor: Lost in Transition. Washington, DC: National Academies Press, 2005.
85. Dewar J. Follow up in breast cancer: A suitable case for reappraisal. *BMJ*. 1995;310:685.

Quality of Life Issues During Adjuvant Endocrine Therapy

Lesley Fallowfield and Valerie Jenkins

Introduction

When the media report the results from studies reporting the latest breakthrough in adjuvant drug treatments, they are usually described in terms of relative rather than absolute benefits. Many women with early stage breast (EBC) cancer may not realise that they do not necessarily require any further adjuvant treatments and that claims for example of a 50% reduction in risk of recurrence does not relate to an individual woman's risk. For many who receive systemic therapy the relative benefits may be small and not outweigh the associated costs of side effects. Until basic science can provide us with a better understanding of how to target treatments to those most likely to derive benefit, we need to collect side-effect data systematically and conduct considerably more research into ameliorative interventions to help patients cope with the worst symptoms. Unrelenting menopausal symptoms, vasomotor complaints in particular, can lead to non adherence with endocrine therapies, which are prescribed for at least 2–5 years.

Acceptability of treatment and long-term adherence is influenced by the actual burdens experienced, the impact of any side effects on quality of life (QoL) and a patient's beliefs and expectations about therapeutic intent [1]. In order for a woman with EBC to make an educated decision about adjuvant treatments, she needs to have clear and consistent verbal and written information provided by all members of the multidisciplinary healthcare team. She would need to know the different treatment options, likely therapeutic gains, and side effect profiles associated with the different therapies. Obviously members of the team can only discuss with patients things that have been systematically studied and recorded. Most of these data result from clinical trials.

L. Fallowfield (✉)
Cancer Research UK Psychosocial Oncology Group, Brighton and Sussex Medical School, University of Sussex, BN1 9QG, tel +441273 873015
e-mail: l.j.fallowfield@sussex.ac.uk

M. Castiglione, M.J. Piccart (eds.), *Adjuvant Therapy for Breast Cancer*, Cancer Treatment and Research 151, DOI 10.1007/978-0-387-75115-3_22,

However the manner in which adverse events and side effects is collected are often unreliable.

Healthcare professionals often underestimate non-life threatening but QoL threatening side effects, making treatments appear more favorable and acceptable during discussions. For example, for over 20 years the selective oestrogen receptor modulator (SERM) tamoxifen, was the primary hormonal treatment choice offered by clinicians to their breast cancer patients. Initially results from the early trials suggested that tamoxifen had few, if any side effects; however the mature, longitudinal data acquired over time now present a truer picture not just of its efficacy, but also its substantial side effect profile. Yet the knowledge that accurate safety and side effect data are usually gathered only after many years of use does not appear to deter some of the media and trialists from extolling the virtues of novel drugs after only 2 or 3 years of use. This has been seen with the aromatase inhibitors (AIs) [2] and other classes of breast cancer drugs such as herceptin.

The focus of this chapter will be on the importance of measuring QoL in terms of side effects, patient preferences and adherence. We will consider these issues particularly in relation to adjuvant hormone treatments for post-menopausal women, SERMS and the AIs and LHRH analogues for the pre-menopausal patient.

How Is Quality of Life Measured?

Several standardised instruments with excellent psychometric properties are available to measure QoL in women receiving breast cancer treatments. Curiously these instruments only ever appear to be used within clinical trials rather than to help monitor and inform the management of patients outside the trial setting and providing further useful data.

Health-related QoL has been evaluated in parallel with efficacy and safety in several clinical trials of adjuvant endocrine therapy in postmenopausal women with EBC, using the Short Form 36-Item Health Survey (SF-36) [3], the Functional Assessment of Cancer Therapy-Breast + Endocrine Subscale (FACT-B + ES) [4, 5], and the Menopause Specific Quality of Life (MENQOL) [6] questionnaires.

SF-36 poses questions about overall health, including energy, fatigue, bodily pain, health-related limitations on physical and social activities, and emotional well-being. The FACT-B + ES is tailored for patients with breast cancer and includes specific questions related to endocrine therapy. The FACT B comprises the FACT-G a general 27 item questionnaire covering 4 QoL domains: physical, functional, social and emotional well-being along with a breast cancer concerns subscale with 9 further questions. The ES subscale comprises 19 items associated with menopausal symptoms such as hot flushes and night sweats. Respondents rate each item on a five point scale from “not at all” to “very much" indicating the extent to which they have been affected in the past 7 days. The ES can be used alone or in combination with the FACT-B.

Another frequently used measure is the generic EORTC QLQ-C30 together with its breast cancer module BR23 [7].

Acceptability of Adjuvant Endocrine Therapy

Until recently, tamoxifen was the gold standard in adjuvant endocrine treatments [8], but despite the efficacy of the drug the serious side effects such as thromboembolic problems, stroke and endometrial cancer limit its use. The treatment also has many side effects that affect QoL including hot flushes, night sweats and vaginal discharge.

It was hoped that the newer third generation AIs, such as anastrozole and letrozole (non-steroidal) and exemestane (steroidal), would not only have better efficacy than tamoxifen but also fewer side effects impacting on QoL. Results from three international trials, which have QoL sub-protocols, are presented to highlight some of the similarities and differences between the endocrine treatments. The ATAC trial compared anastrozole, tamoxifen alone or in combination, IES (the Intergroup Exemestane Study) compared exemestane with tamoxifen in patients who had already received 2–3 years of adjuvant tamoxifen and the MA-17 trial looked at letrozole versus placebo in women who had completed 5 years of tamoxifen. All three trials take patients at different timepoints so are not directly comparable but they do provide some information about the types of side effects experienced and the temporal relationship of treatment starting and symptoms developing. See Fig. 1

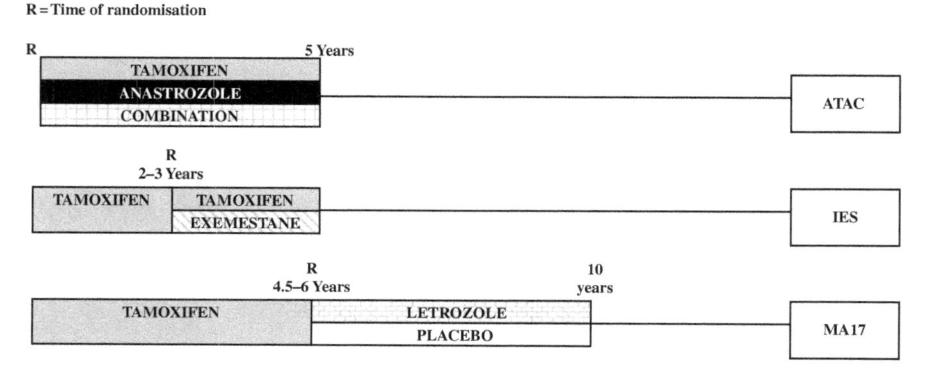

Fig. 1 Recent trials of AIs with QoL

9366 postmenopausal women with localised EBC participated in ATAC and the 5 year completed treatment analysis at a median follow up of 68 months showed that anastrozole was superior in terms of both efficacy and tolerability [9]. The combination arm was discontinued as no efficacy or tolerability benefit was demonstrated compared with either drug alone. In a sub-protocol of the ATAC trial, QoL was investigated prospectively in 1,105 women recruited to the trial; the 2- and 5-year QoL data have been published [10, 11]. The primary objective of the QoL sub-protocol was to compare the difference in overall QoL between the anastrozole and tamoxifen treatment groups as assessed by the FACT-B Trial Outcome Index (TOI). This is the sum of the Physical Well Being (PWB), Functional Well Being (FWB) and Breast Cancer Subscale of the questionnaire. A total of 23 items contribute to the TOI, resulting in a maximum possible score of 92. A high score indicates good QoL and lower scores equate with a poorer QoL. Some items are negatively framed and reversed for analysis. The sample size calculation for this QoL sub-protocol was powered to detect a difference of at least 5 points in the TOI score between anastrozole and tamoxifen groups at the 6-month time point [10]. A change of 5 points in TOI score is considered clinically meaningful [4]. The secondary objectives were to compare the prevalence and severity of specific endocrine symptoms as recorded on the ES inventory, and to compare Emotional Well-Being (EWB) and Social Well Being (SWB) between treatment groups. Also, in order to provide clinically relevant information regarding treatment side effects, patients responses to each ES question were labelled “clinically significant” if they scored “quite a bit” or “very much” and “not clinically significant” if they responded “not at all”, “a little” or “somewhat”.

The 2-year QoL analysis was conducted on 1,021 women: 335 anastrozole, 347 tamoxifen and 339 in the combination arm. Over the 2-year period, 17.8% (182) of patients withdrew from the QoL study, 49 (A), 67 (T), 66 (C); most had withdrawn from the main ATAC trial. There was good compliance from those completing QoL forms, with 85% of questionnaires completed at each post baseline visit. Results showed that all groups improved in TOI from baseline to 3 months: the mean improvements were +1.29 (anastrozole), +2.22 (tamoxifen) and +1.61 (combination arm). Exploratory analysis showed that women who received chemotherapy had lower baseline scores and greater improvements at 3 months compared with women who did not receive chemotherapy. Use of hormone therapy at baseline had no effect on the TOI score. By 24 months the mean improvements were +4.16 (A), +3.49 (T) and +3.73 (C). The proportions of patients showing a clinically significant change in the TOI score at any time point from baseline were 60% (A), 61.9% (T) and 59.8 (C). The proportions who always improved over time were 22.4% (A), 19.5% (T) and 20.5% (C). These two distinctions (ever improved and always improved) provide the least and most conservative estimates, respectively, of the proportion of people who improved from baseline [10].

The ES scores did worsen for all three groups from baseline following 3 months of endocrine treatment but did not differ between groups and subsequently stabilised. There were no significant differences among groups for EWB or SWB scores. The most interesting findings were the post hoc analyses comparing individual endocrine items for the tamoxifen and anastrozole treatment groups. The individual symptoms were categorised into four groups, vasomotor symptoms, neuropsychological problems, gastrointestinal symptoms and gynaecological/sexual problems. The proportions of patients who experienced severe symptoms at each time point are shown in Table 1. There were interesting differences in the reporting of the severity of endocrine symptoms among treatment groups. There was a vasomotor advantage for the anastrozole group, with fewer cold sweats but troublesome gynaecological symptoms, such as vaginal

Table 1 Proportion (%) of patients experiencing "very much" or "quite a bit" ES symptoms from the 2- and 5-year ATAC QoL analyses

	Anastrozole		Tamoxifen	
	2 years	5 years	2 years	5 years
Vasomotor symptoms				
Hot flushes	30.4	26.6	32.7	28.5
Cold sweats	7.8	7.7	10.6	9.1
Night sweats	18.9	17.8	23.9	21.3
Sleeping difficulties	20.1	19.0	19.7	18.8
Neuropsychological symptoms				
Dizziness	3.5	3.1	5.0	5.4
Headaches	4.7	5.1	5.3	5.0
Mood swings	10.8	10.3	11.5	11.3
Irritability	8.6	8.7	9.0	9.1
Lack of energy	16.5	15.9	20.2	18.3
Nervous feeling	6.5	6.6	9.2	8.6
Gastrointestinal symptoms				
Weight gain	21.8	22.6	22.6	20.6
Vomiting	0.5	[a]	0.4	[a]
Diarrhoea	2.9	3.1	1.1	1.3
Bloated feeling	10.9	10.4	11.0	10.9
Nausea	1.3	1.2	2.6	2.2
Gynaecological/sexual symptoms				
Vaginal discharge	1.2	1.2	5.2	5.2
Vaginal itching	2.6	3.4	4.7	5.0
Vaginal bleeding or spotting	0.2	[a]	1.2	[a]
Vaginal dryness	16.3	18.5	8.4	9.1
Pain or discomfort with intercourse	17.8	17.3	7.5	8.1
Loss of interest in sex	15.8	34.0	8.5	26.1
Breast sensitivity	13.0	12.0	13.7	11.6

[a]Data not available due to the very low incidence for these symptoms

dryness and dyspareunia were also more common in this group compared with patients taking tamoxifen.

Over the 5-year study period 17% of expected QoL evaluations were missing and the missing data rate increased particularly in the fifth year of follow up. The results for the QoL profile at 5 years showed a continued improvement for both the anastrozole and tamoxifen groups, continuing a trend from baseline to 2 years. However as the missing data rate increased also, it was not clear whether and to what extent this slight increase reflected the effect of non random missing data, particularly given that some women dropped out from treatment due to side effects [11]. Most patients (67%) regardless of treatment had a clinically meaningful improvement with no differences between the groups. The same improvements applied to the SWB, EWB and ES score. However analysis of the dichotomised ES items suggested some differences between the treatment groups (shown in Table 1). The differences between the treatment groups in terms of side effect profile are evident from these patient reported outcomes (PROs). The importance of such data are that the efficacy benefits of anastrozole in terms of disease free survival and time to recurrence in hormone receptor positive patients was achieved without a detrimental overall impact on QoL. From a clinical point of view women can be informed that most side effects appear within the first 12 weeks of treatment and thereafter either plateau or get slightly better.

Exemestane is an irreversible steroidal AI so it was possible that its side effect profile might differ from anastrozole, a non-steroidal when it too was compared with tamoxifen. The IES used the same QoL instruments to record PROs as used in ATAC, which enables us to conduct some comparison. IES was a double blind randomised controlled study of 4,724 postmenopausal women with primary breast cancer who were disease free after 2–3 years of tamoxifen. Women were randomised to continue tamoxifen until 5 years of treatment had been reached or switch to exemestane. Initial results after a median follow up of 37 months showed significantly fewer recurrences, less contralateral breast cancer and superior disease free survival in patients who were switched to exemestane [12]. The most recent results now show a survival benefit [13].

The QoL subprotocol has published 2 year post-randomisation results from 562 patients, 289 of whom received exemestane and 293 tamoxifen. Attrition rate was low during the 2 year period, with a total of 90 patients (15.5%) withdrawn (exemestane 38, tamoxifen 52). Compliance was good with 85.3% of questionnaires completed at each post baseline visit, similar to ATAC [10]. The analyses performed on the FACT-B and ES questionnaires were the same as for ATAC: That is TOI, ES, EWB, SWB plus differences in individual endocrine symptoms. Again, the results showed no differences between the treatment arms. QoL was generally good and stable over 2 years (by which time most patients had received at least 4 years of endocrine therapy) with no clinically meaningful differences found in TOI or ES between groups. The proportions of patients who maintained a clinically meaningful TOI at all time points were 3.9% (exemestane) and 4.7% (tamoxifen). The proportions of patients who had a clinically meaningful sustained decrease at each time point compared with baseline were 2.5% for exemestane and 3.6% for tamoxifen. Irrespective of treatment, mean ES scores increased over time (i.e. endocrine symptoms decreased). Severe endocrine symptoms were high at trial entry showing that the side-effects of tamoxifen following 2–3 years of treatment are persistent. The most frequently reported symptoms were for vasomotor complaints and sexual problems but the only endocrine symptom showing a significant difference between treatments was vaginal discharge, which was more pronounced with tamoxifen ($p<0.001$) [14].

The results from both the ATAC and IES QoL studies are encouraging. In the former anastrozole compared favourably to tamoxifen whilst having an added clinical benefit. In the latter, clinical benefits for switching to exemestane compared with continuous tamoxifen are achieved without a detrimental effect on QoL. The results from both these sub-studies allow us to begin to compare the profiles of tamoxifen, anastrozole and exemestane, mindful that the IES patients had already received at least 2 years of tamoxifen. Table 2 shows the dichotomised symptom reporting at 24 months for the IES patients (some of whom will have received tamoxifen for 4 or 5 years) and 5 years for ATAC. What is especially interesting to note is that the FACT-ES appears to be a very sensitive instrument and that some tamoxifen symptoms over two different populations of patients at different timepoints remain consistently high. This reinforces an earlier comment that from a clinical point of view, women can be told that the worst endocrine symptoms are apparent by 3 months of treatment' start and that thereafter they stay more or less the same or reduce slightly.

MA-17 compared letrozole with placebo in women with EBC who had already completed 5 years of tamoxifen treatment. The study was stopped early when DFS was found to be better for letrozole than placebo. The most recent update after a median follow-up of 30 months, has shown overall survival to be the same in both arms (HR for death from any cause = 0.82, 95% CI = 0.57–1.19; p = .3) but a survival benefit to women in the letrozole arm among lymph node-positive patients (HR = 0.61, 95% CI = 0.38–0.98; p=.04) [15]. The MA.17 QoL subprotocol used the SF-36 and MENQOL questionnaires. Although large numbers were recruited to the QoL study with 1,799 randomised to placebo and 1,813 to letrozole, few ever completed long term follow up as the trial was stopped early. This is a pity as the study afforded the opportunity to obtain data on the long term consequences of endocrine therapy. However, for those patients who did complete questionnaires some interesting results emerged. There were no differences between groups in mean change scores from baseline for the SF-36 physical and mental summary scores at 6, 12, 24 and 36 months but small statistically significant differences were reported for the SF-36 domains of physical functioning (12 months), bodily pain (6 months) and vitality (6 and 12 months), and the MENQOL vasomotor (6, 12 and 24 months) and sexual domains (12 and 24 months). Using a complicated response analysis, a significant difference was found between groups for the bodily pain (47% placebo vs 51% letrozole;

Table 2 Proportion of patients experiencing "very much" or "quite a bit" ES symptoms from the 2-year IES and 5-year ATAC QoL analyses

	Anastrozole	Tamoxifen (ATAC)	Exemestane	Tamoxifen(IES)
Vasomotor symptoms				
Hot flushes	26.6	28.5	23.5	25.9
Cold sweats	7.7	9.1	8.9	8.7
Night sweats	17.8	21.3	16.8	20.5
Sleeping difficulties	19.0	18.8	16.0	19.6
Neuropsychological symptoms				
Dizziness	3.1	5.4	3.5	5.9
Headaches	5.1	5.0	0.8	1.8
Mood swings	10.3	11.3	8.8	11.0
Irritability	8.7	9.1	6.2	8.1
Lack of energy	15.9	18.3	14.9	12.7
Nervous feeling	6.6	8.6	8.4	9.2
Gastrointestinal symptoms				
Weight gain	22.6	20.6	19.1	28.3
Vomiting	[a]	[a]	0.8	1.3
Diarrhoea	3.1	1.3	5.3	8.2
Bloated feeling	10.4	10.9	8.0	15.1
Nausea	1.2	2.2	1.7	1.8
Gynaecological/sexual symptoms				
Vaginal discharge	1.2	5.2	1.3	8.2
Vaginal itching	3.4	5.0	1.7	4.5
Vaginal bleeding or spotting	[a]	[a]	0	1.8
Vaginal dryness	18.5	9.1	16.0	17.5
Pain or discomfort with intercourse	17.3	8.1	12.0	11.3
Loss of interest in sex	34.0	26.1	34.0	32.0
Breast sensitivity	12.0	11.6	8.0	12.3

[a]Data not available due to the very low incidence for these symptoms

p = .009) and the vasomotor domain (22% placebo vs 29% letrozole; p = .001) [16]. Although overall QoL did not differ significantly between treatment groups, this was a highly selected patient cohort, disease-free after an initial 5 years of tamoxifen and who had volunteered for an additional 5 years of AI therapy. It is plausible that women who had found the menopausal symptoms associated with tamoxifen intolerable had already dropped out of treatment;

thus MA-17 results are from a group of tamoxifen-tolerant women limiting our ability to generalize its results to other populations of patients with early breast cancer.

QoL in the Pre-menopausal Patient

The commonest pituitary down-regulator is the LHRH analogue goserelin. The drug has many advantages over chemotherapy being a more effective means of inducing ovarian ablation than chemotherapy and, because of its reversibility, potential preservation of fertility. It also has fewer unpleasant side-effects than chemotherapy in particular avoidance of alopecia. In the ZEBRA trial of 1640 pre or peri-menopausal women with EBC, adjuvant goserelin showed similar overall survival to CMF in node+ disease after 7.3 years' median follow-up (HR = 0.94; 95%CI: 0.75–1.18) [17].

In another study of 1034 node+/−, receptor+, pre and peri-menopausal patients with early breast cancer randomised to 3 years' goserelin plus 5 years' tamoxifen or to six cycles of CMF, adjuvant goserelin + tamoxifen was 40% more effective for recurrence-free survival. Although adjuvant therapy with anthracyclines is 13% more effective than CMF for reduction of recurrence, there are no direct comparative trials of goserelin +/− tamoxifen vs anthracycline containing chemotherapy.

In the ZEBRA trial, overall quality of life was significantly better with goserelin than with CMF during first 6 months of therapy [18]. Hormonal symptoms improved in goserelin patients at 3 years (1 year after the end of treatment) and were significantly better than CMF patient scores ($p<0.0001$). At 3 years, 1 year after end of goserelin therapy, 77% of CMF patients still had amenorrhea, compared with only 23% of goserelin patients [19].

A recent meta-analysis of 16 trials [20] showed that, together with tamoxifen, goserelin conveys similar benefits to chemotherapy without necessarily affecting fertility or inducing a permanent early menopause with its associated symptoms. These findings are rarely discussed with pre-menopausal women who might well have preferences for treatment other than chemotherapy. In one hypothetical study, 200 healthy pre-menopausal women, were shown profiles describing the administration and side-effects of goserelin and adjuvant chemotherapy; they were then asked which therapy they preferred and why. A total of 78% chose goserelin, 11% chose chemotherapy and 11% were undecided ($p<0.001$). The chemotherapy side effects women most wanted to avoid were alopecia and loss of fertility. Furthermore women regarded goserelin therapy as less disruptive than chemotherapy to their daily life [21].

It seems outrageous that so few young women worldwide are given this information or the option of avoiding chemotherapy especially as patient preferences and choice are meant to be part of the modern era of cancer care.

It is interesting to consider what choices women would make if given the information outlined above.

Patient vs Clinician Reported Side-Effects

Many of the side effects of endocrine therapy are not life threatening but are potentially quality of life threatening. Unresolved side effects may also influence adherence and outcomes so deserve more attention. When reading clinical reports it is very important to consider whether the side-effects and adverse events have been collected by physicians on case report forms or by patients using standardised QoL questionnaires. Treatment-related symptoms, documented by clinicians in medical notes during a clinical trial comparing chemotherapy with or without tamoxifen, differed from those side-effects patients reported in an interview. Hormone related side effects especially hot flushes, night sweats and fatigue were under-reported by the doctors and their severity underestimated [22]. A marked discrepancy in physician-completed CRFs and patient-reported symptoms on QoL forms has been noted in several other hormonal therapy studies. For example, in the IES trial, discordance between physicians and patients was as high as 32% for some side effects with considerable physician under-reporting of vasomotor complaints, vaginal dryness and loss of libido [23]. Likewise, in the ATAC trial it was noted that physicians tended to under-report certain side effects particularly those related to sexual function compared with women. In Canada researchers found that discordance between patient and physician recorded symptoms in breast trials were significant enough to have altered the main study findings [24].

These issues are potentially very serious and require further investigation and explanation as data collected by doctors are used not only to evaluate the effectiveness of drugs in clinical trials but are also important when discussing therapeutic options with patients.

Review of taped interviews between doctors and their patients shows that clinicians tend to monitor only those adverse events that are either potentially life-threatening or those for which they have useful interventions. There is also an ascertainment bias with selective enquiry only about the side effects in areas where problems might be predicted. Few clinicians routinely enquire about such issues as sexual functioning or gynaecological problems other than vaginal bleeding [25]. Another worry about accuracy concerns case report forms being completed by nurses or others transcribing the information written in a patient's medical notes onto the trial forms thus introducing the potential for further error. Finally, women sometime feel embarrassed discussing some symptoms or they may not even realise that they could be associated with the treatment. Without this information about the burdens experienced we are unable to provide patients with facts that might influence their choices between treatment options. Neither can we initiate research into ameliorative interventions [1].

Adherence

Even when patients have a potentially life threatening disease such as cancer it cannot be assumed that they will adhere to treatment. There are some alarming data from a variety of studies in the chemoprevention [26], early breast cancer [27] and even metastatic breast cancer [28, 29] setting that women either forget or deliberately chose not to take their medication particularly if they are getting troubling vasomotor side-effects. Some patients said that they would rather have intramuscular fulvestrant to ensure their own compliance rather than oral drugs [28]. There are physical and psychological explanations for these findings. If a woman stops her medication she 'benefits' from a reduction or cessation of side effects and the constant reminder that she is still at risk of recurrence. If she is asymptomatic she may not feel that the treatment is worthwhile [30] Given the recent work on tamoxifen metabolism and CYP2D6 it may well be the case that the very women who experience hot flushes are those who stand to gain most from medication and need to be helped to take their drugs regularly.

Conclusions

The maturing data from clinical trials of adjuvant hormone therapy in early breast cancer is demonstrating the efficacy of the AIs over tamoxifen. There is reason however to remain vigilant and to question their long term affect upon bone and fracture rates. The AIs appear to be reasonably well tolerated in the trial settings in which they have been tested, but women do have to endure non-life threatening but potentially quality of life threatening side-effects. Vasomotor problems such as hot flushes, night sweats and cold sweats are apparent with all the AIs and with tamoxifen and are bothersome enough to affect adherence.

Vaginal discharge appears greater in tamoxifen but vaginal dryness causing dyspareunia and a loss of libido are probably common to all the AIs. The arthralgias and joint pains are important to monitor especially in the more elderly patients who may well have concomitant osteoarthritis developing. If worries about an increase in the fracture rate materialise then this will have a profoundly detrimental affect upon QoL. Some have expressed concerns about the impact AIs may have on cognition. However, to date the cognitive impairments that have been found with endocrine therapy do not affect all and appear to be specific and subtle in nature. They are unlikely to be more of a problem than that which we have seen with chemotherapy [31, 32].

Finally, we need to invest in much more research on the development of effective ameliorative interventions to help patients cope with quality of life threatening side-effects [33].

References

1. Fallowfield L. Acceptance of adjuvant therapy and quality of life issues. *Breast*. 2005;14(6):612–6.
2. Goodare H, Dimmer C, Page K. ATAC trial: Reporting interim results is not helpful. *BMJ*. 2003;326(7402):1329.
3. Ware JE Jr, Sherbourne CD. The MOS 36-item short-form health survey (SF-36). I. Conceptual framework and item selection. *Med Care*. 1992;30(6):473–83.
4. Brady MJ, Cella DF, Mo F, Bonomi AE, Tulsky DS, Lloyd SR, et al. Reliability and validity of the functional assessment of cancer therapy-breast quality-of-life instrument. *J Clin Oncol*. 1997;15(3):974–86.
5. Fallowfield LJ, Leaity SK, Howell A, Benson S, Cella D. Assessment of quality of life in women undergoing hormonal therapy for breast cancer: Validation of an endocrine symptom subscale for the FACT-B. *Breast Cancer Res Treat*. 1999;55(2):189–99.
6. Hilditch JR, Lewis J, Peter A, van Maris B, Ross A, Franssen E, et al. A menopause-specific quality of life questionnaire: Development and psychometric properties. *Maturitas*. 1996;24(3):161–75.
7. Sprangers MA, Groenvold M, Arraras JI, Franklin J, te Velde A, Muller M, et al. The European Organization for Research and Treatment of Cancer breast cancer-specific quality-of-life questionnaire module: First results from a three-country field study. *J Clin Oncol*. 1996;14(10):2756–68.
8. Early, Breast, Cancer, Trialists', Collaborative, Group. Tamoxifen for early breast cancer: An overview of the randomised trials. *Lancet*. 1998;351:1451–67.
9. Howell A, Cuzick J, Baum M, Buzdar A, Dowsett M, Forbes JF, et al. Results of the ATAC (Arimidex, Tamoxifen, Alone or in Combination) trial after completion of 5 years' adjuvant treatment for breast cancer. *Lancet*. 2005;365(9453):60–2.
10. Fallowfield L, Cella D, Cuzick J, Francis S, Locker G, Howell A. Quality of life of postmenopausal women in the Arimidex, Tamoxifen, Alone or in Combination (ATAC) Adjuvant Breast Cancer Trial. *J Clin Oncol*. 2004;22(21):4261–71.
11. Cella D, Fallowfield L, Barker P, Cuzick J, Locker G, Howell A. Quality of Life of Postmenopausal Women in the ATAC ("Arimidex", Tamoxifen, Alone or in Combination) Trial after Completion of 5 years' Adjuvant Treatment for Early Breast Cancer. Breast Cancer Res Treat 2006;100(3):273–84.
12. Coombes RC, Hall E, Gibson LJ, Paridaens R, Jassem J, Delozier T, et al. A randomized trial of exemestane after two to three years of tamoxifen therapy in postmenopausal women with primary breast cancer. *N Engl J Med*. 2004;350(11):1081–92.
13. Coombes RC, Kilburn LS, Snowdon CF, Paridaens R, Coleman RE, Jones SE, et al. Survival and safety of exemestane versus tamoxifen after 2–3 years' tamoxifen treatment (Intergroup Exemestane Study): A randomised controlled trial. *Lancet*. 2007;369(9561):559–70.
14. Fallowfield LJ, Bliss JM, Porter LS, Price MH, Snowdon CF, Jones SE, et al. Quality of life in the intergroup exemestane study: a randomized trial of exemestane versus continued tamoxifen after 2 to 3 years of tamoxifen in postmenopausal women with primary breast cancer. *J Clin Oncol*. 2006;24(6):910–7.
15. Goss PE, Ingle JN, Martino S, Robert NJ, Muss HB, Piccart MJ, et al. Randomized trial of letrozole following tamoxifen as extended adjuvant therapy in receptor-positive breast cancer: updated findings from NCIC CTG MA.17. *J Natl Cancer Inst* 2005;97(17):1262–71.
16. Whelan TJ, Goss PE, Ingle JN, Pater JL, Tu D, Pritchard K, et al. Assessment of quality of life in MA.17: A randomized, placebo-controlled trial of letrozole after 5 years of tamoxifen in postmenopausal women. *J Clin Oncol*. 2005;23(28):6931–40.
17. Kaufmann M, Jonat W, Blamey R, Cuzick J, Namer M, Fogelman I, et al. Survival analyses from the ZEBRA study. goserelin (Zoladex) versus CMF in premenopausal women with node-positive breast cancer. *Eur J Cancer*. 2003;39(12):1711–7.

18. de Haes H, Olschewski M, Kaufmann M, Schumacher M, Jonat W, Sauerbrei W. Quality of life in goserelin-treated versus cyclophosphamide + methotrexate + fluorouracil-treated premenopausal and perimenopausal patients with node-positive, early breast cancer: The Zoladex Early Breast Cancer Research Association Trialists Group. *J Clin Oncol*. 2003;21(24):4510–6.
19. Jonat W, Kaufmann M, Sauerbrei W, Blamey R, Cuzick J, Namer M, et al. Goserelin versus cyclophosphamide, methotrexate, and fluorouracil as adjuvant therapy in premenopausal patients with node-positive breast cancer: The Zoladex Early Breast Cancer Research Association Study. *J Clin Oncol*. 2002;20(24):4628–35.
20. Cuzick J, Ambroisine L, Davidson N, Jakesz R, Kaufmann M, Regan M, et al. Use of luteinising-hormone-releasing hormone agonists as adjuvant treatment in premenopausal patients with hormone-receptor-positive breast cancer: a meta-analysis of individual patient data from randomised adjuvant trials. *Lancet* 2007;369(9574):1711–23.
21. Fallowfield L, McGurk R, Dixon M. Same gain, less pain: potential patient preferences for adjuvant treatment in premenopausal women with early breast cancer. *Eur J Cancer*. 2004;40(16):2403–10.
22. Fellowes D, Fallowfield LJ, Saunders CM, Houghton J. Tolerability of hormone therapies for breast cancer: How informative are documented symptom profiles in medical notes for 'well-tolerated' treatments? *Breast Cancer Res Treat*. 2001;66(1):73–81.
23. Coombes RC, Bliss J, Hall E, Fallowfield L. Under-reporting of symptoms in patients with early breast cancer who have received tamoxifen treatmentfor 2–3 years. *Proc ASCO*. 2003;22(13):(abs 48).
24. Savage C. He said/she said: How much common agreement is there on symptoms between common toxicity criteria and quality of life ? Proc ASCO. 2002;21(40):(abs 1540).
25. Stead ML, Brown JM, Fallowfield L, Selby P. Lack of communication between healthcare professionals and women with ovarian cancer about sexual issues. *Br J Cancer*. 2003;88(5):666–71.
26. Fallowfield L, Fleissig A, Edwards R, West A, Powles TJ, Howell A, et al. Tamoxifen for the prevention of breast cancer: psychosocial impact on women participating in two randomized controlled trials. *J Clin Oncol*. 2001;19(7):1885–92.
27. Partridge AH. Non-adherence to endocrine therapy for breast cancer. *Ann Oncol*. 2006;17(2):83–4.
28. Fallowfield L, Atkins L, Catt S, Cox A, Coxon C, Langridge C, et al. Patients' preference for administration of endocrine treatments by injection or tablets: results from a study of women with breast cancer. *Ann Oncol*. 2006;17(2):205–10.
29. Atkins L, Fallowfield L. Intentional and non-intentional non-adherence to medication amongst breast cancer patients. *Eur J Cancer*. 2006;42(14):2271–6.
30. Grunfeld EA, Hunter MS, Sikka P, Mittal S. Adherence beliefs among breast cancer patients taking tamoxifen. *Patient Educ Couns*. 2005;59(1):97–102.
31. Jenkins V, Shilling V, Deutsch G, Bloomfield D, Morris R, Allan S, et al. A 3-year prospective study of the effects of adjuvant treatments on cognition in women with early stage breast cancer. *Br J Cancer*. 2006;94(6):828–34.
32. Jenkins V, Atkins L, Fallowfield L. Does endocrine therapy for the treatment and prevention of breast cancer affect memory and cognition? *Eur J Cancer*. 2007;43(9):1342–7.
33. Cella D, Fallowfield L. Recognition and management of treatment related side effects for breast cancer patients receiving adjuvant endocrine therapy. *Breast Cancer Res Treat*. 2008;107(2):167–80.

Fertility

K.J. Ruddy and A.H. Partridge

Introduction

Breast cancer is the most common invasive cancer in women of childbearing age, and the most common cause of cancer-related death in young women. It is estimated that 1 in every 210 women under 40 years old will be diagnosed with breast cancer, and young women represent approximately 5% of new breast cancer patients in the United States [1]. This translates into more than 10,000 women diagnosed annually with breast cancer under age 40 in the United States alone, and over 50,000 young women diagnosed worldwide [1]. Young women with breast cancer face not only the anxieties associated with a potentially life-threatening illness and aggressive treatment, but also several unique medical and psychosocial issues. Future fertility, in particular, has been increasingly recognized as a major concern for many young breast cancer survivors [2, 3].

A diagnosis of breast cancer can compromise a woman's fertility in a number of ways. Optimal breast cancer treatment typically requires that a woman delay pregnancy for at least several months, and often many years. During this time, a woman's fertility is declining naturally with age. Breast cancer treatment, including adjuvant chemotherapy, may also diminish future fertility due to direct cytotoxic effects on the ovary. Concerns that continued menstrual cycling or pregnancy after breast cancer, particularly among women with hormone receptor-positive (HR+) tumors, may increase a woman's risk of recurrence and ultimately decrease her chances of survival complicate these issues. To date, available studies regarding pregnancy after breast cancer have revealed no clear detriment to a woman's survival. Ovarian suppression, however, is a long-standing treatment option for women with HR+ tumors, and retrospective studies have suggested that those who continue to menstruate after chemotherapy may have a greater risk of recurrence of breast cancer compared to women who experience amenorrhea [4–6]. Ongoing studies including the SOFT trial

A.H. Partridge (✉)
Dana-Farber Cancer Institute, 44 Binney St., Boston, MA 02115, USA
e-mail: ahpartridge@partners.org

M. Castiglione, M.J. Piccart (eds.), *Adjuvant Therapy for Breast Cancer*,
Cancer Treatment and Research 151, DOI 10.1007/978-0-387-75115-3_23,

(www.cancer.gov, www.ibcsg.org) should help to elucidate the risks and benefits of ovarian suppression in the era of more modern endocrine therapy, including tamoxifen.

Despite these concerns, future fertility is a vital issue for many young women with breast cancer and their families. Notwithstanding the limitations of available data, patients facing this dilemma are interested in understanding what is known and what is unknown about the risk of infertility, strategies to preserve fertility, and the safety of pregnancy after breast cancer. In the complex treatment decision-making process, patient preferences are critical, especially given the limitations of the data, and some women ultimately may be willing to compromise their therapy in the hope of improving their likelihood of having a biological child in the future [3].

Mechanisms of Ovarian Damage

There are multiple mechanisms by which chemotherapy may cause ovarian damage. The human ovary has a fixed number of primordial follicles, which is maximal at 5 months gestation and declines with age. The rate of decline rises at approximately age 37, preceding menopause by 12–14 years in the average woman. Dividing cells are most vulnerable to the actions of most cytotoxic agents, and drugs may interrupt follicular maturation. Ovarian toxicity from chemotherapy was first reported in 1956, when amenorrhea was described after treatment of a premenopausal woman with busulfan (an alkylating agent) for chronic myelogenous leukemia [7]. Alkylating agents carry the greatest risk of impaired fertility because they are not cell-cycle specific, and may damage cells that are not actively dividing including oocytes and the estrogen-producing granulosa cells and pregranulosa cells of primordial follicles. The alkylating agent cyclophosphamide is the most commonly implicated drug causing infertility, as it is widely used and carries high gonadotoxic potential by inducing inaccurate base pairings, resulting in breaks in DNA strands during replication and inhibiting protein synthesis [8]. Doxorubicin and cisplatin are thought to carry only moderate gonadotoxic potential, while risk from methotrexate and 5-fluorouracil (5-FU) is only mild [9]. The degree of damage to the ovaries will determine whether amenorrhea is temporary or permanent. If fewer oocytes remain after chemotherapy, periods may be irregular and temporary menopausal symptoms may occur. If no oocytes remain viable, periods cease and menopausal symptoms may ensue.

There is some evidence that chemotherapy given during the follicular phase of the menstrual cycle (days 1–14 of an idealized 28-day cycle in which bleeding occurs on days 1–5) is more injurious to ovarian function [10]. In the follicular phase, dividing cells surround a maturing egg until a surge of pituitary hormones induces release of the egg into the fallopian tube, and the remaining follicle becomes the corpus luteum. Drugs that interfere with DNA synthesis may be especially detrimental when given during the phase of rapid follicular cell division prior to ovulation. Some animal research supports this hypothesis [11], but other studies have not supported this finding [12].

Chemotherapy regimen likely interacts with individual patient characteristics including premorbid ovarian reserve and pharmacodynamics to determine the degree of ovarian damage sustained during breast cancer treatment. Age is the conventional surrogate for ovarian reserve, but there is considerable variation among individuals that is not accounted for by age alone. For example, there is some evidence that obese patients may be less likely to develop chemotherapy-related amenorrhea (CRA) than non-obese patients after chemotherapy [12]. Theoretically, this could be a consequence of more fragile ovaries in non-obese patients or of faster metabolism or greater volume of distribution of drugs in the obese patients. Further research to elucidate how obesity and other individual characteristics contribute to the risk of CRA and associated infertility is warranted.

Chemotherapy-Related Amenorrhea with Adjuvant Regimens for Breast Cancer

There are three substantial limitations to the available data regarding ovarian function and fertility among young breast cancer survivors: (1) most studies have used CRA as a surrogate for fertility; (2) studies generally have limited durations of follow-up; (3) patients have been grouped heterogeneously by age making cross study comparisons difficult. Despite these limitations, some generalizations can be made. There is no question that standard adjuvant breast cancer chemotherapy regimens are associated with CRA as well as with a risk of infertility. Risk of CRA increases with age and when greater cumulative dose of alkylating agents are used (see Table 1) [13]. In the International Breast Cancer Study Group (IBCSG) Trial V, 31% of the 188 premenopausal women with node-positive disease who received only one cycle of perioperative cyclophosphamide-methotrexate-fluorouracil (CMF) reported at least 3 months of amenorrhea within the 9 months after surgery, compared with 68% of the 387 similar patients who received 6–7 cycles of CMF [6]. More recently, a prospective study of 25- to 40-year-old women with breast cancer undergoing either doxorubicin-cyclophosphamide (AC, 120 pts), doxorubicin-cyclophosphamide-paclitaxel (ACT, 168 pts), CMF (83 pts), 5-FU-doxorubicin-cyclophosphamide (FAC, 38 pts), doxorubicin-cyclophosphamide-docetaxel (ACD, 19 pts), or another regimen (58 pts) found that menstrual cycles were more likely to persist after the regimens that contained a lower cumulative dose of cyclophosphamide (AC, ACT, or ACD rather than FAC or CMF) [14]. While women who were on CMF were more likely than those on AC, ACT, or ACD to bleed during the one month following chemotherapy (approximately 50% vs 20%, odds ratio 2.9, 95% CI 1.7–5), 1 year later the likelihood of menses was less in the CMF group (OR .37, 95% CI 0.37–0.67). Older age makes higher

Table 1 Risk of amenorrhea with common treatment regimens [5, 14, 18, 25, 74, 75]

Regimen	Age <30	Age 30–40	Age >40
None	~0	<5	20–25
AC × 4	–	13	57–63
CMF × 6	19	31–38	76–96
CAF/CEF × 6	23–47		80–89
TAC × 6		62	
AC × 4, T × 4		38(15% age <40)	

AC = doxorubicin and cyclophosphamide; CMF = cyclophosphamide, methotrexate, 5-fluorouracil; CAF = cyclophosphamide, doxorubicin, 5-fluorouracil; CEF = cyclophosphamide, epirubicin, 5-fluorouracil; TAC = docetaxel, doxorubicin, cyclophosphamide; T = paclitaxel

dose cyclophosphamide particularly damaging. In this study, rates of menstrual bleeding 6 months after completion of chemotherapy were approximately 85% in those <35, 61% in those 35–40, and <25% in those >40.

A meta-analysis of 12 studies confirmed that amenorrhea occurred in approximately 40% of women younger than 40, and in 76% of women older than 40 after CMF chemotherapy [15]. Anthracycline-containing regimens including cyclophosphamide-epirubicin-5-FU (CEF) may be even more gonadotoxic than CMF. In one study, premenopausal women who received CEF had a 51% risk of amenorrhea compared to a 42.6% risk in women who received CMF at 6-month follow-up [5]. However, in this study, rates of amenorrhea were similar in the two groups at 12 months (76% in CEF group, 71% in CMF group), highlighting the importance of longer term follow-up.

The gonadotoxic effect of the addition of a taxane (paclitaxel or docetaxel) to standard anthracycline-based adjuvant chemotherapy for breast cancer remains uncertain as results to date have been conflicting. A small prospective evaluation of 50 premenopausal women revealed hormonal changes in follow-up suggesting that regimens containing a taxane (including paclitaxel or docetaxel) were more gonadotoxic than those that did not [16]. Another retrospective survey of 195 breast cancer patients under age 50 found that only among women aged 40 or younger, the chance of 6 months of CRA beginning within 1 year of the start of chemotherapy was increased by the addition of 3 months of a taxane after AC (40% vs 61%, $p = .04$ in the ≤40 group; 81% vs 84%, $p = .35$ in the >40 group) [17]. In this study, however, many resumed menses in the ≤40 group after this period of CRA (33% in the AC alone group, 43% in the AC → T group). In contrast, a retrospective evaluation of 235 premenopausal women younger than 40 treated with AC followed by a taxane showed a rate of amenorrhea (17%), which was comparable to historic controls treated with AC alone [18]. Similarly, a retrospective study of 403 patients evaluated after treatment with AC or AC followed by paclitaxel every 14 or 21 days revealed no significant increase in amenorrhea at 6 months or later with the addition of paclitaxel (OR 1.45, 95% CI 0.78–2.69) or with giving the treatments more frequently in a "dose dense" fashion (OR 1.61, 95%

CI .74–3.49), when controlling for age and other variables [19]. Prospective recording of menstrual functioning, more specific assays of ovarian function, and fertility outcomes among breast cancer survivors should help to elucidate further the effects of newer chemotherapy regimens.

An additional complicating issue for young women with breast cancer considering their future fertility is that while many will remain premenopausal immediately after treatment, the duration of their premenopausal status and their associated fertility may be shortened by premature ovarian failure. Previous studies have revealed a significantly increased risk of premature menopause among childhood cancer survivors who initially remained premenopausal after treatment compared to age-matched controls [20–22]. A recent retrospective evaluation of long-term follow-up data from IBCSG Trials V and VI showed that the 227 women who remained premenopausal after 6 cycles of adjuvant CMF had high rates of menopause at 5 years even in younger age cohorts [23, 24].

In this study, a woman who was 30 years old at time of diagnosis with continued menstruation after six cycles of CMF had a 37% risk of menopause at age 35 and an 84% risk at age 40. The occurrence of not immediate, but nevertheless premature menopause following adjuvant chemotherapy is not well studied as most studies of amenorrhea have focused on earlier endpoints. However, this has important implications for the duration of fertility of breast cancer survivors and may affect a woman's decisions regarding family planning.

Impact of Hormonally Based Treatments on Fertility

Temporary manipulations of the hormonal axis appear to primarily impact fertility by delaying pregnancies, thereby allowing for natural waning of ovarian function. Previous studies have demonstrated a significant association between amenorrhea in follow-up and the use of tamoxifen [19, 25]. Goodwin and colleagues revealed that use of tamoxifen was independently associated with a small increased risk of amenorrhea at 1 year from diagnosis in a cohort of 183 premenopausal women who were treated for early stage breast cancer [25]. However, this finding likely reflects well-known temporary menstrual abnormalities induced by tamoxifen rather than any permanent ovarian damage.

Gonadotropin-releasing hormone agonists (GNRH-a) and aromatase inhibitor therapy have likewise not been found to impair reproductive function permanently. According to a study by Anderson et al., treatment for breast cancer with GNRH-a reduces estradiol (E2), luteinizing hormone (LH), follicle-stimulating hormone (FSH) and inhibin B almost immediately (after a brief initial flare). After approximately 6 months, AMH also falls [16]. GNRH-a administration downregulates pituitary release of FSH and LH, thereby preventing follicular maturation and associated hormonal changes. However, there is no change in follicular count or ovarian volume during treatment with GNRH-a other than what would be expected with age. Similarly, aromatase inhibitors, which are currently only recommended for premenopausal women in conjunction with GNRH-a in the setting of a clinical trial, may contribute to temporary hormonal changes but probably not permanent ovarian damage. There is little data on their long-term effects in the younger group of breast cancer patients, but they are unlikely to impair fertility directly.

Measuring Fertility

One of the major limitations of available information regarding fertility is the use of ongoing menses or CRA as surrogates for fertility or infertility, respectively, among breast cancer survivors. Interruptions in menstrual cycles are not entirely sensitive or specific for infertility. Some women who experience amenorrhea during or after chemotherapy later recover menses and are able to conceive. Women who menstruate after chemotherapy may still have impaired fertility. The fact that menstruation is a poor surrogate for fertility status is evident in the general population in the low rates of conception of women over 45 despite the fact that many menstruate into their 50s. Women may be infertile for 5–10 years before menses cease. In addition, hormonal treatments like tamoxifen may cause menstrual irregularities, making the presence or absence of menses even less accurate a reflection of reproductive potential. Assessment of the ability to conceive a child after treatment for breast cancer based on actual fertility outcomes including pregnancy and live births is complicated by an array of medical and psychosocial factors. Thus, many survivors are interested in better predictors and surrogate measures of fertility.

Serum levels of hormones may be better indicators of fertility than ongoing menses. E2 is produced by granulosa cells in functioning ovaries, and levels drop after menopause. After ovarian cycling stops, because estradiol provides negative feedback to FSH and LH release from the pituitary gland, FSH and LH levels rise. In general, an FSH <20 mIU/mL by radioimmunoassay, LH <20 mIU, and E2 >20 pg suggest that ovulation is still possible, and thus fertility may be preserved, even if periods are absent. Even within the normal premenopausal range of these hormones, there may be a correlation between higher levels and poorer chance of conception [26]. Furthermore, cycle length is important, as those with decreased ovarian reserve often have shorter more regular cycles due to accelerated follicle development. Pregnancy years into CRA is rare, though it is likely that many women retain some ovarian function for months to years after amenorrhea develops. There are case reports of patients becoming pregnant many years into CRA, with previous menopausal-level FSH and estradiol measurements [27].

Several other markers of ovarian reserve have been evaluated including serum inhibin levels, anti-mullerian hormone (AMH), and measurements of antral follicle count (AFC) and ovarian volume. Inhibin A is primarily secreted during the luteal phase of the ovarian cycle, while inhibin B is primarily secreted during the follicular phase. Blumenfeld et al. report that levels of both decrease during chemotherapy but return to normal range in those who eventually resume menses [28, 29]. AMH is produced by early stage ovarian follicles, so AMH level reflects ovarian reserve present in quiescent primordial follicles [30]. Antral follicle count as measured by transvaginal ultrasound during the early follicular phase (on days 2–4) of the menstrual cycle is an excellent predictor of fertility in non-cancer populations [31]. Ultrasound is usually preferable to ovarian biopsy because a biopsy specimen may inaccurately estimate the density of follicles in other areas of the ovary because distribution is very heterogeneous [32].

Ideally, these measurements of ovarian reserve should be done before women begin adjuvant hormonal therapy including tamoxifen, because hormonal manipulation can have a major impact on these values. E2 can be elevated fivefold and FSH can be markedly reduced due to long-term tamoxifen use. Because FSH is needed to stimulate follicular development, antral follicle counts while on tamoxifen may not accurately reflect potential fertility. Because AMH is produced by very early follicles and is not influenced by menstrual cycle phase [33], it may be a better indicator of ovarian reserve in a woman who has been on tamoxifen, although there are only limited available data.

Fertility Preservation Considerations in Women with Breast Cancer

Choice of Chemotherapy

For women for whom chemotherapy is necessary, but who are interested in retaining fertility, treatment with the most effective, and least gonadotoxic regimen may be prudent. It is also reasonable to consider foregoing chemotherapy in some women with low risk disease for whom the benefits may be small, and concerns about and likelihood of ovarian toxicity are high. However, for those women who do require chemotherapy and are at risk of future infertility, there are several strategies that have been explored for fertility preservation (see Table 2).

Hormonal Manipulation

Hormonal manipulation to stop ovarian cycling through treatment is one method that has been considered in order to preserve fertility. Oral contraceptive pills (OCPs), which are generally comprised of either combined estrogen and progestin or progestin alone, downregulate FSH and LH levels such that follicular growth is halted. Because fewer cells are dividing in the ovary under the influence of OCPs, it is plausible that fewer cells would be vulnerable to chemotherapeutic damage. To date, results regarding the efficacy of OCPs in reducing damage from chemotherapy are mixed, and have focused on

Table 2 Strategies for fertility preservation in women with breast cancer

Method	Risks	Efficacy
OCPs	• Theoretical stimulus to growth and development of breast cancer	Efficacy unknown
GNRH-a	• Menopausal symptoms and bone thinning	Efficacy unknown, studies ongoing
GNRH-antagonists	• Menopausal symptoms and bone thinning	Efficacy untested
Embryo cryopreservation	• Requires sperm source • Ethically problematic if patient dies • Delay in treatment • Concern that hormones may adversely impact prognosis	20–30% pregnancy rate per transfer of two or three embryos
Oocyte cryopreservation	• Concern that hormones may adversely impact prognosis	Approximately 2% pregnancy rate per thawed oocyte
Ovarian tissue cryopreservation	• Invasive • Potential for reintroduction of malignant cells at reimplantation	Case report level evidence (few babies born to date)

non-breast cancer populations. One older study (of only 44 patients) found no protective effect of oral contraceptives in women who received MVPP for Hodgkin's disease [34]. However, a survey sent to all Hodgkin's patients treated in Germany between 1994 and 1998 revealed that, of the 405 who were under age 40, those who had not been taking oral contraceptives during chemotherapy had a 44.1% rate of amenorrhea at the time of the survey, while those who had been taking them (but were no longer) only had an amenorrhea rate of 10% ($p<.0001$) [35]. Although interesting, this result could reflect the fact that younger women with better ovarian function at the time of diagnosis were more likely to have taken oral contraceptives. At present, data are too limited to recommend this approach broadly and there is limited enthusiasm for this approach for women with breast cancer due to concerns about the effects of exogenous hormones among women with hormone receptor positive disease, and uncertainty about their role in the development and promotion of hormone receptor-negative disease.

There is more interest in studying GNRH-a as ovarian protectants because they do not carry the potential risk of stimulation of cancer growth. There are multiple mechanisms by which GNRH-a are purported to protect the ovaries from chemotherapy and most animal studies do support their efficacy [36, 37]. After causing an initial flare in FSH and LH, recruiting more follicles and potentially briefly heightening sensitivity to gonadotoxic chemotherapy, GNRH-a suppresses further FSH and LH spikes, thereby interrupting the ovarian-pituitary feedback loop. If chemotherapy is given after GNRH-a administration, GNRH-a should prevent the release of FSH and LH from the pituitary in response to a fall in inhibin and estrogen concentrations when ovarian cells are killed by chemotherapy. If no FSH and LH spike occurs, maturation of more follicles is halted. If fewer follicles are maturing, fewer may be vulnerable to damage by the gonadotoxic drugs. In addition, GNRH-a treatment induces a low estrogen environment in which blood flow to ovaries and uterus may be reduced, decreasing delivery of chemotherapies to the ovaries. Furthermore, GNRH-a may bind directly to ovarian cells, decreasing apoptosis. In an ovarian carcinoma cell line in vitro, activating GNRH-I and II receptors has been found to prevent cell death [38].

Although several small clinical trials have failed to show that giving GNRH-a before and during chemotherapy for lymphoma improves rate of return of menses [39, 40], other small clinical trials do conclude that these agents may increase the likelihood of ovarian cycling after chemotherapy (see Table 3) [41, 42]. Previous single-arm studies of women with breast cancer suggest potential efficacy in this population. Recchia et al. administered goserelin monthly to 64 premenopausal women (median age 42) with early breast cancer (44% ER+). Eighteen patients received CMF, 46 received an anthracycline-based regimen, and 9 received an autologous stem cell transplant. Of these patients, 86% resumed normal menses by 12 months after they completed chemotherapy [43]. In another study, 24 premenopausal patients (median age 35) with early-stage breast cancer were given leuprolide before and during treatment [44]. Menses resumed in 23/24 by 12 months after chemotherapy (mean 5.7 months). Of the 21 not lost to follow up or death, at a mean of 34 months, 5 women had been pregnant (1 twice), with 3 of these 6 pregnancies requiring assisted reproduction techniques. To elucidate further the effects of GNRH-a for preservation of menstrual functioning and ovarian reserve in young women with breast cancer, the Southwestern Oncology Group is conducting a randomized trial among women with hormone receptor negative Stage I–IIIA breast cancer to receive or not receive goserelin through treatment (www.cancer.gov/clinicaltrials/SWOG-S0230). In the UK, the ongoing OPTION trial is similar, but also includes women with hormone receptor positive disease (www.isdscotland.org/isd/1663.html).

Because GNRH-antagonists would suppress FSH and LH release without causing an initial flare in LH and FSH levels, it has been hypothesized that these would be more efficacious ovarian protectors. However, these agents are new and very expensive, and studies have not yet evaluated their effect in women undergoing chemotherapy. It is unclear how they would directly affect the cells' apoptotic pathways. Mouse studies have not been consistent in their findings regarding efficacy of GNRH-antagonists in protection of primordial follicles [45, 46]. Another very experimental class of drugs are the anti-apoptotic agents such as sphingosine-1-phosphate. The anti-apoptotic action of GNRH-a may occur via upregulation of sphingosine-1-phosphate, an inhibitor of ceramide, a pro-apoptotic second messenger [47]. Therefore, there is interest in developing these compounds to assist in protecting gonadal tissue from chemotherapy damage.

Table 3 Evidence on efficacy of GNRH-agonists

Study	Subjects	N	Result
Recchia (2002) [43]	Early breast cancer (average 42 years old, 44% ER+) given GNRHa before/during chemo	64	86% resumed menses by 12 months after chemo
Fox (2003) [44]	24 women (average 35 years old) with early breast cancer given GNRHa before/during tx	24	23 resumed menses by 12 months (mean 5.7 months), 5 had been pregnant by 34 months, 3 had been unable to conceive despite assisted reproduction
Blumenfeld and Eckman (2005) [41]	GNRHa given to women (average 25.5 years old) receiving cytoxan for leukemia, lymphoma, or other dx compared to similarly treated pts (average 26.7 years old)	202	Premature ovarian failure in 6.7% of GNRHa treated group, but in 53.7% of the group who received chemotherapy alone ($p < .01$)
Castelo-Branco (2007) [76]	Women aged 14–45 w/ Hodgkin's were given GNRH-a plus HRT 1–2 wks pre-chemo and compared to control group who did not want to postpone chemo for GNRH-a	56	Significant differences found in FSH ($p < .001$), LH ($p < .001$), E2 ($p < .05$), inhibin A ($p < .01$) and B ($p < .05$), all suggesting better reproductive function in GNRH-a/HRT arm. No difference in bone mineral density between groups.
Pereyra Pacheco (2001) [42]	Girls aged 14.7–20 given GNRHa during tx for leukemia and lymphoma	12	100% recovered menses, two became pregnant.
Waxman (1987) [39]	Premenopausal women receiving cytoxan were randomized to buserelin or not	17	At 3 years, no difference in rates of amenorrhea (4/8 vs 5/9).

Embryo Cryopreservation

Embryo cryopreservation is the most well-established method for the treatment of infertility in the general population. For older women especially, it is the most reliable fertility preservation technique in the breast cancer patient population. Although success rates are slightly lower than with transfer of fresh embryos, women who have a partner or want to use donor sperm can freeze embryos in order to plan pregnancy after cancer treatment is completed. One persistent controversy is whether the presence of cancer limits the feasibility of in vitro fertilization (IVF) by impairing oocyte development. One small cohort study found that eight women with cancer of various types who underwent in IVF prior to treatment had fewer high quality mature oocytes retrieved than did an age-matched non-cancer group [48]. Also, stimulated cycles carry the theoretical risk that drugs used to induce ovulation may also encourage tumor growth. Estradiol levels during traditional stimulated IVF cycles are 2,000 pg/mL, while levels are only 200 pg/mL in the normal menstrual cycle. Although natural cycle IVF is an option, natural cycle IVF has a much lower efficacy than stimulated IVF. It is difficult to assess how much risk IVF poses to breast cancer prognosis. There is interest in using tamoxifen and aromatase inhibitors to prevent breast cancer proliferation during an IVF cycle prior to adjuvant therapy. Oktay et al. compared 12 women with breast cancer who were stimulated with 40–60 mg tamoxifen daily for their IVF to a retrospective control group of 5 breast cancer patients who had natural cycle IVF. Embryos were produced from all twelve tamoxifen-stimulated women, but only from three out of five of the women who underwent natural-cycle IVF [49]. Although peak estradiol level was higher in the tamoxifen group, one might expect that tamoxifen would block the effects on potential micrometastatic disease.

Letrozole either alone or in combination with FSH is another option for ovulation induction. It has been shown to be effective either 2.5–5 mg on days 3–7 of the menstrual cycle or in a 20 mg one-time dose on day 3 [50]. Oktay et al. compared several IVF regimens in 29 nonmetastatic breast cancer patients aged 24–43: tamoxifen alone, tamoxifen plus FSH, and letrozole plus FSH [51]. Tamoxifen plus FSH produced higher estradiol levels than the other two regimens. Letrozole plus FSH produced the most mature oocytes. After approximately 1.5 years, cancer had recurred in 3 of the 29 patients who had undergone IVF (not obviously different from the rate in 31 similar patients who had not received IVF). Future research to elucidate the risks and efficacy of these strategies is warranted.

Other important issues that may arise when a woman undergoes IVF in the setting of adjuvant therapy for breast cancer is the ethical dilemma that may result if a patient dies prior to the use of the resultant embryos. Consideration of this issue in the decision-making process may be prudent. Furthermore, IVF requires a 2- to 6-week delay in treatment (depending on when in the menstrual cycle a woman presents to a reproductive specialist), which may be prohibitive in some disease settings.

Oocyte Cryopreservation

Oocyte cryopreservation is another experimental strategy for fertility preservation, particularly for patients who do not have a partner and do not wish to create embryos using a sperm donor. The Practice Committee of the American Society for Reproductive Medicine recommends that oocyte cryopreservation only be offered to cancer patients as part of a research protocol because it is not yet well-studied. Technical difficulties include crystal formation causing cytoplasmic damage, sensitivity to temperature changes, depolymerization of meiotic spindle by cryoprotectants leading to aneuploidy, and hardening of the zona pellucida. Success rates are only approximately 1.6% live births per frozen oocyte, 3–4 times lower than standard embryo cryopreservation [2]. The concerns about hormonal stimulation on breast tissue apply, just as they do in traditional IVF. However, ethical issues are less problematic than when embryos are stored.

The standard technique for oocyte cryopreservation is termed "slow freeze-rapid thaw," but vitrification (use of highly concentrated cryoprotectant solution and rapid cooling to prevent ice formation) appears to improve pregnancy rate from 1.52% to 1.7% per thawed oocyte. New technologies allowing transplant of germinal vesicle oocytes may improve outcomes because of the absence of the easily damaged spindle apparatus and zona pellucida, abundant germ cells, a nuclear membrane to protect chromosomes, and less delay (only 2–5 days). However, germinal vesicle oocyte retrieval and maturation are still fraught with difficulties, so the final yield of mature oocytes may be no better than with the standard technique [9].

Ovarian Tissue Cryopreservation

Ovarian tissue cryopreservation is another novel and not yet well-tested method for allowing pregnancy after gonadotoxic treatments. Theoretically, it could allow preservation of hundreds of primordial follicles prior to chemotherapy without any need for ovarian stimulation and the associated concerns about hormonal surges, and treatment delays, as menstrual phase is irrelevant. In comparison to more mature oocytes, primordial follicles are less vulnerable to freezing-related damage due to their smaller size, slower metabolic rates, and lack of zona pellucida [9]. Limitations to the efficacy of ovarian tissue cryopreservation arise primarily from the difficulty of maturing these follicles into oocytes that are ready for fertilization. The safety of ovarian tissue cryopreservation in cancer patients has been demonstrated in several case reports; however, there are theoretical concerns about the reintroduction of cancer cells hiding in the ovary during reimplantation [52–54]. However, the rarity of ovarian-only metastases makes this fear less than overwhelming. Success rates in older patients are unclear, but in younger patients it appears that approximately 70% of follicles survive. Concerns over ischemia-reperfusion injury persist despite improving techniques. Although orthotopic placement is the only method that allows natural conception, heterotopic placement of ovarian tissue into the arm is a less invasive procedure. Xenotransplantation is not yet in use because of concerns regarding transmission of infections and abnormal oocyte development. In the future, this may facilitate repeat grafting and easy access for IVF. At present, however, this technique should be considered highly experimental and only conducted at experienced centers under IRB-approved protocols.

For some patients, a combination of these options may be the best choice. For example, a woman could have an IVF cycle or an ovarian tissue removal for cryopreservation and then start on GNRH-a before chemotherapy begins. If she regains ovulatory function after chemotherapy ends, she might attempt natural conception and only turn to the embryos or ovarian tissue she froze if she is unsuccessful. Prompt referral of any patient who expresses interest in fertility preservation is essential to allowing every woman access to the best options available to her.

Safety of Pregnancies After Breast Cancer

Outcomes of Offspring

Previous studies among select populations have suggested that 5–15% of young women with breast cancer will have a subsequent pregnancy [44, 55, 56]. Although an increased rate of birth defects might be expected in offspring conceived using eggs exposed to potentially mutagenic drugs, none has been found. In 3 large studies including nearly 4,000 offspring of survivors of childhood cancer, when clearly hereditary cancers like retinoblastoma were excluded, no statistically significant increase in cancers or malformations was detected in the offspring [57]. Some women and their families may consider preimplantation genetic testing in the setting of cancers associated with known mutations in the germ line (i.e., a BRCA 1 or 2 mutation).

Maternal Outcomes

In breast cancer, fertility preservation is more complex than in many other cancers because of concerns that hormone-receptor positive tumors will grow under the influence of high hormonal levels surrounding a pregnancy. To date, however, there is no clear evidence for a negative effect of subsequent pregnancy on the prognosis of young women with breast cancer. Several retrospective studies have evaluated the safety of pregnancy after breast cancer, comparing breast cancer survivors who had a subsequent pregnancy to those who did not (See Table 4). These studies suggest that subsequent pregnancy itself does not appear to impair prognosis of women with early stage breast cancer, and in some studies, pregnancy appears to have a protective effect [56, 58–69]. It is likely that this protective effect reflects at least to some degree a "healthy mother" effect, in which only the healthiest women attempt to and are able to become pregnant after cancer treatment [70]. However, there may also be a biological effect by which pregnancy protects against breast cancer recurrence. Conventionally, high dose estrogen and progestins have been used as a treatment modality for breast cancer. There has also been an anti-tumor effect

Table 4 Safety of pregnancy after breast cancer

First author of study (year of publication)	# Breast cancer survivors with subsequent pregnancy	# Controls	Relative risk (95% CI) of recurrence or death
Sankila(1994) [70]	91	471	0.20 (0.10–0.50)
Von Schoultz (1995) [60]	50	2,119	0.48 (0.18–1.29)
Kroman (1997) [58]	173	5,514	0.55 (0.28–1.06)
Valentgas (1999) [63]	53	265	0.80 (0.30–2.30)
Gelber (2001) [66]	94	188	0.44 (0.21–0.46)
Mueller (2003) [68]	438	2,775	0.54 (0.41–0.71)
Blakely (2004) [69]	47	323	0.70 (0.25–1.95)
Ives (2007) [56]	123	2,416	0.59 (0.37–0.95)

seen in in vitro and animal models, possibly due to signaling via the insulin growth factor pathway [71]. Nonetheless, available studies are all limited by significant biases and concerns remain for some women and their physicians regarding the safety of pregnancy after breast cancer [61]. Conducting a randomized controlled trial to answer this question more definitively would obviously be unethical. Ongoing prospective studies may help to elucidate further the potential risks and benefits of pregnancy after breast cancer.

A common recommendation is that that women wait at least 2 years after treatment is completed before attempting conception, primarily because this is the time of highest rate of aggressive recurrence, and treatment for a breast cancer may be quite complicated during a pregnancy. However, it is unclear whether a shorter wait has any effect on prognosis in a patient who does not plan to take pregnancy-prohibitive treatment such as tamoxifen during that time. Ives et al. reviewed records from women under 45 years old in Western Australia who conceived after breast cancer treatment between 1982 and 2000, finding that 123 out of 2,539 (5%) conceived, and only 50 (41%) of these had received chemotherapy [56]. Of the 123 women, 62 conceived earlier than 2 years after diagnosis. They found that women who had a pregnancy after breast cancer had better breast cancer outcomes than those who did not have such a pregnancy. This seemingly protective effect was stronger among women who became pregnant at least 2 years after diagnosis, but also present if the pregnancy was only 6 months after diagnosis. This study highlights the fact that the 2-year wait recommendation is somewhat arbitrary, especially given that rates of recurrence are significant long beyond the 2-year point and conception becomes more and more difficult with time.

Conclusion

Fertility after breast cancer is one of the most complex and difficult issues facing young women with breast cancer, their families, and their clinicians. There is some evidence, however, that more attention should be paid to this important survivorship issue. According to a survey of 166 premenopausal breast cancer patients under 50 years old, only 34% recalled a discussion with a physician about fertility, though 68% recalled a discussion about menopause [72]. In another study of 228 women under age 40 at diagnosis of breast cancer, 71% of patients recalled discussing fertility issues with a health professional as part of oncologic care [73]. A survey of 657 premenopausal women with breast cancer revealed that 57% described fertility as a major concern, and 51% said that fertility issues had been adequately addressed by their caregivers [3]. In 2006, guidelines published by the American Society of Clinical Oncology recommended that oncologists address the possibility of infertility with all patients with cancer treated during their reproductive years and be prepared to discuss possible fertility preservation options or refer interested patients to reproductive specialists as early as possible [2]. References that physicians may provide to patients include websites such as www.plwc.org, http://www.BreastCancer.Org/fertility_pregnancy_adoption.html and http://www.fertilityandcancerproject.org. Another resource is Fertile Hope (www.fertilehope.org), a nonprofit organization that provides cancer patients with reproductive information as well as emotional and financial support to facilitate infertility treatments.

Because a short delay before chemotherapy is not likely to impair outcomes in breast cancer (unlike in leukemia), avenues for fertility protection are particularly relevant in this disease. For a woman interested in assisted reproduction, early referral to an infertility specialist may be critical to avoid excessive treatment delays. However, in breast cancer patients, the issue of ovarian damage due to chemotherapy is complicated by the fact that post-treatment amenorrhea correlates with improved survival in hormone-receptor positive disease [5]. Data are limited, partly due to obstacles to randomization to fertility-preservation strategies and due to the impossibility of randomizing women to pregnancy. Nonetheless, future research is needed to empower patients to make decisions best suited to their preferences and values. Discussions of fertility should be tailored to each patient's individual priorities and risks for recurrence and infertility.

References

1. Jemal A, Siegel R, Ward E, et al. Cancer statistics, 2007. *CA Cancer J Clin.* 2007;57:43–66.
2. Lee SJ, Schover LR, Partridge AH, et al.American Society of Clinical Oncology Recommendations on Fertility Preservation in Cancer Patients. *J Clin Oncol.* 2006;24(18):2917–31.
3. Partridge AH, Gelber S, Peppercorn J, et al. Web-based survey of fertility issues in young women with breast cancer. *J Clin Oncol.* 2004;22:4174–83.
4. Pagani O, O'Neill A, Castiglione M, et al. Prognostic impact of amenorrhoea after adjuvant chemotherapy in premenopausal breast cancer patients with axillary node involvement: results of the International Breast Cancer Study Group (IBCSG) Trial VI. *Eur J Cancer.* 1998;34:632–40.
5. Parulekar WR, Day AG, Ottaway JA, et al. Incidence and prognostic impact of amenorrhea during adjuvant therapy in high-risk premenopausal breast cancer: analysis of a

National Cancer Institute of Canada Clinical Trials Group Study–NCIC CTG MA.5. *J Clin Oncol.* 2005;23:6002–8.
6. Goldhirsch A, Gelber RD, Castiglione M. The magnitude of endocrine effects of adjuvant chemotherapy for premenopausal breast cancer patients. The International Breast Cancer Study Group. *Ann Oncol.* 1990;1:183–8.
7. Louis J, Limarzi LR, Best WR. Treatment of chronic granulocytic leukemia with Myleran. *Arch Int Med.* 1956;97:299–308.
8. Falcone T, Attaran M, Bedaiwy MA, et al. Ovarian function preservation in the cancer patient. *Fertil Steril.* 2004;81:243–57
9. Marhhom E, Cohen I. Fertility preservation options for women with malignancies. *Obstet Gynecol Surv.* 2007;62:58–72.
10. Di Cosimo S, Alimonti A, Ferretti G, et al. Incidence of chemotherapy-induced amenorrhea depending on the timing of treatment by menstrual cycle phase in women with early breast cancer. *Ann Oncol.* 2004;15:1065–71.
11. Hrushesky WJ, Vyzula R, Wood PA. Fertility maintenance and 5-fluorouracil timing within the mammalian fertility cycle. *Reprod Toxicol.* 1999;13:413–20.
12. Mehta RR, Beattie CW, Das Gupta TK. Endocrine profile in breast cancer patients receiving chemotherapy. *Breast Cancer Res Treat.* 1992;20:125–32
13. Walshe JM, Denduluri N, Swain SM. Amenorrhea in premenopausal women after adjuvant chemotherapy for breast cancer. *J Clin Oncol.* 2006;24:5769–79.
14. Petrek JA, Naughton MJ, Case LD, et al. Incidence, time course, and determinants of menstrual bleeding after breast cancer treatment: A prospective study. *J Clin Oncol.* 2006;24:1045–51.
15. Bines J, Oleske DM, Cobleigh MA. Ovarian function in premenopausal women treated with adjuvant chemotherapy for breast cancer. *J Clin Oncol.* 1996;14:1718–29.
16. Anderson RA, Themmen AP, Al-Qahtani A, et al. The effects of chemotherapy and long-term gonadotrophin suppression on the ovarian reserve in premenopausal women with breast cancer. *Hum Reprod.* 2006;21:2583–92.
17. Kramer R, Tham YL, Sexton K, et al. Chemotherapy-induced amenorrhea is increased in patients treated wtih adjuvant doxorubicin and cyclophosphamide (AC) followed by a taxane (T). *J Clin Oncol, ASCO Annual Meeting Proceedings* 2005;23:651.
18. Fornier MN, Modi S, Panageas KS, et al. Incidence of chemotherapy-induced, long-term amenorrhea in patients with breast carcinoma age 40 years and younger after adjuvant anthracycline and taxane. *Cancer.* 2005;104:1575–9.
19. Abusief ME, Missmer SA, Ginsburg ES, et al. Chemotherapy-related amenorrhea in women with early breast cancer: The effect of paclitaxel or dose density. Journal of Clinical Oncology, *ASCO Annual Meeting Proceedings* (Post-Meeting Edition). 2006;24:10506.
20. Byrne J, Fears TR, Gail MH, et al. Early menopause in long-term survivors of cancer during adolescence. *Am J Obstet Gynecol.* 1992;166:788–93.
21. Chiarelli AM, Marrett LD, Darlington G. Early menopause and infertility in females after treatment for childhood cancer diagnosed in 1964–1988 in Ontario, Canada. *Am J Epidemiol.* 1999;150:245–54.
22. Sklar CA, Mertens AC, Mitby P, et al. Premature menopause in survivors of childhood cancer: A report from the childhood cancer survivor study. *J Natl Cancer Inst.* 2006;98:890–6.
23. Partridge A, Gelber S, Gelber R, et al. Delayed premature menopause following chemotherapy for early stage breast cancer: Long-term results from IBCSG Trial V. *Proc Am Soc Clin Oncol.* 2005;23:50s (abstract 687)
24. Partridge A, Gelber S, Gelber R, et al. Age of menopause among women who remain premenopausal following treatment for early breast cancer: long-term results from International Breast Cancer Study Group Trials V and VI. *Eur J Cancer*. In press
25. Goodwin PJ, Ennis M, Pritchard KI, et al. Risk of menopause during the first year after breast cancer diagnosis. *J Clin Oncol.* 1999;17:2365–70.

26. Weghofer A, Margreiter M, Fauster Y, et al. Age-specific FSH levels as a tool for appropriate patient counselling in assisted reproduction. *Hum Reprod.* 1005;20:2448.–52
27. Bath LE, Tydeman G, Critchley HOD, et al. Spontaneous conception in a young woman who had ovarian cortical tissue cryopreservation before chemotherapy and radiotherapy for a Ewing's sarcoma of the pelvis: Case report. *Hum Reprod.* 2004;19:2569–72.
28. Blumenfeld Z, Ritter M, Shen-Orr Z, et al. Inhibin A concentrations in the sera of young women during and after chemotherapy for lymphoma: Correlation with ovarian toxicity. *Am J Reprod Immunol.* 1998;39:33–40
29. Blumenfeld Z. Preservation of fertility and ovarian function and minimalization of chemotherapy associated gonadotoxicity and premature ovarian failure: The role of inhibin-A and -B as markers. *Mol Cell Endocrinol.* 2002;187:93–105.
30. van Rooij IA, Broekmans FJ, te Velde ER, et al. Serum anti-Mullerian hormone levels: A novel measure of ovarian reserve. *Hum Reprod.* 2002;17:3065–71
31. Scheffer GJ, Broekmans FJ, Looman CW, et al. The number of antral follicles in normal women with proven fertility is the best reflection of reproductive age. *Hum Reprod.* 2003;18:700–6.
32. Schmidt KL, Byskov AG, Nyboe Andersen A, et al. Density and distribution of primordial follicles in single pieces of cortex from 21 patients and in individual pieces of cortex from three entire human ovaries. *Hum Reprod.* 2003;18:1158–64.
33. Cook CL, Siow Y, Taylor S, et al. Serum mullerian-inhibiting substance levels during normal menstrual cycles. *Fertil Steril.* 2000;73:859–61.
34. Whitehead E, Shalet SM, Blackledge G, et al. The effect of combination chemotherapy on ovarian function in women treated for Hodgkin's disease. *Cancer.* 1983;52:988–93.
35. Behringer K, Breuer K, Reineke T, et al. Secondary amenorrhea after Hodgkin's lymphoma is influenced by age at treatment, stage of disease, chemotherapy regimen, and the use of oral contraceptives during therapy: A report from the German Hodgkin's Lymphoma Study Group. *J Clin Oncol.* 2005;23:7555–64.
36. Ataya K, Rao LV, Lawrence E, et al. Luteinizing hormone-releasing hormone agonist inhibits cyclophosphamide-induced ovarian follicular depletion in rhesus monkeys. *Biol Reprod.* 1995;52:365–72.
37. Letterie GS. Anovulation in the prevention of cytotoxic-induced follicular attrition and ovarian failure. *Hum Reprod.* 2004;19:831–7.
38. Grundker C, Emons G. Role of gonadotropin-releasing hormone (GnRH) in ovarian cancer. *Reprod Biol Endocrinol.* 2003;1:65.
39. Waxman JH, Ahmed R, Smith D, et al. Failure to preserve fertility in patients with Hodgkin's disease. *Cancer Chemother Pharmacol.* 1987;19:159–62
40. Dann EJ, Epelbaum R, Avivi I, et al. Fertility and ovarian function are preserved in women treated with an intensified regimen of cyclophosphamide, adriamycin, vincristine and prednisone (Mega-CHOP) for non-Hodgkin lymphoma. *Hum Reprod.* 2005;20:2247–9.
41. Blumenfeld Z, Eckman A. Preservation of fertility and ovarian function and minimization of chemotherapy-induced gonadotoxicity in young women by GnRH-a. *J Natl Cancer Inst Monogr.* 2005;40–3
42. Pereyra Pacheco B, Mendez Ribas JM, Milone G, et al. Use of GnRH analogs for functional protection of the ovary and preservation of fertility during cancer treatment in adolescents: A preliminary report. *Gynecol Oncol.* 2001;81:391–7
43. Recchia F, Sica G, De Filippis S, et al. Goserelin as ovarian protection in the adjuvant treatment of premenopausal breast cancer: A phase II pilot study. *Anticancer Drugs.* 2002;13:417–24.
44. Fox KR, Scialla J, Moore H. Preventing chemotherapy-related amenorrhea using leuprolide during adjuvant chemotherapy for early-stage breast cancer [abstract 50]. *Proc ASCO.* 2003;22:13.

45. Danforth DR, Arbogast LK, Friedman CI. Acute depletion of murine primordial follicle reserve by gonadotropin-releasing hormone antagonists. *Fertil Steril.* 2005;83:1333–8
46. Meirow D, Assad G, Dor J, et al. The GnRH antagonist cetrorelix reduces cyclophosphamide-induced ovarian follicular destruction in mice. *Hum Reprod.* 2004;19:1294–9.
47. Morita Y, Perez GI, Paris F, et al. Oocyte apoptosis is suppressed by disruption of the acid sphingomyelinase gene or by sphingosine-1-phosphate therapy. *Nat Med.* 2000;6:1109–14.
48. Pal L, Leykin L, Schifren JL, et al. Malignancy may adversely influence the quality and behaviour of oocytes. *Hum Reprod.* 1998;13:1837–40.
49. Oktay K, Buyuk E, Davis O, et al. Fertility preservation in breast cancer patients: IVF and embryo cryopreservation after ovarian stimulation with tamoxifen. *Hum Reprod.* 2003;18:90–5.
50. Mitwally MF, Casper RF. Single-dose administration of an aromatase inhibitor for ovarian stimulation. *Fertil Steril.* 2005;83:229–31.
51. Oktay K, Buyuk E, Libertella N, et al. Fertility preservation in breast cancer patients: A prospective controlled comparison of ovarian stimulation with tamoxifen and letrozole for embryo cryopreservation. *J Clin Oncol.* 2005;23:4347–53.
52. Kim SS, Radford J, Harris M, et al. Ovarian tissue harvested from lymphoma patients to preserve fertility may be safe for autotransplantation. *Hum Reprod.* 2001;16:2056–60.
53. Donnez J, Dolmans MM, Demylle D, et al. Restoration of ovarian function after orthotopic (intraovarian and periovarian) transplantation of cryopreserved ovarian tissue in a woman treated by bone marrow transplantation for sickle cell anaemia: case report. *Hum Reprod.* 2006:21:183–8.
54. Donnez J, Dolmans MM, Demylle D, et al. Livebirth after orthotopic transplantation of cryopreserved ovarian tissue. *Lancet.* 2004;364:1405–10.
55. Partridge A, Gelber S, Peppercorn J, et al. Fertility outcomes in young women with breast cancer: A web-based survey. *Proc ASCO.* 2004;23:538 [abstract #6085].
56. Ives A, Saunders C, Bulsara M, et al. Pregnancy after breast cancer: Population based study. *BMJ.*2007;334:194.
57. Hawkins MM. Pregnancy outcome and offspring after childhood cancer. *BMJ.* 1994;309:1034.
58. Kroman N, Jensen MB, Melbye M, et al. Should women be advised against pregnancy after breast-cancer treatment? *Lancet.* 1997;350:319–22.
59. Sankila R, Heinavaara S, Hakulinen T. Survival of breast cancer patients after subsequent term pregnancy: "Healthy mother effect". *Am J Obstet Gynecol.* 1994;170:818–23.
60. von Schoultz E, Johansson H, Wilking N, et al. Influence of prior and subsequent pregnancy on breast cancer prognosis. *J Clin Oncol.* 1995;13:430–4.
61. Petrek JA. Pregnancy safety after breast cancer. *Cancer.* 1994;74:528–31.
62. Gemignani ML, Petrek JA. Pregnancy After Breast Cancer. *Cancer Control.* 1999;6:272–6.
63. Velentgas P, Daling JR, Malone KE, et al. Pregnancy after breast carcinoma: Outcomes and Influence on Mortality. *Cancer.* 1999;85:2424–32.
64. Dow KH. Having children after breast cancer. *Cancer Pract.* 1994;2:407–13.
65. Higgins S, Haffty BG. Pregnancy and lactation after breast-conserving therapy for early stage breast cancer. *Cancer.* 1994;73:2175–80.
66. Gelber S, Coates AS, Goldhirsch A, et al. Effect of pregnancy on overall survival after the diagnosis of early-stage breast cancer. *J Clin Oncol.* 2001;19:1671–5.
67. Upponi SS, Ahmad F, Whitaker IS, et al. Pregnancy after breast cancer. *Eur J Cancer.* 2003;39:736–41.
68. Mueller BA, Simon MS, Deapen D, et al. Childbearing and survival after breast carcinoma in young women. *Cancer.* 2003;98:1131–40.
69. Blakely LJ, Buzdar AU, Lozada JA, et al. Effects of pregnancy after treatment for breast carcinoma on survival and risk of recurrence. *Cancer.* 2004;100:465–9.

70. Sankila R, Heinavaara S, Hakulinen T. Survival of breast cancer patients after subsequent term pregnancy: "Healthy mother effect". *Am J Obstet Gynecol.* 1994;170:818–23.
71. Yuri T, Tsukamoto R, Miki K, et al. Biphasic effects of zeranol on the growth of estrogen receptor-positive human breast carcinoma cells. *Oncol Rep.* 2006;16:1307–12.
72. Duffy CM, Allen SM, Clark MA. Discussions regarding reproductive health for young women with breast cancer undergoing chemotherapy. *J Clin Oncol.* 2005;23:766–73.
73. Thewes B, Meiser B, Taylor A, et al. Fertility- and menopause-related information needs of younger women with a diagnosis of early breast cancer. *J Clin Oncol.* 2005;23:5155–65.
74. Burstein HJ, Winer EP. Primary care for survivors of breast cancer. *N Engl J Med.* 2000;343:1086–94.
75. Martin M, Pienkowski T, Mackey J, et al. Adjuvant docetaxel for node-positive breast cancer. *N Engl J Med.* 2005;352:2302–13.
76. Castelo-Branco C, Nomdedeu B, Camus A, et al. Use of gonadotropin-releasing hormone agonists in patients with Hodgkin's disease for preservation of ovarian function and reduction of gonadotoxicity related to chemotherapy. *Fertil Steril.* 2007;87:702–5.

Cognitive Function in Breast Cancer Survivors

Janette Vardy

Cancer survivors have coined the terms "chemobrain" and "chemofog" to refer to the problems that patients experience with their memory and/or concentration during and after completing chemotherapy. A number of studies have confirmed that some breast cancer survivors suffer cognitive impairment after chemotherapy [1–8], although recent studies have found that some women's cognitive impairment may predate the chemotherapy [9], and hormonal treatment may also impact on cognitive function [8, 10]. For most women the problem appears subtle and often improves after ceasing chemotherapy; however, for a subset of survivors, the symptoms are sustained and can impact significantly on their quality of life and ability to function in their everyday activities [7, 11, 12].

Cognitive studies in cancer patients who have received chemotherapy are inconsistent in describing the types of neuropsychological dysfunction found, although commonly affected cognitive domains are attention/concentration, verbal and visual memory, and processing speed [1–8, 13]. Similar types of cognitive impairment have been identified in patients with early stage human immunodeficiency virus (HIV) infection [14, 15], Huntington's disease [16], Parkinson's disease [17] and multiple sclerosis [18]. In each of these diseases, when cognitive dysfunction occurs, it is generally subtle, "spotty" and variable from one patient to the next [14, 19]. A number of neuropsychologists believe that the deficits found are generally more consistent with sub-cortical abnormality [14, 15, 20–23] as distinct from the cortical deficits seen in dementias.

Age, intelligence quotient (IQ) and education are all factors that can influence cognitive function [24, 25] and are often corrected for in standard neuropsychological tests. Other variables that may affect cognitive function, particularly in the context of a cancer diagnosis, but are more difficult to correct

J. Vardy (✉)
Sydney Cancer Centre, Concord Repatriation General Hospital, Department of Medical Oncology, The University of Sydney, Cancer Institute NSW, Concord, Australia
e-mail: jvardy@med.usyd.edu.au

M. Castiglione, M.J. Piccart (eds.), *Adjuvant Therapy for Breast Cancer*, Cancer Treatment and Research 151, DOI 10.1007/978-0-387-75115-3_24,

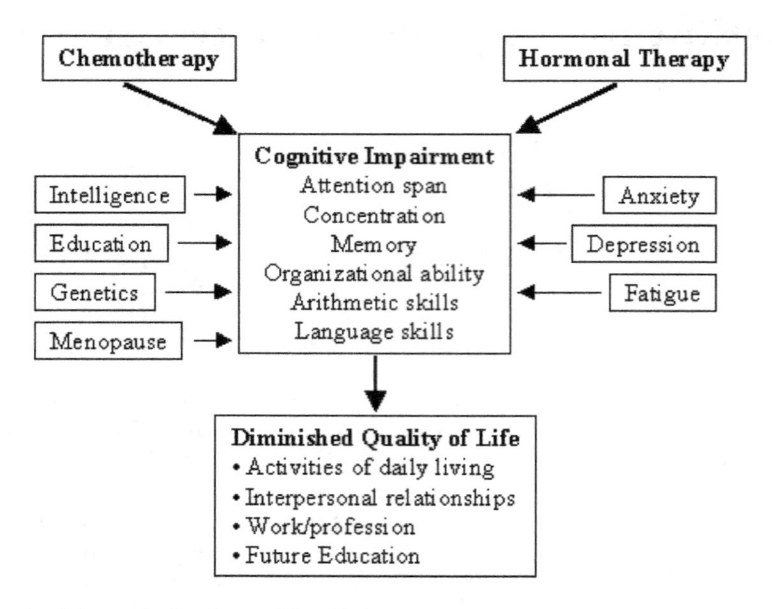

Reprinted with permission from: Olin JJ. Cognitive function after systemic therapy for breast cancer. *Oncology*, 15, Number 5, 2001

Fig. 1 Effect of Chemohormonal Therapy on Cognitive Function and Quality of Life

for, include fatigue, anxiety and depression [25, 26]. Information on these variables (summarised in Fig. 1 and discussed below) needs to be included in cognitive studies in order to be able to determine their impact on neuropsychological function.

Overview of the Literature

The earliest reports of cognitive dysfunction in relation to chemotherapy were by Weiss and colleagues and appeared in 1974 [27, 28]. A limited number of small studies evaluating cognitive impairment after chemotherapy in breast cancer patients was published in the subsequent 25 years [29–35], but it has only been in the last 10 years that larger studies have been published [1–6, 8, 9, 13, 36–44]. There has been very little research performed investigating cognitive function in non-breast cancer survivors, and there are still more reviews of cognitive impairment post-chemotherapy [7, 11, 13, 25, 26, 30, 34, 36, 45–80] than original studies.

Table 1 summarises the main cognitive studies that have been published in breast cancer survivors and the incidence of cognitive impairment found. The major studies will be discussed below.

Table 1 Summary of cognitive articles in breast cancer survivors

First author (year)	Study design	Sample size	Patient groups ± controls	Neuropsychological assessments	Mean time from start of CT	% Overall cognitive impairment/comments
Van Dam (1998) [3]	Cross sectional	34	BC post-high dose CT	Traditional battery (2 h)	2 years	32
		36	BC post-standard CT (FEC)			17
		34	BC no CT			9
Schagen (1999) [4]	Cross sectional	39	BC post–CT (CMF)	Traditional battery	>6 months	28
		34	BC no CT	(2 h)	~ 2 years	12
Schagen (2002) [42]	Cross sectional (Follow up of previous studies)	22	BC post-high dose CT	Traditional battery (2 h)	~4 years	14
		23	BC post-standard CT (FEC)			9
						13
		31	BC post-standard CT (CMF)			
		27	BC No CT			11
Ahles (2002) [2]	Cross sectional	71	BC or lymphomapost–CT	Traditional battery (2 h)	10 years	39
		57	BC or lymphoma No CT			14
Brezden (2000) [1]	Cross sectional	31	BC on CT	HSCS	On CT	48
		40	BC post–CT	(25 min)	2 years	50
		36	Healthy controls		-	11
Tchen (2003) [6]	Cross sectional	100	BC on CT	HSCS	On CT	16
		100	Healthy controls	Trails A & B CCP	-	4
Mar Fan (2005) [40]	Cross sectional	91	BC post-CT (1 year)	HSCS	1 yr	4.4
	(1 and 2 years follow up of Tchen Study)	83	Healthy controls (1 year)	Trails A & B CCP	2 yr	3.6
		83	BC post-CT (2 years)			3.8
		81	Healthy controls (2 years)			0

Table 1 (continued)

First author (year)	Study design	Sample size	Patient groups ± controls	Neuropsychological assessments	Mean time from start of CT	% Overall cognitive impairment/comments
Vardy (2006) [125]	Longitudinal	31	BC and CRC assessed three times Healthy controls	HSCS Coghealth (18 min) Headminder (30 min)	On CT or within 2 years	N/A Cancer group on HSCS: 30% time 1 5% time 2 6% time 3
Wienneke (1995) [81]	Cross sectional	28	BC post-CT	Traditional battery (2.5–3 h)	~6 months post-CT	75
Wefel (2004) [9]	Cross sectional	84	BC pre CT	Traditional batteries: 5–14 tests	Pre CT	35
Wefel (2004) [44]	Prospective longitudinal 0, 6 and 18 months	18	BC to receive CT baseline	Traditional batteries: 14 tests	Pre CT 6 months 18 months	33 61% decline Most stable or improved
Castellon (2004) [8]	Cross sectional	36 19 19	BC post-CT BC no CT Healthy controls	Traditional battery and computer test (~2 h)	2–5 years 2–5 years -	N/A CT group worse than non-CT but not different to controls
Jacobsen (2004) [167]	Longitudinal	77	Mixed solid tumors (10% BC)	Battery 7 tests	Pre CT Pre C4	N/A
Donovan (2005) [38]	Cross sectional	60 83	BC post-CT BC no CT	Traditional battery 9 tests	~1 year	N/A No difference between groups
Freeman (2002) [13]	Cross sectional	8 9	BC on CT BC post-CT	Traditional battery 20 tests (3 h)	On CT 6–12 months post-CT	N/A CT worse than post-CT
O'Shaugh-nessy (2005) [112]	Longitudinal	47 47	BC on CT on epoetin alpha BC on CT on placebo	EXIT 25 CLOK (20 min)	0, pre cycle 4 and 6 months post-CT	N/A No difference in groups at 6 months

Table 1 (continued)

First author (year)	Study design	Sample size	Patient groups ± controls	Neuropsychological assessments	Mean time from start of CT	% Overall cognitive impairment/comments
Shilling (2005) [85]	Longitudinal (preliminary analysis of Jenkins article)	50 43	BC pre CT Healthy controls baseline	Traditional battery 14 tests	0 and 6 months	Decline in 34% on CT vs 19% controls
Jenkins (2006) [39]	Longitudinal	85 43 49	BC who will have CT BC not for CT Healthy controls	Traditional battery 9 tests	0, 6 and 18 months	Decline in 20% on CT at 6 mo, 18% at 18 mo vs 26%/14% no CT & 18%/11% healthy controls
Bender (2005) [37]	Longitudinal	19 15 12	BC who will have CT BC for CT and tamoxifen DCIS	Battery (90 min)	0, 6 & 18 months	Worse memory in CT groups
Scherwath (2006) [43]	Cross sectional	24 23 29	BC post-high dose CT BC post-standard dose CT BC no CT	Traditional battery and computer test (<2 h)	5 years post-CT	8 13 3
Cimprich 1998 [222]	Longitudinal	74	BC pre surgery BC post-surgery	Attention battery 4 tests	Pre-surgery and post-surgery	N/A Older women only showed decline post Surgery

Table 1 (continued)

First author (year)	Study design	Sample size	Patient groups ± controls	Neuropsychological assessments	Mean time from start of CT	% Overall cognitive impairment/comments
Cimprich (2001) [223]	Longitudinal	47 48	Elderly BC Controls with no BC	Attention battery	Pre surgery, 2 weeks and 3 months post-surgery for BC. For non BC: post-MMG and 3/12 later	N/A Cancer group scored worse than controls at baseline, no change at 2 weeks.
Cimprich (2005) [84]	Cross sectional	184	BC pre-surgery	Attention battery	18 days pre surgery	N/A Mean scores within normal range
Gottschalk (2003) [224]	Longitudinal	12	BC	Computerised speech analysis	Pre and immediately post-CT on C1, C3 and post-C4	N/A
Servaes (2002) [100]	Cross sectional	150 78	BC <50 years old at diagnosis (heterogenous treatments) Age matched healthy controls	Reaction time Digit symbol	Mean 28 months post-treatment	N/A BC survivors worse slower reaction time

BC = Breast cancer; DCIS = Ductal carcinoma in situ; CRC = Colorectal cancer; CT = Chemotherapy; RT = Radiotherapy; PCI = Prophylactic cranial irradiation; SD = Standard deviation; HSCS = High Sensitivity Cognitive Screen; CCP = Conner's Continuous Performance Test; RCI = Reliable Change Index; ANOVA = Analysis of Variance; Sx = Surgery; OR = Odds ratio; MMG = Mammogram; Pt = Patient; Mo = Months; EXIT25 = Executive Interview

Wieneke and Dienst first used comprehensive neuropsychological tests to evaluate cognitive impairment in women with breast cancer 3–18 months post-chemotherapy (predominantly cyclophosphamide, methotrexate and 5-fluorouracil [CMF]) and compared the results to published normative data. As many as 75% of women were reported to have cognitive impairment based on a definition of >2 standard deviations (SD) below the normative mean in at least 1 of 16 tests [81]. No association was found between cognitive impairment and chemotherapy regimen, time from treatment, or depression, although increased duration of chemotherapy was associated with worse cognitive impairment. The main domains affected were concentration and memory. This paper stimulated further research, although thankfully this high degree of impairment has not been found in subsequent studies. The main weaknesses of this study are that normative data only was used for comparison, the sample size was small, and the definition for cognitive impairment required impairment on only one test.

The Dutch group, led by van Dam, published a study in 1998 that compared lymph node positive breast cancer patients randomised to either standard dose chemotherapy (5-fluorouracil, epirubicin and cyclophosphamide [FEC]) plus tamoxifen or high dose chemotherapy (FEC-cyclophosphamide, thiotepa, carboplatin (CTC) with peripheral blood stem cell transplant) plus tamoxifen, vs a control group with stage 1 disease, who did not receive chemotherapy. Patients were a mean of 2 years post-chemotherapy. A comprehensive neuropsychological battery was used to assess seven cognitive domains, and cognitive impairment was defined as greater than 2 SD below the control group mean for individual tests and below the fifth percentile of controls overall. They showed that 32% of those receiving high dose chemotherapy had cognitive impairment, compared to 17% of those who received standard dose chemotherapy, and 9% of women who received local treatment only ($p = 0.043$) [3]. This study was important both for its methodology, and in demonstrating a likely dose dependent relationship for cognitive impairment.

A subsequent study compared patients who were lymph node positive and received CMF chemotherapy with the same control group from the previous study (lymph node negative patients not receiving chemotherapy). Cognitive impairment in the chemotherapy arm was 28% as compared to 12% for those receiving only local treatment, with memory and concentration the main domains affected. This study demonstrated a significant difference between two groups in which all subjects had breast cancer, albeit with a difference in severity of disease, and had all been through the stress of diagnosis and local treatment (surgery and radiotherapy) approximately 2 years previously (OR 6.4, 95% CI 1.5–27.6, $p = 0.013$) [4].

Follow up of patients from both of the above studies showed improvement in cognitive function in all chemotherapy groups, with mild deterioration in the control group, approximately 4 years post-treatment. No significant difference was found between the groups in the incidence of cognitive impairment, although more of the high dose chemotherapy group were not assessed due to disease progression. There was no difference in anxiety, fatigue or depression between the arms [42].

The Toronto group, led by Tannock, published a pilot study in 2000 in which they found substantial cognitive impairment in 48% of patients receiving chemotherapy (mainly CMF), compared with 50% of patients that had received chemotherapy more than 1 year previously, and 11% of healthy controls ($p<0.002$) [1]. This was followed by the largest published study to date, which compared 100 patients receiving adjuvant chemotherapy (mainly anthracycline-based) with age-matched controls nominated by the patients, and evaluated cognitive function, fatigue and menopausal symptoms. Large and highly significant differences in fatigue and menopausal symptoms were found between patients and controls, with moderate-severe cognitive impairment in 16% of patients compared to 4% of the controls ($p = 0.008$) on the High Sensitivity Cognitive Screen (HSCS). A strong correlation was found between fatigue, menopausal symptoms and quality of life, but none were significantly associated with cognitive dysfunction [82]. The patients and controls were re-evaluated 1 and 2 years later and cognitive function appeared to improve to within normal range in most subjects [40], although this may be due to practice effect associated with the use of the HSCS [83] (see below).

Ahles and his colleagues assessed breast cancer and lymphoma survivors a minimum of 5 years post-treatment and compared survivors who had received chemotherapy with those who had received local treatment only. Of chemotherapy patients, 39% had cognitive impairment (below the 25th percentile on Z score in at least 3/9 domains) compared with 14% who received local treatment only ($p<0.002$). Although the cognitive impairment was global, verbal memory and executive function domains were the most affected [2].

Wefel and colleagues combined data from three separate studies assessing 84 breast cancer patients after either surgery or core-needle biopsy and prior to any chemotherapy. They found that 35% had cognitive impairment, based on impairment in at least 1 of up to 14 tests. The main domains affected were verbal learning (18%) and memory (25%) [9]. The same group published the first prospective longitudinal study in which 18 breast cancer patients were assessed pre-chemotherapy, at approximately 6 months post-baseline (>3 weeks post-chemotherapy) and again at 18 months. Prior to chemotherapy, 33% of patients had cognitive impairment; at 6 months, 61% had cognitive decline in at least one domain; and at 18 months, 50% of those with decline had improved and 50% remained stable (although below baseline) [44]. The main domains affected were attention, learning speed and information processing speed. At baseline and 6 months there was no association found between cognitive impairment and age, education, menopausal status, radiotherapy, hormone replacement therapy history or tumour stage. There was no correlation between cognitive function and depression or anxiety at any time point.

Despite methodological problems, the Wefel studies raise the important question as to whether there is a higher rate of cognitive impairment pre-chemotherapy than previously appreciated, which might have been attributed to the effects of chemotherapy in the cross-sectional studies. Another study, albeit with a limited neuropsychological battery, suggests that post-diagnosis, but prior to surgery, cognitive function is not impaired in women with breast cancer [84]. A longitudinal study by Bender and colleagues evaluated 46 women at baseline (post-surgery and pre-chemotherapy) with assessments at approximately 6 and 18 months; only 21 women completed the 18-month assessment. Patients with breast cancer receiving chemotherapy and tamoxifen were compared with patients receiving chemotherapy alone, and with women with ductal carcinoma in situ (DCIS) who did not receive chemotherapy or hormonal treatment. Those who received chemotherapy and tamoxifen had decline on visual and verbal working memory at 18 months, whilst women who received chemotherapy alone had deterioration in verbal working memory only. The healthy controls had improvement in cognitive scores, consistent with practice effect [37]. Both the above longitudinal studies (albeit with small sample sizes) support the findings of the majority of the cross-sectional studies that a subset of patients experience a decline in cognitive impairment with chemotherapy, and help to define domain specific deficits.

By contrast, the larger longitudinal study by Jenkins and colleagues found that only a non-significant minority of patients experienced decline in cognitive function after chemotherapy [39, 85]. Their study evaluated 85women with breast cancer who were to receive chemotherapy (predominantly FEC), 43 who were to have local treatment only (hormone treatment and/or radiotherapy) and 49 healthy controls. Subjects were assessed at baseline (pre-chemotherapy), at 6 months (post-chemotherapy), and at 18 months. Although more women with cancer had a decline on multiple measures than healthy controls there was no statistically significant difference in cognitive decline between the three groups, with 20% of the chemotherapy group, 26% of the hormone group and 18% of the controls having declined at 6 months, and 18%, 14% and 11% respectively at 18 months. Women who had a treatment-induced menopause had a trend to more cognitive decline at 6 months (OR 2.6, 95% CI 0.82–8.3, $p = 0.09$). There was no association of objective cognitive function with self reported impairment, quality of life or psychological distress, although the later three variables were significantly intercorrelated [39].

Determining if Cognitive Impairment Is Present

A major difficulty in evaluating cognitive function is determining what constitutes impairment. There is no consistency in the definition of cognitive dysfunction used in the cancer studies or in the neuropsychological literature. Most cognitive tests report their results as Z (mean = 0; SD = 1) or T (mean = 50; SD = 10) scores, thus indicating how many standard deviations (SD) an observation is from the mean for a "normal" population. A definition of cognitive impairment is usually based on cut-off scores for the various tests.

Subtle cognitive impairment is most commonly defined as >1 SD below the mean, while more severe impairment is defined by a cut-off at 1.5–2 SD below the mean [22, 86]. The definition of cognitive impairment is complex because neuropsychological batteries include several tests, which are scored individually. If an abnormal result on any single test is used to define cognitive impairment, the probability of falsely classifying a subject as impaired increases with the number of neuropsychological tests, such that with 20 tests and a significance level of 5%, the probability of at least one significant result given no true difference is 0.64 [87]. Most studies require impairment on more than one measure to classify a subject's performance as abnormal, but false positives and negatives will still occur.

One way to mitigate the problem of multiple tests is to compute a summary score or a neuropsychological impairment score to reflect overall performance [88]. Deficit scores can be calculated for each domain and then an average computed: they are weighted by both the number and severity of deficits and have been used widely to define cognitive impairment [19, 20, 89].

Of paramount importance to the survivor is whether her cognitive function has deteriorated in comparison to pre-morbid status. The major limitation of the cross-sectional studies is the lack of evaluation of cognitive function prior to chemotherapy and no longitudinal data. Lack of pre-chemotherapy or pre-surgery baseline assessments means that women who were functioning at a high level prior to diagnosis may have had a substantial decline in cognitive function but still formally score within normal limits so that the degree of their cognitive decline is not recognised [25, 90, 91]. Conversely, lack of baseline assessments can mean that impairment that was already present prior to chemotherapy is being incorrectly assumed to be secondary to chemotherapy [25, 91]. However, baseline evaluations have their own limitations, as they may be confounded by the stress related to a new life-threatening diagnosis, anaesthesia and surgery.

Neuropsychological Tests

Neuropsychological tests should be valid, reliable and have good sensitivity and specificity. The test battery selected needs to be able to identify correctly subjects who do and do not have cognitive impairment [92]. An individual's cognitive function is likely to decline initially during chemotherapy and then either stabilize or improve after ceasing treatment. Tests that are administered to the same subjects more than once need to be responsive; that is, to detect change when it occurs [93]. Unless the cognitive battery is responsive, and testing is performed at appropriate time intervals, the decline may be missed. Responsiveness is confounded by practice effect, whereby subjects perform better on subsequent tests, and this needs to be accounted for in longitudinal studies which must differentiate between true change in performance, practice effect and chance variation.

Most neuropsychologists recommend a comprehensive battery of neuropsychological tests as the "gold standard" for assessing cognitive function, but vary in opinion as to which tests, and how many, should be incorporated into a battery. A test battery should include assessment of the full range of psychological functions, both general and specific, allow comparison to a control group or normative data, and include validated tests with good sensitivity and specificity [94]. Extensive batteries take several hours [15, 95], and require a trained psychometrist to administer, and a neuropsychologist to interpret them [96]. An 8-h battery has been recommended for subjects with Human Immunodeficiency Virus (HIV) [15], but is not feasible for large trials or for patients about to receive chemotherapy, many of whom have had a recent diagnosis of cancer and major surgery.

Testing of cognitive function is a compromise between extensive batteries, which are likely to be more sensitive and detect more subtle impairment, and shorter tests that are more practical for serial assessment of patients receiving chemotherapy. The latter seek to determine if impairment is present, and to indicate whether in-depth testing is warranted. However, very brief screening tests are unlikely to provide helpful information and in particular the Mini Mental State Examination is not a useful screening test for subtle cognitive impairment [97].

Computerised tests have been developed to replicate traditional tests and to provide briefer screens. Potential advantages are there is less variance in administration and scoring, greater reaction time precision, they can be less language dependent, are able to be administered by less experienced staff and can generate immediate results. However, despite considerable overlap with tests, they do not necessarily provide the same information as traditional tests [89, 98].

Self-Reported Cognitive Impairment

Multiple studies have reported no significant association between objective cognitive impairment after chemotherapy and patients' self-report of their cognitive function: the patient's perception of cognitive impairment is generally worse than that detected on objective assessment [2–4, 7, 8, 38, 99–101]. This apparent dissociation between subjective and objective cognitive function has been described in patients with other medical illnesses [102–107].

Reasons for the discrepancy may be due to limitations of neuropsychological tests to evaluate cognitive function under relevant conditions [8, 102, 108, 109]. Survivors frequently report that their cognitive problems are most noticeable on multitasking and become more apparent when they resume their daily work [7, 12]. Despite attempts at using more ecologically valid tests it is possible that patients are not being evaluated under the conditions most likely to reproduce their problems. Also, the cross sectional studies do not detect as impaired people who were previously high functioning and then declined to within normal limits, although the individual would be very aware of the difference [7, 8, 90]. Other possible explanations are that people reclassify pre-existing cognitive problems as due to the cancer and its treatment, and/or that the perceived impairment is secondary to increased emotional stress/anxiety, which may be more apparent in everyday situations than in a controlled test situation [7, 60, 109].

The literature indicates consistently that perceived cognitive impairment is more strongly related to affective problems than objective impairment [37, 110], with a strong association between perceived cognitive impairment and fatigue, anxiety and/or depression [3, 4, 8, 12, 39, 84, 109, 111] (see below).

Incidence of Cognitive Impairment After Chemotherapy

Despite their methodological problems [7, 36, 45, 47, 62, 80, 91], most studies report a 15–50% incidence of cognitive impairment in breast cancer patients who have received chemotherapy [1, 2, 4, 6, 7, 40, 112] (see Table 1). In addition to the study of Jenkins [39, 85], one cross-sectional breast cancer study reported evidence against a causative role for chemotherapy with respect to cognitive impairment, but it had methodological limitations [38]. Six months after completing treatment, 60 women who received chemotherapy and radiotherapy for localised breast cancer were compared with 83 women who received radiotherapy alone. No significant difference was found between the two groups in mean cognitive performance or prevalence of impairment [38]. However, the radiotherapy group was significantly older and a higher proportion was receiving hormonal agents, which might have contributed to the negative result.

Shilling and colleagues have highlighted the interpretive difficulties caused by different definitions of cognitive impairment and methods of analysis by comparing data from breast cancer patients 4 weeks post-chemotherapy with healthy controls and reanalysing the data using seven different criteria selected from the literature. They found that the incidence differed substantially depending on the method of analysis used, with "cognitive impairment" ranging from 12 to 68% in the chemotherapy group, and 5 to 64% in the control group [91]. The odds ratio of being classified with cognitive impairment post-chemotherapy ranged from 1.21 to 3.68 compared to either controls or normative data, depending on which criteria and method were used [91].

Effect Sizes and Cognitive Domains Affected: Results of Meta-analyses

An overview of the studies suggests that cognitive deficits are diffuse, spotty within domains, and most frequently involve the domains of attention/concentration, verbal and visual memory, and processing speed [1–5]. There have been four meta-analyses of the cancer literature [77–80], with each using different selection criteria, and combining different cancer populations. Two of these were restricted to adjuvant breast cancer survivors [78, 80]. Methods of comparison depended on the original study design, and included comparison with normative data, controls, or the patient's own baseline performance. Each calculated an effect size to compare the magnitude of a treatment effect between the studies: the effect size is intended to convey clinical as opposed to statistical significance. However the clinical significance of any effect size on an individual's everyday functioning is unknown [79, 80].

Both the breast cancer meta-analyses showed a small overall effect size on cognitive function. Stewart reported that the cognitive domains with the greatest effect size were language (−0.37), short-term memory (−0.31) and spatial abilities (−0.30) [80] and Faletti reported the effect size being greatest for spatial ability (but the sample size was small in this domain), language and motor function [78]. Possible reasons for an apparent lack of a significant effect are that the neuropsychological tests may not be sensitive to subtle cognitive impairment; many studies had small sample sizes, and many of the individual studies had methodological limitations [78, 79].

Establishing a Causal Relationship Between Chemotherapy and Cognitive Impairment

It can be difficult to establish causation but the presence of the following criteria are generally regarded as evidence that an association is more likely to be a true cause and effect rather than an association due to chance, confounding, bias or an effect-cause relationship: appropriate timing between the exposure and effect, strength of the association, a dose response relationship, consistency of the association, biological plausibility and specificity of the association [113, 114].

Animal Studies

Support for a causal relationship between cognitive dysfunction and chemotherapy can be derived from animal studies investigating the effect of chemotherapy on cognitive function. Our own cognitive studies in mice have demonstrated that mice randomised to receive intraperitoneal methotrexate and 5-fluorouracil (5-FU) performed worse on spatial memory, non-spatial memory and conditional rule learning than mice randomised to receive normal saline [115]. A mouse model of cognitive dysfunction associated with a single administration of high dose chemotherapy has been developed by Koolhas et al. [7]. They demonstrated that post-chemotherapy, mice had difficulties with spatial learning and exhibited problems with retaining new information.

A second mouse model developed by Lee et al. did not support a causal effect of chemotherapy on cognition, with the chemotherapy group performing better than controls at 2 months post-chemotherapy; no difference was seen at 8 months [116].

Brain Imaging

Structural and functional brain imaging studies with magnetic resonance imaging (MRI) and positron emission tomography (PET) support a causal relationship for chemotherapy and cognitive impairment. Changes seen in chemotherapy-treated breast cancer survivors, compared with healthy controls include reductions in grey matter, and regions of locally decreased white matter [61]. One study showed smaller regional brain volume in grey and white matter in breast cancer patients at 1 year post-chemotherapy compared to women who did not receive chemotherapy, although this difference did not persist at 3 years post-treatment [117]. Studies using functional MRI (fMRI) with participants performing a working memory task have shown increased activation in the cingulate area in patients who received chemotherapy compared to controls [61, 118]. Our own preliminary fMRI studies show modified brain activation after chemotherapy, with lower levels in the parietal region and increased superior to the cingulate gyrus in women who had chemotherapy who self report cognitive impairment compared to those who do not [119]. PET scans of breast cancer survivors who received adjuvant chemotherapy 5–10 years previously have shown greater cerebral activation in the inferior frontal gyrus when performing a mental task compared to women who had not received chemotherapy. There were also differences in blood flow in the frontal cortex and cerebellum. Women who had received chemotherapy and tamoxifen had decreased metabolism in the basal ganglia compared to those who received chemotherapy alone or no chemotherapy [120].

Neurophysiological Studies

Studies by the Dutch group have demonstrated changes on neurophysiological evaluation between patients receiving high and standard dose chemotherapy and cancer controls [121]. Event related potential (ERP) and electroencephalograms (EEG) with asymmetry of alpha rhythm >0.5 Hz (considered to be pathological) were reported in 42% of the high dose chemotherapy patients, 12.5% of the standard dose and none of patients who received only local treatment [121]. No correlation was found between neuropsychological test results and the EEG results. Two studies by Kruekels et al. found that breast cancer patients who received chemotherapy had reduced amplitude in the P3 component (thought to be related to decreased activity in the norepinephrine system and important for attention) as compared to cancer patients not receiving chemotherapy [122, 123].

Chemotherapy Studies

The lack of pre-chemotherapy assessments in most studies makes the establishment of a causal relationship between cognitive dysfunction and chemotherapy difficult. As discussed above, support for a causal relationship comes from the studies by Schagen et al. [4] and Ahles et al. [2] which both showed greater cognitive deficits in patients treated with chemotherapy than in those patients who had not received chemotherapy. There are limited longitudinal studies, and sample sizes are generally small. Large longitudinal studies with appropriate control groups not receiving chemotherapy are underway and these, together with other mechanistic studies, will be required to determine definitively whether chemotherapy causes cognitive impairment, or whether it is secondary to the cancer per se or other aspects of treatment.

Chemotherapy Regimen and Dose Related Toxicity

Chemotherapy Intensity and Duration

It is probable that the chemotherapy regimen used, and the dose and duration of chemotherapy, influence the incidence and severity of cognitive dysfunction. The study by Van Dam et al. supports a dose effect with patients receiving high dose chemotherapy having worse impairment than those receiving standard doses. The risk of cognitive impairment was 8.2 times greater for high dose chemotherapy than for local treatment alone (95% CI 1.8–38, $p = 0.006$) and 3.5 times greater than for standard chemotherapy (95% CI 1.0–12.8, $p = 0.06$) [3]. In contrast, a recent study found no statistical difference in cognitive impairment between high dose and standard dose chemotherapy 5 years after treatment [43]. The study of Ahles et al. found an association with cognitive impairment and the number of cycles of chemotherapy received [2].

Chemotherapy Regimens

The probability of impairment appears to be higher following cyclophosphamide, methotrexate and 5-fluorouracil (CMF) chemotherapy than after anthracycline-containing regimens [7, 73, 124]. This may account for the higher incidence of impairment in breast cancer survivors reported in the earlier studies, in which CMF was generally used, than in the later studies in which methotrexate was generally replaced by doxorubicin or epirubicin.

Duration of Cognitive Impairment

The duration of cognitive impairment after anti-cancer treatment is uncertain. Ahles et al. reported cognitive dysfunction in patients up to 10 years post systemic treatment [2]. Schagen et al. found such impairment in patients at a median of 1.9 years after chemotherapy [4], but no difference between groups at 4 years post-treatment [42]. In the study of Mar Fan et al. using the High Sensitivity Cognitive Screen (HSCS) there was no statistically significant difference between chemotherapy patients and healthy controls at 2 years post-treatment [40]. However, subsequent research has shown that the HSCS has a marked practice effect [125] and it is possible that the improvement seen, in both controls and patients, is a reflection of practice effect rather than true improvement in cognitive function [83, 125]. Large, longitudinal studies with long term follow up are required to determine the duration of cognitive impairment post-chemotherapy, but will need to account for practice effect.

Potential Confounders

Fatigue

Cancer related fatigue is described by the National Comprehensive Cancer Network expert panel as "a common, persistent, and subjective sense of tiredness related to cancer, or to treatment for cancer, that interferes with usual functioning." [126].

In contrast with normal fatigue, cancer-related fatigue results in tiredness and weakness despite adequate rest or sleep [127]. It is estimated that 75–96% of cancer patients suffer chemotherapy-induced fatigue [128–133] that may last well beyond the treatment period [6, 127, 128, 130, 132, 134–137]. It has become recognised as the most common and most disabling symptom associated with chemotherapy [12, 133, 138] and can have a marked deleterious effect on quality of life [6, 40, 132]. As fatigue is a subjective state it needs to be assessed by patient-report measures [129, 139]. Mechanisms leading to fatigue are largely unknown but are thought to be multifactorial. A fall in haemoglobin and sleep disturbance may contribute, but account for a relatively small component of fatigue [127].

Although there is a strong association between fatigue and perceived cognitive impairment, studies have not shown a significant association between fatigue and objective neuropsychological testing [2–4, 6, 8, 37, 39, 40, 85, 100, 123]. For example, Mar Fan et al.'s follow up study showed that fatigue gradually improved during the 2 years after treatment but it remained significantly worse than in healthy controls at 1 ($p<0.0001$) and 2 years ($p<0.01$). There was a non-significant trend for women receiving hormonal treatment to have worse fatigue than those breast cancer patients not receiving it at 2 years (p = 0.02) [40]. At 1 and 2 years post-chemotherapy, fatigue was strongly associated with menopausal symptoms and overall quality of life, but not with chemotherapy regimen or duration or with the presence of cognitive impairment.

Anxiety, Depression and Stress

The diagnosis of a life-threatening disease is stressful, but there is no consensus on the incidence of pathological anxiety or depression in cancer patients. Studies suggest an incidence of depression ranging from no difference compared to the general population (approximately 6%) [140, 141] to greater than four times higher, with the greatest rates of major depression in those with advanced cancer (40–50%) [142–145]. The strongest predictor of depression in survivors was found to be ongoing cancer-related symptoms [146]. The study of Jenkins et al. found that 55% of breast cancer patients about to commence adjuvant chemotherapy had psychological distress (on the General Health Questionnaire), compared with 62% waiting to start local treatment, and 16% in healthy controls; at 6 months the incidence was 51, 24 and 18% respectively [39].

Only one study has reported any association between objective cognitive testing and affective stress, and this was found on only one (of up to 14) cognitive test, and using one of 6 measure of affective stress [9], so that it may well be due to chance alone. All the other cognitive studies which have measured psychological distress have found no correlation between objective cognitive performance and depression, anxiety and/or mood [1–4, 6, 8, 37, 39, 40, 44, 81, 84, 99, 147, 148]. However, as discussed above, many studies have found a strong association between perceived cognitive impairment and anxiety and/or depression [3, 8, 39, 84, 99, 111].

Hormonal Agents

Approximately 60% of women with breast cancer have oestrogen receptor positive disease, and almost all of these receive hormonal treatment for at least 5 years after completing chemotherapy, or after surgery if they do not require chemotherapy [149]. A thorough review of the impact of hormonal treatment on cognitive function is beyond the scope of this chapter but hormonal treatment either in the form of hormone replacement therapy (HRT) or anticancer hormone treatment might affect cognition [150–155]. Oestrogen receptors are located throughout the brain and central nervous system (CNS) [156]. Although decreased oestrogen levels are often implicated in cognitive impairment [47], the Women's Health Initiative did not find a cognitive function benefit in post-menopausal women randomised to receive HRT compared with placebo [157]. Three studies found no cognitive difference in patients on chemotherapy and tamoxifen compared to chemotherapy alone [2, 4, 6] but Castellon et al.'s study showed that patients who received tamoxifen after chemotherapy had worse cognitive impairment [8]. Paganini-Hill and Clark performed limited neuropsychological testing in 1,163 breast cancer patients, of whom 710 had received tamoxifen. They found that current tamoxifen users reported seeing their physician more often for memory problems, and performed worse than women who had never received tamoxifen on a task assessing narrative writing [158].

Shilling et al. reviewed cognitive performance from 94 breast cancer patients on the Arimidex, Tamoxifen, Alone or in Combination (ATAC) Trial. Women receiving these hormonal agents had specific impairments on verbal memory and information processing speed tasks in comparison to a group of healthy controls [10].

The above findings suggest that some of the cognitive impairment seen in breast cancer studies might be due to hormonal agents. If so, hormonal therapy may be an important confounder, affecting both patients who have had chemotherapy and women with cancer in the control groups of many previous studies. Studies in other cancer populations not using hormonal treatments may give additional insight.

Other Medications

Most breast cancer patients at the time of surgery receive opioids for analgesia; patients then take anti-emetics during chemotherapy, including glucocorticosteroids for control of nausea and vomiting. Glucocorticosteroids have been shown to decrease capillary permeability of the blood brain barrier and decrease cerebral blood flow [61]. Complementary and alternative therapies are also employed by a large proportion of cancer patients (mean 36%, range up to 70%), particularly women with breast cancer (45%) [159]. It is unknown if any of these agents have an impact on long-term cognitive function.

Potential Mechanisms

The aetiology of cognitive impairment in cancer patients is unknown but it is likely multifactorial [47]. Possible mechanisms by which chemotherapy might lead to cognitive dysfunction include direct neurotoxic effects (e.g. injury to neurons or surrounding cells, altered neurotransmitter levels) [61, 66, 160], oxidative damage [68, 161], indirect effects such as induced hormonal changes [76], immune dysregulation with release of cytokines [68, 162], blood clotting in small vessels of the CNS and anaemia and reduced delivery of oxygen to the CNS. Some individuals may have a genetic predisposition [61, 163].

Chemotherapy can cause direct neurotoxic damage, with a higher concentration of anticancer drugs crossing the blood brain barrier than had previously been recognized, including methotrexate, 5FU and cisplatin [66, 160]. Noble's group have reported that carmustine, cisplatin and cytosine arabinoside are toxic to CNS progenitor cells and oligodendrocytes in vitro and in animal studies with increased cell death and decreased cell division in the subventricular zone, the hippocampus and corpus callosum [164]. It is hypothesised that chemotherapy may affect the microglia, oligodendrocytes and neuronal axons, causing demyelination or alterations in water content [61, 160]. Free radicals are metabolic by-products of oxidative stress and are known to cause accumulative damage to blood vessels in the CNS [68]. Changes in neurotransmitter levels have also been reported [165].

Women with breast cancer often experience early menopause secondary to chemotherapy [130, 166]. It is hypothesised that an early abrupt menopause induced by chemotherapy might contribute to cognitive impairment, secondary to decreased oestrogen, which is thought to be neuroprotective [47, 61]. The study of Tchen et al. showed profound changes in women's levels of sex hormones after chemotherapy but did not find a significant correlation between hormone level or menopausal symptoms with cognitive dysfunction, although it may have been underpowered to detect a weak association [82].

Anaemia is a common side effect of cancer and/or chemotherapy that can cause fatigue and decreased cerebral oxygenation [26, 56]. Jacobsen reported that patients with greater levels of anaemia performed worse on visual memory and executive function tasks than those with normal haemoglobin or mild anaemia; however the effect was associated with fatigue [167]. This mechanism may account for acute problems with cognitive function but is less likely to account for cognitive impairment with increased duration from chemotherapy when haemoglobin levels have normalised. The administration of erythropoietin has been found to increase haemoglobin levels during chemotherapy. Two randomised controlled trials have been performed looking at differences in breast cancer patients randomised to receive erythropoietin or placebo during adjuvant chemotherapy. One assessed cognitive function from 12 to 30 months post-chemotherapy and found no difference in cognitive function between the two groups at any time point [168]. The second study reported improved executive functioning during chemotherapy (prior to cycle 4) in the erythropoietin group, but no difference in cognitive function at 6 months follow up in comparison to the placebo group [112].

Chemotherapy can damage blood vessels and interfere with blood perfusion and flow to the small vessels of the CNS, either by direct effects, from damage due to the by-products of oxidative stress [11, 68, 161, 169, 170], or from increased blood coagulation [171]. Thrombin-anti-thrombin complex (TAT), prothrombin fragment-1 & -2, and d-dimers have been found to be elevated in patients with breast cancer receiving chemotherapy, and might be involved in thromboembolic events [172]. High circulating homocysteine concentrations are associated with cardiovascular disease, stroke, Alzheimer's disease and vascular dementia, and with poor performance on some cognitive tests in healthy elderly men and women [173, 174]. It is possible that patients with greater homocysteine levels are predisposed to greater cognitive impairment secondary to cerebral vascular changes.

One hypothesis is that either the cancer and/or chemotherapy cause activation of the immune system with proinflammatory cytokines. Inflammatory cytokines such as interleukin (IL)-1, IL-6 and tumour necrosis factor alpha (TNF-α) cross the blood-brain barrier and have been associated with cognitive impairment and/or fatigue in other disease states [175–179]. Support for this cytokine-immunologic prototype is seen in animal models where "sickness behaviour" is found after injecting infectious or inflammatory agents or some cytokines [180, 181]. It is also seen in cancer patients and others treated with cytokine therapy (e.g. interferon, IL-1), in whom the rate limiting toxicity is often severe fatigue, depressed mood, cognitive disturbance and flu-like symptoms [181–184].

Meyers et al. reported that higher IL-6 levels were associated with poorer executive function, whereas higher levels of IL-8 were associated with better memory performance in patients with acute myelogenous leukaemia or myelodysplastic syndrome [179]. Studies by Collado-Hidalgo et al. have reported an association between increased monocyte production of IL-6 and TNFα, decreased monocyte cell-surface IL-6 receptor, and decreased frequencies of activated T lymphocytes and myeloid dendritic cells in the peripheral blood of breast cancer survivors with prolonged fatigue compared to those without fatigue [185]. Our ongoing studies show that serum levels of several cytokines are elevated in breast cancer survivors (and colorectal cancer patients) compared to healthy subjects and remain elevated at 5 years post-treatment [119, 186]. There is a trend to cytokine levels being higher in women who had not received chemotherapy for their breast cancer and a strong trend to elevated cytokine levels being associated with greater cognitive impairment on neuropsychological testing [119, 186].

The apolipoprotein E gene is polymorphic with three common alleles, APOϵ2, -ϵ3 and -ϵ4, which produce six genotype combinations [25]. People with APOϵ4 alleles are more vulnerable to cognitive impairment after head trauma [187] and cardiac bypass surgery [188] and have a higher risk of dementia [189], possibly due to reduced microvascular and neuronal repair processes [190]. One study suggests greater cognitive impairment after chemotherapy in people with APOϵ4 genotypes, which is also associated with changes in MRI images of the brain [7].

It is also hypothesised that other genetic polymorphisms may increase the risk of some individuals to cognitive impairment after chemotherapy due to a predisposition to some of the above mechanisms [163]. For example, by decreasing the effectiveness of the blood-brain-barrier due to less efficient efflux pumps or changes in transporters, [164, 191, 192] decreased DNA or neuronal repair mechanisms, [170, 193] decrease in neurotransmitters, [194, 195] shorter telomere length or less telomerase, [196, 197] and cytokine dysregulation [163].

Interventions

There are no proven interventions to prevent cognitive impairment or to treat it once it has developed. It is difficult to develop rational treatments until the mechanisms have been elucidated, but the following interventions have been either evaluated or are undergoing evaluation.

The use of erythropoietin has not been shown to improve cognitive function after completing chemotherapy (see above). Improved cognitive impairment in other disease states has been seen with methylphenidate, the herb Ginkgo Biloba, and anti-cholinesterase inhibitors such as donepezil. Methylphenidate has been widely used in children and adults to treat attention-deficit/hyperactivity disorder (ADHD) and narcolepsy. Methylphenidate has also been used to treat cognitive impairment in childhood survivors of cancer [198], patients with brain tumours [199] and in two placebo-controlled RCT in solid tumour patients. One trial randomised women receiving adjuvant chemotherapy for breast cancer to receive methylphenidate or placebo as prophylaxis for fatigue and cognitive dysfunction, but the study closed early due to poor accrual with 57 of a planned 170 patients entered. No difference was found in either fatigue or cognitive function between the two groups [200]. The second study used methylphenidate in a heterogeneous cancer population, which included patients with metastases from any primary excluding brain or patients with known CNS involvement. Although reported by the authors as positive, cognitive function was only improved in the memory component of the HSCS with no difference in overall HSCS score between the groups [201].

Ginkgo biloba has been evaluated in randomised placebo controlled trials in patients with other types of acquired cognitive impairment, particularly in elderly people with dementia. Although there are some conflicting results, most studies show a modest benefit for gingko biloba, particularly in people with milder forms of cognitive impairment [202–204]. A Cochrane review has concluded that gingko biloba improves cognition and mood, with no increase in side effects, in patients with acquired cognitive impairment including dementia [205]. Studies in healthy younger volunteers have shown improved cognition in subjects treated with daily gingko ± ginseng compared to placebo [206–208]. The Mayo group are assessing gingko biloba in a placebo-controlled RCT in breast cancer patients.

Cholinesterase inhibitors, such as donepezil, have been widely investigated and found to improve cognitive function across a variety of disease states, particularly dementia [209–212]. However, a recent Cochrane review shows no evidence to support the use of donepezil in patients with mild cognitive impairment without a diagnosis of dementia [213].

Based on the hypotheses about mechanisms of cognitive dysfunction, other pharmacological agents that could be considered for future trials are antiplatelet agents (e.g. aspirin, anti-inflammatory non-steroidal agents or low dose warfarin), anti-inflammatories and anti-oxidants.

Cognitive rehabilitation has been shown to be effective in treating non-cancer patient groups with cognitive impairment [214–217]. The majority of methods focus on either restoration of a specific cognitive function or compensatory training to help patients adapt to the presence of deficits [214, 216, 218, 219]. In view of the strong association of anxiety and depression with perceived cognitive impairment it is also important to treat the psychological distress in affected patients [216, 219]. Psychosocial programs have been found to help improve non-cancer patients' coping with cognitive problems, to increase understanding of their difficulties and to improve well-being [216, 220]. Education about brain injury has also been found to result in improved self-reports of psychosocial function in other patient populations [221]. Studies are underway to assess whether cognitive behavioural programmes or psychosocial support programmes would be beneficial for cancer survivors with either objective or subjective cognitive impairment [7, 25].

Summary

Studies have found consistently that a subset of cancer survivors have cognitive sequelae that persist after cancer treatment. Most evidence suggests an association with chemotherapy, although other factors associated with the diagnosis and treatment of cancer may contribute. For most cancer survivors the objective impairment is subtle, although patients self-report a greater degree of impairment than is found on current neuropsychological testing. Even mild cognitive dysfunction can have substantial impact on a patient's daily activities and quality of life.

References

1. Brezden CB, Phillips KA, Abdolell M, et al. Cognitive function in breast cancer patients receiving adjuvant chemotherapy. *J Clin Oncol.* 2000;18:2695–701.
2. Ahles TA, Saykin AJ, Furstenberg CT, et al. Neuropsychologic impact of standard-dose systemic chemotherapy in long-term survivors of breast cancer and lymphoma. J Clin Oncol. 2002;20:485–93.
3. van Dam FS, Schagen SB, Muller MJ, et al. Impairment of cognitive function in women receiving adjuvant treatment for high-risk breast cancer: high-dose versus standard-dose chemotherapy. J Natl Cancer Inst. 1998;90:210–8.
4. Schagen SB, van Dam FS, Muller MJ, et al. Cognitive deficits after postoperative adjuvant chemotherapy for breast carcinoma. Cancer. 1999;85:640–50.
5. Wieneke MH, Dienst E. Neuropsychological assessment of cognitive functioning following chemotherapy for breast cancer. *Psycho-oncology*. 1995;4:61–6.
6. Tchen N, Juffs HG, Downie FP, et al. Cognitive function, fatigue, and menopausal symptoms in women receiving adjuvant chemotherapy for breast cancer. *J Clin Oncol.* 2003;21:4175–83.
7. Tannock IF, Ahles TA, Ganz PA, van Dam FS. Cognitive impairment associated with chemotherapy for cancer: Report of a Workshop. *J Clin Oncol.* 2004;22:2233–9.

8. Castellon SA, Ganz PA, Bower JE, et al. Neurocognitive performance in breast cancer survivors exposed to adjuvant chemotherapy and tamoxifen. *J Clin Exp Neuropsychol.* 2004;26:955–69.
9. Wefel JS, Lenzi R, Theriault R, et al. 'Chemobrain' in breast carcinoma?: A prologue. *Cancer.* 2004;101:466–75.
10. Shilling V, Jenkins V, Fallowfield L, et al. The effects of hormone therapy on cognition in breast cancer. *J Steroid Biochem Mol Biol.* 2003;86:405–12.
11. Ahles TA, Saykin A. Cognitive effects of standard-dose chemotherapy in patients with cancer. *Cancer Invest.* 2000;19:812–20.
12. Downie FP, Mar Fan HG, Houede-Tchen N, et al. Cognitive function, fatigue, and menopausal symptoms in breast cancer patients receiving adjuvant chemotherapy: Evaluation with patient interview after formal assessment. *Psychooncology.* 2006;15:921–30.
13. Freeman JR, Broshek DK. Assessing cognitive dysfunction in breast cancer: What are the tools? *Clin Breast Cancer.* 2002; 3(Suppl 3):S91–9.
14. Carey CL, Woods SP, Rippeth JD, et al. Initial validation of a screening battery for the detection of HIV-associated cognitive impairment. *Clin Neuropsychol.* 2004;18:234–48.
15. Butters N, Grant I, Haxby J, et al. Assessment of AIDS-related cognitive changes: Recommendations of the NIMH Workshop on Neuropsychological Assessment Approaches. *J Clin Exp Neuropsychol.* 1990;12:963–78.
16. Cummings JL, Benson DF. Subcortical dementia. Review of an emerging concept. *Arch Neurol.* 1984;41:874–9.
17. Massman PJ, Delis DC, Butters N, et al. Are all subcortical dementias alike? Verbal learning and memory in Parkinson's and Huntington's disease patients. *J Clin Exp Neuropsychol.* 1990;12:729–44.
18. Rao SM, Leo GJ, Bernardin L, et al. Cognitive dysfunction in multiple sclerosis. I. Frequency, patterns, and prediction. *Neurology.* 1991;41:685–91.
19. Heaton RK, Kirson D, Velin D, RA. Grant I. and the HNRC Group: The Utility of Clinical Ratings for Detecting Cognitive Change in HIV Infection, in Grant IM, A. (ed) *Neuropsychology of HIV Infection.* New York: Oxford University Press, 1994, pp.188–206.
20. Heaton RK, Grant I, Butters N, et al. The HNRC 500–neuropsychology of HIV infection at different disease stages. HIV Neurobehavioral Research Center. *J Int Neuropsychol Soc.* 1995;1:231–51
21. Carey CL, Woods SP, Gonzalez R, et al. Predictive validity of global deficit scores in detecting neuropsychological impairment in HIV infection. *J Clin Exp Neuropsychol.* 2004;26:307–19.
22. Martin EM, Sullivan TS, Reed RA, et al. Auditory working memory in HIV-1 infection. *J Int Neuropsychol Soc.* 2001;7:20–6.
23. Durvasula RS, Miller EN, Myers HF, et al. Predictors of neuropsychological performance in HIV positive women. *J Clin Exp Neuropsychol.* 2001;23:149–63.
24. Wechsler D. Manual for the Wechsler Adult Intelligence Scale. 3rd ed. New York: The Psychological Corporation; 1997
25. Ferguson RJ, Ahles TA. Low neuropsychologic performance among adult cancer survivors treated with chemotherapy. *Curr Neurol Neurosci Rep.* 2003;3:215–22.
26. Minisini A, Atalay G, Bottomley A, et al. What is the effect of systemic anticancer treatment on cognitive function? *Lancet Oncol.* 2004;5:273–82.
27. Weiss HD, Walker MD, Wiernik PH. Neurotoxicity of commonly used antineoplastic agents (second of two parts). *N Engl J Med.* 1974;291:127–33
28. Weiss HD, Walker MD, Wiernik PH. Neurotoxicity of commonly used antineoplastic agents (first of two parts). *N Engl J Med.* 1974;291:75–81.

29. Oxman TE, Silberfarb PM. Serial cognitive testing in cancer patients receiving chemotherapy. *Am J Psychiatry*. 1980;137:1263–5.
30. Silberfarb PM, Philibert D, Levine PM. Psychosocial aspects of neoplastic disease: II. Affective and cognitive effects of chemotherapy in cancer patients. *Am J Psychiatry*. 1980;137:597–601.
31. Kaasa S, Olsnes BT, Thorud E, et al. Reduced short-term neuropsychological performance in patients with nonsmall-cell lung cancer treated with cisplatin and etoposide. *Antibiot Chemother*. 1988;41:226–31.
32. Meyers CA, Abbruzzese JL. Cognitive functioning in cancer patients: Effect of previous treatment. *Neurology*. 1992;42:434–6.
33. Meyers CA, Byrne KS, Komaki R. Cognitive deficits in patients with small cell lung cancer before and after chemotherapy. *Lung Cancer*. 1995;12:231–5.
34. Silberfarb PM. Chemotherapy and cognitive defects in cancer patients. *Annu Rev Med*. 1983;34:35–46.
35. Komaki R, Meyers CA, Shin DM, et al. Evaluation of cognitive function in patients with limited small cell lung cancer prior to and shortly following prophylactic cranial irradiation. *Int J Radiat Oncol Biol Phys*. 1995;33:179–82.
36. Phillips KA, Bernhard J. Adjuvant breast cancer treatment and cognitive function: Current knowledge and research directions. *J Natl Cancer Inst*. 2003;95:190–7.
37. Bender CM, Sereika SM, Berga SL, et al. Cognitive impairment associated with adjuvant therapy in breast cancer. *Psychooncology*. 2006;15:422–30.
38. Donovan KA, Small BJ, Andrykowski MA, et al. Cognitive functioning after adjuvant chemotherapy and/or radiotherapy for early-stage breast carcinoma. *Cancer*. 2005;104:2499–507.
39. Jenkins V, Shilling V, Deutsch G, et al. A 3-year prospective study of the effects of adjuvant treatments on cognition in women with early stage breast cancer. *Br J Cancer*. 2006.
40. Mar Fan H, Houédé-Tchen N, Yi Q-L, Chemerynsky I, Downie FP, Sabate K, Tannock I.F. Fatigue, menopausal symptoms and cognitive function in women following adjuvant chemotherapy for breast cancer: One and two year follow-up of a prospective controlled study. *J Clin Oncol*. 2005;23:8025–32.
41. O'Shaughnessy JA, Vukelja SJ, Holmes FA, et al. Feasibility of quantifying the effects of epoetin alfa therapy on cognitive function in women with breast cancer undergoing adjuvant or neoadjuvant chemotherapy. *Clin Breast Cancer*. 2005;5:439–46.
42. Schagen SB, Muller MJ, Boogerd W, et al. Late effects of adjuvant chemotherapy on cognitive function: a follow-up study in breast cancer patients. *Ann Oncol*. 2002;13: 1387–97.
43. Scherwath A, Mehnert A, Schleimer B, et al. Neuropsychological function in high-risk breast cancer survivors after stem-cell supported high-dose therapy versus standard-dose chemotherapy: Evaluation of long-term treatment effects. *Ann Oncol*. 2006;17:415–23.
44. Wefel JS, Lenzi R, Theriault RL, et al. The cognitive sequelae of standard-dose adjuvant chemotherapy in women with breast carcinoma: results of a prospective, randomized, longitudinal trial. *Cancer*. 2004;100:2292–9.
45. Ganz PA. Cognitive dysfunction following adjuvant treatment of breast cancer: A new dose-limiting toxic effect? *J Natl Cancer Inst*. 1998;90:182–3.
46. Ahles TA, Saykin AJ. Breast cancer chemotherapy-related cognitive dysfunction. *Clin Breast Cancer*. 2002;3(Suppl 3):S84–90.
47. Bender CM, Paraska KK, Sereika SM, et al. Cognitive function and reproductive hormones in adjuvant therapy for breast cancer: A critical review. *J Pain Symptom Manage*. 2001;21:407–24.
48. Cimprich B. Symptom management: Loss of concentration. *Semin Oncol Nurs*. 1995;11: 279–88.

49. McAllister TW, Ahles TA, Saykin AJ, et al. Cognitive effects of cytotoxic cancer chemotherapy: predisposing risk factors and potential treatments. *Curr Psychiatry Rep.* 2004;6:364–71.
50. Weitzner MA, Meyers CA. Cognitive functioning and quality of life in malignant glioma patients: A review of the literature. *Psychooncology.* 1997;6:169–77.
51. Meyers CA. Neurocognitive dysfunction in cancer patients. *Oncology* (Williston Park). 2000;14:75–9;discussion 79,81–2,85.
52. Meyers CA, Scheibel RS. Early detection and diagnosis of neurobehavioral disorders associated with cancer and its treatment. *Oncology* (Williston Park). 1990;4:115–22;discussion 122,126–7,130.
53. Meyers CA, Weitzner M, Byrne K, et al. Evaluation of the neurobehavioral functioning of patients before, during, and after bone marrow transplantation. *J Clin Oncol.* 1994; 12:820–6.
54. Meyers CA, Weitzner MA. Neurobehavioral functioning and quality of life in patients treated for cancer of the central nervous system. *Curr Opin Oncol.* 1995;7:197–200.
55. Olin JJ. Cognitive function after systemic therapy for breast cancer. *Oncology* (Williston Park). 2001;15:613–8;discussion 618,621–4.
56. O'Shaughnessy J. Chemotherapy-related cognitive dysfunction in breast cancer. *Semin Oncol Nurs.* 2003;19:17–24.
57. O'Shaughnessy JA. Chemotherapy-induced cognitive dysfunction: A clearer picture. *Clin Breast Cancer.* 2003;4(Suppl 2):S89–94.
58. Peterson LG, Popkin MK. Neuropsychiatric effects of chemotherapeutic agents for cancer. *Psychosomatics.* 1980;21:141–53.
59. Redd WH, Silberfarb PM, Andersen BL, et al. Physiologic and psychobehavioral research in oncology. *Cancer.* 1991;67:813–22.
60. Rugo HS, Ahles T. The impact of adjuvant therapy for breast cancer on cognitive function: current evidence and directions for research. *Semin Oncol.* 2003;30:749–62.
61. Saykin AJ, Ahles TA, McDonald BC. Mechanisms of chemotherapy-induced cognitive disorders: Neuropsychological, pathophysiological, and neuroimaging perspectives. *Semin Clin Neuropsychiatry.* 2003;8:201–16.
62. Schagen SB, Muller MJ, Boogerd W, et al. Cognitive dysfunction and chemotherapy: Neuropsychological findings in perspective. *Clin Breast Cancer.* 2002;3(Suppl 3): S100–8.
63. Oxman TE, Schnurr PP, Silberfarb PM. Assessment of cognitive function in cancer patients. *Hosp J.* 1986;2:99–128 .
64. Silberfarb PM, Oxman TE. The effects of cancer therapies on the central nervous system. *Adv Psychosom Med.* 1988;18:13–25.
65. Tope DM, Ahles TA, Silberfarb PM. Psycho-oncology: Psychological well-being as one component of quality of life. *Psychother Psychosom.* 1993;60:129–47.
66. Troy L, McFarland K, Littman-Power S, et al. Cisplatin-based therapy: A neurological and neuropsychological review. *Psychooncology.* 2000;9:29–39.
67. Morse R, Rodgers J, Verrill M, et al. Neuropsychological functioning following systemic treatment in women treated for breast cancer: A review. *Eur J Cancer.* 2003;39:2288–97.
68. Barton D, Loprinzi C. Novel approaches to preventing chemotherapy-induced cognitive dysfunction in breast cancer: the art of the possible. *Clin Breast Cancer.* 2002;3(Suppl 3): S121–7.
69. Matsuda T, Takayama T, Tashiro M, et al. Mild cognitive impairment after adjuvant chemotherapy in breast cancer patients–evaluation of appropriate research design and methodology to measure symptoms. *Breast Cancer.* 2005;12:279–87.
70. Raffa RB, Duong PV, Finney J, et al. Is 'chemo-fog'/'chemo-brain' caused by cancer chemotherapy? *J Clin Pharm Ther.* 2006;31:129–38.
71. Kayl AE, Wefel JS, Meyers CA. Chemotherapy and cognition: effects, potential mechanisms, and management. *Am J Ther.* 2006;13:362–9.

72. Castellon SA, Silverman DH, Ganz PA. Breast cancer treatment and cognitive functioning: current status and future challenges in assessment. *Breast Cancer Res Treat.* 2005;92:199–206.
73. Wefel JS, Kayl AE, Meyers CA. Neuropsychological dysfunction associated with cancer and cancer therapies: A conceptual review of an emerging target. *Br J Cancer.* 2004;90: 1691–6.
74. Baumgartner K. Neurocognitive changes in cancer patients. *Semin Oncol Nurs.* 2004;20: 284–90.
75. Paraska K, Bender CM. Cognitive dysfunction following adjuvant chemotherapy for breast cancer: Two case studies. *Oncol Nurs Forum.* 2003;30:473–8.
76. Ahles TA. Do systemic cancer treatments affect cognitive function? *Lancet Oncol.* 2004; 5:270–1.
77. Anderson-Hanley C, Sherman ML, Riggs R, et al. Neuropsychological effects of treatments for adults with cancer: A meta-analysis and review of the literature. *J Int Neuropsychol Soc.* 2003;9:967–82.
78. Falleti MG, Sanfilippo A, Maruff P, et al. The nature and severity of cognitive impairment associated with adjuvant chemotherapy in women with breast cancer: A meta-analysis of the current literature. *Brain Cogn.* 2005;59:60–70.
79. Jansen CE, Miaskowski C, Dodd M, et al. A metaanalysis of studies of the effects of cancer chemotherapy on various domains of cognitive function. *Cancer.* 2005;104:2222–33.
80. Stewart A, Bielajew C, Collins B, et al. A meta-analysis of the neuropsychological effects of adjuvant chemotherapy treatment in women treated for breast cancer. *Clin Neuropsychol.* 2006;20:76–89.
81. Wieneke MH, Dienst ER. Neuropsychological assessment of cognitive functioning following chemotherapy for breast cancer. *Psycho-oncology.* 1995;4:61–6.
82. Tchen N JH, Downie F, Yi Q, Hu H, et al. Cognitive function, fatigue, and menopausal symptoms in women receiving adjuvant chemotherapy for breast cancer. *J Clin Oncol.* 2003;22(22):4175–83.
83. Mar Fan H, Vardy J, Xu W, Tannock IF. Does cognitive impairment after chemotherapy improve over time or does practice make perfect? In reply. *J Clinl Oncol.* 2006;24:5171–2.
84. Cimprich B, So H, Ronis DL, et al. Pre-treatment factors related to cognitive functioning in women newly diagnosed with breast cancer. *Psychooncology.* 2005;14:70–8.
85. Shilling V, Jenkins V, Morris R, et al. The effects of adjuvant chemotherapy on cognition in women with breast cancer–preliminary results of an observational longitudinal study. *Breast.* 2005;14:142–50.
86. Symes E, Maruff P, Ajani A, et al. Issues associated with the identification of cognitive change following coronary artery bypass grafting. *Aust N Z J Psychiatry.* 2000;34: 770–84.
87. Ingraham L, Aiken, CB. An empirical approach to determining criteria for abnormality in test batteries with multiple measures. *Neuropsychology.* 1996;10:120–4.
88. Bornstein R. Methodological and conceptual issues in the study of cognitive change in HIV infection, in Grant IM A. ed. *Neuropsychology of HIV Infection.* New York: Oxford University Press; 1994
89. Gonzalez R, Heaton RK, Moore DJ, et al. Computerized reaction time battery versus a traditional neuropsychological battery: Detecting HIV-related impairments. *J Int Neuropsychol Soc.* 2003;9:64–71.
90. Vardy J. Cognitive impairment postchemotherapy. Review. *American Journal of Oncology.* 2004;3:568–70.
91. Shilling V, Jenkins V, Trapala IS. The (mis)classification of chemo-fog – methodological inconsistencies in the investigation of cognitive impairment after chemotherapy. *Breast Cancer Res Treat.* 2005;1–5.

92. Taylor MJ, Heaton RK. Sensitivity and specificity of WAIS-III/WMS-III demographically corrected factor scores in neuropsychological assessment. *J Int Neuropsychol Soc.* 2001;7:867–74.
93. Fletcher RH, Fletcher SW, Wagner EH. Responsiveness, In: Satterfield T ed. Clinical epidemiology: the essentials 2nd ed. Baltimore: Williams & Wilkins; 1988, pp. 71–72.
94. Reitan RM, Wolfson, D. The Halstead-Reitan Neuropscyhological Test Battery: *Theory and Clinical Interpretation* 2nd ed. Tucson, Arizona: Neuropsychology Press, 1993.
95. White DA, Heaton RK, Monsch AU. Neuropsychological studies of asymptomatic human immunodeficiency virus-type-1 infected individuals. The HNRC Group. HIV Neurobehavioral Research Center. *J Int Neuropsychol Soc.* 1995;1:304–15.
96. Miller EN, Wilkie FL. Computerized Testing to Assess Cognition in HIV-Positive Individuals, In Grant I, Martin A ed. *Neuropsychology of HIV Infection.* New York: Oxford University Press; 1994, pp. 161–75.
97. Meyers CA, Wefel JS. The use of the mini-mental state examination to assess cognitive functioning in cancer trials: no ifs, ands, buts, or sensitivity. *J Clin Oncol.* 2003;21: 3557–8.
98. Miller EN, Satz P, Visscher B. Computerized and conventional neuropsychological assessment of HIV-1-infected homosexual men. *Neurology.* 41:1608–16.
99. Cull A, Hay C, Love SB, et al. What do cancer patients mean when they complain of concentration and memory problems? *Br J Cancer.* 1996;74:1674–9.
100. Servaes P, Verhagen CA, Bleijenberg G. Relations between fatigue, neuropsychological functioning, and physical activity after treatment for breast carcinoma: Daily self-report and objective behavior. *Cancer.* 2002;95:2017–26.
101. Poppelreuter M, Weis J, Kulz AK, et al. Cognitive dysfunction and subjective complaints of cancer patients. A cross-sectional study in a cancer rehabilitation centre. *Eur J Cancer.* 2004;40:43–9.
102. Sbordone RJ. Limitations of neuropsychological testing to predict the cognitive and behavioral functioning of persons with brain injury in real-world settings. *NeuroRehabilitation.* 2001;16:199–201.
103. Radziwillllowicz W, Radziwillllowicz, P. Subjective and objective assessment of memory functions in endogenous depression. *Arch Psych Psychother.* 2000;2:33–41.
104. Vermeulen J, Aldenkamp AP, Alpherts WC. Memory complaints in epilepsy: Correlations with cognitive performance and neuroticism. *Epilepsy Res.* 1993;15:157–70.
105. Vercoulen JH, Swanink CM, Galama JM, et al. The persistence of fatigue in chronic fatigue syndrome and multiple sclerosis: Development of a model. *J Psychosom Res.* 1998;45:507–17.
106. Sunderland A, Watts K, Baddeley AD, et al. Subjective memory assessment and test performance in elderly adults. *J Gerontol.* 1986;41:376–84.
107. Millikin CP, Rourke SB, Halman MH, et al. Fatigue in HIV/AIDS is associated with depression and subjective neurocognitive complaints but not neuropsychological functioning. *J Clin Exp Neuropsychol.* 2003;25:201–15.
108. Heaton RK, Marcotte TD, Mindt MR, et al. The impact of HIV-associated neuropsychological impairment on everyday functioning. *J Int Neuropsychol Soc.* 2004;10:317–31.
109. Shilling V, Jenkins V. Self-reported cognitive problems in women receiving adjuvant therapy for breast cancer. *Eur J Oncol Nurs.* 2007;11:6–15.
110. Booth-Jones M, Jacobsen PB, Ransom S, et al. Characteristics and correlates of cognitive functioning following bone marrow transplantation. *Bone Marrow Transplant.* 2005;36:695–702.
111. Cimprich B. Pretreatment symptom distress in women newly diagnosed with breast cancer. *Cancer Nurs.* 1999;22:185–94;quiz 195.
112. O'Shaughnessy JA. Effects of epoetin alfa on cognitive function, mood, asthenia, and quality of life in women with breast cancer undergoing adjuvant chemotherapy. Clin *Breast Cancer.* 2002;3(Suppl 3):S116–20.

113. Newman T, Browner WS, Hulley SB. Enhancing causal inference in observational studies, Designing clinical research: An epidemiologic approach 2nd ed. Philadelphia, Pa., Lippincott: Williams & Wilkins; 2000, pp. 125–38.
114. Fletcher R, Fletcher SW, Wagner EH. Cause, in Satterfield T ed. Clinical Epidemiology 3rd ed. Baltimore: Lippincott Williams & Wilkins; 1996, pp. 228–48.
115. Winocur G, Vardy J, Binns MA, et al. The effects of the anti-cancer drugs, methotrexate and 5-fluorouracil, on cognitive function in mice. *Pharmacol Biochem Behav*. 2006;85:66–75.
116. Lee GD, Longo DL, Wang Y, et al. Transient improvement in cognitive function and synaptic plasticity in rats following cancer chemotherapy. *Clin Cancer Res*. 2006;12: 198–205.
117. Inagaki M, Yoshikawa E, Matsuoka Y, et al. Smaller regional volumes of brain gray and white matter demonstrated in breast cancer survivors exposed to adjuvant chemotherapy. *Cancer*. 2007;109:146–56.
118. Saykin AJ, Ahles TA, Schoenfeld J.D. et al. Gray matter reduction on voxel-based morphometry in chemotherapy-treated cancer survivors. *J Int Neuropsych Soc*. 2003;9:246.
119. Booth CM, Vardy J, Crawley A, et al. Cognitive impairment associated with chemotherapy for breast cancer: An exploratory case-control study. *J Clin Oncol* (Meeting Abstracts). 2006;24:8501.
120. Silverman DH, Dy CJ, Castellon SA, et al. Altered frontocortical, cerebellar, and basal ganglia activity in adjuvant-treated breast cancer survivors 5–10 years after chemotherapy. *Breast Cancer Res Treat*. 2007;103:303–11.
121. Schagen SB, Hamburger HL, Muller MJ, et al. Neurophysiological evaluation of late effects of adjuvant high-dose chemotherapy on cognitive function. *J Neurooncol*. 2001; 51:159–65.
122. Kreukels BP, Schagen SB, Ridderinkhof KR, et al. Effects of high-dose and conventional-dose adjuvant chemotherapy on long-term cognitive sequelae in patients with breast cancer: An electrophysiologic study. *Clin Breast Cancer*. 2006;7:67–78.
123. Kreukels BP, Schagen SB, Ridderinkhof KR, et al. Electrophysiological correlates of information processing in breast-cancer patients treated with adjuvant chemotherapy. *Breast Cancer Res Treat*. 2005;94:53–61.
124. Vezmar S, Becker A, Bode U, et al. Biochemical and clinical aspects of methotrexate neurotoxicity. *Chemotherapy*. 2003;49:92–104.
125. Vardy J, Wong K, Yi QL, et al. Assessing cognitive function in cancer patients. *Support Care Cancer*. 2006;14:1111–8.
126. Mock V, Atkinson A, Barsevick A, et al. NCCN Practice Guidelines for Cancer-Related Fatigue. *Oncology* (Huntington). 2000;14:151–61.
127. Cella D, Davis K, Breitbart W, et al. Cancer-related fatigue: Prevalence of proposed diagnostic criteria in a United States sample of cancer survivors. *J Clin Oncol*. 2001;19: 3385–91.
128. Yellen SB, Cella DF, Webster K, et al. Measuring fatigue and other anemia-related symptoms with the Functional Assessment of Cancer Therapy (FACT) measurement system. *J Pain Symptom Manage*. 1997;13:63–74.
129. Stone P, Richards M, Hardy J. Fatigue in patients with cancer. *Eur J Cancer*. 1998;34:1670–6.
130. Knobf MT. Physical and psychologic distress associated with adjuvant chemotherapy in women with breast cancer. *J Clin Oncol*. 1986;4:678–84.
131. Stone P, Richardson A, Ream E, et al. Cancer-related fatigue: inevitable, unimportant and untreatable? Results of a multi-centre patient survey. Cancer Fatigue Forum. *Ann Oncol*. 2000;11:971–5,
132. Stone P, Ream E, Richardson A, et al. Cancer-related fatigue–a difference of opinion? Results of a multicentre survey of healthcare professionals, patients and caregivers. *Eur J Cancer Care* (Engl). 2003;12:20–7.

133. Ashbury FD, Findlay H, Reynolds B, et al. A Canadian survey of cancer patients' experiences: are their needs being met? *J Pain Symptom Manage.* 1998;16:298–306.
134. Stone P. The measurement, causes and effective management of cancer-related fatigue. *Int J Palliat Nurs.* 2002;8:120–8.
135. Broeckel JA, Jacobsen PB, Horton J, et al. Characteristics and correlates of fatigue after adjuvant chemotherapy for breast cancer. *J Clin Oncol.* 1998;16:1689–96.
136. Bower JE, Ganz PA, Desmond KA, et al. Fatigue in breast cancer survivors: Occurrence, correlates, and impact on quality of life. *J Clin Oncol.* 2000;18:743–53
137. Jacobsen PB, Stein K. Is Fatigue a Long-term Side Effect of Breast Cancer Treatment? *Cancer Control.* 1999;6:256–63.
138. Richardson A. Fatigue in cancer patients: A review of the literature. *Eur J Cancer Care* (Engl). 1995;4:20–32.
139. Jacobsen PB. Assessment of fatigue in cancer patients. *J Natl Cancer Inst Monogr.* 2004;93–7.
140. Massie M. Depression, in Holland J, Rowland ed. *Handbook of Psycho-oncology.* New York: Oxford University Press; 1990, pp.283–90.
141. Keating NL, Norredam M, Landrum MB, et al. Physical and mental health status of older long-term cancer survivors. *J Am Geriatr Soc.* 2005;53:2145–52.
142. Honda K, Goodwin RD. Cancer and mental disorders in a national community sample: Findings from the national comorbidity survey. *Psychother Psychosom.* 2004;73:235–42.
143. Hewitt M, Rowland JH. Mental health service use among adult cancer survivors: Analyses of the National Health Interview Survey. *J Clin Oncol* 2002;20:4581–90.
144. Fallowfield L, Ratcliffe D, Jenkins V, et al. Psychiatric morbidity and its recognition by doctors in patients with cancer. *Br J Cancer.* 2001;84:1011–15.
145. Derogatis LR, Morrow GR, Fetting J, et al. The prevalence of psychiatric disorders among cancer patients. *JAMA.* 1983;249:751–7.
146. Deimling GT, Kahana B, Bowman KF, et al. Cancer survivorship and psychological distress in later life. *Psychooncology.* 2002;11:479–94.
147. Eberhardt B, Dilger S, Musial F, et al. Short-term monitoring of cognitive functions before and during the first course of treatment. *J Cancer Res Clin Oncol.* 2006; 132:234–40.
148. Eberhardt B, Dilger S, Musial F, et al. Medium-term effects of chemotherapy in older cancer patients. *Support Care Cancer.* 2006;14:216–22.
149. Tamoxifen for early breast cancer: An overview of the randomised trials. Early Breast Cancer Trialists' Collaborative Group. *Lancet.* 1998;351:1451–67.
150. Eberling JL, Wu C, Tong-Turnbeaugh R, et al. Estrogen- and tamoxifen-associated effects on brain structure and function. *Neuroimage.* 2004;21:364–71.
151. Ernst T, Chang L, Cooray D, et al. The effects of tamoxifen and estrogen on brain metabolism in elderly women. *J Natl Cancer Inst.* 2002;94:592–7.
152. Resnick SM, Maki PM, Rapp SR, et al. Effects of combination estrogen plus progestin hormone treatment on cognition and affect. *J Clin Endocrinol Metab.* 2006;91:1802–10.
153. Espeland MA, Rapp SR, Shumaker SA, et al. Conjugated equine estrogens and global cognitive function in postmenopausal women: Women's Health Initiative Memory Study. *JAMA.* 2004;291:2959–68.
154. Yaffe K, Lui LY, Grady D, et al. Cognitive decline in women in relation to non-protein-bound oestradiol concentrations. *Lancet.* 2000;356:708–12.
155. Barrett-Connor E, Goodman-Gruen D. Cognitive function and endogenous sex hormones in older women. *J Am Geriatr Soc.* 1999;47:1289–93.
156. Ciocca DR, Roig LM. Estrogen receptors in human nontarget tissues: Biological and clinical implications. *Endocr Rev.* 1995;16:35–62.

157. Rapp SR, Espeland MA, Shumaker SA, et al. Effect of estrogen plus progestin on global cognitive function in postmenopausal women: The Women's Health Initiative Memory Study: A randomized controlled trial. *JAMA*. 2003;289:2663–72.
158. Paganini-Hill A, Clark LJ. Preliminary assessment of cognitive function in breast cancer patients treated with tamoxifen. *Breast Cancer Res Treat*. 2000;64:165–76.
159. Molassiotis A, Fernadez-Ortega P, Pud D, et al. Use of complementary and alternative medicine in cancer patients: A European survey. *Ann Oncol*. 2005;16:655–63.
160. Tuxen MK, Hansen SW. Neurotoxicity secondary to antineoplastic drugs. *Cancer Treat Rev*. 1994;20:191–214.
161. Joseph JA, Denisova N, Fisher D, et al. Age-related neurodegeneration and oxidative stress: Putative nutritional intervention. *Neurol Clin*. 1998;16:747–55.
162. Fillit HM, Butler RN, O'Connell AW, et al. Achieving and maintaining cognitive vitality with aging. *Mayo Clin Proc*. 2002;77:681–96.
163. Ahles TA, Saykin AJ. Candidate mechanisms for chemotherapy-induced cognitive changes. *Nat Rev Cancer*. 2007;7:192–201.
164. Dietrich J, Han R, Yang Y, et al. CNS progenitor cells and oligodendrocytes are targets of chemotherapeutic agents in vitro and in vivo. *J Biol*. 2006;5:22.
165. Madhyastha S, Somayaji SN, Rao MS, et al. Hippocampal brain amines in methotrexate-induced learning and memory deficit. *Can J Physiol Pharmacol*. 2002;80:1076–84.
166. Ganz PA, Greendale GA, Petersen L, et al. Breast cancer in younger women: reproductive and late health effects of treatment. *J Clin Oncol*. 2003;21:4184–93.
167. Jacobsen PB, Garland LL, Booth-Jones M, et al. Relationship of hemoglobin levels to fatigue and cognitive functioning among cancer patients receiving chemotherapy. *J Pain Symptom Manage*. 2004;28:7–18.
168. Mar Fan H, Yi Q-L, Park A, Braganza S, Chang J, Couture F, Tannock IF. The influence of erythropoietin on cognitive function in women following adjuvant chemotherapy for breast cancer. San Antonio Breast Cancer Symposium. San Antonio, Texas, 2004 Abstract No. 3075
169. Ramassamy C, Averill D, Beffert U, et al. Oxidative damage and protection by antioxidants in the frontal cortex of Alzheimer's disease is related to the apolipoprotein E genotype. *Free Radic Biol Med*. 1999;27:544–53.
170. Fishel ML, Vasko MR, Kelley MR. DNA repair in neurons: So if they don't divide what's to repair? *Mutat Res*. 2007;614:24–36.
171. Lee AY, Levine MN. Venous thromboembolism and cancer: Risks and outcomes. *Circulation*. 2003;107:I17–21.
172. Falanga A, Levine MN, Consonni R, et al. The effect of very-low-dose warfarin on markers of hypercoagulation in metastatic breast cancer: Results from a randomized trial. *Thromb Haemost*. 1998;79:23–7.
173. Kuller LH, Evans RW. Homocysteine, vitamins, and cardiovascular disease. *Circulation*. 1998;98:196–9.
174. Shea TB, Lyons-Weiler J, Rogers E. Homocysteine, folate deprivation and Alzheimer neuropathology. *J Alzheimers Dis*. 2002;4:261–7.
175. Moss RB, Mercandetti A, Vojdani A. TNF-alpha and chronic fatigue syndrome. *J Clin Immunol*. 1999;19:314–16.
176. Mantovani G, Maccio A, Madeddu C, et al. Quantitative evaluation of oxidative stress, chronic inflammatory indices and leptin in cancer patients: Correlation with stage and performance status. *Int J Cancer*. 2002;98:84–91.
177. Banks WA, Farr SA, Morley JE. Entry of blood-borne cytokines into the central nervous system: Effects on cognitive processes. *Neuroimmunomodulation*. 2003;10: 319–27.
178. Pusztai L, Mendoza TR, Reuben JM, et al. Changes in plasma levels of inflammatory cytokines in response to paclitaxel chemotherapy. *Cytokine* 2004;25:94–102.

179. Meyers CA, Albitar M, Estey E. Cognitive impairment, fatigue, and cytokine levels in patients with acute myelogenous leukemia or myelodysplastic syndrome. *Cancer*. 2005; 104:788–93.
180. Lee BN, Dantzer R, Langley KE, et al. A cytokine-based neuroimmunologic mechanism of cancer-related symptoms. *Neuroimmunomodulation*. 2004;11:279–92.
181. Cleeland CS, Bennett GJ, Dantzer R, et al. Are the symptoms of cancer and cancer treatment due to a shared biologic mechanism? A cytokine-immunologic model of cancer symptoms. *Cancer*. 2003;97:2919–25.
182. Valentine AD, Meyers CA. Neurobehavioral effects of interferon therapy. *Curr Psychiatry Rep*. 2005;7:391–5.
183. Scheibel RS, Valentine AD, O'Brien S, et al. Cognitive dysfunction and depression during treatment with interferon-alpha and chemotherapy. *J Neuropsychiatry Clin Neurosci*. 2004;16:185–91.
184. Meyers CA. Mood and cognitive disorders in cancer patients receiving cytokine therapy. *Adv Exp Med Biol*. 1999;461:75–81.
185. Collado-Hidalgo A, Bower JE, Ganz PA, et al. Inflammatory biomarkers for persistent fatigue in breast cancer survivors. *Clin Cancer Res*. 2006;12:2759–66.
186. Vardy J, Booth C, Pond GR, Galica J, Zhang H, Dhillon H, Clarke SJ, Tannock IF. Cytokine levels in patients with colorectal cancer and breast cancer and their relationship to fatigue and cognitive function. American Society of Clinical Oncology. Chicago, 2007
187. Liberman JN, Stewart WF, Wesnes K, et al. Apolipoprotein E epsilon 4 and short-term recovery from predominantly mild brain injury. *Neurology*. 2002;58:1038–44.
188. Tardiff BE, Newman MF, Saunders AM, et al. Preliminary report of a genetic basis for cognitive decline after cardiac operations. The Neurologic Outcome Research Group of the Duke Heart Center. *Ann Thorac Surg*. 1997;64:715–20.
189. Roses AD, Saunders AM. ApoE, Alzheimer's disease, and recovery from brain stress. *Ann N Y Acad Sci*. 1997; 826:200–12.
190. Ahles TA, Saykin AJ, Noll WW, et al. The relationship of APOE genotype to neuropsychological performance in long-term cancer survivors treated with standard dose chemotherapy. *Psychooncology*. 2003;12:612–9.
191. Jamroziak K, Robak T. Pharmacogenomics of MDR1/ABCB1 gene: The influence on risk and clinical outcome of haematological malignancies. *Hematology*. 2004;9:91–105.
192. Kreb R. Implications of genetic polymorphisms in drug transporters for pharmacotherapy. *Cancer Lett*. 2006;234:4–33.
193. Blasiak J, Arabski M, Krupa R, et al. Basal, oxidative and alkylative DNA damage, DNA repair efficacy and mutagen sensitivity in breast cancer. *Mutat Res*. 2004;554: 139–48.
194. Morley KI, Montgomery GW. The genetics of cognitive processes: Candidate genes in humans and animals. *Behav Genet*. 2001;31:511–31.
195. Savitz J, Solms M, Ramesar R. The molecular genetics of cognition: Dopamine, COMT and BDNF. *Genes Brain Behav*. 2006;5:311–28.
196. Schroder CP, Wisman GB, de Jong S, et al. Telomere length in breast cancer patients before and after chemotherapy with or without stem cell transplantation. *Br J Cancer*. 2001;84:1348–53.
197. Vasa-Nicotera M, Brouilette S, Mangino M, et al. Mapping of a major locus that determines telomere length in humans. *Am J Hum Genet*. 2005;76:147–51.
198. Thompson SJ, Leigh L, Christensen R, et al. Immediate neurocognitive effects of methylphenidate on learning-impaired survivors of childhood cancer. *J Clin Oncol*. 2001;19:1802–8.
199. Meyers CA, Weitzner MA, Valentine AD, et al. Methylphenidate therapy improves cognition, mood, and function of brain tumor patients. *J Clin Oncol*. 1998;16:2522–7.

200. Mar Fan HG, Chemerenysky I, Xu W, Clemons M, Tannock IF. A randomised, placebo-controlled double-blind trial of the effects of d-methylphenidate therapy on fatigue and cognitive dysfunction in women undergoing adjuvant chemotherapy, Canadian Breast Cancer Research Alliance Reasons for Hope 4th Scientific Conference. Montreal, 2006 Abstract M156.
201. Lower E, Fleishman S, Cooper A, et al. A phase III, randomized placebo-controlled trial of the safety and efficacy of d-MPH as new treatment of fatigue and "chemobrain" in adult cancer patients. *J Clin Oncol* (Meeting Abstracts). 23:8000.
202. Le Bars PL, Kieser M, Itil KZ. A 26-week analysis of a double-blind, placebo-controlled trial of the ginkgo biloba extract EGb 761 in dementia. *Dement Geriatr Cogn Disord.* 2000;11:230–7.
203. Le Bars PL. Response patterns of EGb 761 in Alzheimer's disease: influence of neuropsychological profiles. *Pharmacopsychiatry*. 2003;36(Suppl 1):S50–5.
204. Kleijnen J, Knipschild P. Ginkgo biloba for cerebral insufficiency. *Br J Clin Pharmacol.* 1992;34:352–8.
205. Birks J, Grimley EV, Van Dongen M. Ginkgo biloba for cognitive impairment and dementia. *Cochrane Database Syst Rev:CD003120*. 2002.
206. Wesnes KA, Ward T, McGinty A, et al. The memory enhancing effects of a Ginkgo biloba/Panax ginseng combination in healthy middle-aged volunteers. *Psychopharmacology (Berl)*. 2000;152:353–61.
207. Kennedy DO, Scholey AB, Wesnes KA. The dose-dependent cognitive effects of acute administration of Ginkgo biloba to healthy young volunteers. *Psychopharmacology (Berl)*. 2000;151:416–23.
208. Subhan Z, Hindmarch I. The psychopharmacological effects of Ginkgo biloba extract in normal healthy volunteers. *Int J Clin Pharmacol Res*. 1984;4:89–93
209. Birks J. Does donepezil improve well-being for dementia due to Alzheimer's disease? *Neuroepidemiology*. 2005;24:168–9.
210. Birks J. Cholinesterase inhibitors for Alzheimer's disease. *Cochrane Database Syst Rev:CD005593*. 2006.
211. Christodoulou C, Melville P, Scherl WF, et al. Effects of donepezil on memory and cognition in multiple sclerosis. *J Neurol Sci*. 2006;245:127–36.
212. Krupp LB, Christodoulou C, Melville P, et al. Donepezil improved memory in multiple sclerosis in a randomized clinical trial. *Neurology*. 2004;63:1579–85.
213. Birks J, Flicker L. Donepezil for mild cognitive impairment. *Cochrane Database Syst Rev 3:CD006104*. 2006.
214. Eslinger PJ. Neuropsychological Interventions: Clinical Research and Practice. New York: Guilford Press; 2002.
215. Sohlberg MM, Mateer CA. Introduction to Cognitive Rehabilitation: Theory and Practice. New York: Guilford Press; 1989.
216. Sohlberg MM, Mateer CA. Cognitive Rehabilitation: An Integrative Neuropsychological Approach. New York: Guilford Press; 2001
217. Cicerone KD, Dahlberg C, Kalmar K, et al. Evidence-based cognitive rehabilitation: Recommendations for clinical practice. *Arch Phys Med Rehabil.* 2000;81:1596–615.
218. Carney N, Chesnut RM, Maynard H, et al. Effect of cognitive rehabilitation on outcomes for persons with traumatic brain injury: A systematic review. J Head Trauma *Rehabil*. 1999;14:277–307.
219. Consensus conference. Rehabilitation of persons with traumatic brain injury. NIH Consensus Development Panel on Rehabilitation of Persons with Traumatic Brain Injury. *JAMA*. 1999;282:974–83.
220. Mateer CA, Sira CS, O'Connell ME. Putting Humpty Dumpty together again: The importance of integrating cognitive and emotional interventions. *J Head Trauma Rehabil*. 2005;20:62–75.

221. Sohlberg MM, McLaughlin KA, Pavese A, et al. Evaluation of attention process training and brain injury education in persons with acquired brain injury. *J Clin Exp Neuropsychol*. 2000;22:656–76.
222. Cimprich B. Age and extent of surgery affect attention in women treated for breast cancer. *Res Nurs Health*. 1998;21:229–38.
223. Cimprich B, Ronis DL. Attention and symptom distress in women with and without breast cancer. *Nurs Res*. 2001;50:86–94.
224. Gottschalk LA, Holcombe RF, Jackson D, et al. The effects of anticancer chemotherapeutic drugs on cognitive function and other neuropsychiatric dimensions in breast cancer patients. *Methods Find Exp Clin Pharmacol*. 2003;25:117–22.

Costs of Adjuvant Breast Cancer Treatments

Nina Oestreicher

Introduction

Breast cancer is the leading incident cancer and the second highest cause of cancer mortality in the U.S. In 2004, breast cancer treatment expenditures were $8.1 billion [1], and may account for as much as 1% of healthcare expenditures in the U.S. [2]. Increased early detection has led to a shift towards diagnosis of early stage cancer and with the array of adjuvant therapies available, average survival has improved over time [3]. Primary therapy for early breast cancer is commonly surgery. Following surgery, chemotherapy and endocrine therapy are used alone or in combination to kill cancer cells that have spread throughout the body, because a high percentage of patients with localized disease have undetectable metastases [4]. This treatment choice depends on stage and progression of disease, tumor characteristics, presence of hormone receptors, side effect profile, and patient age, menopausal status, and comorbidities [2, 5]. Because of the strong demonstrated survival benefit of adjuvant therapy (chemotherapy and endocrine therapy) in early stage breast cancer (summarized in [4, 6]), NIH and National Comprehensive Cancer Network guidelines recommend the use of adjuvant chemotherapy for the majority of these patients and endocrine therapy to those women whose tumors express hormone receptor protein [5, 7].

The use of endocrine therapy and chemotherapy is common and has been increasing over time [8] for almost all stages and ages, suggesting that the results of clinical trials are disseminated fairly rapidly to community-based physicians and their patients. Treatments are also getting more expensive. As a result of the increasing utilization of and expense associated with adjuvant therapy, it has become important to understand the economic burden on the healthcare system and on patients placed by the use of these therapies. In addition, in recent years,

N. Oestreicher (✉)
School of Pharmacy, University of California San Francisco, CA, Genentech, Inc., South San Francisco, CA, USA
e-mail: hill.nina@gene.com

M. Castiglione, M.J. Piccart (eds.), *Adjuvant Therapy for Breast Cancer*, Cancer Treatment and Research 151, DOI 10.1007/978-0-387-75115-3_25,

economic modeling has become a popular method for evaluating costly healthcare technologies (drugs and devices) in oncology that are arriving on the market. For example, genetic tests have been developed that predict prognosis (with or without the use of endocrine therapy) in patients with breast cancer [9, 10] and would presumably spare some women unwarranted chemotherapy. The costs of chemotherapy have been an important driver of economic analyses of these technologies [11, 12], so it is especially important to have accurate chemotherapy cost estimates to inform such analyses. Another example where costs of adjuvant therapy have been used in economic modeling is in a cost-effectiveness analysis comparing aromatase inhibitors to tamoxifen as adjuvant endocrine therapy [13].

Economic studies in breast cancer have varied widely in design and focus. The common goal, however, has been to arrive at an estimate of opportunity costs, or the health benefits lost due to the next best alternative not being selected [14]. Reimbursements [15], provider charges [16], or, more rarely, accounting costs [17], have all been used in studies as proxy measures of opportunity costs, although reimbursements are a better estimate of opportunity costs than are charges, which tend to overestimate costs. The parameters that differentiate cost studies include healthcare setting, years over which the study was conducted, analytic method for costing, characteristics of the study population, time horizon, components of care included in costs, and cost perspective. Also, discounting of results to present day monetary values may or may not be performed. Differences in these design elements may dramatically affect cost estimates and may also make comparisons of costs between studies difficult. Several examples of parameters by which studies may differ are discussed in the following section.

Calendar Years of Study

Many new and expensive targeted chemotherapies, endocrine agents, and supportive care agents are being developed for use, shifting the treatment paradigm and causing an increase in the overall level of cancer treatment costs. One such example is the use of taxanes (docetaxel, paclitaxel) as adjuvant therapy. Therefore, costs may vary widely depending upon the time period in which costs were evaluated. Indeed, few studies have been performed from 2000 onward to take costs of these new therapies into account (e.g., [13, 18]).

Characteristics of the Study Population

Personal and clinical characteristics such as age, menopausal status, stage and insurance status may also influence costs. For example, older patients may cost less because they tend to receive less aggressive therapy than younger patients, and patients with more advanced stage disease at diagnosis tend to receive more aggressive therapies and cost more than those with earlier stage disease. Despite these known phenomena, there are few studies that stratify costs by these characteristics (e.g., [15, 17, 19]).

Time Horizon

The chosen time horizon for the analysis may affect results because patients may, for example, take longer than usual to complete all the cycles of a chemotherapy regimen due to temporary stoppage because of side effects. If the chosen time horizon is relatively short, it may not fully capture the costs of these patients. In addition, adjuvant endocrine therapy may be taken for 5 years after the initial cancer diagnosis [7]. However, if the time horizon is relatively long, costs may not only include those of adjuvant therapy but may also include treatment costs for women with aggressive cancers who experience an early recurrence.

Cost Perspective

Studies may adopt different viewpoints from which to evaluate costs. Common perspectives are the healthcare system payer perspective or the societal perspective. The payer perspective evaluates only direct medical costs. The societal perspective includes all costs from the payer perspective and also may include direct non-medical costs (e.g., lost productivity from time spent in treatment) or place an economic value on caregiver burden, an indirect cost.

Methods

Since the early 1990s, there has been an emerging trend of using payer administrative claims databases to estimate cancer treatment costs because of the convenience of obtaining large amounts of data on relatively large study populations in a relatively short timeframe. However, some of the greatest challenges in evaluating cancer treatment costs using these secondary data sources are (1) the lack of clinical data which may be an important predictor of cancer costs and (2) determining which costs are attributable to the cancer itself vs to some other condition. The lack of clinical data can be overcome if an investigator is fortunate to have access to a cancer registry (such as the Surveillance, Epidemiology and End Results (SEER) registry) to which the administrative records of patients with a cancer diagnosis who are enrollees of a health plan can be linked to their cancer diagnosis record in the cancer registry for a complement of clinical, utilization and economic data. This approach has been used successfully in several economic studies of breast cancer [15, 17, 19].

Most important of all aspects of economic evaluation in breast cancer, the rigor and methods of estimating costs are critical to producing reliable results. There are two predominant techniques used to evaluate costs, namely attributable costing (e.g., [15, 19, 20]) and microcosting (e.g., [21, 22]). There are various other empirical estimation methods for costs that are not well defined, which appear in various studies.

Attributable Costing

To overcome the challenge associated with attributing individual cost elements to the cancer vs to some other condition, studies have used the attributable costing method. Attributable costing is an indirect estimation approach which avoids this attribution issue. This method estimates cancer-related costs as the difference in total healthcare costs for breast cancer cases and age- and gender-matched controls without breast cancer, and assumes that cancer-related costs are additive to the costs of existing comorbid conditions [23]. Attributable costing has the advantage of generating estimates that take into account the full range of possible treatment outcomes and costs, but carries with it the limitations of potential selection bias in the study groups, violating the assumptions of similarities between the case and control groups and making the interpretation of results difficult.

Microcosting

In contrast, microcosting takes into account a narrower range of treatment costs and outcomes. First, a typical course of therapy is determined based on clinical guidelines, clinical trial regimens [21], expert opinion, or review of patient medical records, and then a cost is applied to each line item in this treatment protocol. Treatment of complications and treatment discontinuation may not consistently be taken into account. In general, accounting for heterogeneity in patient experience is limited with this method, and evaluations of RCT-based treatment regimens generally have poor external generalizability [24]. Although published guidelines exist for the appropriate use of adjuvant therapies, in community practice these guidelines are not necessarily followed [25], and may depend on the type of insurance a patient has [26] which will affect costs.

Types of Costs

Breast cancer treatment costs can be separated into direct costs (both medical and non-medical), morbidity costs (indirect) and mortality costs [27]. Direct medical costs are expenditures for medical procedures and services associated with care for the breast cancer. Direct non-medical costs, such as time spent in treatment and transportation costs, may also be included. Morbidity costs encompass lost income due to inability to work, caregiver burden and lost time to engage in leisure activities. Mortality cost is lost income associated with premature death.

For analyses relevant to payers, generally only direct medical costs are included, whereas for analyses from the societal perspective, direct non-medical and indirect costs may be included as well. For economic modeling exercises such as cost-effectiveness analysis, which may be useful for policymaking, the inclusion of indirect costs is less common. It is also potentially important to account for patient copayment if it is desirable to estimate the full costs of the drug (economic burden of disease) and not just costs to the payer.

Studies of Breast Cancer Treatment Costs

Studies of breast cancer treatment costs in the U.S. have focused on a variety of phases of treatment, treatment modalities and healthcare settings and have used various proxies for costs. For example, some studies have identified the costs incurred during the initial, continuing and terminal phases of treatment, for both a Medicare population [28] and at an HMO [17]. Costs have also been compared between specific breast cancer treatment procedures at the same HMO [29]. Other, informal analyses were based on charges rather than costs [16, 30] or included costs unrelated to cancer [31].

In addition, there are few studies that specifically address the costs of adjuvant therapy in a U.S. healthcare setting. In a review of adjuvant therapy cost studies published in 1999, van Enckevort and colleagues commented how few studies had been published from 1980 to 1997 [32]. The same is true of the present time. Hillner and Smith performed some early economic analyses of chemotherapy costs [16, 33–35], but these analyses considered treatment regimens from the 1990s. The types of adjuvant therapy regimens used and associated costs have changed dramatically since that time so results may no longer be applicable. For example, the cyclophosphamide/methotrexate/fluorouracil regimen standard at the time of these analyses is less popular now, with the availability of other regimens such as the adriamycin/cyclophosphamide regimen recommended by current guidelines [5].

Perhaps because of the predominance of single payer health systems outside of the U.S., international studies, especially in European countries, of adjuvant therapy costs (e.g., [36–42]) or overall breast cancer treatment costs [42] have been more common than studies in the U.S. In contrast to Europe, there are few population-based resources available to identify breast cancer costs in the U.S. [28]. However, applying results from ex-U.S. studies to a U.S. healthcare setting may not be straightforward, as considerable variation would be expected in costs and practices between the U.S. and other countries, such as differences in aggressiveness of treatment approaches, administration of healthcare in these systems and differences in cost structures between single payer systems and the more diffuse payer system in the U.S. Also, most European studies addressed costs in the healthcare systems of the early 1990s and, as discussed above, treatment options have changed since then. Thus these estimates may not be useful for healthcare decision-making today, in the U.S. or elsewhere. In the coming sections, results of ex-U.S. economic analyses are reported infrequently, mainly in circumstances where there is a dearth of literature from U.S. healthcare systems.

Costs of Chemotherapy

Current NIH consensus guidelines [5] recommend adjuvant chemotherapy for breast cancer patients with lymph node metastases or primary tumor size larger than 1 cm. Because most women who are diagnosed with breast cancer have tumors larger than 1 cm, adjuvant chemotherapy is recommended for the majority of patients, including those with early stage disease. Adjuvant chemotherapy use in community practice in patients less than 50 years of age with early stage disease has been reported to be in the range of 45–86%, depending on lymph node and hormone receptor status [25, 43] and has been increasing over time [8]. As chemotherapy use increases, it has become critical to understand the economic burden of this treatment on the healthcare system. At the same time, genetic tests have been developed that predict prognosis in breast cancer patients and would spare some women from unwarranted chemotherapy (and spare medical resources). The costs of chemotherapy have been an important driver of economic analyses of these technologies [11, 12], so it is especially important to have accurate chemotherapy cost estimates to inform such analyses.

Chemotherapy cost per cycle is highly dependent on the type of chemotherapy administered. The type of chemotherapy administered can depend on factors such as the stage of disease, tumor characteristics, presence of hormone receptors, side effect profile and the patient's menopausal status [2], and CMF, because it is an older regimen, is generally the least costly chemotherapy regimen. A chemotherapy regimen usually combines several drugs. For example, one regimen is referred to as "CMF" combines cyclophosphamide (a DNA damaging agent), and methotrexate and fluorouracil (which interfere with the metabolism of cancer cells). Cyclophosphamide may also be combined with doxorubicin ("AC" regimen) and a taxane. However, it is difficult to compare the costs of chemotherapy regimens solely by examining the cost per cycle, as number of cycles may vary by regimen and regimens may not be completed due to side effects.

Chemotherapy cost studies have varied on factors such as cost estimation methods, assumptions about the risk of chemotherapy-induced complications, the years over which the study was conducted, and characteristics of the study population. Due to these design differences, there has been wide variation in costs reported in studies. A 2005 study [44] by Naiem et al. estimated costs of adjuvant chemotherapy regimens, including treatment of side effects, using Medicare Average Wholesale Price (AWP) and the less conservative Medicare Public Health Service price that pharmaceutical manufacturers offer to facilities with a disproportionate share of indigent patients. Naiem and colleagues found that using Medicare AWP, costs ranged from $4568 for a six-cycle CMF regimen to $12,320 for an AC regimen (including the cost of 5 years of tamoxifen use). Although there is not an extensive description of methods, it appears that microcosting methods were used, with assumptions about the risk of chemotoxicity during therapy. In a recent study of trial-based chemotherapy protocols for node-positive patients in Canada, costs ranged over twofold from $3,557 for a fluorouracil/epirubicin/cyclophosphamide regimen to $8,266 for a docetaxel/doxorubicin/cyclophosphamide combination (costs in U.S. dollars), including the costs of supportive care agents [45] (Table 1).

Table 1 Treatment costs and health care utilization of selected regimens for node-positive breast cancer patients (from Trudeau et al. 2005) [45]

	FEC100	Oral CEF	TAC	AC60 then P175	AC60 then P225	Dose dense AC then P175
Administration cost	$216	$347	$239	$221	$221	$221
Chemotherapy acquisition cost per treatment	$3,162	$3,860	$6,825	$4,072	$5,185	$4,072
Protocol-driven supportive drug cost per treatment	...	$159	$92	$11	$11	$7,412
Incidental supportive-care cost per treatment	$179	$486	$1,110	$36	$248	$36
Total treatment cost	$3,557	$4,852	$8,266	$4,340	$5,665	$11,741
Monthly clinic visits	1.3	2	1.3	1.3	1.3	2
Overall clinic visits	6	12	6	8	8	8
Total time on treatment (months)	4.5	6	4.5	6	6	4
Total chair time (h)	9.0	5.4	14.0	21.6	21.6	21.6

FEC100 = fluorouracil, epirubicin 100 mg/m^2, and cyclophosphamide; CEF = cyclophosphomide, epirubicin, and fluorouracil; TAC = docetaxel, doxorubicin, and cyclophosphamide; AC60 then P175 = doxorubicin 60 mg/m^2 and cyclophosphamide then paclitaxel 175 mg/m^2; AC60 then P225 = doxorubicin 60 mg/m^2 and cyclophosphamide then paclitaxel 225 mg/m^2; Dose dense AC then P175 = dose dense doxorubicin 60 mg/m^2 and cyclophosphamide then paclitaxel 175 mg/m^2

Few studies of the costs of adjuvant chemotherapy have focused on premenopausal women [15, 46], and one of these was conducted outside of the

U.S. [46]. A study by Oestreicher et al. was the first known U.S. study to focus on premenopausal women. It was also the first study to examine costs of adjuvant chemotherapy stratified by age, stage, type of surgery, and comorbidity status in a community oncology setting and found total costs to be $23,019 in the overall group. This study was notable in that it was the only one that utilized an attributable cost methodology to specifically estimate costs of chemotherapy. Not surprisingly, the cost of adjuvant chemotherapy reported by Oestreicher and colleagues was higher than what had been found previously using different costing methods, because this method accrues costs arising from the true clinical experiences of the patients, as opposed to, for example, costing a trial-based chemotherapy regimen, which may have poor generalizability to community practice. The study by Oestreicher et al. did not estimate costs for specific chemotherapy regimens. However, the authors performed a preliminary evaluation of the incremental costs of taxanes when compared to the costs of adjuvant therapy pooled over all regimens ($23,019), and found they increased chemotherapy costs by $8,328 per patient when included as part of treatment.

There are some older articles that specifically estimate chemotherapy costs but some of these articles are too low to be applicable to modern healthcare systems. For example, in one of these studies [47], the costs of chemotherapy and supportive care agents amounted to no more than $1,500. As previously mentioned, CMF was the standard regimen at the time of these analyses, but an AC regimen is recommended by current guidelines and taxanes are often used in conjunction with AC [5]. A 1995 study by Kattlove et al. [30] notable for its public health significance, evaluated the costs of a CMF regimen at $2,523, including nine cycles of chemotherapy, administration of antiemetics, supplies, blood cell counts, and physician visits. They estimated these costs with the goal of developing a basic benefit package for detection and treatment of early breast cancer by evaluating the effectiveness and costs for screening mammography, primary surgery, adjuvant therapy, and follow-up care. Messori et al. [48] estimated the costs of a CMF regimen for a cost-effectiveness model at $1,595, which included administration costs but did not include costs of supportive care agents for treating toxicities. Irvin and Kuhn [22] costed trial-based regimens and found that costs (represented as charges) varied from $2,026 for six cycles of CMF to $9,316 for six cycles of fluorouracil/doxorubicin/cyclophosphamide and includes costs of antiemetics as supportive care agents. In addition to these cost estimates pertaining to practice patterns from the 1990s, they were also derived from charges to the insurer and were protocol-based so may not be realistic representations of the current economic burden of these regimens. Lokich et al. [49] estimated costs of $5,300 for an AC regimen, excluding hospital visit and radiology charges and the cost of treating drug toxicity. The healthcare setting in which costs were evaluated for this study was unclear. The highest chemotherapy cost estimate from studies prior to 2000 was by Hillner et al. [16], who reported a cost of approximately $16,000, including complications from chemotherapy, although it is not clear what other medical resource utilization is included in this estimate. In any case, results from these studies are difficult to interpret because they were conducted too long ago to represent the economic burden of current chemotherapy regimens, were sometimes based on trial-based regimens with poor generalizability to community practice and used charges as a proxy for costs.

Costs of Endocrine Therapy

Breast cancer is considered to be a hormone-dependent cancer and endocrine therapy deprives cancer cells of the estrogen that some of them need to grow. Cells in the breast contain estrogen and progesterone receptors that allow tissue to grow or change in response to changing hormone levels and if the levels of these receptors are high enough, the cancer may be amenable to anti-estrogen treatment. As of 1998, 78% of invasive breast cancers were estrogen receptor positive and 68% were progesterone receptor positive [50]. For these types of tumors, the primary treatments have been oral medication, most commonly tamoxifen, which has been approved since 1977 for treatment of breast cancer. Newer agents are the aromatase inhibitors, anastrozole, letrozole and exemestane, that specifically target aromatase-mediated production of estrogen. The Arimidex, Tamoxifen Alone or in Combination (ATAC) trial resulted in a statistically significant increase in progression-free survival compared to tamoxifen [51]. Based on results from the ATAC and other studies, aromatase inhibitors are now recommended as adjuvant endocrine therapy, either as initial therapy or after treatment with tamoxifen, for postmenopausal women [7, 52]. Aromatase inhibitors are also being prescribed more frequently because tumors may become resistant to tamoxifen over time and also because of the serious side effects of tamoxifen, such as thromboembolism and endometrial carcinoma [2, 13].

Tamoxifen has been available as a generic agent since 2003. In contrast, anastrozole, the first aromatase inhibitor to be developed, was approved by the FDA for use in the adjuvant setting in 2002. The prices of these two agents that have been reported reflect their relative maturity in the market. Hillner et al. reported a fivefold price difference between tamoxifen and anastrozole ($1.25 vs $6.75 per day), based on 2004 estimates from drugstore.com in their cost-effectiveness model of anastrozole vs tamoxifen based on results from the ATAC trial [13]. International estimates of the costs of endocrine therapy have been as parameters in economic models, including a recent one for letrozole therapy [53], although the costs are given per cycle as opposed to for the entire treatment period. Another study performed in Norway did include annual costs of tamoxifen and letrozole, at $200 and $1,727, respectively (in U.S. dollars) [54]. Finally, analyses performed from the perspective of a health-care payer in Brazil again suggest high costs for aromatase inhibitors [55]. Extended adjuvant letrozole therapy after 5 years of tamoxifen use in postmenopausal women would cost approximately $2,735, $2,650, $2,572, and $2,467 in years 1–4 following tamoxifen therapy, respectively.

Costs of Supportive Care Agents

Both chemotherapy and endocrine therapy may lead to complications requiring treatment with supportive care agents. Side effects associated with chemotherapy are common and may include nausea, alopecia, hematologic toxicities, cardiotoxicity, menopausal symptoms, fatigue, decrements in cognitive function, and weight gain [56]. For endocrine therapy, side effects of tamoxifen may include endometrial cancer and vaginal bleeding [2, 13], whereas aromatase inhibitors commonly lead to brittle bones and fractures.

Chemotherapy Supportive Care Agents

There is a host of supportive care agents available to address chemotherapy complications. Hematological side effects of chemotherapy, anemia, neutropenia, and thrombocytopenia are common to all chemotherapy regimens and are usually the most costly side effect to treat, because they may become life-threatening and require hospitalization. These hematological complications can be prophylaxed or treated with granulocyte colony stimulating factors (G-CSF). National Comprehensive Cancer Network (NCCN) guidelines suggest G-CSFs should be used prophylactically with dose dense AC/paclitaxel chemotherapy regimens [7]. Febrile neutropenia is a severe and costly side effect that can result in infection and sometimes death [45]. Economic analyses have suggested that about 10% patients may require G-CSFs during their chemotherapy regimen for low white blood cell counts and 3% would require hospitalization for neutropenia [44]. Monitoring and treatment of cardiotoxicity, a side effect for anthracyclines, particularly for doxorubicin/paclitaxel in combination [45], can be costly. Nausea may be treated with antiemetics such as serotonin 5-HT3 receptor antagonists, ondansetron, and granisetron.

Costs of supportive care agents for chemotherapy have been examined directly in the metastatic setting [57], but little such work has been performed in the adjuvant setting. Data from a recent study suggest that protocol-driven supportive care agents can vary from $47 for an AC60 then P175 regimen to $7,448 for the dose dense counterpart of this regimen [45] (Table 1). Oestreicher et al. [15] included the costs of supportive care agents in the overall cost of chemotherapy and also broke out the incremental costs of these supportive care agents as separate line items. They estimated costs of $2,833 per patient treated with erythropoietin or darbepoetin for anemia, $3,682 per patient treated with G-CSFs for neutropenia and $1,040 for antiemetics. Hospitalizations for complications costed an extra $6,945 per patient. Guidelines for the use of CSFs [58] suggest that the routine use of CSFs for primary prophylaxis cannot be justified on the basis of cost savings unless the risk of febrile neutropenia is greater than 40% (based on a hospitalization cost of $10,000), but no routine regimens have rates greater than 15%. If the hospitalization costs were lower, the risk of neutropenia would have to be even higher to offset the costs of G-CSFs.

Endocrine Therapy Supportive Care Agents

It is important to note that endocrine therapies may be taken over a long period of time, up to 5 years after the initial course of adjuvant therapy [7]. Because of the long duration of treatment, there is a high probability of side effects in the patient. Bisphosphonates are substances that inhibit the resorption of bone and also may prevent bone metastases. Even though bisphosphonates are not inexpensive, they are being used to prevent osteoporosis and fractures in patients treated with aromatase inhibitors. Lonning et al. [54] reported annual costs of $484 for use of oral alendronate, a bisphosphonate used to prevent osteoporosis and bone metastases, which is far smaller than the costs of a hip fracture ($33,000) or hip replacement ($16,600). These costs were derived from a clinical trial [59].

Costs of Targeted Therapies: Trastuzumab and Lapatinib

As oncology as a field progresses and gets more molecular in nature, drug development has evolved to design agents that act on specific molecular targets in carcinogenesis, leading to more intensive and expensive modes of therapy. Trastuzumab was the first monoclonal antibody specifically targeted for HER2-overexpressing breast cancer. Trastuzumab was approved in 2006 for use in the adjuvant treatment of HER2+, node-positive breast cancer as part of a treatment regimen containing doxorubicin, cyclophosphamide and paclitaxel, after having been used in the metastatic setting since 1998. There are now therapies being developed with the goal of avoiding chemotherapy and its concurrent toxicities. Lapatinib, although not FDA-approved for the adjuvant setting, is already being used off-label for this purpose. Lapatinib was only recently approved by the FDA for use in women with HER2+ metastatic breast cancer who received prior therapy in the form of anthracycline, taxanes or trastuzumab, in combination with capecitabine [60]. There are no cost data available for lapatinib in the metastatic setting since it was only recently approved for use.

Since trastuzumab had not been approved until recently for the adjuvant setting, there are no known published economic analyses of its use in article form, although one article in the metastatic setting suggests its costs are $21,209, including the cost of the fluorescent in situ hybridization (FISH) as the diagnostic test for HER2 status. Its cost is $17,395 if FISH is not used [61]. In recently disseminated economic modeling exercises of trastuzumab in the adjuvant setting from the payer perspective, average costs of trastuzumab were estimated at $47,278 (Canadian dollars) in one such exercise, as compared to $26,648 for the treatment of metastatic disease [62]. These estimates included the costs supportive medications, diagnostics and health resources utilization attributable to the use of trastuzumab. It is not explicitly stated whether the costs of monitoring for cardiotoxicity associated with trastuzumab are included in estimates. Garrison et al. [18] also estimated the costs of adjuvant trastuzumab when added to a standard regimen of doxorubicin, cyclophosphamide and paclitaxel for a cost-effectiveness model, at $46,300. This estimate included HER2 testing, monitoring and treatment for cardiotoxicity, treatment for recurrence and end-of-life costs for dying patients. Costs are likely overestimated because Garrison et al. used a 20-year time horizon for their cost-effectiveness model, whereas adjuvant treatment occurs in a much shorter timeframe.

Differences in Costs by Age, Stage and Other Characteristics

As previously mentioned, many clinical and personal characteristics are considered in the choice of adjuvant therapy. One example of this is that although tamoxifen is indicated for ER+ tumors, not all patients with ER+ breast cancer receive tamoxifen [10]. In general, cancer treatment tends to be more intensive in younger patients and in more aggressive cancers, so these factors need to be taken into account when evaluating treatment costs in real world studies of breast cancer patients. Not surprisingly, age and stage gradients have been found in cancer care [15, 17, 19] (negative age-cost gradient and positive stage-cost gradient). For example, younger women can tolerate more aggressive regimens which also have greater side effects, leading to higher treatment costs. Baker et al. [20] showed that the total costs of breast cancer care increase with stage and decrease with age using an attributable cost approach. Tollestrup et al. found differences in total costs of care by age using an attributable cost approach [63] when cases of in situ disease were compared to regional distant disease for women under age 50 years ($17,093 vs $5,089) and about twice as great for women over 50 years. Oestreicher [15] found similar effects for costs of adjuvant chemotherapy (Table 2). Costs for women <50 years, 50–59 years and 60+ years were $26,834, $19,889, and $17,098, respectively. In the Oestreicher et al. study [15], for local stage disease, costs were $12,659 and for regional stage they were almost threefold greater ($36,076). Interestingly, costs of care were not substantially influenced by level of comorbidities as measured by the Charlson Index, adapted to utilize International Classification of Diseases (ICD-9-CM) diagnosis and procedure codes [64, 65].

Table 2 Adjuvant Chemotherapy Attributable Costs Stratified by Age, Stage and Comorbidity (from Oestreicher et al, 2005)[a]

	Breast Cancer Attributable Costs With Chemotherapy	Breast Cancer Attributable Costs With Chemotherapy	Chemotherapy Attributable Costs	95% ConfidentceInterval Lower Bound	Upper Bound
Age at diagnosis					
<50 yr	$47,034	$20,199	$26,834	$22,234	$31,434
50–59 yr	$42,819	$22,929	$19,889	$14,269	$25,510
60 +	$36,421	$19,322	$17,098	$10,055	$24,142
Stage Stratified by Age					
Local Stage					
Age <50	$34,651	$20,443	$14,208	$10,359	$18,058
Age 50–59	$34,983	$23,259	$11,724	$6,101	$17,348
Age 60 +	$28,787	$19,593	$9,194	-$215	$18,602
All Ages	$34,175	$21,516	$12,659	$9,416	$15,902
Regional Stage					
Age <50	$59,756	$15,949	$43,806	$33,213	$54,400
Age 50–59	$50,405	$18,032	$32,374	$20,801	$43,946
Age 60 +	$40,913	$17,150	$23,763	$13,119	$34,407
All Ages	$53,376	$17,300	$36,076	$30,609	$41,544
Charison Index Stratified by Age					
0 Comorbidities					
Age <50	$47,000	$20,482	$26,517	$21,506	$31,529
Age 50–59	$43,051	$22,752	$20,299	$14,102	$26,496
Age 60 +	$36,984	$20,080	$16,904	$8,528	$25,280
All Ages	$45,012	$21,406	$23,606	$19,804	$27,407
>= ***1 Comorbidities***					
Age <50	$43,534	$16,444	$27,091	$17,077	$37,104
Age 50–59	$45,281	$24,246	$21,035	$9,629	$32,440
Age 60 +	$34,796	$17,023	$17,773	$7,010	$28,536
All Ages	$42,037	$20,697	$21,340	$14,599	$28,081
Charlson Index Stratified by Stage					
0 Comorbidities					
Local Stage	$34,552	$21,611	$12,941	$9,480	$16,402
Regional Stage	$55,488	$18,817	$36,671	$29,072	$44,269
All Stages	$45,012	$21,406	$23,606	$19,804	$27,407
>= **1 Comorbidities**					
Local Stage	$34,877	$21,688	$13,188	$4,526	$21,851
Regional Stage	$46,440	$10,901	$35,539	$26,826	$44,252
All Stages	$42,037	$20,697	$21,340	$14,599	$28,081

Direct Non-medical, Indirect and Out of Pocket Costs

Few studies have been performed to estimate the indirect costs of cancer, such as the economic burden on the family for their care of the patient [66–68] and the effect of cancer survivorship on employment [69–71]. Also, direct non-medical costs, such as lost wages due to time spent in cancer treatment and out of pocket costs to the patient are seldom included in economic analyses, which often are performed from the payer perspective. Although there has been little literature on the effect of adjuvant therapy on ability to work after breast cancer, a recent study [70] suggests that adjuvant treatments do not appear to play a role in breast cancer survivors' cessation of employment. Adjuvant treatments did not appear to predict work cessation 3 years after breast cancer diagnosis, although the authors acknowledge other aspects of having breast cancer may have influenced the decision to reduce work effort after diagnosis of the disease. Other studies [69, 71, 72] have had similar findings.

Even for women who are insured, out of pocket costs to the patient from their breast cancer care can be substantial [73], as much as 98% of household income for women with annual household incomes below $30,000. Out of pocket costs were estimated at $1,455 in a recent study [73], including medications not fully covered by insurance and transportation (an average of 36 miles roundtrip for clinic visits at an average of 4.5 visits per month [72]). Other studies have also reported on these costs [68, 74]

Methodologic Challenges

Despite the large recognized economic burden of adjuvant therapy for breast cancer there is only a limited literature quantifying this burden. As previously mentioned, claims databases are becoming a popular source of data for cost analyses. It is possible that the lack of depth in the literature is due to the extensive methodologic challenges in performing these analyses in administrative claims databases. However, because of the decentralized healthcare system of the U.S., there are few population-based alternatives available to identify breast cancer treatment costs [28]. There are challenges around identifying the use of chemotherapy or other treatments in administrative databases and algorithms are often developed to identify these treatments in claims data. Although, investigators who have used such algorithms in breast cancer patients have found reasonable accuracy (88% sensitivity) [75]. These inaccuracies can still affect results. For example, Oestreicher et al. found trastuzumab users in their population of breast cancer patients undergoing adjuvant therapy, well before it was approved for use in the adjuvant setting [15]. With these algorithms it may be possible to identify whether a patient received chemotherapy or endocrine treatment, but it may be more difficult to identify the type of treatment received. Specific treatment modalities might not even be accurately identified by cancer registries such as SEER which are more focused on disease characteristics than treatment.

Claims-based data also have several other important limitations. First, there may be selection bias among patients who did and did not receive chemotherapy. In other words, important differences may exist between these two groups beyond the treatment itself and if results are not stratified by these characteristics they may be misleading. Age is a good example of where multiple aspects of selection bias may be acting on costs. In the Oestreicher et al. study [15], women treated with chemotherapy were younger and tended to have more severe disease than women not treated with chemotherapy, leading to higher costs. On the other hand, peri-/post-menopausal women may be experiencing conditions such as depression, hot flashes, insomnia, and endometrial bleeding, which may potentially increase their health care costs. We would expect these phenomena to affect not only the decision to administer chemotherapy, but also other treatment decisions and health conditions in the adjuvant therapy period following diagnosis. Furthermore, premenopausal women may elect to have different procedures than older women. For example, premenopausal women with early stage breast cancer are more likely to forego mastectomy and undergo breast-conserving therapy than older women [29]. In the Oestreicher et al. study [15], chemotherapy attributable costs for mastectomy patients ($31,075) were almost twice as large as for patients who had breast conserving surgery, and it is expected that some of this difference would be due to the cost difference between the two types of surgery, in addition to any cost differences due to the chemotherapy itself. Because of potential selection bias, cost estimates pooled over subgroups may be difficult to interpret, and the analyses stratified by age, stage, type of surgery, and comorbidities may be more informative for decision-making.

Conclusion

As healthcare costs continue to rise and technology-based therapies so common in oncology play a role, payers and patients will need estimates of the economic burden of these new therapies. Costs of adjuvant therapy are high and make a substantial contribution to economic burden in cancer care. The treatment of breast cancer is evolving constantly and new approaches, especially in the area of targeted therapies, are being explored. There can now be a variety of active regimens designed to deal with the diversity of patient characteristics, and economic information will be an important contributor to cost-benefit analyses of these agents for policymaking. In this era of increasing financial constraints and where new therapies are generally more expensive than existing ones, policy allocation decisions may need to be made, especially for a disease as common as breast cancer. Increasing use and availability of electronic sources of data for analyses may increase the knowledge base around this large economic burden and help policymakers make better decisions around resource allocation. Costs can be useful information on their own, but may also serve to inform policy-oriented models in oncology, such as evaluating the cost-effectiveness of using the results of DNA microarray analysis to inform chemotherapy decisions in early stage patients [11, 12].

An important defining characteristic of a reliable cost analysis is the rigor of its methods. Even if the analytic methods are adequate to address the research question, it is important for the consumer of these analyses to critically interpret the results of any economic study, especially because of the dramatic differences in study results that can be produced by differences in study parameters. Other caveats are that costs may only generalize to the institution or type of institution in which they were studied, and thus may only be useful to decision makers at that institution.

There are several areas in evaluation of the costs of adjuvant therapy in which further study is needed. First, it is important to perform up to date cost analyses which take into account the costs of newer chemotherapies and endocrine agents which are quickly coming onto the market and changing the treatment paradigm for early stage breast cancer. Second, further investigation is merited as to the important contributors to costs of adjuvant therapies in breast cancer, and differences in treatment patterns among recipients and non-recipients of various types of adjuvant therapy that may bias results. Finally, little work has been done to investigate the indirect costs of cancer and the economic burden of cancer care to patients. In conclusion, in order to make decisions about resource allocation in oncology taking into account the stakeholders for these decisions, patients, payers and physicians, it is critical to accurately identify economic burden to the payer, and to the patient.

Acknowledgment

I would like to thank my husband, Dale Hill, for his review of the chapter.

References

1. National Cancer Institute. Cancer trends progress report – 2005 update.
2. Radice D, Redaelli A. Breast cancer management: Quality-of-life and cost considerations. *Pharmacoeconomics*. 2003;21(6):383–96.
3. Ries LAG, Eisner MP, Kosary CL, Hankey BF, Miller BA, Clegg LX, et al. SEER Cancer Statistics Review, 1975–2003 Bethesda, MD: National Cancer Institute, 2006.
4. Early Breast Cancer Trialists' Collaborative Group. Polychemotherapy for early breast cancer: An overview of the randomised trials. *Lancet*. 1998;352(9132):930–42.
5. Eifel P, Axelson JA, Costa J, Crowley J, Curran WJ Jr, Deshler A, et al. National Institutes of Health Consensus Development Conference Statement: Adjuvant therapy for breast cancer, November 1–3, 2000. *J Natl Cancer Inst*. 2001;93(13):979–89.

6. Early Breast Cancer Trialists' Collaborative Group. Tamoxifen for early breast cancer: An overview of the randomised trials. *Lancet.* 1998;351(9114):1451–67.
7. Carlson R, Anderson B, Burstein H, et al. National Comprehensive Cancer Network Clinical Practice Guidelines in Oncology: Breast Cancer: National Comprehensive Cancer Network, 2007.
8. Mariotto A, Feuer EJ, Harlan LC, Wun LM, Johnson KA, Abrams J. Trends in use of adjuvant multi-agent chemotherapy and tamoxifen for breast cancer in the United States: 1975–1999. *J Natl Cancer Inst.* 2002;94(21):1626–34.
9. van 't Veer LJ, Dai H, van de Vijver MJ, He YD, Hart AA, Mao M, et al. Gene expression profiling predicts clinical outcome of breast cancer. *Nature.* 2002;415(6871):530–6.
10. Habel L, Quesenberry C, Jacobs M, Greenberg D, Fehrenbacher L, Alexander C, et al. Gene expression and breast cancer mortality in Northern California Kaiser Permanente Patients: A large population-based case control study *American Society for Clinical Oncology Annual Meeting.* 2005.
11. Oestreicher N, Ramsey SD, Linden HM, McCune JS, van't Veer LJ, Burke W, et al. Gene expression profiling and breast cancer care: what are the potential benefits and policy implications? *Genet Med.* 2005;7(6):380–9.
12. Hornberger J, Cosler LE, Lyman GH. Economic analysis of targeting chemotherapy using a 21-gene RT-PCR assay in lymph-node-negative, estrogen-receptor-positive, early-stage breast cancer. *Am J Manag Care.* 2005;11(5):313–24.
13. Hillner BE. Benefit and projected cost-effectiveness of anastrozole versus tamoxifen as initial adjuvant therapy for patients with early-stage estrogen receptor-positive breast cancer. *Cancer.* 2004;101(6):1311–22.
14. Gold ME, Russell LB, Siegel JE, Weinstein ME. Cost-effectiveness in Health and Medicine New York: Oxford University Press, 1996.
15. Oestreicher N, Ramsey SD, McCune JS, Linden HM, Veenstra DL. The cost of adjuvant chemotherapy in patients with early-stage breast carcinoma. *Cancer.* 2005;104(10):2054–62.
16. Hillner BE, Smith TJ. A model of chemotherapy in node-negative breast cancer. *J Natl Cancer Inst Monogr.* 1992(11):143–9.
17. Taplin SH, Barlow W, Urban N, Mandelson MT, Timlin DJ, Ichikawa L, et al. Stage, age, comorbidity, and direct costs of colon, prostate, and breast cancer care. *J Natl Cancer Inst.* 1995;87(6):417–26.
18. Garrison L, Perez E, Dueck A, Lalla D, Paton V, Lubeck D. Cost-effectiveness analysis of trastuzumab in the adjuvant setting for treatment of HER2 + breast cancer. *J Clin Oncol.* 2006;24(18S):6023.
19. Fireman BH, Quesenberry CP, Somkin CP, Jacobson AS, Baer D, West D, et al. Cost of care for cancer in a health maintenance organization. *Health Care Financ Rev.* 1997;18(4):51–76.
20. Baker MS, Kessler LG, Urban N, Smucker RC. Estimating the treatment costs of breast and lung cancer. *Med Care.* 1991;29(1):40–9.
21. Lober J, Sogaard J, Mouridsen HT, Jorgensen J. Treatment costs of adjuvant cytotoxic therapy in premenopausal breast cancer patients. *Acta Oncol.* 1988;27(6A):767–71.
22. Irvin R, Kuhn J. Financial considerations in the use of adjuvant chemotherapy. In: Henderson I, ed. *Adjuvant Therapy of Breast Cancer.* Boston: Kluwer Academic Publishers, 1992.
23. Hartunian NS, Smart CN, Thompson MS. The incidence and economic costs of cancer, motor vehicle injuries, coronary heart disease, and stroke: a comparative analysis. *Am J Public Health.* 1980;70(12):1249–60.
24. Johnston K, Gerard K, Brown J. Generalizing costs from trials. Analyzing center selection bias in a breast screening trial. *Int J Technol Assess Health Care.* 1998;14(3):494–504.
25. Du XL, Key CR, Osborne C, Mahnken JD, Goodwin JS. Discrepancy between consensus recommendations and actual community use of adjuvant chemotherapy in women with breast cancer. *Ann Intern Med.* 2003;138(2):90–7.

26. Harlan LC, Greene AL, Clegg LX, Mooney M, Stevens JL, Brown ML. Insurance status and the use of guideline therapy in the treatment of selected cancers. *J Clin Oncol.* 2005;23(36):9079–88.
27. Brown ML, Lipscomb J, Snyder C. The burden of illness of cancer: Economic cost and quality of life. *Annu Rev Public Health.* 2001;22:91–113.
28. Warren JL, Brown ML, Fay MP, Schussler N, Potosky AL, Riley GF. Costs of treatment for elderly women with early-stage breast cancer in fee-for-service settings. *J Clin Oncol.* 2002;20(1):307–16.
29. Barlow WE, Taplin SH, Yoshida CK, Buist DS, Seger D, Brown M. Cost comparison of mastectomy versus breast-conserving therapy for early-stage breast cancer. *J Natl Cancer Inst.* 2001;93(6):447–55.
30. Kattlove H, Liberati A, Keeler E, Brook RH. Benefits and costs of screening and treatment for early breast cancer. Development of a basic benefit package. *JAMA.* 1995;273(2):142–8.
31. Riley GF, Potosky AL, Lubitz JD, Kessler LG. Medicare payments from diagnosis to death for elderly cancer patients by stage at diagnosis. *Med Care.* 1995;33(8):828–41.
32. van Enckevort PJ, TenVergert EM, Schrantee S, Rutten FF, de Vries EG. Economic evaluations of systemic adjuvant breast cancer treatments: Methodological issues and a critical review. *Crit Rev Oncol Hematol.* 1999;32(2):113–24.
33. Hillner BE, Smith TJ. Efficacy and cost effectiveness of adjuvant chemotherapy in women with node-negative breast cancer. A decision-analysis model. *N Engl J Med.* 1991;324(3):160–8.
34. Hillner BE, Smith TJ, Desch CE. Assessing the cost effectiveness of adjuvant therapies in early breast cancer using a decision analysis model. *Breast Cancer Res Treat.* 1993;25(2):97–105.
35. Smith TJ, Hillner BE. The efficacy and cost-effectiveness of adjuvant therapy of early breast cancer in premenopausal women. *J Clin Oncol.* 1993;11(4):771–6.
36. Friedlander ML, Tattersall MH. Counting the costs of cancer therapy. *Eur J Cancer Clin Oncol.* 1982;18(12):1237–41.
37. Wolstenholme JL, Smith SJ, Whynes DK. The costs of treating breast cancer in the United Kingdom: Implications for screening. *Int J Technol Assess Health Care.* 1998;14(2):277–89.
38. Koopmanschap MA, van Roijen L, Bonneux L, Barendregt JJ. Current and future costs of cancer. *Eur J Cancer.* 1994;30A(1):60–5.
39. Kruijshaar ME, Barendregt JJ. The breast cancer related burden of morbidity and mortality in six European countries: the European Disability Weights project. *Eur J Public Health.* 2004;14(2):141–6.
40. Remak E, Brazil L. Cost of managing women presenting with stage IV breast cancer in the United Kingdom. *Br J Cancer.* 2004;91(1):77–83.
41. Will BP, Berthelot JM, Le Petit C, Tomiak EM, Verma S, Evans WK. Estimates of the lifetime costs of breast cancer treatment in Canada. *Eur J Cancer.* 2000;36(6):724–35.
42. McArdle CS, Calman KC, Cooper AF, Hughson AV, Russell AR, Smith DC. The social, emotional and financial implications of adjuvant chemotherapy in breast cancer. *Br J Surg.* 1981;68(4):261–4.
43. Harlan LC, Abrams J, Warren JL, Clegg L, Stevens J, Ballard-Barbash R. Adjuvant therapy for breast cancer: Practice patterns of community physicians. *J Clin Oncol.* 2002;20(7):1809–17.
44. Naeim A, Keeler EB. Is adjuvant therapy for older patients with node (+) early breast cancercost-effective?*. *Breast Cancer Res Treat.* 2005;94(2):95–103.
45. Trudeau M, Charbonneau F, Gelmon K, Laing K, Latreille J, Mackey J, et al. Selection of adjuvant chemotherapy for treatment of node-positive breast cancer. *Lancet Oncol.* 2005;6(11):886–98.
46. Norum J. Adjuvant cyclophosphamide, methotrexate, fluorouracil (CMF) in breast cancer – is it cost-effective? *Acta Oncol.* 2000;39(1):33–9.

47. Butler JR, Furnival CM, Hart RF. The costs of treating breast cancer in Australia and the implications for breast cancer screening. *Aust N Z J Surg*. 1995;65(7):485–91.
48. Messori A, Becagli P, Trippoli S, Tendi E. Cost-effectiveness of adjuvant chemotherapy with cyclophosphamide + methotrexate + fluorouracil in patients with node-positive breast cancer. *Eur J Clin Pharmacol*. 1996;51(2):111–6.
49. Lokich JJ, Moore CL, Anderson NR. Comparison of costs for infusion versus bolus chemotherapy administration – Part two. Use of charges versus reimbursement for cost basis. *Cancer*. 1996;78(2):300–3.
50. Li CI, Daling JR, Malone KE. Incidence of invasive breast cancer by hormone receptor status from 1992 to 1998. *J Clin Oncol*. 2003;21(1):28–34.
51. Baum M. The ATAC (Arimidex, Tamoxifen, Alone or in Combination) adjuvant breast cancer trial in postmenopausal patients: factors influencing the success of patient recruitment. *Eur J Cancer*. 2002;38(15):1984–6.
52. Winer E, Hudis C, Burstein H, et al. Use of aromatase inhibitors as adjuvant therapy for postmenopaual women with hormone receptor-positive breast cancer: Status report 2004: *ASCO*. 2006.
53. Ouagari KE, Karnon J, Delea T, Talbot W, Brandman J. Cost-effectiveness of letrozole in the extended adjuvant treatment of women with early breast cancer. *Breast Cancer Res Treat*. 2007;101(1):37–49.
54. Lonning PE. Comparing cost/utility of giving an aromatase inhibitor as monotherapy for 5 years versus sequential administration following 2–3 or 5 years of tamoxifen as adjuvant treatment for postmenopausal breast cancer. *Ann Oncol*. 2006;17(2):217–25.
55. Calabro A, Garcia M, Portella M. A budget impact analysis of extended adjuvant letrozole following 5 years of tamoxifen in postmenopausal women with early breast cancer *American Society of Clinical Oncology Annual Meeting*. 2006.
56. Longman AJ, Braden CJ, Mishel MH. Side effects burden in women with breast cancer. *Cancer Pract*. 1996;4(5):274–80.
57. De Cock E, Hutton J, Canney P, Body JJ, Barrett-Lee P, Neary MP, et al. Cost-effectiveness of oral ibandronate versus IV zoledronic acid or IV pamidronate for bone metastases in patients receiving oral hormonal therapy for breast cancer in the United Kingdom. *Clin Ther*. 2005;27(8):1295–310.
58. Ozer H, Armitage J, Bennett C, et al. Update of recommendations for the use of hematopoietic colony-stimulating factors: Evidence-based clinical practice guidelines. *J Clin Oncol*. 2000;18:3558–85.
59. Hillner B, Ingle J, Chlebowski R, et al. 2003 ASCO update on the role of bisphosphonates and bone health issues in women with breast cancer, 2006.
60. GlaxoSmithKline. Tykerb® website. www.tykerb.com. Accessed April 1, 2007.
61. Neyt MJ, Albrecht JA, Clarysse B, Cocquyt VF. Cost-effectiveness of Herceptin: a standard cost model for breast-cancer treatment in a Belgian university hospital. *Int J Technol Assess Health Care*. 2005;21(1):132–7.
62. Drucker A, Virik K, Skedgel C, Payson D, Sellon M, Younis T. The cost burden of trastuzumab and bevacizumab monoclonal antibody therapy in solid tumors: Can we afford it? *J Clin Oncol*. 2006;24(18S):6044.
63. Tollestrup K, Frost FJ, Stidley CA, Bedrick E, McMillan G, Kunde T, et al. The excess costs of breast cancer health care in Hispanic and non-Hispanic female members of a managed care organization. *Breast Cancer Res Treat*. 2001;66(1):25–31.
64. Charlson ME, Pompei P, Ales KL, MacKenzie CR. A new method of classifying prognostic comorbidity in longitudinal studies: Development and validation. *J Chronic Dis*. 1987;40(5):373–83.
65. Deyo RA, Cherkin DC, Ciol MA. Adapting a clinical comorbidity index for use with ICD-9-CM administrative databases. *J Clin Epidemiol*. 1992;45(6):613–9.
66. Given BA, Given CW, Stommel M. Family and out-of-pocket costs for women with breast cancer. *Cancer Pract*. 1994;2(3):187–93.

67. Grunfeld E, Coyle D, Whelan T, Clinch J, Reyno L, Earle CC, et al. Family caregiver burden: Results of a longitudinal study of breast cancer patients and their principal caregivers. *CMAJ*. 2004;170(12):1795–801.
68. Lauzier S, Maunsell E, De Koninck M, Drolet M, Hebert-Croteau N, Robert J. Conceptualization and sources of costs from breast cancer: findings from patient and caregiver focus groups. *Psychooncology*. 2005;14(5):351–60.
69. Bouknight RR, Bradley CJ, Luo Z. Correlates of return to work for breast cancer survivors. *J Clin Oncol*. 2006;24(3):345–53.
70. Drolet M, Maunsell E, Mondor M, Brisson C, Brisson J, Masse B, et al. Work absence after breast cancer diagnosis: a population-based study. *CMAJ*. 2005;173(7):765–71.
71. Chirikos TN, Russell-Jacobs A, Cantor AB. Indirect economic effects of long-term breast cancer survival. *Cancer Pract*. 2002;10(5):248–55.
72. Moore KA. Breast cancer patients' out-of-pocket expenses. *Cancer Nurs*. 1999;22(5):389–96.
73. Arozullah AM, Calhoun EA, Wolf M, Finley DK, Fitzner KA, Heckinger EA, et al. The financial burden of cancer: estimates from a study of insured women with breast cancer. *J Support Oncol*. 2004;2(3):271–8.
74. Secker-Walker RH, Vacek PM, Hooper GJ, Plante DA, Detsky AS. Screening for breast cancer: time, travel, and out-of-pocket expenses. *J Natl Cancer Inst*. 1999;91(8):702–8.
75. Warren JL, Harlan LC, Fahey A, Virnig BA, Freeman JL, Klabunde CN, et al. Utility of the SEER-Medicare data to identify chemotherapy use. *Med Care*. 2002;40(8 Suppl):IV-55–61.

Social Issues: Marital Support

Louise Picard

The cancer's appearance awakens a shared anxiety about the possible ending of the conjugal relationship. For many couples, this anxiety leads to a re-evaluation of the depth of their attachment and commitment and of the importance of the other person in their life. The goal of this chapter is to present two dimensions crucial to the deepening of the intimate bond in cases where the female partner has breast cancer: the establishment of open, emotional communication and the development of exchanges based on mutuality. They will be commented on in terms of their contribution to marital well-being or marital distress. Implications for psychosocial intervention and research will be discussed.

Introduction

The development of a body of knowledge on psychosocial oncology in recent decades has highlighted the fact that the appearance of breast cancer in women does not merely constitute a medical event, but also a social event. Its occurrence profoundly disrupts the family system, especially the conjugal system. The stressors connected to the illness and its treatment and the emotional upheavals that they cause in both individual and conjugal life are liable to provoke changes in the type of communication, sexual intimacy, and the exercise of roles and responsibilities [1–3].

More fundamentally, the cancer's appearance awakens a shared anxiety about the possible ending of the conjugal relationship. For many couples, this anxiety leads to a re-evaluation of the depth of their attachment and commitment and of the importance of the other person in their life. The entire universe of the couple's relationship is suddenly disrupted and brought to the forefront [4].

On the other hand, marital support seems to play a role in protecting against cancer-related stress. Some studies recognize the quality of marital support as a

L. Picard (✉)
Faculté des sciences sociales, École de service social, Pavillon Charles-De-Koninck, Université Laval, Québec (Québec), Canada GIK 7P4
e-mail: louise.picard@svs.ulaval.ca

M. Castiglione, M.J. Piccart (eds.), *Adjuvant Therapy for Breast Cancer*, Cancer Treatment and Research 151, DOI 10.1007/978-0-387-75115-3_26,

determinant of the degree to which both spouses adjust to breast cancer. The quality of exchanges within a couple's intimate relationship is increasingly viewed as a crucial aspect to consider with respect to the quality of support [4–8].

For Laurenceau and Kleimann [9], intimacy is "a personal, subjective (and often momentary) sense of connectedness that is the outcome of an interpersonal, transactional process consisting of self-disclosure and partner responsiveness." Intimacy is conceived as an interpersonal process that rests on two determining facets: the personal revelation of significant information (feelings, thoughts) and the sincere and immediate response of the partner, who communicates his or her affection and comprehension of needs and confirms the personal value of the other. Reis and Shaver [10] add a third determinant: the perception of the response. They observe that despite the intention to give a sincere and understanding response and confirm personal value, the person receiving the response may not perceive it as such.

These authors underline the importance of ensuring correspondence between the information disclosed, the understanding transmitted, and the perception of this response for developing a sense of intimacy within exchanges. Intimate exchanges are said to have a beneficial effect, insofar as they contribute to improving mutual comprehension, validating the other person's sense of value and nourishing the bond of trust within the marital relationship. The feeling of being supported in a marital relationship is said to stem from this intimate sense of being connected, understood and accepted by the other [10]. The mutual understanding that emerges from these intimate exchanges is thought to help guide the type of support to be given on both sides [4]. However, while the intimate conjugal relationship can be a haven of security, affection, and well-being that attenuates the uncertainty surrounding the continuity of the attachment bond, it can also become a source of tension and generate feelings of loneliness, resentment, and insecurity if the partners do not provide each other with the kind of support that fosters the deepening of this intimate bond.

The goal of this chapter is to present two dimensions crucial to the deepening of the intimate bond in cases where the female partner has breast cancer: the establishment of open, emotional communication and the development of exchanges based on mutuality. These two dimensions are presented in succession for purposes of clarity, but within the conjugal dynamic, they coexist and influence each other. They will be commented on in terms of their contribution to marital well-being or marital distress. Finally, we will draw implications for psychosocial intervention and for the development of future research.

Open and Healing Communication

Communication based on self-disclosure is thought to play an important role in the development and maintenance of the intimacy bond between couples [6, 11–13]. Greene et al. [14] define self-disclosure as "an interaction between at least two individuals where one intends to deliberately divulge something personal to another." Self-disclosure gives access to personal feelings and thoughts regarding the self and the intimate relation in which the partners are engaged. It permits a deeper knowledge of each person's personal experience, the real self, and the status of the relationship. On the other hand, the decision to disclose personal information is a complex process that presupposes reflection about a certain number of questions: *what* will be revealed and *how, when* and *where* the disclosure will take place. The question of *why* constitutes a key factor for positively orienting the process of personal disclosure. The motivations for disclosure considered most likely to lead to positive outcomes are those associated with the desire and willingness to improve relational intimacy and emotional support. Beyond this, the benefits of self-disclosure are also said to depend in part on the other person's reactions to what is disclosed [14]. It is viewed as beneficial insofar as it leads to an understanding and confirmation of identity and personal value. In the opposite situation, however, it can lead to a deterioration of the intimacy bond. Self-disclosure thereby requires discernment regarding timing (which moment makes most sense), the setting, and the manner in which to proceed. It calls upon communication skills as well as adequate knowledge of the feelings of each person and the areas of vulnerability the couple faces. This knowledge may not always be present in the absence of open and appropriate communication concerning the various aspects affected within the intimate relationship.

Adopting open intimate communication can be uncomfortable for a couple confronted with breast cancer. Encounters with couples in clinical practice reveal that one of the first tasks confronting women and their partners is to resolve their personal discomfort regarding what they can or wish to communicate about their experience. They will often express their discomfort in dichotomous terms: for example, as a matter of talking openly or not about emotions provoked by the disease and the tensions it introduces to their relationship. The reasoning behind the choice to talk or not often reveals the magnitude of their disarray as well as their own personal style of dealing with their personal suffering and the suffering of those they love. The decision to open up completely or partially or to remain closed will largely be influenced by their capacity to assess and endure their own distress as well as that of their partner in the search for individual and mutual well-being. It also reveals their beliefs regarding the most appropriate way of giving support in such an emotionally charged context.

Despite the growing recognition of the benefits of open emotional communication [5, 6, 11, 12, 15], the belief most often encountered among couples is that hiding one's worries is a way to protect the other [16, 17]. This protective attitude translates into the suppression of negative feelings and the need to keep up an optimistic facade at all times so as to minimize impact, avoid conflict or discussion about the illness. Both partners feel fragile and feel a legitimate need to protect themselves by diminishing the emotional repercussions for themselves and for those around them. Each is afraid of further upsetting the other and the relationship if they open up regarding their needs, thoughts and negative feelings (fears, frustrations, etc.).

However, this fear discourages the adoption of open communication regarding issues related to the illness (loss, fears of death and recurrence of the disease, disruption of sex life, overburden of responsibilities, etc.). Limiting self-expression or silencing one's concerns and emotions is generally harmful and prevents people from resolving sources of anxiety and sharing plans for the future [13]. A facade of assurance has been shown to block rather than facilitate marital communication [18]. Moreover, the protective attitude of the male spouse may be interpreted by his partner as insensitivity and leave her with feelings of isolation, abandonment, and rejection [19].

In this context, one of the relational issues for the couple becomes precisely that of adopting a type of communication that favours the nuanced disclosure of feelings, thoughts, and needs. Intervention with couples often reveals that emotional distance arises from the partners' inability to share their feelings and needs, and from the adoption of an inappropriate pattern of conflict resolution based primarily on an attitude of protection [20]. Better understanding of feelings and needs is reported to facilitate the resolution of problems and conflicts. The problem is not so much the presence of conflicts, but rather the manner in which they are resolved [19]. Constructive resolution of conflict based on open communication and commitment to the other is reported to lead to greater harmony in the couple and a greater understanding of specific individual, as well as relationship, needs.

General knowledge regarding the resolution of conjugal conflict indicates that suitable resolution is more closely associated with open communication and a genuine interest in understanding the feelings of one's partner. On the other hand, patterns of demand-withdraw (one partner presses to discuss a problem and the other withdraws and refuses to talk about it) and avoidance are problematic for conflict resolution [21]. Moreover, prolonged exposure to conflict in the context of ineffective conflict resolution erodes the positive aspects of an intimate relationship and is reported to expose the couple to tensions and ultimately to marital break-up. An ineffective pattern of communication is thought to often precede the development of marital distress [22].

In a context of distress such as that generated by the development of breast cancer, establishing and maintaining open marital communication that is comforting and healing and adopting a constructive process of conflict resolution can prove difficult tasks. Stronger communication skills are required to be able to formulate problems and needs clearly, and to solicit or provide support, while physical, cognitive, and affective resources are likely to be considerably affected and solicited [23, 24]. However, a significant percentage of couples seem to rise to the challenge and maintain the quality of their intimate relationship [25]. Couples possessing the skills for establishing open communication before the diagnosis will have more chances of avoiding this pitfall and experiencing an increase in closeness.

Unfortunately, intervention with couples undergoing unusual hardship often reveals that a lack of understanding of the needs, concerns, and meaning of support behaviours can rapidly become a source of tension and lead to emotional distancing. Couples who considerably limit the expression of their needs, concerns, and feelings or express them poorly during the initial crisis and the months that follow risk developing an emotional distance between themselves. With time, this distance may increase even further because they possess insufficient and sometimes erroneous knowledge of how they respectively function, both personally and as a couple, in a situation of mutual suffering. The knowledge they do have is based on presuppositions, unvoiced ideas and, sometimes worse, misunderstandings. Lack of communication or a communication deficit (light, medium, severe) is often revelatory of their difficulties in establishing open intimate communication. Progressively and without realizing it, they lose sight of each other and become increasingly at risk of experiencing conflicts that have no real resolution.

For some couples, the return to harmony comes with the development of skills for coping with the reactions of their partner and clearly communicating their specific concerns and need for support. Simultaneously, they must come to terms with their own distress and learn to deal with intimate communication that may upset them further in the short term. Otherwise, emotional distance may set in, undermining the attachment bond and making them vulnerable during other episodes of the illness.

Mutuality within the Relationships

A second major issue for developing well-being within the intimacy bond is the reinforcement or development of a couple's mutuality. Mutuality relates specifically to reciprocity of exchanges within the intimate relationship. The presence or lack of mutuality within the relationship depends on the partners' capacity for empathy, i.e., their capacity to be mutually affected by one another. It rests essentially on an attitude of receptivity to differences and active mutual engagement [26, 27]. Mutuality thus presupposes the emotional availability needed for understanding one another within each partner's system of reference as well as a commitment to undertaking, if necessary, a change in response patterns for the sake of the partner's well-being, as well as one's own.

Mutuality involves the recognition of the other person's uniqueness and respect for his or her autonomy and different experiences. In situations where empathy or commitment is lacking on the part of one or both of the partners, the development of mutuality within the couple may be compromised. For Jordan [27], the principal obstacles to mutuality are discomfort with revealing oneself, reluctance to allow the partner to have an emotional impact, withdrawal into oneself, and decreasing interest in the partner's world due to depression.

Research increasingly highlights the beneficial effects of mutual support in cases where the female partner is affected by breast cancer. An empathetic response oriented towards confirmation and personal acceptance of the other favours greater adjustment in the two partners. The sentiment of being heard, understood, and validated, both for the woman and her partner, is associated with a greater feeling of intimacy and greater satisfaction with the relationship. The presence of mutuality in exchanges also promotes constructive resolution of conflicts and the use of positive joint strategies of adaptation. It ensures better relational support and the pursuit of the most normal interactions possible in the context of crisis [5–8, 28, 29].

Another aspect of mutuality is constructing the meaning of the experience. According to the results of a qualitative study by Skerrett [30], couples that coped best with the cancer experience reportedly demonstrated a capacity to experience it as 'Our' problem. They were shown capable of redefining their identity as a couple—the 'We'—by reconciling the demands introduced by the illness and the other aspects of their daily lives. This redefinition provided direction for their coping efforts. In contrast, couples that were having difficulty coping were shown to exhibit a deficit in the formulation of the mutual meaning of their experience. The development of the sense of 'We' is an important aspect of marital support and coping. Skerrett proposes a type of intervention that helps couples develop dialogue promoting a more acute awareness of this feeling of togetherness. The efforts of the couple are guided towards a greater awareness of the history of the evolution of their intimacy bond, at its genesis, during and following their experience of the illness.

These few studies corroborate certain clinical observations and provide evidence of the importance of a mutual attitude of empathy and engagement in ensuring support that has significant affective scope and connects to partner concerns, worries and needs. This receptivity to what the other person is going encourages active listening to his or her needs and subjective experience, and thereby fosters marital cohesion in resolving problems and conflicts and defining the future of the couple. This mutual understanding ensures a clearer articulation of needs and the responses they engender. Support based on the harmonization of needs and responses to these needs is seen as most beneficial. Empathy and active commitment to the other are two key elements to be achieving this harmonization [31]. Thus, the positive or negative effects of support within the intimacy bond are not linked solely to the use of specific communication strategies; the affective tone and related commitment are equally determinant.

Finally, exchanges based on mutuality foster the construction of a healing dialogue that nurtures the sense of connectedness. This dialogue is founded on listening to the real self and respecting the uniqueness of the other in his or her difference [30]. From this point of view, we could argue that a rigid protective attitude constitutes a sizeable obstacle to the establishment of this dialogue. Conversely, the establishment of open communication receptive to the intersubjective experience of the couple will favour a further deepening of the intimacy bond. As a result, the bond of intimacy will be able to play its full protective role against individual and conjugal suffering when the female partner is going through the experience of breast cancer.

Conclusion

Interest in better understanding what occurs within couples' intimate relationships when the female partner is diagnosed with breast cancer is still a recent phenomenon. Current developments in knowledge highlight the importance of taking into account the relational aspects of marital support. More and more studies indicate that the establishment of intimate and open communication and the development of exchanges founded on mutuality are crucial for marital support during the cancer experience. These issues appear to be sufficiently important to determine whether couples develop a sense of well-being or marital distress within their intimate relationships. However, other studies are necessary to further document and deepen our understanding of the relational processes at work with respect to marital support in the event of breast cancer. For example, studies are needed to address how the presence or absence of feelings of intimacy affects the relationship and the repercussions this has for the couple's adjustment process. It would also be useful to understand better the conditions and circumstances in which the intimacy bond interferes negatively or positively with the process of adjustment for couples confronted with breast cancer. More studies are required on exchanges within couples and their positive or negative effects on the development of the intimacy bond. Cancer also affects the manner in which couples perceive their evolution and future. The way they assimilate the experience, and the meaning they give to it, will have an impact on how their bond of intimacy evolves. More specifically, research needs to delve deeper into the existential dimension of couples' experiences of cancer.

The studies presented in this chapter show how important it is for health professionals to support couples in a way that takes into account issues of communication and mutuality related to the deepening of the bond of intimacy. First and foremost, they highlight the importance of offering a support programme that includes a preventive and educational component as well as support for couples in difficulty. A preventive and educational intervention should be offered immediately upon diagnosis of cancer to make couples aware of the dimensions of their intimacy bond that may be affected and constitute normal aspects of their cancer experience. This intervention should also aim at helping them review and adjust their beliefs about the best way to support each other and acquire communications and relationship skills that promote the development or maintenance of their intimacy bond as well as marital adjustment. For example, it is important to dispel the belief that a protective attitude and unidirectional support will always have the positive effect desired. It would also be useful to lead them to open up to different communication strategies that promote the maintenance and deepening of the intimacy bond. This intervention should help them increase their response repertoire. Interest in what the other person is going through and the desire to 'be with and together' can express themselves in diverse ways [4]. All couples have their own personal style of manifesting their love and commitment. They sometimes need help rediscovering their love relationship and nourishing it positively [30]. Furthermore, the possibility of developing a standard early intervention to promote awareness would help reach the greatest number of couples and prevent the possible development of marital distress.

Finally, couples in difficulty should be subject to special attention. It is important that they receive more sustained support so as to better understand how they have evolved within their intimate relationship and acquire skills to nurture it positively. Marital support is thought to be more effective with empathetic communication, which develops feelings of being connected, loved, accepted, and understood. Intervention models oriented towards dyadic coping and the development of mutual emotional support are currently emerging in both clinical and scientific circles. These models are of interest for applications and validation in different contexts [8, 30, 32]. They generally aim to improve individual coping, marital communication, and problem and conflict resolution skills. At the same time, evaluative studies are necessary to establish better which interventions are most effective in helping couples provide each other with mutual support. Parallel to this, screening tools adapted to the context of breast cancer will have to be designed to identify more quickly couples at risk, based among other things on the two fundamental dimensions of their intimacy bond—communication and mutuality. Detecting problems before they become irreparable is preferable for preventing potential marital breakdown.

In the years ahead, research and clinical facilities must join forces in developing and deepening knowledge of relationship issues linked to marital support that appear fundamental for reinforcing the intimate relationship of couples dealing with breast cancer. Meetings with such couples often reveal that when the bond of intimacy is nourished in a positive way, it can help protect against the loss of meaning provoked by suffering from this devastating experience.

References

1. Hilton BA. Issues, Problems, and Challenges for Families Coping with Breast Cancer. *Seminars in Oncology Nursing*. May 1993;9(2):88–100.
2. Lethborg CE. It's Not the Easy Part: The Experience of Significant Others of Women with Early Stage Breast Cancer, at Treatment Completion. *Social Work in Health Care*. 2003;37(1):63–85.
3. Manne S. Couples Coping with Cancer: Research Issues and Recent Findings. *Journal of Clinical Psychology in Medical Settings*. 1994;1(4):317–30.
4. Picard L, Dumont S, Gagnon P, et al. Coping Strategies Among Couples Adjusting to Primary Breast Cancer. *Journal of Psychosocial Oncology*. 2005;23(2/3):115–35.
5. Manne SL, Ostroff J, Norton TR, et al. Cancer-Related Relationship Communication. Couples Coping with Early Stage Breast Cancer. *Psycho-Oncology*. 2006;15:234–47.
6. Manne S, Ostroff J, Rini C, et al. The Interpersonal Process Model of Intimacy: The role of self-disclosure, partner disclosure, and partner responsiveness in interactions between breast cancer patients and their partners. *J Fam Psychol*. 2004;18(4):589–99.
7. Feldman B, Broussard CA. The Influence of Relational Factors on Men's Adjustment to Their Partners' Newly-Diagnosed Breast Cancer. *Journal of Psychosoc Oncol*. 2005;23(2/3):23–43.

8. Kayser K. Enhancing dyadic coping during a time of crisis: A theory-Based intervention with breast cancer patients and theirs partners. Revenson T, Kayser K, Bodenmann G, eds. Couples coping with stress: Emerging perspectives on dyadic coping. Washington: American Psychological Association, 2005:175–94.
9. Laurenceau J-P, Kleinman BM. Intimacy in Personal Relationships. Vangelisti and Perlaman, eds. The Cambridge Handbook of Personal Relationships. New York: Cambridge University Press, 2006:637–53.
10. Reis HT, Shaver P. Intimacy as an Interpersonal Process. Duck S, ed. *Handbook of Personal relationships*, Chichester, England: Wiley; 1988:367–89.
11. Manne S, Ostroff J, Sherman M, et al. Couples' Support-Related Communication, Psychological Distress, and Relationship Satisfaction Among Women With Early Stage Breast Cancer. *Journal of Consulting and Clinical Psychology*. 2004;72(4):660–70.
12. Figueiredo M, Fries E, Ingram KM. The Role of Disclosure Patterns and Unsupportive Social Interactions. The Well-Being of Breast Cancer Patients. *Psycho-Oncology*. 2004;13:96–105.
13. Spiegel D, Bloom JR, Gottheil E. Family Environment as a Predictor of Adjustment to Metastatic Breast Carcinoma. *Journal of Psychosocial Oncology*. Spring, 1983;1(1):33–44.
14. Greene K, Derlega VJ, Mathews A. Self-Disclosure in Personal Relationships. Vangelisti and Perlman, eds. The Cambridge Handbook of Personal Relationships. New York: Cambridge University Press; 2006:409–27.
15. Mesters I, et al. Openness to Discuss Cancer in the Nuclear Family: Scale, Development, and Validation. *American Psychosomatic Society*. May/June, 1997;59(3):269–79.
16. Manne S, Dougherty J, Veach S, et al. Hiding Worries from One's Spouse: Protective Buffering Among Cancer Patients and their Spouses. *Cancer Research Therapy and Control*. 1999;8:175–88.
17. Worthman CB, Dunkel-Schetter C. Interpersonal relationships and cancer: A theoretical analysis. *Journal of Social Issues*. 1979;35(1):120–55.
18. Sabo D, Brown J, Smith C. The Male Role and Mastectomy: Support Groups and Men's Adjustment. Journal of Psychosocial Oncology Spring/Summer 1986;4(1/2):19–31.
19. Giese-Davis J, Hermanson K, Koopman C, et al. Quality of Couples' Relationship and Ajustment to Metastatic Breast Cancer. *J Fam Psychol*. 2000;14(2):251–66.
20. Holmberg S, Scott LL, William A, et al. Relationship Issues of Women With Breast Cancer. *Cancer Nursing*. 2001;24(1):53–60.
21. Kline GH, Pleasant ND, Whitton SW, et al. Understanding Couple Conflict. Vangelisti and Perlman, editors. The Cambridge Handbook of Personal Relationships. New York: Cambridge University Press, 2006:445–62.
22. Pasch LA, Bradbury TN. Social support, Conflict, and the Development of Marital Dysfunction. *J Consult Clin Psychol*. 1998;66(2):219–30.
23. Cutrona CE. Social Support in Couples. Marriage as a Resource in Times of Stress. Thousand Oaks. California: Sage Publications; 1996,150.
24. Neff LA, Karney BR. How does context affect intimate relationship? Linking external stress and cognitive processes within marriage. *Pers Soc Psycho Bul*. February 2004;30(2):134–48.
25. Dorval M, Guay S, Mondor M, et al. Couples who get closer after breast cancer: Frequency and predictors in a prospective investigation. *J Clin Onco*. May 2005;23(15):3588–96.
26. Genero NP, Miller JB, Surrey J, et al. Measuring perceived Mutuality in Close Relationships: Validation of the Mutual Psychological Development Questionnaire. *J Fam Psychol*. 1992;6(1):36–48.
27. Jordan JV. The meaning of mutuality. Jordan JV, Kaplan AG, Miller JB, et al. Women's growth in connection: writings from Stone Center. New York: Guilford Press, 1991:81–96.

28. Wimberley SR, Carver CS, Laurenceau J-P, et al. Perceived Partner Reactions to Diagnosis and Treatment of Breast Cancer: Impact on Psychosocial and Psychosexual Adjustment. *J Consult Clin Psychol.* 2005;73(2):300–11.
29. Sormanti M, Kayser K. Partner support and changes in relationships during life-threatening illness: Women's perspectives. *J Psychosocl Oncol.* 2000;18(3):45–66.
30. Skerrett K. Couple Dialogues with illness: Expanding the "We". *Families, Systems Health.* 2003;21(1):69–80.
31. Cutrona CE, Russell DW. Type of social support and specific stress: Toward a theory of optimal matching. Sarason BR, Sarason IG, Pierce Gregory R, eds. Social Support: An Interactional View. New York: A Wiley-Interscience Publication, 1990:319–66.
32. Widmer K, Cina A, Charvoz L, et al. A Model Dyadi-Coping Intervention. Revenson T, Kayser K, Bodenmann G, eds. Couples coping with stress: Emerging perspectives on dyadic coping. Washington: *American Psychological Association.* 2005:159–74.

The View and Role of Breast Cancer Advocacy

Stella Kyriakydes

Breast Cancer – The Journey

A diagnosis of breast cancer finds no woman prepared. Despite the increasing levels of awareness surrounding this disease, one never actually expects to hear this diagnosis when it involves one's own self. It appears that human beings have an inborn defense mechanism which frequently allows one to push undesirable or difficult life events into dark areas of ones brain, or, when actually faced with the potential reality, one still feels it is almost magically going to go away. How often do human beings project onto others experiences which they are afraid will touch upon themselves?

Breast cancer is a disease that is known not only to affect the body of the woman diagnosed but also to have a huge psychological impact affecting all aspects of her psyche, impacting on her concept of femininity, sexuality and "motherhood".

However, more than this, it brings the woman in touch with possibly one of the most basic fears of the human being, the fear of death. No matter the amount of information or support, the patient is always aware that facing a cancer diagnosis is always potentially a life threatening situation. One is thrown into a world of uncertainty, a world taken over by medical and other interventions; the feeling is one of suddenly finding oneself in the deep sea and finding out if the skills you thought you had in terms of surviving will now serve you well. It is characteristically expressed by a woman patient that, following her diagnosis, she felt as if she had been swept away by a tsunami, but that it was not one alone but a series of tsunamis that washed over her over and over again until she finally saw calmer waters and felt safe.

It is a long and often difficult journey, from the moment of diagnosis, through the treatment, and then forward with living a life with changed and often unknown realities. It is a journey that has many different intense

S. Kyriakydes (✉)
Past President of EUROPA DONNA Cyprus, 28 Prodromou street, Engomi, Nicosia, Cyprus
e-mail: cysky@cytanet.com.cy

M. Castiglione, M.J. Piccart (eds.), *Adjuvant Therapy for Breast Cancer*, Cancer Treatment and Research 151, DOI 10.1007/978-0-387-75115-3_27,

emotions, emotions that at times overtake you like a dam breaking out of its walls, but at other times seem to freeze within you like the snow on a glacier. Emotions that alternate between anger-denial-depression-fear-leading hopefully to acceptance, not necessarily in this order and not necessarily one at a time. Much has been written about these stages. Elisabeth Kubler-Ross has been instrumental in increasing our understanding of how the patient and family feels, but the experience itself gives an insight that is at times daunting. Daunting because it is almost wondrous actually to be part of this emotional journey and then realize that this is a journey shared by thousand of others, thus creating an almost universal awareness of being travelers on this road together.

In writing this chapter it is, for a patient advocate, impossible to stand away from the experience of the disease in addressing the role and meaning of advocacy. It is part of this life experience and is part of the concept of where this journey, this road can lead. A journey that leads to travels into worlds initially unknown, strange and frightening, but that along the way have their own meaning, become familiar and strangely inspiring.

This stems from the premise that, when faced with a difficult life reality, one has fundamentally two choices – to go on in life feeling sorry for oneself while angrily asking "why me" questions, or to try to integrate this experience into your own life pattern and thus transform this experience into something that is creative, productive and dynamic. Into a movement that can lead to change and progress, to strength and solidarity. This is the passion behind advocacy.

The Meaning Of Advocacy

Advocating for a cause has been part of people behavior for centuries. Joining voices to promote a cause has been advocated by Martin Luther King Jr among others who once said that "an individual has not started living until he can rise above the individual confines of his individualistic experience."

This is what is entailed in moving away from personal experience to advocating for a cause that is far broader. The role of advocacy is in fact to effect change. This is never to be seen as a static process but is a journey that involves many changing emotions and pathways.

When advocating for a cause, one needs to define clearly the goals and the process, and one needs to have a very clear view of the cause itself. It is of paramount importance to have an understanding of the end points, what are the challenges involved and the roads to get to ones goals. Advocacy involves the belief that one can bring about actual changes and frequently this may also involve a political process. Advocacy can also lead to the changing of attitudes, of beliefs, of society standards, of legislations. This can only be done by building a common base of the cause in question-by creating a movement that has a wider pertinence and acceptance.

Following the Universal Declaration of Human Rights there began to be a change in the way that individuals looked at their own position in society and this had a direct impact in the promotion of patient rights. The emphasis on the right to equality and the right to dignity are fundamental issues that have been advocated by patients.

Of course, patient rights differ across countries and across jurisdictions depending on prevailing social and cultural norms. The roles that are assigned to doctors and their relationship with patients are forever changing and are not in any way predefined in the practical sense.

Advocating for patient rights has, however, brought about a fundamental change – it has allowed individuals to have dignity and equality as key issues and it has in some cases enabled patients to be able to participate in the decision making processes. Advocacy is in itself an art – it is the art of changing political opinions, it is the art of dialogue between citizens and public officials, it is the art of shaping policy making and, finally, it is the art of collective action. This creates a momentum for change – this has led to the promotion of patient rights, to the breakdown of taboos and stigmas, to changing the face of a cancer diagnosis.

The aims of cancer advocacy are varied – it is fundamental to work towards minimizing the disparities between countries in terms of diagnosis and treatment, to equalize standards, quality and access to services and to dispel the myths around cancer. Advocates need to be well informed and well educated and this knowledge needs to be disseminated in order to maintain the strength in collective actions.

Patient advocacy is about the building of partnerships. Patients slowly develop effective voices which are not threatening to physicians, while other professions also become involved as equal partners.

Breast cancer has been one of the most dynamic fields where patient advocacy has resulted in changing the face of this disease. In fact, one could say there has been a revolution in breast cancer in the last 20–30 years .A revolution that is still ongoing, and as with many revolutions, only when one looks back into the pages of history can one truly understand the magnitude of what has taken place.

Cancer – The Fear

Cancer has always been a disease that evokes fear. There was always a stigma attached to this diagnosis, it was little understood and at times thought even to be contagious. Cancer patients were treated in separate hospitals, many patients felt that this diagnosis was equivalent to a death sentence, and many kept their diagnosis a secret.

The fear of death is a very primitive fear, it brings an individual in touch with the reality of ones own mortality. It was a disease that at times was considered to be best left untreated and that spread in almost devious and unpredictable ways. With the progress of science, the understanding on the nature of this disease changed, and with this change in the understanding came the introduction of concepts of reality that allowed those affected to have a new perspective, that of hope. Research redefined the ideas behind early diagnosis, treatment and care; cancer became understood not as a single entity but as a multitude of entities each with their own outcomes.

The word "cancer" suddenly does not have one meaning but a multitude of meanings generating a multitude of emotions – the emotional rollercoaster of a diagnosis is still very much there – but it is now not only characterized by fear but by hope, power, and a changing feeling of control. Possibly the greatest element evoking fear in diagnosis is the loss of control over ones body, over ones life – breast cancer advocacy had added new ingredients into this life event and this has allowed many a patients to achieve a sense of control and thus have less fear and helplessness.

Diagnosis of Breast Cancer

Breast cancer has evoked its own fears, and in many ways has brought different psychological issues to the forefront. The breasts are a part of the female body that have swept and inspired the imagination of artists and sculptors, that have been associated with basic female characteristics that have to do with motherhood, with sexuality, with femininity. The breasts as the source of milk for breast feeding are a source of life. It is of little wonder when a disease is associated with a threat to life and has as its "source" the female breast that this gave rise to fear, to stigma, to taboo, to silence. Women felt guilty that their bodies were not only failing them but that the part of their bodies that is associated with everything that is life giving is in fact life threatening. In many cultures women were almost blamed for this; in many parts of the world women still hide their diagnosis, while others still shy away from having the necessary routine examinations almost in denial that their breasts could ever be the source of disease.

Breast cancer is however not a disease that affects only the patient herself – it is a disease that affects the whole family, the surroundings. It has an impact that is life changing, and needs to be addressed at this multi-varied level by teams of professionals. Many women are not aware of this, many women do not allow themselves to think that they should be sharing their experience, out of fear and out of guilt. It is a journey that can be extremely lonesome in some societies, while in others it is one that can lead to a sense of belonging to a greater cause.

It is a strongly emotive powerful personal journey, one that starts from the moment of diagnosis. The confirmation of a breast cancer diagnosis throws the woman into a world of uncertainty. It is the beginning of a long road that is often frightening and confusing. It is the beginning of a journey that involves the whole family. As this diagnosis can come at any age in a woman's adult life it often finds children in the centre of this family journey. Children are affected differently at different ages. In some cultures children are protected from the knowledge of disease and a diagnosis of any type of cancer is even more prone to silence and foreboding. For this to be effectively dealt with, adults need to have an understanding of the situation, myths need to be dispelled and realities faced.

Breast cancer is indeed a changing disease. The knowledge pertaining to its diagnosis and treatment are dramatically changing; terminology is becoming not simpler but more and more complex. A woman, or man, diagnosed with this is often faced with medical terms used by those treating that make the situation even more frightening and confusing. Terms that were never heard before need not only to be understood but treatment decisions need to be made based on these. And these are situations that at the same time are full of anxiety and uncertainty, where the human defense mechanisms are on full alert, thus bringing denial and projection into play.

The breast cancer revolution has not only impacted in the decisions that need to be made concerning treatment – it has impacted on life styles in terms of prevention, it has impacted in the need for screening and the optimal screening methods, it has impacted in the surgical methods, in the introduction of new concepts such as breast reconstruction, in the understanding of long term treatments and their side effects; in fact, the list is never ending and ever changing. It is indeed a revolution that has not yet run its course – one that is a challenge to all, especially breast cancer advocates.

The Personal Becomes Political

This is the ethos of breast cancer advocacy. It is using ones own personal experience with this disease to create energy that is dynamic, creative and even positive. When one has to face any difficult and painful life event, one has two fundamental choices – either to proceed through life feeling angry and asking "why me?" or to incorporate this difficult life event into ones personal realities and use it into becoming creative. This is exactly what breast cancer advocates do – but, more than this, they use their personal experience into bringing about change that will affect woman and men across the world. It is about the joining of voices, of individuals not only affected by the disease but women and men who believe that this will create a new momentum for change and progress.

Breast cancer advocacy has raised awareness of this disease. However, no woman believes that this will be a diagnosis that will directly affect herself. Even when faced with confirmation of the diagnosis, women often describe the feeling of wanting to "wake up from a nightmare", or of almost being part of a film that is not part of the real world. This comes from the difficulty of integrating this painful experience into the self. The personal experience with breast cancer is a life changing event. In many parts of the world women still hide after diagnosis, frightened by the reality of the situation, and often feeling alone not aware of the many other women and men affected by this disease. This feeling of isolation in fact puts patients in greater danger as they are not able to pursue their rights to optimal care. Additionally, traditional relationships between doctors and patients often put patients in a position of absolute dependency where they are concerned that asking for information or explanations will in fact threaten this relationship. The doctor patient relationship is the centre point of the breast cancer journey – the need to challenge and the right to question is part of a changing concept of the characteristics of communication – patients need more written information, they need to be allowed time, they need to be treated always with respect and individuality. The growing demands have now led to the development of multi-disciplinary teams so that the different patient needs are met by a team of trained professionals. This is not to say that the doctor–patient relationship has taken second place – when dealing with the diagnosis of a potentially life threatening disease, the most important single factor is individual survival. However, communication skills have in fact led to the strengthening of this relationship, breaking new ground that is of benefit to all.

Following initial diagnosis, the patient is faced with many different treatment options. Many of these are difficult to comprehend. Clinical trial options create further confusion with many patients believing that entering a clinical trial will in fact place them at a disadvantage. The various surgical options create added anxiety. Until recently better outcome was directly associated with more aggressive surgery. This has led to many women having to live with mutilating surgery with little or no option to breast reconstruction. When diagnosed with breast cancer, many women feel that the only way forward is to have the cancer removed, and many do not consider the long term impact this will have on their future body image. It is in fact only after the initial fear has subsided that other worries and concerns come to the surface. Women describe how difficult it is to allow their partners or children to see their body, sexual relationships are thrown off balance, and there is a feeling of guilt as if the woman brought the cancer on herself.

Informing ones children, in the case of a mother being diagnosed, is approached differently across cultures and even within societies and families. Issues that are now related to breast cancer and pregnancy or having children after having had breast cancer are all new and constantly changing. Information is difficult to access and there are many wrong and inaccurate concepts that concern these areas.

Breast cancer is therefore an overwhelming personal experience that affects the individual patient, the family, and the surroundings. It is a disease that one does not have to learn about as a past reality but it is a disease that someone has to learn to live with. It is part of the life reality that involves follow up and, unfortunately, in many cases recurrence or even loss of life. It is an experience that has to be shared and not dealt with through silence and fear. It is a disease whose treatment is undergoing a revolution, thus creating an even greater need for better understanding and care. And this is where the power of the advocacy movement has come to rise to the many challenges and changing realities.

Advocates Join Forces

The breast cancer advocacy movement started in the early 1970s and tracing the first successes one could say that these were realized first in the United States. There, women joined forces and voices to lobby government to provide funding for research and to allocate funds from the defense budget towards this cause. Other continents followed, with various degrees of success and empowerment. The power of the advocacy movement was enhanced by inspired scientists, doctors and other professionals who saw that building partnerships would strengthen the voice and the goals would only be achieved if this was possible.

Breast cancer advocacy covers a spectrum of targets, goals, and inspirations. It involves advocating for more research in finding the cure, the best treatment for this disease; it involves advocating for access to optimal care, to accede to early diagnostic procedures and methods. It involves advocating for the right to access to information and the promotion of guidelines. It involves advocating towards the promotion and respect for patient rights at all stages of the disease process; it involves advocating for the right of families, for the right to secure employment, for the right of equality and not to be discriminated because of this diagnosis.

Breast cancer advocacy is a commitment to change the world and realities of a disease that affects thousands of women, and men, to change the realities for the generations that will follow. However, is the joining of this power of voice and building partnership enough to lead to change?

Advocacy and Politics

Bringing about change can be achieved at different levels. Raising awareness is a fundamental first step. One needs to be aware of the problem and even to have proposed solutions. This can only be achieved if advocacy is strong at the grassroots level. It is this spreading voice that can lead to effective and long term change. One of the largest problems faced world wide by advocacy movements, not least in the field of breast cancer, is not creating the movement but maintaining the momentum. Maintaining the momentum is a challenge that is achieved if the grassroots strength is maintained. If this is not done, many advocacy movements remain small, limited groups that do not lead to effective progress. This is where breast cancer advocacy can build on its successes. It has achieved a global nature, one that has moved men and women across countries and that has allowed the scientific revolution in the world of breast cancer to reach as many citizens as possible.

The breast cancer advocates have learnt that having a strong and effective voice can only be achieved if they are well educated and informed. Having had experience of the disease does not necessarily mean effective advocacy – the personal experience cannot stand and maintain a reliable advocacy movement if this is based solely on emotion. Breast cancer advocates have fought to achieve a seat at the table where decisions about them are made, but the battle is maintaining that seat and convincing all other partners that this is an effective and valid voice and representation.

This voice can only be powerful if there is partnership with the media. The role of the media is of paramount importance because media can create and change attitudes and beliefs in a society. Over the last few decades, the role of the media in raising awareness in breast cancer and enhancing the breast cancer advocacy movement cannot be understated. However, media can also have a negative effect by giving false hope, by creating false expectations. Working effectively with the media is only one portion of the many delicate balances that advocates need to master.

This changing face of advocacy has led to the voice leading to political change. It has led to legislations that have safeguarded patient rights, that have led to the aims and goals placed by breast cancer advocacy movements being translated into governmental policies and decisions. It has led to lobbying at country and other levels, thus laying the foundations for cementing all that is being achieved by the breast cancer revolution.

All type of discrimination, whether this has to do with access to optimal care, to the latest clinical trials, to employment, to privacy, to screening, need to be fully supported by legislative changes. In this way there is dissemination of the achievements, and new goals and targets can be placed. Advocacy is never static – it is a changing journey that aims at genuinely impacting positively on all those affected by this disease.

Final Thoughts

Is this a role then that is clearly defined? Is it a role that has an inherent power? Is breast cancer advocacy really making a difference? Making a difference is only measurable in terms of the realities that are changing for patients across the world. In some countries these changes are happening very slowly, frustratingly so due to the direct relationship with the economic realities of the country and its social welfare state. In other countries, there is still a loud silence, a stigma, while in others breast cancer awareness months have become extraordinary media events.

Whether the steps are big or small, whether they are quick or slow, the important fact is that worldwide steps are being made, breast cancer advocates are no longer those that have been through the disease fighting the battle alone, but they are advocacy partners together with all who are committed to making the difference. This is the power of the breast cancer advocacy voice.

Breast cancer advocacy has as its mission to:

- Inform
- Empower
- Represent
- Link together individuals and groups sharing similar issues and experiences
- Develop and strengthen partnerships with media, clinicians, scientists, politicians

Advocacy works at many levels including the political and the systemic to improve the diagnosis, management, care, and the future world of breast cancer patients.

"So long as some women are still misdiagnosed, or poorly managed, so long as the number of breast cancer diagnoses increases, so long as so many women die from this disease, it is vital that breast cancer remains on the political agenda across the world – this is a global effort. There is still much work to be done."

The Voice of a Special Patient

Stefan Aebi

What is the meaning of "special" in the context of breast cancer or, in particular, of this book? Dictionary definitions encompass *distinguished from what is ordinary or usual, of a distinct or particular kind or character, particularly valued, having a particular function or purpose*, or simply *additional; extra* [1]. The title of this chapter was proposed by the editor but I do not feel "special" in any of the above senses, and I do not intend to use my author privilege, only to give an additional testimony of my coping with breast cancer.

The reader may recognize that the adjective "special" is derived from the Latin root "specio", an archaic word meaning "I see" or "I look at." "Species", a derived Latin noun with female grammatical gender, is usually translated by "sight, appearance", "kind" or "type". In addition to "special", a large number of derived words are commonly used in contemporary English, such as suspicious, perspective, respect, spectrum, conspicuous, aspect, specimen, prospective, auspices, expect, spectacular, speculative, and many more [2]. The word "spice" for delicacies like lemongrass or chili peppers obviously evolved from the same linguistic origin. The Latin word, in turn, has Indo-German roots, presumably characterized by the letters SPC and – by metathesis – SCP; therefore, some reference works indicate that certain words derived from Greek such as "micro*scop*e" and "*sk*e*p*tical" share the same origin [3]. Thus, this family of words, gravitating around the concept of seeing, covers many aspects of today's practice of medicine.

Special. A superficial look at the above definitions might lead to the conclusion that, being a man, I might somehow be distinct among other persons suffering from breast cancer. But in addition to men, who represent about 0.8% of newly diagnosed cases of breast cancer [4], there are many other patients whose characteristics make them belong to rare subgroups of persons with breast cancer. Some of these particular populations have been appropriately

S. Aebi (✉)
Associate Professor of Medical Oncology, Breast and Gynecological Cancer Center, Departments of Medical Oncology and Gynecology, University Hospital, Inselspital, 3010 Berne, Switzerland

M. Castiglione, M.J. Piccart (eds.), *Adjuvant Therapy for Breast Cancer*, Cancer Treatment and Research 151, DOI 10.1007/978-0-387-75115-3_28,

addressed in the present volume, such as patients who are diagnosed with cancer during pregnancy, and in many regards, a man with breast cancer is not more "special" than one of those patients. Further, even without the promise of highly individualized medicine based on molecular properties of the cancer and its host, patients have always been unique individuals such that being special is not "special" after all.

Suspicious. Of course, I was very worried when the chest strap of my Polar heart rate monitor started to hurt, leading me to discover a lump. A biopsy a few days later confirmed it as carcinoma. I asked the multidisciplinary team I always work with to take care of my surgery and adjuvant therapy. I still think that this was a wise decision, as it gave me a fresh view of my own service from the patient's perspective. In spite of long-lasting efforts to the contrary, the patient's or consumer's perspectives of the achievements of medical and nursing sciences tend to receive little attention in professional education and thus in the thinking of physicians and nurses, men and women alike. If I were asked to name the single most important aspect of my experience as a patient, it would be the respect for my concerns and values that should be and usually was central to the communication with my physicians and nurses.

Spectrum. Little is known about breast cancer in men, although men do profit from the huge research efforts that women with breast cancer have agreed to participate in. Breast cancer in men occurs at an average age of 65–70 years, so I was at least 20 years below the average. Its incidence has been increasing in the past few years in the United States and likely in other Western countries [5]. The occurrence of breast cancer in a man is an indication for genetic counseling as there is a substantial probability of germline mutations of BRCA2 [6–8] and other genes [9]. The surgical therapy in men should be similar to that in women, including sentinel lymph node biopsy [10, 11], and the indications for radiation therapy are likely the same as in women although traditionally, postmastectomy radiation was considered more essential in men than in women. Stage by stage, the prognosis after breast cancer is similar in men and in women [12]. The biological characteristics of breast cancer in men are slightly different from those in women: the vast majority of cancers express estrogen receptors [5] and the amplification and overexpression of the HER-2/neu gene may be relatively uncommon [13, 14].

Auspices. The adjuvant therapy of breast cancer in men has never been investigated in prospective trials. Thus, the merits of chemotherapy and hormonal therapy are unknown, although it is reasonable to conjecture that tamoxifen is effective adjuvant therapy based on non-controlled studies. The efficacy of chemotherapy is less certain although, by tradition, men have been treated with the same regimens as women [15]. The adjuvant use of aromatase inhibitors has not been investigated, and they may be less effective in men as the suppression of circulation estrogen is less complete than in women [16–19]. The worth of the suppression of testicular androgen production to therapeutically target the frequent expression of androgen receptors or to facilitate the use of aromatase inhibitors is unknown. However, the experience with metastatic breast cancer in men suggests that androgen deprivation could be effective adjuvant therapy [20–22]. Advanced disease is treated according to the same general principles as in women with an emphasis on endocrine therapies; letrozole has been used successfully in a small number of patients [23, 24], whereas anastrozole induced no remissions in a small series of five patients [25]. The efficacy of the suppression of testicular androgens in conjunction with aromatase inhibition is being investigated [26].

Spices. Given the uncertainties outlined above, I consulted a small number of excellent medical oncologists and finally opted for anthracycline-containing chemotherapy followed by adjuvant radiation therapy and hormonal therapy with tamoxifen. I have tolerated the chemotherapy, the radiation therapy, and the hormonal therapy with no major adverse effects. This is not to say that I had no grade 3 or 4 toxicity according to the "Common Terminology Criteria for Adverse Events", but the grading of severity reflects the concerns of the regulatory authorities, the pharmaceutical industry, and the physicians rather than those of the patients. For instance, a mild hand-foot-syndrome induced by doxorubicin and possibly sports ("Moderate to brisk erythema; patchy moist desquamation, mostly confined to skin folds and creases; moderate edema" [27]) was much worse than a short episode of grade 4 neutropenia. A frequent, harmless but annoying effect of chemotherapy is a disturbance of taste. In my case, I developed a taste for spicy food, such as found in Thai cuisine because this tasted almost normal and was for a couple of weeks the only kind of food that I truly enjoyed.

Prospects. Quality of life and life style are important, but many aspects are poorly investigated and are hard to investigate in terms of generalizable knowledge. Quality of life at the time of diagnosis does not predict the outcome of breast cancer in women [28, 29]. Exercise is likely to reduce the fatigue associated with chemotherapy [30] and may diminish the risk of recurrence [31]. The importance of different aspects of work, such as responsibilities and social contacts, or psychological "stress" have been poorly investigated. A Medline search using "Quality of Life"[MeSH] AND "Work"[MeSH] AND ("Breast Neoplasms"[MeSH] OR "Breast Neoplasms, Male"[MeSH]) retrieved zero articles. Stress is difficult to conceptualize, but a systematic review concluded that psychological stress does not cause breast cancer in women [32]. A retrospective study suggested an adverse relation between severe life events and relapse of breast cancer [33], but a more extensive prospective evaluation by the same authors did not confirm the initial findings [34], and other authors also failed to associate stressful life events with the risk of breast cancer recurrence [35, 36]. I do not see an argument against extrapolating these conclusions from women to men with breast cancer. In my case, I think that the results of such research have helped me to keep up my work and exercise habits during chemotherapy, although at a reduced level of around 70% of my usual activities, and they have motivated me to resume my normal life soon after the end of chemotherapy. I also conclude that it is appropriate to approach the normal changes in mood, perceived quality of life, and the stressful events of everyday life with serenity as I am convinced that these factors will not jeopardize my medical prognosis.

Perspectives. It is encouraging that the NCI Clinical Trial web site lists 99 trials that are accessible to men with breast cancer [37]. At last, affected men can contribute to the progress of certain breast cancer research projects. However, only one trial is listed that specifically targets men [26]. Maybe gender-specific research will be obsolete in the future if the progress in the molecular understanding of breast cancer makes individually targeted therapies possible. In the meantime, at least endocrine questions deserve to be investigated specifically in men with breast cancer. The current research environment discourages the design of clinical trials targeting small populations [38], especially if the evaluation includes drugs that are already registered for breast cancer in women. Thus the role of patient advocacy organizations such as the John Nick Foundation (http://www.johnwnickfoundation.org) or Y-ME (http://www.y-me.org/information/male_breast_cancer) is crucial to raise men's awareness to the condition and to encourage scientific research in the field of breast cancer in men.

Introspection. Did my experience make me a better doctor, and more specifically a better breast cancer physician? I doubt it, even though a patient who had found out that I was being treated for breast cancer came to my consultation saying "now you are one of us". There are new chances and challenges in communicating with patients. The chances are obvious: I have learnt a few lessons on being a patient, like having to have confidence in a surgeon, a nurse, and other health professionals. I know that it is hard to wait for test results, while at the same time desiring that the tests be conducted according to the highest standards of quality. And, yes, I do have a personal experience with some therapies commonly used to treat patients with breast cancer, an advantage that I share with very few oncologists. Thus, I think that I have a deeper understanding and empathy for the concerns of the patients than I had before. But the challenges must not be overlooked. For instance, it is trivial that the physiological, psychological, and social meaning of the breast differs between men and women; the changes in body image might be less dramatic for a man than for a woman, although this hypothesis has not been investigated to date [39]. I did not have to cope with anything resembling iatrogenic menopause. Thus, contrary to a superficial appearance, I do not have a first-hand experience of everything related to early breast cancer. Indeed, the "emotional labor" of clinical empathy [40] has become even more demanding than it was: Personal empathy could cause an inappropriate professional distance, too close and too distant being equally possible, and result in flawed diagnostic and therapeutic reasoning. Thus, I try to profit from the advantages of my special experience while avoiding the numerous new pitfalls.

Is it necessary to have had cancer in order to communicate adequately with and treat a patient with cancer? Certainly not, just as an oncologist need not be a man to treat a man nor a woman to treat a woman. However, sympathy and mutual respect are the essential ingredients of the special partnership between health professionals and patients.

Reference

1. Random House. "special". In: Costello RB, ed. Random House Webster's College Dictionary. 1995 ed. New York: Random House, Inc.; 1995:1284–5.
2. Ernout A, Meillet A. Dictionnaire étymologique de la langue latine – Histoire des mots. In. 4 ed. Paris: Editions Klincksieck; 1985:639–41.
3. Walde A, Hofmann JB. *Lateinisches etymologisches Wörterbuch*. Heidelberg: Carl Winter's Universitätsbuchhandlung; 1938.
4. Jemal A, Siegel R, Ward E, et al. Cancer Statistics, *CA Cancer J Clin*. 2006;56(2):106–30.
5. Giordano SH, Cohen DS, Buzdar AU, Perkins G, Hortobagyi GN. Breast carcinoma in men: A population-based study. *Cancer*. 2004;101(1):51–7.
6. Friedman LS, Gayther SA, Kurosaki T, et al. Mutation analysis of BRCA1 and BRCA2 in a male breast cancer population. *Am J Hum Genet*. 1997;60(2):313–9.
7. Thorlacius S, Sigurdsson S, Bjarnadottir H, et al. Study of a single BRCA2 mutation with high carrier frequency in a small population. *Am J Hum Genet*. 1997;60(5):1079–84.
8. Basham VM, Lipscombe JM, Ward JM, et al. BRCA1 and BRCA2 mutations in a population-based study of male breast cancer. *Breast Cancer Res*. 2002;4(1):R2.
9. Fentiman IS, Fourquet A, Hortobagyi GN. Male breast cancer. *Lancet*. 2006;367(9510):595–604.
10. Cimmino VM, Degnim AC, Sabel MS, Diehl KM, Newman LA, Chang AE. Efficacy of sentinel lymph node biopsy in male breast cancer. *J Surg Oncol*. 2004;86(2):74–7.
11. Goyal A, Horgan K, Kissin M, et al. Sentinel lymph node biopsy in male breast cancer patients. *Eur J Surg Oncol*. 2004;30(5):480–3.
12. Cutuli B, Lacroze M, Dilhuydy JM, et al. Male breast cancer: Results of the treatments and prognostic factors in 397 cases. *Eur J Cancer*. 1995;31A(12):1960–4.
13. Bloom KJ, Govil H, Gattuso P, Reddy V, Francescatti D. Status of HER-2 in male and female breast carcinoma. *Am J Surg*. 2001;182(4):389–92.
14. Muir D, Kanthan R, Kanthan SC. Male versus female breast cancers. A population-based comparative immunohistochemical analysis. *Arch Pathol Lab Med*. 2003;127(1):36–41.
15. Giordano SH, Perkins GH, Broglio K, et al. Adjuvant systemic therapy for male breast carcinoma. *Cancer*. 2005;104(11):2359–64.
16. Mauras N, O'Brien KO, Klein KO, Hayes V. Estrogen suppression in males: Metabolic effects. *J Clin Endocrinol Metab*. 2000;85(7):2370–7.
17. Leder BZ, Rohrer JL, Rubin SD, Gallo J, Longcope C. Effects of aromatase inhibition in elderly men with low or borderline-low serum testosterone levels. *J Clin Endocrinol Metab*. 2004;89(3):1174–80.
18. de Boer H, Verschoor L, Ruinemans-Koerts J, Jansen M. Letrozole normalizes serum testosterone in severely obese men with hypogonadotropic hypogonadism. *Diabetes Obes Metab*. 2005;7(3):211–5.
19. Mauras N, Lima J, Patel D, et al. Pharmacokinetics and dose finding of a potent aromatase inhibitor, aromasin (exemestane), in young males. *J Clin Endocrinol Metab*. 2003;88(12):5951–6.
20. Labrie F, Dupont A, Belanger A, et al. Complete response to combination therapy with an LHRH agonist and flutamide in metastatic male breast cancer: A case report. *Clin Invest Med*. 1990;13(5):275–8.
21. Lopez M, Natali M, Di Lauro L, Vici P, Pignatti F, Carpano S. Combined treatment with buserelin and cyproterone acetate in metastatic male breast cancer. *Cancer*. 1993;72(2):502–5.
22. Doberauer C, Niederle N, Schmidt CG. Advanced male breast cancer treatment with the LH-RH analogue buserelin alone or in combination with the antiandrogen flutamide. *Cancer*. 1988;62(3):474–8.

23. Zabolotny BP, Zalai CV, Meterissian SH. Successful use of letrozole in male breast cancer: A case report and review of hormonal therapy for male breast cancer. *J Surg Oncol.* 2005;90(1):26–30.
24. Italiano A, Largillier R, Marcy PY, et al. [Complete remission obtained with letrozole in a man with metastatic breast cancer]. *Rev Med Interne.* 2004;25(4):323–4.
25. Giordano SH, Valero V, Buzdar AU, Hortobagyi GN. Efficacy of anastrozole in male breast cancer. *Am J Clin Oncol.* 2002;25(3):235–7.
26. Phase II study of goserelin and anastrozole in men with estrogen receptor – or progesterone receptor-positive recurrent or metastatic breast cancer. *SWOG S-0511.* 2005; Available at http://clinicaltrials.gov/ct/show/NCT00217659. Accessed January 14, 2007
27. Common Terminology Criteria for Adverse Events v3.0 (CTCAE). 2006. Available at http://ctep.cancer.gov/reporting/ctc_v30.html. Accessed December, 7 2006.
28. Efficace F, Therasse P, Piccart MJ, et al. Health-Related Quality of Life Parameters As Prognostic Factors in a Nonmetastatic Breast Cancer Population: An International Multicenter Study. *J Clin Oncol.* 2004;22(16):3381–8.
29. Goodwin PJ, Ennis M, Bordeleau LJ, et al. Health-Related Quality of Life and Psychosocial Status in Breast Cancer Prognosis: Analysis of Multiple Variables. *J Clin Oncol.* 2004;22(20):4184–92.
30. Markes M, Brockow T, Resch KL. Exercise for women receiving adjuvant therapy for breast cancer. *Cochrane Database Syst Rev.* 2006(4):CD005001.
31. Holmes MD, Chen WY, Feskanich D, Kroenke CH, Colditz GA. Physical activity and survival after breast cancer diagnosis. *JAMA.* 2005;293(20):2479–86.
32. Nielsen NR, Gronbaek M. Stress and breast cancer: A systematic update on the current knowledge. *Nat Clin Pract Oncol.* 2006;3(11):612–20.
33. Ramirez AJ, Craig TK, Watson JP, Fentiman IS, North WR, Rubens RD. Stress and relapse of breast cancer. *BMJ.* 1989;298(6669):291–3.
34. Graham J, Ramirez A, Love S, Richards M, Burgess C. Stressful life experiences and risk of relapse of breast cancer: Observational cohort study. *BMJ.* 2002;324(7351):1420–23.
35. Barraclough J, Pinder P, Cruddas M, Osmond C, Taylor I, Perry M. Life events and breast cancer prognosis. *BMJ.* 1992;304(6834):1078–81.
36. Maunsell E, Brisson J, Mondor M, Verreault R, Deschenes L. Stressful Life Events and Survival After Breast Cancer. *Psychosom Med.* 2001;63(2):306–15.
37. Clinical Trials. Available at http://www.cancer.gov/clinicaltrials. Accessed January 14, 2007.
38. Hearn J, Sullivan R. The impact of the 'Clinical Trials' directive on the cost and conduct of non-commercial cancer trials in the UK. *Eur J Cancer.* 2007;43(1):8–13.
39. Iredale R, Brain K, Williams B, France E, Gray J. The experiences of men with breast cancer in the United Kingdom. *Eur J Cancer.* 2006;42(3):334–41.
40. Larson EB, Yao X. Clinical empathy as emotional labor in the patient-physician relationship. *JAMA.* 2005;293(9):1100–6.

Final word

The preparation of a book is always a very demanding task that needs to be accomplished within the daily work of every one of the contributors.

We therefore particularly appreciate the effort of all of the contributors and their attempt to keep the deadlines despite their numerous other activities as scientist, physician, spouse, mother and daughter. Thanks to all!

We are also particularly grateful to Stefan Aebi, the only man "allowed" to participate in this project, who had the amiability and the courage to report on his experience as a male breast cancer patient.

Laura Walsh, the editor at Springer, deserves special thanks: her support was continuous, firm and friendly and even during difficult moments she never lost her wonderful balance and her sense of humor.

Index

D

CPSIA information can be obtained
at www.ICGtesting.com
Printed in the USA
LVHW080734180520
655866LV00001B/7